Complications in
VASCULAR SURGERY

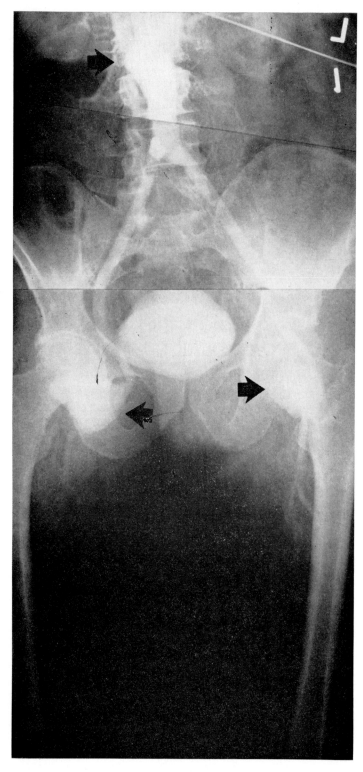

A translumbar aortogram showing three false aneurysms at the sites of anastomosis of an aortofemoral bypass graft placed 8 years previously using silk suture material.

Complications in
VASCULAR SURGERY

Edited by

Hugh G. Beebe, M.D.
The Virginia Mason Medical Center
Seattle, Washington

J. B. Lippincott Company
Philadelphia and Toronto

ISBN 0–397–50269–9

Library of Congress Catalog Card Number 73–7978

Printed in the United States of America

1   3   4   2

Library of Congress Cataloging in Publication Data

Beebe, Hugh G.
    Complications in vascular surgery.

    Includes bibliographical references.
    1. Cardiovascular system—Surgery—Complica-
tions and sequelae.   I. Title.   [DNLM: 1. Vascular surgery—Adverse effects.   WG168 B414c
1973]
RD598.B38   617′.413′01   73–7978
ISBN 0–397–50269–9

Dedication

TO OUR PATIENTS: As we have been their physicians, so have we also been their pupils as they have taught us to strive to overcome the limitations of science, of art, and of ourselves.

Contributors

HUGH G. BEEBE, M.D.
The Virginia Mason Medical
Center;
Clinical Instructor in Surgery,
School of Medicine,
University of Washington,
Seattle, Washington

**F. WILLIAM BLAISDELL,
M.D.**
Chief of Surgery,
San Francisco General Hospital;
Professor of Surgery,
University of California School
of Medicine,
San Francisco, California

**THEODORE J. CASTELE,
M.D.**
Senior Clinical Instructor,
Department of Radiology,
Case Western Reserve
University School of Medicine,
Cleveland, Ohio

RICHARD H. DEAN, M.D.
Instructor in Surgery,
School of Medicine,
Vanderbilt University,
Nashville, Tennessee

JAMES A. DeWEESE, M.D.
Professor of Surgery,
School of Medicine and
Dentistry,
University of Rochester,
Rochester, New York

**EDWARD B. DIETHRICH,
M.D.**
Director and Chief of
Cardiovascular Surgery,
Arizona Heart Institute,
Phoenix, Arizona

THOMAS J. FOGARTY, M.D.
Clinical Assistant Professor of
Surgery,
Stanford University School of
Medicine,
Palo Alto, California

JOHN H. FOSTER, M.D.
Professor of Surgery,
School of Medicine,
Vanderbilt University,
Nashville, Tennessee

**H. EDWARD GARRETT,
M.D.**
Clinical Associate Professor of
Surgery,
School of Medicine,
University of Tennessee,
Memphis, Tennessee

LUCIUS D. HILL, M.D.
Chief of Surgery,
The Virginia Mason Medical
Center,
Seattle, Washington

JERE W. LORD, JR., M.D.
Professor of Clinical Surgery,
New York University,
New York, New York

**T. CRAWFORD McASLAN,
M.D.**
Professor of Anesthesia,
School of Medicine,
University of Maryland,
Baltimore, Maryland

WILLIAM H. MORETZ, M.D.
President and
Professor of Surgery,
Medical College of Georgia,
Augusta, Georgia

**CORNELIUS OLCOTT IV,
M.D.**
Department of Surgery,
University of California School
of Medicine,
San Francisco, California

J. CUTHBERT OWENS, M.D.
Professor of Surgery,
School of Medicine,
University of Colorado,
Denver, Colorado

FRED R. PLECHA, M.D.
Assistant Professor of Surgery,
Case Western Reserve University
School of Medicine,
Cleveland, Ohio

WALTER J. PORIES, M.D.
Chief of Surgery,
Cuyahoga County Hospitals;
Professor and Associate
Director,
Department of Surgery,
Case Western Reserve University
School of Medicine,
Cleveland, Ohio

NORMAN M. RICH, M.D.
Chief, Peripheral Vascular
Surgery,
Walter Reed Army Medical
Center,
Washington, D.C.

CHARLES G. ROB, M.D.
Professor and Chairman,
Department of Surgery,
School of Medicine and
Dentistry,
University of Rochester,
Rochester, New York

**SEYMOUR I. SCHWARTZ,
M.D.**
Professor of Surgery,
School of Medicine and
Dentistry,
University of Rochester,
Rochester, New York

WILLIAM H. STRAIN, Ph.D.
Director of Surgical
Laboratories,
Cleveland Metropolitan General
Hospital;
Consultant,
Department of Surgery,
Case Western Reserve University
School of Medicine,
Cleveland, Ohio

CHARLES H. WRAY, M.D.
Associate Professor of Surgery
and Acting Chairman,
Department of Surgery,
Medical College of Georgia,
Augusta, Georgia

Preface

Sir Astley Cooper, a pupil of John Hunter's, asked with surprise one day whether Hunter had stated an opinion the year before directly contradicting what he was now saying. Hunter, one of the founders of vascular surgery, replied, "Very likely I did; I hope I grow wiser every year." Vascular surgery remains a dynamic field, and change in the understanding and treatment of its complications is a certainty. Therefore, this work should be thought of as a consolidation of present information upon which improvements can be made.

Information about complications is sometimes difficult to acquire by means other than personal experience. Every physician and surgeon who accepts the challenge of treating vascular disease will encounter complications, but all too often complications seem to be just the reverse of the weather—everyone does something about it, but no one talks about it.

It is intended that this text will serve to improve the lot of the patient with vascular disease. The authors have had three objectives: To prevent complications where their causes are known and can be anticipated; to provide a clear guide to management of complications while avoiding a restrictive, rigid view of therapeutic alternatives; and to establish a foundation of information from which the clinician can deal logically and effectively with problems that have not been described.

Over the past decade vascular surgery has matured as a surgical discipline. A measure of this maturity is seen in the widespread inclusion of training in the management of disorders of blood vessels in all surgical training programs. Secondly, while it is true that improvements in vascular surgery techniques are sought and needed, it is also true that a degree of stability in procedures has been acquired.

These two observations have generated interest in producing this collection of information about the particular complications of surgical treatment of vascular disease. The first observation demands such a work, while the second permits it.

HUGH G. BEEBE

Acknowledgements

Many surgeons whose names do not appear in this text have contributed to this collection of information by sharing their thoughts with the authors. Special acknowledgement is due the late Doctor Robert Buxton, then Chairman of the Department of Surgery of the University of Maryland and to Doctor George Yeager, of the same institution, for their encouragement of the project at its inception.

Particular appreciation is offered to Mrs. Patience Smith Echols for her able editorial assistance and cheerful assumption of the major secretarial burden of preparing the text. Also, our thanks are extended to Mrs. Anne P. Hug for her many contributions to revision of the manuscript.

The editorial staff of J. B. Lippincott Company, particularly Mr. George F. Stickley and Mr. J. Stuart Freeman, Jr., have patiently understood the manifold problems of preparing a book written by busy clinicians with many other demands on their time, and continually helped overcome these problems.

Finally, the editor expresses his deepest thanks to the contributing authors, who agreed to add to already overburdened schedules and share their understanding and experience with their colleagues.

Contents

Walter J. Pories, M.D.
Fred R. Plecha, M.D.
Theodore J. Castele, M.D.
William H. Strain, Ph.D.

Arteriography and Phlebography

Introduction

Arteriography and phlebography have become essential procedures in the diagnosis of vascular lesions, hemorrhagic sites, and certain neoplastic diseases. The complications associated with the surgical procedures, the reactions to the contrast media, and the radiographic techniques should be completely understood by all members of the angiographic team. Complications from mechanical trauma predominate in the surgical procedures, from chemical or pharmacologic reactions in the injection of the contrast media, and from electrical and radiologic hazards in the radiography. A well-designed suite for angiography is essential to minimize complications. The facility should be completely equipped with all necessary surgical accessories, anesthesia equipment, contrast media, drugs for resuscitation, and physiologic monitors. Provision should also be made for intraoperative angiography in the operating room prior to wound closure because this procedure may reveal unsuspected vascular problems.[1] The technical details of vascular radiology are covered completely in the monographs cited at the end of this chapter. The two publications edited by Schobinger and Ruzicka,[2] and by Abrams,[3] are especially useful.

Arteriography and phlebography, the two divisions of angiography, have complication rates of 1-2 percent. In the early stages of development, the reported mortality ranged up to 16.0 percent, and morbidity up to 27.2 percent,[4] but these rates have decreased greatly with the passage of time. There have been remarkable improvements in techniques and contrast media since the first human venogram in 1923 with strontium bromide by Berberich and Hirsch[5] and arteriogram in 1924 with aqueous sodium iodide by Brooks.[6] These early efforts have been summarized in a monograph by Moniz[7] who developed cerebral angiography and phlebography, but who unfortunately employed radioactive thorotrast as the contrast medium. Seldinger[8] reported 8,000 angiograms by the femoral route without mortality, and only one of his patients required surgical intervention for bleeding. From a survey of 13,207 lumbar aortograms performed in various centers in the United States, McAfee[9] in 1957 found a mortality of 0.28 percent and a morbidity of 0.74 percent, as summarized in Table 1-1. In 1964, Beall and associates[10] reported two deaths in 4,613 translumbar aortograms, a mortality of 0.05 percent. More recently, Robertson, Dyson, and Sutton[11] performed 1,750 renal angiograms by the Seldinger technique without mortality.

Arteriography and phlebography are usually performed on high-risk patients comprised mainly of elderly people with advanced degenerative disease and infants with birth defects. The procedures should be

TABLE 1-1. COMPLICATIONS ASSOCIATED WITH 13,207 ABDOMINAL AORTOGRAMS, CHIEFLY TRANSLUMBAR*

Complications	Fatal	Serious Nonfatal
Renal	12	27
Neurologic	5	24
Hemorrhage	5	8
Cardiovascular	5	8
Gastrointestinal	5	5
General anesthetic	3	7
Retroperitoneal sepsis	1	2
Dissecting aneurysm	1	0
Respiratory	0	11
Catheter insertion	0	5
Gangrene of skin	0	1
TOTAL	37 (0.28%)	98 (0.74%)
COMBINED TOTAL		135 (1.02%)

* From McAfee[9]

scheduled only after the patient has been thoroughly evaluated and provisions have been made to minimize any complications that may arise. It is generally accepted that the incidence of complications decreases sharply with the increasing experience and judgment of the angiographer.

The complications of angiography are frequently due to advanced arteriosclerosis. These include strokes, cardiac arrhythmia and infarction, renal failure, fracture of plaques with peripheral embolization, subintimal dissection, and uncontrolled hemorrhage due to the poor elasticity of the injured vessel. In special procedures, such as adrenal venography, the excessive pressure during the injection may rupture the delicate vasculature.[12] Other complications are due to technical errors such as traumatic puncture, guide wire fracture, catheter embolization, failure to control hemorrhage, and peripheral nerve injury, as illustrated by the data of Lang[13] in Table 1-2, Halpern[14] in Table 1-3, and Seidenberg and Hurwitt[15] in Table 1-4. Adverse reactions to the contrast media account for additional mortality and morbidity. Fatalities and traumatic experiences from electrical shocks and radiation are relatively uncommon.

Complications of Arteriography

Excellent technique, careful attention to detail, and mature clinical judgment are the hallmarks of safe angiography. In general, the approaches to the arterial tree can be divided into direct percutaneous injections and the indirect, but often more accurate, Seldinger techniques.

Direct Carotid Arteriography

Although Broadbent[16] described extracranial arterial occlusive disease in 1875, it was not until 1951 that occlusion of the internal carotid artery was recognized to be a significant cause of cerebral infarction by Fisher.[17] Carotid arteriography has developed slowly. Moniz[6] first injected contrast media into the carotid artery following surgical exposure of the vessel in 1927. Percutaneous puncture of the common carotid artery was described by Loman and Myerson[18] in 1936, and improved by Turnbull[19] in 1939. The carotid percutaneous forward catheterization technique of Donald et al.[20] has fallen into disuse because of the requirement of a large bore needle and the consequent danger of hemorrhage.

The advantages and disadvantages of the direct injection of the carotid and vertebral arteries have been outlined by Hinck and Dotter.[21] The advantages include a minimum of special equipment and contrast medium. The disadvantages are multiple punctures when several arteries are studied, the failure to demonstrate the proximal portions of vessels, and the frequent need for general anesthesia. The puncture techniques are difficult, especially in the vertebral artery, and positioning of the neck is sharply limited by the presence of the needle.

Determination of the complication rate for direct percutaneous carotid angiography is difficult. Decker[22] claimed only one residual neurologic deficit for every 1-2,000 examinations. Hinck and Dotter,[21] however, pointed out that "the more general experience indi-

TABLE 1-2. COMPARISON OF SELDINGER PROCEDURES AND TRANSLUMBAR AORTOGRAMS

Complications	Fatal	Serious Nonfatal	Minor
Complications Associated with 11,402 Seldinger Procedures			
Arterial thrombosis	3	47	
(with secondary loss of limb)		(6)	
Perforation of major vessels		13	22
Arterial embolism		9	
Broken tip of guide wire or catheter		5	
Bowel ileus or necrosis		5	
Renal		2	
Cardiovascular	1		
Venous thrombosis and pulmonary infarction	1		
Intramural or subintimal medium injection	1		136
Local hematomas		1	167
Other	1		
TOTAL	7 (0.06%)	82 (0.7%)	325 (3%)
Complications Associated with 3,240 Translumbar Aortograms			
Retroperitoneal hemorrhage and dissecting aneurysm		4	34
Bowel necrosis, mesenteric thrombosis, and ileus		2	
Hemorrhagic pancreatitis		1	
Renal damage		1	1
Thrombosis of aorta		1	
Pneumohemochylothorax		1	
Hypertensive crisis		1	
Extravasations and intramural injections			97
Allergic reactions			2
Unspecified	1		
TOTAL	1 (0.03%)	11 (0.3%)	134 (4%)

* Data from Lang[13]

TABLE 1-3. COMPLICATIONS ASSOCIATED WITH 1,000 PERCUTANEOUS TRANSFEMORAL ARTERIOGRAMS*

Complications	Serious Nonfatal	Minor
Hematoma	2	12
Bleeding		3
Thrombosis	4	1
False aneurysm	1	
Broken guide wire tip	2	
Intramural passage of catheter		2
TOTAL	9 (0.9%)	18 (1.8%)

* Data from Halpern[14]; no fatal complications

TABLE 1-4. COMPLICATIONS ASSOCIATED WITH 1,500 RETROGRADE FEMORAL SELDINGER AORTOGRAMS*

Complications	Fatal	Serious Nonfatal
Arterial thrombosis		11
(with loss of limb)		(1)
Uncontrolled bleeding		5
False aneurysm	1	4
Massive hematoma		2
Aortic perforation		2
Fractured guide wire		1
TOTAL	1 (0.07%)	25 (1.7%)

* Data from Seidenburg and Hurwitt[15]

cates that death and permanent complications can be expected in from 1 to 5 or more percent of examinations, with risk higher in older people and in those with hypertensive or occlusive cerebral vascular disease." Allen, Parera and Potts[23] reported 21 complications in 538 direct carotid arteriograms (3.9 percent) with one death and one case of permanent hemiplegia. When four attempts at arterial puncture were necessary, the incidence of complications rose to 9.6 percent. In the whole series, subintimal or extraluminal injections occurred in 7.1 percent of all patients, but in the 21 patients with complications, the incidence of subintimal injection was 62 percent. Bergstrom and Lodin[24] reported three cases of vertebral arteriovenous fistula, resulting from the trauma of direct arterial puncture.

In the British survey of radiologic complications, Ansell[25] reviewed the experience of 265 radiologists during the year 1965. Three deaths were reported following carotid arteriography: two due to unexplained respiratory arrest after satisfactory recovery from the general anesthetic and a third unexplained death in a moribund patient. Blindness of six days' duration followed bilateral vertebral angiography complicated by extraluminal injection in a 51-year-old housewife. In the survey there were six cases of hemiplegia. One followed hypotension due to myocardial infarction, another occurred after multiple injections of contrast medium. The third was due to an embolism from the tip of the catheter. The fourth followed a subintimal dissection with 10 ml. of contrast medium, but with almost immediate recovery. The fifth resulted from the injection of Conray 420 rather than Conray 280. The sixth case of hemiparesis developed after a normal arteriogram and was unexplained.

Craigmile[26] reported 717 carotid angiograms from 1960-1968 with only seven significant complications, an incidence of 1 percent. These included three instances of transitory contralateral hemiparesis, a persistent increase in a pre-existent hemiparesis, a

proximal extension of an internal carotid artery occlusion, a focal motor seizure in a man with a tumor, and increasing respiratory distress in an obtunded elderly man.

Microemboli. The injection of microemboli of foreign material accounts for a surprisingly large number of complications in direct carotid arteriography and perhaps in other types of arteriograms. Chason, Landers, and Swanson[27] found ten cases of cotton fiber microembolisms in autopsies following cerebral angiography, and Adams, Olin and Kosek[28] reported four additional cases. The sources of microemboli appear to be the release of cotton fibers from the equipment into the bowls of saline used for irrigation and these fibers are flushed into the artery between injections of the contrast medium. This complication can be avoided by the use of a closed system. Similarly, talcum powder and corn starch from glove powder, or small clots from the system, may be other sources of microemboli.

It is not clear whether the volume of the injection may also be a cause of complications. Bouzarth, Goldfedder, and Shenkin[29] reported two cases with immediate hemiplegia following the accidental injection of up to 80 ml. of diluted 20 percent sodium diatrizoate. Intravenous infusion of 20 percent mannitol reversed the hemiplegia and resulted in complete recovery in both cases.

Precautions. Most complications from direct cerebral arteriography are avoidable. The excessive use of contrast medium can be controlled by using 10 ml. syringes and keeping careful record of the volumes administered. Excellent pulsatile flow through the needle is required to insure that the injection will be wholly into the lumen of the vessel. Subintimal injections are avoidable if good flow is achieved through the needle and if the needle is well stabilized. The disruption of a plaque at the bifurcation can usually be prevented by employing a short needle inserted low into the common carotid artery. The injection of air bubbles and other microemboli can be avoided by insuring that the closed system is completely free of air.

Hemorrhage into the visceral space of the neck may occasionally produce difficulties in maintaining an airway. It is hard to compress the carotid vessels after the withdrawal of the needle and, in fact, it may even be hazardous. Use of small, sharp needles modified by the method of Craigmile[26] prevents this frightening complication. The procedure should not be used in patients too sick to tolerate anesthesia, considerable manipulation, prolonged immobilization, unsupervised transport through hospital corridors and elevators, or with sickle-cell anemia.[30]

Today, there is a trend away from direct carotid arteriography to selective retrograde techniques. This preference is due in part to the multiple injections required for direct extracranial artery visualization. The retrograde approach can provide simultaneous visualization of the aortic arch and the origins of the innominate, carotid and subclavian arteries.

Direct Vertebral Arteriography

The vertebral artery has also been injected directly through the exposed vertebral approach. This was first described by Olivecrona[31] in 1935, and later by Takahashi[32] in 1940. These percutaneous techniques have almost been abandoned in favor of selective retrograde catheter angiography.

Direct Translumbar Aortography

Translumbar aortography is a widely used method of visualizing the abdominal aorta and the vessels of the lower extremities. The procedure is rapid, does not require sophisticated equipment, and can be used when the Seldinger approach would be difficult or impossible. This method is particularly useful in patients with total peripheral aortic occlusion or obstructive lesions in the brachial or iliac artery.

The indications and techniques for direct translumbar aortography have been well reviewed by Sanders and Ramirez.[33] Since the direct injection of a sizable bolus of contrast medium may be more difficult than with the retrograde catheter technique, opacification of the peripheral blood vessels may not be as satisfactory. Even so, the run-off can usually be visualized to 6 to 8 inches below the trifurcation without great difficulty. Usually, it is possible to insert the needle into the lumbar aorta on the first attempt, but the

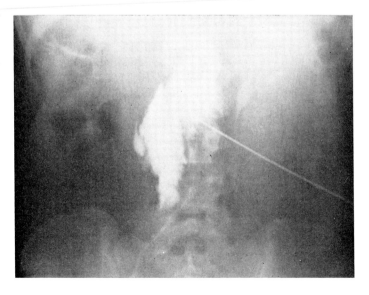

FIG. 1-1. Extravasation of contrast media during a translumbar aortogram. The patient experienced significant right flank pain, but no hemorrhage or visceral ischemia.

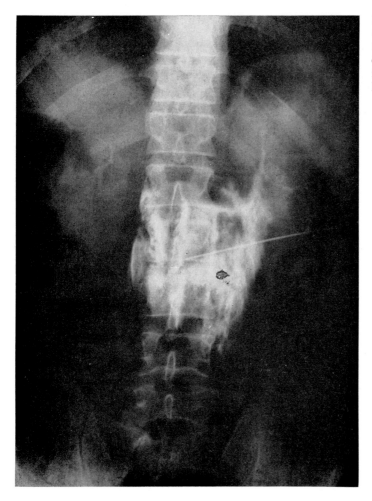

FIG. 1-2. Blind injection of contrast medium into the aorta may result in the nearly complete extravasation shown, if the needle is not within the lumen of the artery.

position of the needle should always be checked by means of a 5-ml. test dose to avoid subintimal injection. Typical complications of this type of blind needle approach are illustrated in Figures 1-1 and 1-2, which show extravasation of the contrast medium, and in Figure 1-3, which demonstrates intramural injection. Other complications associated with blind injection are illustrated in Figures 1-4 to 1-6.

The most common hazard in intraabdominal aortography is retroperitoneal hemorrhage. Generally, hemorrhage of 300-500 ml. is self-limited, and does not cause much difficulty. Whether puncture of an abdominal aortic aneurysm may lead to its rupture has not been adequately reported. At present, it seems prudent to avoid this approach when an aortic aneurysm is suspected.

Embolization due to fragmentation of atheromata would be expected to be common, but seems to be quite rare. The fragmentation is illustrated by the report of a death by Lonni, Matsumoto and Lecky[34] in a patient subjected to translumbar aortography followed by a Seldinger approach. At autopsy, large areas of aortic fragmentation and erosion were seen along the intimal surface, and emboli were found in the small arteries of the kidney, spleen, liver, pancreas, stomach, and colon. Retinal embolization,

FIG. 1-3. Intramural injection of contrast medium occurs fairly frequently in lumbar aortography. Accordingly, a test dose of 5 ml. should be injected to check the position of the point of the needle.

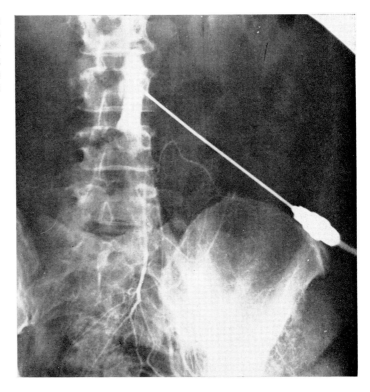

FIG. 1-4. A translumbar aortogram attempt with injection directly into the right renal artery. Fortunately, this patient did not demonstrate impaired renal function.

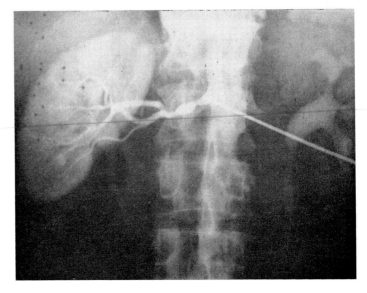

as described by Haney and Preston,[35] may be present, in addition to a characteristic skin rash, livedo reticularis.

Intramural injection of contrast medium occurs in about 10 percent of lumbar aortograms,[36] but significant aortic dissections have not been reported frequently. Coran and Tyler[37] reviewed the literature and published a classic picture of angiographic dissection. Their patient experienced back pain during the injection and the arteriograms demonstrated occlusion of the lower aorta

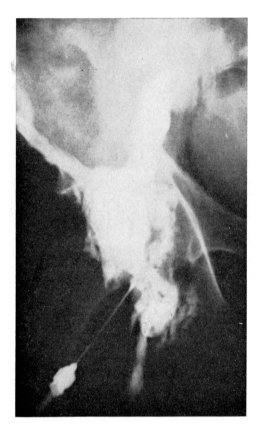

Fig. 1-5. Extravasation of contrast medium outlining inguinal ligament and retroperitoneal space as a result of improper positioning of needle during femoral arteriography. Checking blood flow and use of test injecton should prevent this painful complication.

in spite of the pre-angiographic clinical impression that the significant pathology was limited to below the groins. At exploration, dissection of the right common iliac artery and the aortic bifurcation were found, and endarterectomy yielded an excellent clinical result.

Paraplegia following abdominal aortography is fortunately rare. McAfee[9] reported an incidence of 0.22 percent of neurologic complications in his series of abdominal aortograms, with a somewhat higher incidence when either spinal or general anesthesia was used. Although the incidence of neurologic complications seems to have decreased, it still occurs with the newer contrast media. Ansell[25] reported two cases, one with diatrizoate sodium, and the other with metrizoate sodium, and both patients were found to be paraplegic on recovery from general anesthesia.

The neurotoxic effects of aortography have been well studied and documented in dogs by Margolis.[38] Profound hemorrhagic necrosis of the lumbar spinal cord of a dog is shown in Figure 1-7 six hours following retrograde aortography with Hypaque 70% under norepinephrine vasopressor stimulus. Figure 1-8 illustrates the severe histologic change seen five hours after passage of a vasotoxic concentration of this contrast agent. Margolis emphasized that peripheral resistance is a major determinant in the distribution of the radiopaque agents. He also pointed out that "Because of significant differences in basal tonus and reactivity of the neural and extraneural vascular beds, vasopressor stimuli favor neuripetal, and vasodepressor stimuli neurifugal, flow in an arterial injection mass."

When the needle is introduced too far cephalad during translumbar aortography, intrathoracic complications may ensue. Poulias and Stergiou[39] reported two patients with such complications. One had a pulmonary infarct with a true hemothorax and another a massive intrathoracic hemorrhage. Both patients had hypertension. This rare complication was also reported by McAfee[9] who had one incidence of hemothorax in his review of 12,832 translumbar aortographies. In both patients reported by Poulias and Stergiou, the puncture occurred at the level of the 11th and 12th thoracic vertebrae, and both recovered completely following conservative management.

Infection may also follow aortography. Candy, Grainger, and Guyer[40] reported the case of a 46-year-old woman with persistent backache after a translumbar aortogram. Seventeen days later, an emergency laparotomy was performed for massive hematemesis, but the patient died. Autopsy revealed an infected hematoma with an aortoduodenal fistula.

FIG. 1-6. Direct injection of abdominal aortic aneurysm with resultant 1000 ml. retroperitoneal hematoma which was confirmed during operation.

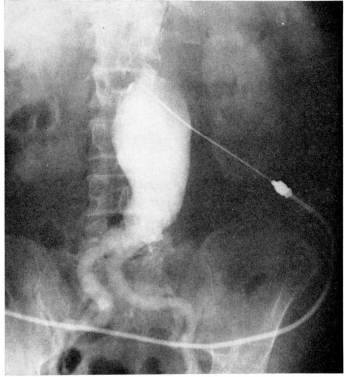

FIG. 1-7. Typical anatomic lesions induced in the spinal cord of a dog as a result of injecting contrast media in toxic concentrations. The hemorrhagic necrosis was observed six hours following retrograde aortography with "70% Hypaque." (Margolis, G.: *Invest. Radiol.*, 5:398, 1970)

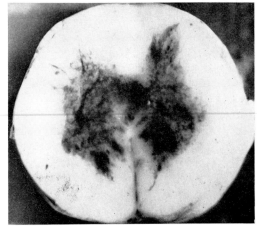

FIG. 1-8. The gray matter of the spinal cord of the dog shows a striking hydropic degeneration of neurones and sattelite glia five hours after passage of vasotoxic concentrations of contrast media. Edema of the parenchyma is also manifested. (Margolis, G.: *Invest. Radiol.*, 5:399, 1970)

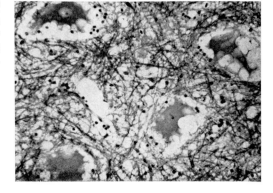

The intestinal vasculature can be injected with small amounts of contrast media without serious consequences. The needle tip should not be placed near the orifice of an intestinal artery during translumbar aortography, to avoid injections of large volumes of radiopaque solutions into the mesenteric circulation. The incidence of mass injection into the inferior mesenteric has been reported to vary between 0.03 percent by McAfee[9] and 0.2 percent by Szilagyi.[4] The bowel is much less sensitive to contrast media than the kidney.

Injuries to the colon secondary to abdominal aortography have been reported. Killen, Sewell, and Foster[41] reviewed 15 clinical injuries and found that the damage resulted from the inadvertent injection of contrast medium into the inferior mesenteric artery. Intense opacification of the inferior mesenteric artery was observed in ten patients. There was persistent staining of the colon wall in seven patients, indicating extravasation of the medium or arrest of the capillary circulation of the colon wall. Necrosis of the colon occurred in 11 patients. Two, who were treated nonoperatively, passed necrotic segments of the colon per rectum and survived. In nine patients, the colonic necrosis was extensive and emergency resection was performed in seven with survival. Andersen[42] reported a case of ischemic colitis caused by angiography which was treated by defunctioning colostomy and healed with stricture formation in the rectum, requiring later resection.

Even massive amounts of concentrated contrast media were well tolerated by the canine colon, as demonstrated by Killen and co-workers.[41] They concluded that the complications are more likely to be due to mechanical trauma than to toxicity of contrast media, and that selective arterial studies of the colon could probably be performed safely.

Susceptibility of the small bowel to direct infusion of contrast media was also studied by Killen and co-workers.[41] Their review revealed eight deaths out of 17 cases of small bowel injury due to abdominal aortography. The fatalities were primarily associated with the older more toxic contrast media. Thrombosis of the superior mesenteric artery was implicated in nine patients, but was verified at laparotomy or autopsy in only three cases. It is doubtful that the incidence of these small bowel complications exceeds 0.05 percent of all arteriograms. Gangrene of the small bowel was the cause of death in all patients. Sewell, Killen and Foster[43] felt that the newer contrast media were better tolerated by the small bowel and that the complications were almost exclusively due to mechanical trauma from the injections.

Patients with pheochromocytomas tolerate translumbar aortography poorly. Rossi, Young, and Panke[44] reviewed 99 cases and described in detail three deaths and eight nonfatal major complications due to massive retroperitoneal hemorrhage following 18 translumbar examinations. In the group of 99 patients studied by both techniques, all deaths occurred with translumbar techniques and none followed the transfemoral approach.

Direct Percutaneous Femoral Arteriography

Percutaneous femoral arteriography continues to be widely applied to the visualization of arteries of the lower extremity. This technique is another method of selective angiography, and, therefore, permits the use of small amounts of contrast media. The hazards of hemorrhage are reduced because, in contrast to carotid angiography, the femoral artery can be compressed until good hemostasis has been obtained. Hemorrhage, hematoma, false aneurysm, infection, thrombosis, distal embolization, and dissection have been observed following this technique, but the actual incidence is difficult to determine from the literature. The advantages of percutaneous femoral arteriography are simplicity, and the ability to perform the examination without sophisticated equipment. Femoral arteriography can be done with portable x-ray machines, and is particularly useful in the operating room. It is the best technique for the visualization of vessel detail below the knees. Femoral arteriography can also be used to demonstrate iliac and lower aortic pathology by injecting the contrast material briskly upstream.

Ansell[25] in his survey of radiologic complications in Britain reported two deaths during femoral arteriography due to coronary thrombosis. Both patients had been under general anesthesia. In another case, cardiac arrest was successfully reversed by external massage. He also reported three other complications including peripheral embolization, excessive bleeding, and dislodgement of a plaque requiring immediate arterial grafting.

Direct Brachial and Axillary Arteriography

The brachial and axillary arterial system has obvious advantages for arteriography. The vessels are infrequent sites of atheroma, can easily be compressed against the bones of the arm, and usually have excellent collateral circulation. Pneumothorax is an unusual complication and the massive loss of blood encountered by other approaches is rare.

The vessels of the arm have been used for three approaches: (1) a direct percutaneous technique for visualization of the vessels of the upper extremity, (2) a percutaneous or open retrograde Seldinger approach with the introduction of a catheter into the aorta, and (3) a percutaneous noncatheter left brachial technique where the bolus is rapidly injected in a retrograde fashion into the upper aorta and then observed in the distal tree. Caine, Kedar, and Schwartz[45] reported 100 cases of satisfactory renal angiography by this third technique, and demonstrated excellent visualization without serious complications.

The major disadvantage of this approach is the likelihood and seriousness of neurologic injury. The axillary artery and the brachial plexus are contained within the axillary sheath, and even a small hematoma within this rigid envelope may produce nerve damage, by pressure or by interrupting the segmental blood supply to the nerves. The neurologic complications include loss of sensation of the palmar surface of the index and middle fingers with thenar atrophy, limitation of flexion in the interphalangeal joints of the index finger or thumb, and failure of thumb adduction.

Only five cases of brachial plexus injury following axillary percutaneous arteriograms have been reported,[46] but it is likely that this complication is considerably more frequent. To avoid this complication, care must be taken to puncture the artery only once, and to avoid hematomas by application of pressure for at least ten minutes after withdrawal of the needle. It is probably wise to immobilize the arm by means of a sling and swath for 24 hours. The patient should be warned about the possible appearance of pain, numbness or paralysis so that such symptoms will prompt early operative intervention to evacuate the hematoma.

Thrombosis of the axillary or brachial artery is usually the result of multiple punctures with elevation of an intimal flap, the use of a too large catheter, or overly enthusiastic pressure on the vessel. The incidence of thrombosis after brachial arteriography is unknown, but it is high following cardiac catheterization by this route. Armstrong and Parker,[47] in a review of the literature, state that the complication rate following brachial arteriotomy for cardiac catheterization is from 4 to 28 percent, and that almost all of these complications are due to thrombotic occlusions of the vessel. In their own prospective series of 70 brachial arteriotomies, they observed an overall complication rate of 16 percent with 10 percent of the patients having diminished arterial pulsation in the follow-up period. They described their approach to the management of these complications, including the appropriate use of Fogarty catheters, heparinization, infusion of low molecular weight dextran, close clinical follow-up, and occasional re-exploration with good results.

The complications in their own series of brachial arteriograms on 1,202 patients were reviewed in 1972 by Feild, Lee, and

TABLE 1-5. MILD, SEVERE, AND FATAL
COMPLICATIONS ASSOCIATED WITH
1,202 BRACHIAL ARTERIOGRAMS*

Complications	Cases
Mild:	
Transient motor deficit	11
Novocain reaction	1
Seizure or irritative reaction	2
Sensitivity reaction (rash)	4
Cardiovascular	1
Transient loss of radial pulse	12
Aneurysm (brachial artery)	1
Transient visual symptoms and/or signs	5
Subintimal injection	
carotid	4
brachial	4
Shocklike state (transient)	2
Tracheotomy secondary to carotid arteriogram	1
Miscellaneous complaints secondary to arteriogram	
vertigo	1
laryngospasm	1
chest pain	2
confusion	1
guide wire break	1
delayed hemorrhage in arm	2
TOTAL	56 (4.7%)
Severe:	
Brain stem lesion	2
Seizure & hyperthermia	1
TOTAL	3 (0.25%)
Fatal:	
Myocardial infarction during arteriogram	1
Ruptured aneurysm	2
Completion of stroke	1
Brain stem lesion with aspiration pneumonia	1
TOTAL	5 (0.42%)

* Data from Feild, Lee, and McBurney[48]

McBurney.[48] This extensive summary showed one serious complication per 152 arteriograms (0.66 percent). Where carotid vascular disease was present, the rate was 2.70 percent; basilar artery disease, 6.4 percent; and cerebral vascular disease, 12.17 percent. The distribution of the mild, severe, and fatal complications associated with these 1,202 brachial arteriograms are shown in Table 1-5. The overall fatality rate in this large series was 0.42 percent.

The Seldinger Technique

Seldinger[50] devised a method of arteriography in 1953 which has proved to be one of the breakthroughs for diagnosis and surgery of arterial disease. This method has made it possible to study even very small vessels with extraordinary clarity and safety. The technique is based on arterial puncture with a specially designed needle, followed consecutively by introduction of a thin flexible-tip guide wire, removal of the needle, and subsequent passage of a catheter into the vessel over the wire. Since the catheter is larger than the needle hole in the artery, a snug fit and minimal hemorrhage during the procedure is assured. In addition, selective positioning catheterization increases the safety of arteriography by the use of much smaller dosages of contrast media. General anesthesia is usually not necessary for the Seldinger approach although it is used in children and in unusually anxious individuals.

The safety of the Seldinger technique varies with angiographers. As mentioned earlier not a single death occurred in Seldinger's own series of 8,000 angiograms, and only one patient required operation to arrest hemorrhage. In Lang's[13] survey of complications in 11,402 Seldinger procedures for arteriography, 7 (0.06 percent) fatalities, 82 major complications and 325 minor complications were reported. Arterial thrombosis occurred in 47 patients, and asymptomatic intramural or subintimal injections and perforation of major vessels without late sequelae were found in 136 patients, as shown in the data of Table 1-2. Ranniger and Saldino[51] discovered 14 patients with absent pulses in a series of 2,197 percutaneous femoral angiograms, with 5 requiring surgery. In 1,000 consecutive examinations, Halpern[14] experienced 2.4 percent significant complications with thrombosis in 0.5 percent. Mortensen[52] found a 4.4 percent incidence of major complications.

Robertson, Dyson, and Sutton[11] examined

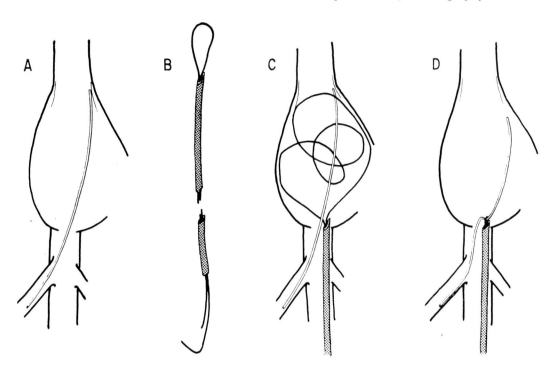

Fig. 1-9. Use of the redundant loop snare for percutaneous transluminal retrieval of a catheter embolism to the right atrium. (*A*) An 8-cm. fragment in right atrium and hepatic vein is recovered with a homemade loop snare (*B*) prepared by threading a 4-Fr loop through a 12-Fr outer sleeve, both of radiopaque Teflon. One convolution of the redundant loop has caught the foreign body (*C*) and the fragment is secured (*D*) for removal via inferior vena cava and right femoral vein. (Dotter, C. *et al.*: *Am. J. Roentgenol., 111*:467, 1971)

2,000 patients by the Seldinger technique for renal angiography and had no mortality or major complications. In Ansell's[25] survey of radiologic complications in Britain, two cases were described of femoral artery occlusion following Seldinger catheterization requiring amputation in both cases for gangrene. Three cases of false aneurysm of the femoral artery and one of the external iliac artery were found in a series of 800 transfemoral procedures in one unit. There were two cases of severe hematoma, one of which involved the scrotum and resulted in unilateral testicular atrophy.

Using a technique of catheterization by a translumbar approach, Haut and Amplatz,[53] reported 242 cases of transaortic catheterization with a complication rate of 0.8 percent compared to complications with a transfemoral approach of 1.8 percent. They felt that better results were due to the decrease in vascular complications by their technique.

The serious complication rate should not exceed 1 percent with experienced angiographers.

The Seldinger approach has proved to be particularly useful for the demonstration of the extracranial and intracerebral vasculature. Takahashi and Kawanami[54] reported 422 Seldinger retrograde cerebral angiograms with two hypotensive reactions, thrombosis of a femoral artery, and hemorrhage from the femoral puncture site. There were seven neurologic complications, of which four were transient and three long lasting. Carotid angiograms were successfully performed in 97.4 percent with selective internal carotid angiograms in more than 85 percent of all studies. The rate of success in selective vertebral angiography was better than 95 percent. Obsenchain and his coworkers[55] demonstrated that cerebral angiography by the Seldinger technique can also be done in children with a 5 percent com-

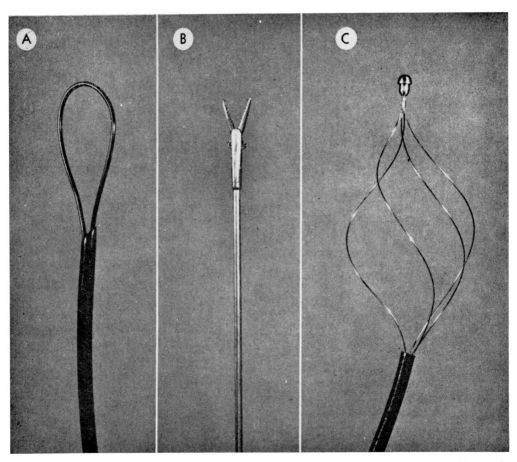

Fig. 1-10. Three devices used with success by Dotter, Rösch, and Bilbao[56] in the cardiovascular system for retrieval of catheter and guide fragments. (*A*) Homemade opaque Teflon adjustable loop snare, which can also be made with the gentle curve at the end of the outer catheter. (*B*) Bronchoscopic grasping forceps, which has limited use because of rigidity and shortness. (*C*) A larger version of the basket stone catcher, which can be modified to serve as an all-purpose transluminal extractor of particular value in catching nonopaque tubing and nontubular foreign bodies. (Dotter, C. *et al.*: *Am. J. Roentgenol.*, *111*:467, 1971)

plication rate. The pediatric patients were done under ketamine anesthesia and premedication consisted of 0.1 to 0.3 mg. of scopolamine. Complications included hematomas, one case with loss of a pedal pulse which returned without therapy within 24 hours, and one death. The death was apparently not due to the angiogram, but was related to a rapidly fulminating posterior fossa tumor complicated by tuberculous meningitis. There was no increase in complications as the volume of contrast agent was increased.

The guide wire may be the cause of complications. Arterial perforation by guide wire was reported by Ansell[25] in three patients, but was probably much more frequent. It is unusual for such perforations to cause any major clinical difficulty. The wire hole seems to close readily although it is certain that a small amount of hemorrhage must occur. The flexible leader of the Seldinger guide wire became detached and embolized in two patients in the British survey.[25] Although one was removed, one was left in place without ill effects. Dotter, Rösch, and Bilbao[56] have emphasized the frequency of fracture of wires and catheters and described several approaches (Figs. 1-9, 10) for removing these fragments from the

FIG. 1-11. This right external iliac artery occlusion was noted 2 weeks after a right retrograde femoral carotid arteriogram. Thromboendarterectomy was successful.

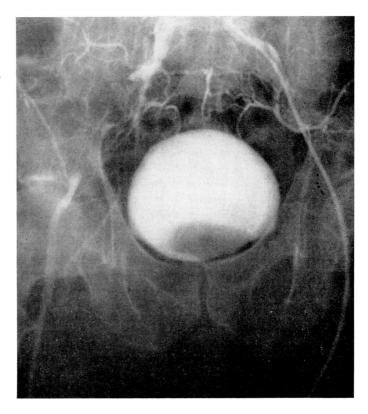

heart and great vessels. From their review and experience of 29 cases, they agree that catheter emboli to the heart and great vessels can and should be promptly removed by the percutaneous transluminal route, usually with the loop snare catheter. Curry[57] reviewed a useful technique with a modified side arm catheter irrigator which provides a closed system.

It is important to test the integrity of the leader by "twist and pull" prior to introduction. Sheiner and associates[58] fragmented a plastic wire during catheterization of the internal carotid artery from the common carotid. The fragment was lodged in the internal carotid artery just proximal to the carotid syphon and was removed with great difficulty through an arteriotomy with the help of a small suction device.

Intimal injury is common, but rarely has serious effects. Gudbjerg and Christensen[36] found a 9.9 percent incidence of intimal injury in 419 examinations, but without serious damage. Kocandrle, Kittle, and Petasnick[59] reviewed the incidence of intimal injuries

from retrograde dissections reported by various authors and described a case of their own. They point out that these cases can usually be handled conservatively, and that they are normally caused by the patient's intrinsic arterial disease. The catheter slides underneath an intimal plaque allowing the blood to carry on the remaining dissection or a forceable subintimal injection produces the injury which is then propagated by the blood stream. Kocandrle's case was unusual because the aorta was normal, yet it appeared that the blood flow had separated the intima over a large portion of the vessel. The patient recovered well after the dissected intima was excised and the arteriotomy repaired. A death due to aortic dissection following Seldinger femoral aortogram was also reported by Ansell.[25] The patient developed an aortic aneurysm at the level of L3-L5 which ruptured into the peritoneum causing death.

Although intimal dissection is one of the major complications of the Seldinger retrograde technique, this approach is also the

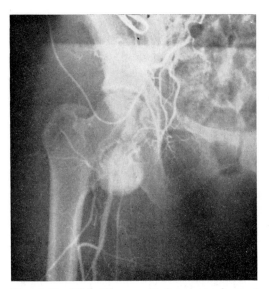

FIG. 1-12. This 53-year-old female underwent a right retrograde femoral arch aortogram 6 weeks prior to this arteriogram, which demonstrates a false aneurysm at the site of the femoral puncture. The false aneurysm was successfully corrected.

best method of diagnosing dissecting aortic aneurysms and has been used repeatedly and freely for this diagnosis. Kirschner and co-workers[60] with an extensive experience of over 200 cases, feel that retrograde femoral aortography is the definitive diagnostic method of choice for dissecting aneurysms of the aorta. The site of dissection and re-entry may be clearly demonstrated, injections into the true and false lumens may be made, and serious complications do not result from the technique. Shuford, Sybers, and Weens[61] also confirmed the safety of retrograde aortography in the diagnosis of dissecting aneurysms of the aorta. In their series of 44 patients, 23 had dissecting aneurysms and were examined without complications or rupture. Harrington, Sommers, and Kassirer[62] described two cases in which renal arteriography had produced progressive renal failure by multiple atheromatous emboli; both the patients died. Nawar and his co-workers[63] reported a death due to massive hemorrhagic necrosis of the bowel from multiple atheromatous emboli after Seldinger abdominal aortography.

Iatrogenic arterial lesions appear to be the principal sources of complications. Moore and co-workers[64] have pointed out that the major complications of retrograde catheter arteriography are thrombosis and hemorrhages, and the minor are false aneurysms and arteriovenous fistulas. Hall[65] has editorialized that as much as possible should be learned about the manner in which these lesions are produced so that their incidence may be reduced to a minimum. There is general agreement that the common etiologic factors include excessive manipulation of the catheter, prolonged procedure time, large catheters, multiple arterial punctures, and excessive digital pressure on the artery at the conclusion of the study. Complications associated with retrograde catheter arteriography are illustrated in Figures 1-11 to 1-14.

The site of insertion of the catheter is important. The vessels in the legs are preferable to those in the arms, although the superficial femoral artery may be narrowed by athersclerotic disease and is therefore liable to injury. The external iliac artery dives deeply into the pelvis just above the groin, and may be difficult to compress after removal of the needle. It has been our choice to use a common femoral artery because of its easy accessibility, general sparing from atherosclerosis until late in the disease, easy control of hemorrhage, and accessibility for postangiographic examination.

Siegelman, Caplan, and Annes[66] described a "pull-out" angiogram as a method to determine the presence or absence of thrombosis after a Seldinger retrograde catheter examination. They pointed out that all patients with objective evidence of decreased circulation, either by oscillometry or decrease in pulses, in the extremity on a day following the procedure, had a 2.5 mm. or larger filling defect in the pull-out arteriogram.

The prompt recognition of arterial complications must be insured by careful pre- and postoperative assessment of peripheral pulses, vital signs, observations for swelling or hematoma at the arterial puncture sites, and signs of ischemia such as pain, coldness, and blueness. The pull-out technique of arteriography may be a help in predicting

Fig. 1-13. Extraluminal passage of retrograde femoral catheter with retroperitoneal extravasation of contrast media.

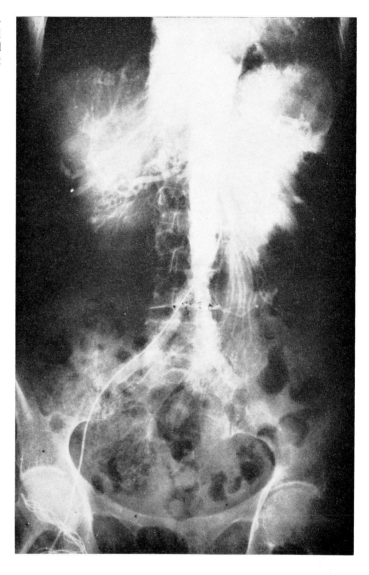

which patients will have difficulty post-arteriographically. Delays must be avoided and arterial complications should be treated promptly without long delays by injections of Papaverine, heparin, or procaine in valiant efforts to avoid surgery. Instead, repeat arteriography and exploration of the involved arteries, usually under local anesthesia, with the use of Fogarty catheters, will generally provide a good result. Generally, the immediate intended arterial repair is often the best approach and the complication and the patient's original disease are thereby corrected at the same time.

The contraindications to the Seldinger technique have been outlined by Pollard and Nebesar.[67] These include low cardiac output, oliguria, allergy to iodinated contrast agents, and bleeding tendencies, although angiography has been successfully performed on patients with prothrombin levels as low as 20 per cent or platelet counts as low as 50,000. Absence of the pulse distal to a proposed puncture site is a relative contraindication to the use of that site, and an absent pulse or local infection of the proposed site of puncture precludes its use. Evidence of emboli in the fundus of the eye

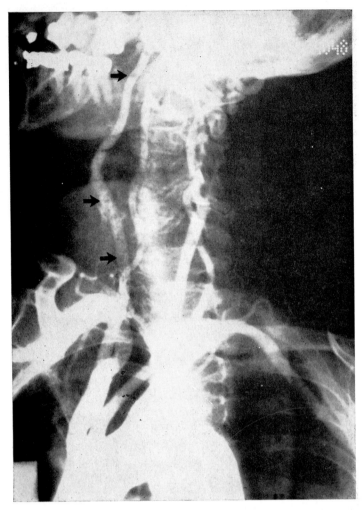

FIG. 1-14. Arch aortogram during which 40 ml. of air and 20 ml. of contrast media were injected under pressure. The patient died immediately. Multiple large air bubbles are seen in all four major vessels.

or elsewhere prohibits catheter angiography, and previous anaphylactic reaction is an absolute contraindication.

Phlebography

Phlebography, like arteriography, has become one of the most useful tools in the diagnostician's armamentarium. The venous system can be visualized either by direct injection into the venous flow or into bone. Additionally, it can be demonstrated in the later phases of arteriography. Both the systemic veins and the portal tree can be studied by these techniques.

Peripheral Phlebography

Although phlebography was described in 1923 by Berberich and Hirsch,[5] it was not until 1958 that the procedure was revived by DeWeese and Rogoff[68] in describing the long film technique, the semi-erect position, and the larger volumes of contrast media. Their descriptions in this, and in a later paper,[69] of the angiographic criteria of thrombosis have become classic contributions. The indications for performing peripheral phlebography include: evaluation of leg swelling, seeking the source of pulmonary emboli, establishing or eliminating the diagnosis of thrombophlebitis, evaluation of deep circulation in patients with varicose veins, and following the progress of anticoagulant or surgical therapy of thrombophlebitis. In addition, venography has been expanded to find tumor patterns throughout the body, to demonstrate the portal system, and to visual-

FIG. 1-15. Bilateral phlebogram illustrating the result of poor contrast medium injection technique. The left leg was injected properly and shows an essentially normal venous system. The right leg was injected improperly and only the sheath of the saphenous vein is delineated. Severe local discomfort and a nondiagnostic examination resulted.

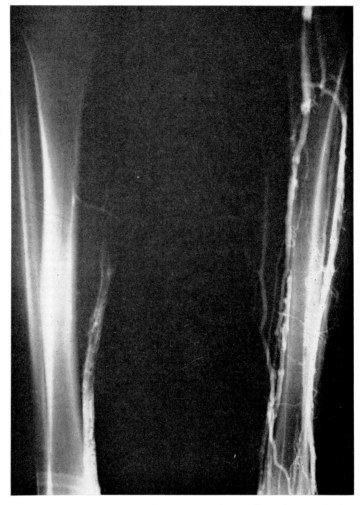

ize the venous anatomy of a number of normal and abnormal organ systems.

In most institutions, phlebography is carried out by cannulating a superficial vein of the foot, as described by DeWeese and Rogoff.[68,69] The following technique has proved useful and trouble-free: the dorsum of the foot is prepared with Betadine with the leg dependent. A tourniquet is applied above the ankle and a superficial vein is selected as the injection site close to the metatarsal head level of the foot. Better deep venous filling is obtained if the vein is not cannulated too close to the ankle level. A 1 percent plain Xylocaine wheal is infiltrated adjacent to the vein, and a 20-gauge, "butterfly" type needle is inserted and securely taped in place. A 250 ml. bottle of dextran or 5 percent dextrose solution is adjusted to run continuously before and after the contrast medium injection. For a single leg phlebogram, approximately 35 ml. of 50-60 percent contrast medium are injected over a two-minute period with double tourniquets above the ankle and 45 to 60 degrees of leg dependency, as described by DeWeese and Rogoff. Double amounts of contrast agent are injected for bilateral studies. After contrast medium injection, the intravenous solution is allowed to run continuously until the bottle is empty, and then the needle is removed. A flexible, disposable, Teflon cannula with mandrin and stopcock in place of the steel needle reportedly reduces extravasation from 60-78 percent to 4.5-18 percent.[70] A bilateral phlebogram contrasting the results of good versus poor injection technique is shown in Figure 1-15.

Complications from venography of the lower extremities include calf pain and cramping immediately after the injection, but this generally resolves rapidly. Some patients complain of dizziness, burning in the throat, or nausea, which may be due to the elevation of the head of the table. In a series described by Sanders and Glaser[71] three of 200 patients developed mild superficial thrombophlebitis in localized segments of the dorsal foot vein and the saphenous vein, but none developed deep venous thrombosis. No report of deep venous thrombosis following phlebography has been found in the literature, but we have had a patient whose pre-existing thrombophlebitis extended rapidly immediately after the examination. Lea Thomas[72] described two patients in a series of 400 who developed gangrene of the skin of their toes after phlebography. In one, a girl of 13, the skin slough was followed by complete healing, but in the other patient, a 21-year-old postpartum woman with preeclamptic toxemia and a cardiac arrest during delivery, there was a fatal outcome three weeks later. At postmortem examination, the forefoot was gangrenous with deep and superficial venous thrombosis of the right foot and calf, but the arterial tree was normal.

Osseous Phlebography

Phlebography of the extremities can also be carried out by the osseous injection of up to 50 ml. of 50-60 percent contrast medium as described, for example, by Schobinger[73] and by Wegner and co-workers.[74] Infectious processes near the bone and coagulation dyscrasias are contraindications to this method. Local anesthetics must be used prior to the injection because patients have discomfort both from the injection and extravasation of contrast media. No serious sequelae have been reported, nor has there been clinical evidence of embolization. Random urinalyses monitoring for fat and serum lipase levels have not given evidence of fat embolism. Wegner and associates had no postprocedure thrombophlebitis, but have

had one staphylococcal infection at the puncture site. Sanders, Ramirez, and Kortz[75] also noted superficial phlebitis in an undisclosed number of their patients, but denied the presence of any deep venous thrombophlebitis or extension of the process. Lea Thomas[76] has also used an intraosseous technique for pelvic phlebography through the femoral trochanter when percutaneous techniques were not possible. Three of 134 patients investigated by this technique experienced pain at the site of injection, but other complications were not recorded.

Complications of Phlebography

Phlebography is now widely employed to demonstrate virtually all parts of the systemic venous tree. Although most examinations are directed toward demonstration of pathology in the lower extremities, venography of the upper extremities has clarified a variety of problems in the arms and shoulders. Similarly, venacavography has led to the recognition of the frequency of venacaval thrombosis and has been useful in the demonstration of paracaval lymph nodes or tumor infiltration.[77] The complication rates for each of these procedures seem to be low and are related either to local hematomas or reactions to the contrast media.

Although phlebography has proved to be a generally safe procedure in almost every part of the body, a curiously high incidence of complication has been reported following adrenal venography. Bookstein, Conn, and Reuter[12] reported that adrenal venography was a safe and reliable procedure in over 80 patients, except in those with primary aldosteronism. In this disease, the intra-adrenal veins are apparently uniquely fragile and adrenal venography frequently results in intra-adrenal extravasation and hemorrhage. In addition, the method frequently fails to demonstrate the causative lesion. Of the 83 patients, nine adrenals were studied in suspected primary aldosteronism and of these, gross extravasation occurred in four cases, and minimal extravasation in one case. Extravasation was not seen by these authors with any other problem, and similar reports have been published by others. Bayliss and his associates[78] reviewed 349 cases of venograms of the adrenal veins and found that complications occurred in about 5 percent. They reported an additional case in which both adrenals were infarcted after successful left and unsuccessful right adrenal venography.

Splenoportography

The first successful splenoportogram in a human was performed by Leger[79] in 1951. This technique has since found wide application for the delineation of the portal system, especially in patients with portal hypertension or hepatic tumors. Recently, selective catheterization of the celiac axis or of the superior mesenteric artery with venous phase radiography has proved to be another useful approach for delineation of this anatomic system.[81]

Hemorrhage is the chief danger of splenoportography, and it is common to find as much as 500 ml. of blood within the peritoneal cavity if the patient is explored afterwards. Even if the stage one prothrombin time is greater than 50 percent of normal and the platelet count is more than 1,000,000/ml., the most common complication of splenoportography is intraperitoneal bleeding. This can be expected in 1 to 2 percent of patients, and the hemorrhage is usually apparent within three days of the procedure. Panke[82] reported 2 percent of his series of 172 splenoportograms required 500 to 2,000 ml. of blood replacement.

It is important that the needle be placed squarely within the center of the spleen, that the patient be able to cooperate by holding his breath for a reasonably prolonged period of time, and that an excellent flow of blood be obtained through the needle before the injection is carried out. There should, of course, be no hesitation about an exploratory laparotomy if active bleeding from the spleen is suspected. Bleeding may also occur into the spleen, causing subcapsular hematoma. Hemothorax and hydrothorax have

also been reported, possibly due to laceration of diaphragmatic-intercostal venous collaterals associated with portal hypertension.

Limits of Phlebography

The limits of phlebography seem to be only the ingenuity of man. Even sublingual venography has been described by Damascelli[83] for studying the cervical circulation successfully in 15 out of 18 patients. Hematomas developed in two patients but, apparently, no long-term complications were observed.

Contrast Media

Four principal types of water-soluble contrast media are employed today for arteriography and phlebography. These aqueous solutions are mixtures of the meglumine (methylglucamine), sodium, and other salts of four iodinated benzoic acid derivatives (I-IV) which are usually stabilized with small amounts of calcium edetate and buffered with phosphate salts. The solutions used for angiography usually have an iodine content ranging from 30 to 48 percent. The formulas and generic names of the contrast media are given in structural formulas I-IV, and the product names are listed in Tables 1-6 to 1-9. As is evident, the contrast media are supplied under various product names in different countries throughout the world. Occasionally, the product name can be confusing because the same name is used for different contrast media in different countries.

Generic Names. Concerted efforts have been made by national and international health and medical organizations to systematize the nomenclature for the generic names. The American Medical Association and the United States Pharmacopoeia have set up the AMA-USP Cooperative Program. A joint nomenclature committee facilitates the adoption of acceptable nonproprietary names for drugs, which are known as the United States Adopted Names (USAN). The World Health Organization (WHO) has also established a subcommittee for International Nonproprietary Names. This subcommittee con-

A

Methylglucamine Diatrizoate: 3,5-Diacetamido-2,4,6-triiodobenzoic Acid Methylglucamine Salt (47.1% I); 30%, 60%, 70%, and 85% w/v solutions

B

Sodium Diatrizoate: 3,5-Diacetamido-2,4,6-triiodobenzoic Acid Sodium Salt (59.9% I); 25%, 45%, and 50% w/v solutions

I. DIATRIZOIC ACID SALTS

TABLE 1-6. DIATRIZOATE CONTRAST MEDIA FOR ANGIOGRAPHY

Contrast Medium	Percent Diatrizoate Salt MG	Na	Iodine mg./ml.	Source Country-Firm
Angiografin	65.00	—	310	W. Germany-Schering AG
Cardiografin	85.00	—	400	U.S.-Squibb
Hypaque 45%	—	45.00	270	Gt. Britain-Winthrop
Hypaque 65%	50.00	15.00	325	Gt. Britain-Winthrop
Hypaque 85%	56.67	28.33	437	Gt. Britain-Winthrop
Hypaque sodium 50%	—	50.00	300	U.S.-Winthrop
Hypaque Meglumine 60%	60.00	—	282	Canada-Winthrop
Hypaque-M, 75%	50.00	25.00	385	U.S.-Winthrop
Hypaque-M, 90%	60.00	30.00	462	U.S.-Winthrop
Natriumjoddiazoate 45%	—	45.00	270	Denmark-Winthrop
Natriumjoddiazoate 90%	60.00	30.00	462	Denmark-Winthrop
Neo-urografin	66.00	10.00	370	Near East-Schering AG
Odiston 60%	60.00	—	282	Rumania-Terapia
Odiston 76%	76.00	—	357	Rumania-Terapia
Pielograf	63.00	9.30	353	Spain-Juste
Renografin 60	52.00	8.00	288	U.S.-Squibb
Renografin 76'	66.00	10.00	370	U.S.-Squibb
Reno=m=60	60.00	0.00	282	U.S.-Squibb
Renovist II	28.50	29.10	310	U.S.-Squibb
Triombrin 45%	—	45.00	270	USSR
Urografin 45%	39.00	6.00	218	Gt. Brit. Pharmethicals
Urografin 60%	52.00	8.00	290	W. Germany-Schering AG
Urografin 76%	66.00	10.00	370	W. Germany-Schering AG
Urografina 76%	66.00	10.00	370	Italy-Schering AG
Urografine 76%	66.00	10.00	370	W. Germany-Schering AG
Uromiro 60%	54.40	6.70	296	Italy-Bracco
Uromiro 75%	68.00	8.30	370	Italy-Bracco
Urotrast 60%	52.10	7.90	290	Yugoslavia-KRKA
Urotrast 75%	65.10	9.90	370	Yugoslavia-KRKA
Urovison	18.00	40.00	325	W. Germany-Schering AG
Verografin 60%	52.10	7.90	290	Czechoslovakia-Spofa
Verografin 76%	66.00	10.00	370	Czechoslovakia-Spofa
Visotrast "290"	52.00	8.00	290	E. Germany-Fahlberg-List
Visotrast "370"	66.00	10.00	370	E. Germany-Fahlberg-List
Yrigrafub	39.00	6.00	218	Pakistan-Schering AG

A

Iodamide Meglumine: 3-Acetamido-5-(acetamidomethyl)-2,4,6-triiodobenzoic Acid Methylglucamine Salt (46.3% I)

B

Iodamide Sodium: 3-Acetamido-5-(acetamidomethyl)-2,4,6-triiodobenzoic Acid Sodium Salt (59.9% I)

II. IODAMIDE SALTS

TABLE 1-7. IODAMIDE CONTRAST MEDIA FOR ANGIOGRAPHY

Contrast Medium	Percent of Iodamide Salt MG	Na	Iodine mg./ml.	Source Country-Firm
Angiomiron	70.00	9.70	380	Latin America-Schering AG
Conraxin H	70.00	9.70	380	Japan-Takeda
Conraxin L	65.00	—	300	Japan-Takeda
Iodamid(e) 300	65.00	—	300	W. Germany-Köhler
Iodamid(e) 380	70.00	9.70	380	W. Germany-Köhler
Iodoradiopaque 300	65.00	—	300	France-Heuprophax
Iodoradiopaque 380	70.00	9.70	380	France-Heuprophax
Jodamid(e) 300	65.00	—	300	Italy-Schering AG W. Germany-Köhler
Jodamid(e) 380	70.00	9.70	380	Italy-Schering AG W. Germany-Köhler
Jodomiron 300	65.00	9.70	300	Scandinavia-Erco
Jodomiron 380	70.00	9.70	380	Scandinavia-Erco
Urombrine 65%	65.00	—	300	Netherlands-Dagra
Urombrine 80%	70.00	9.70	380	Netherlands-Dagra
Uromiro 300	64.9	—	300	Distributors II*
Uromiro 340	18.30	43.40	340	Italy-Bracco
Uromiro 380	70.00	9.70	380	Distributors II*
Uromiron 300	64.90	—	300	Portugal-Remedius
Uromiron 380	70.00	9.70	380	Portugal-Remedius
Uromiron para inyeccion intravenosa	64.90	—	300	Latin America-Schering AG

* Distributors II: Austria-Gerot; Ethiopia, Italy, Libya, Somalia-Bracco; India-Pharmed; S. Africa-Satab; Spain-Vinas, S.A.; Switzerland-Tripharma; W. Germany-Köhler

siders submitted names, and those approved are printed in the WHO Chronicle as a Proposed International Nonproprietary Name (INN). If no objections are registered within four months, the name is published as a Recommended International Nonproprietary Name, and may be adopted by any or all countries. There are other national and international bodies who act on such names, such as the British Pharmacopoeia Committee, the French Codex, and the Nordic Pharmacopoeia. Through the action of these official bodies, the acceptability of a nonproprietary name is evaluated on an international basis. These generic names are given under the structural formulas.

Product Names. The product, or proprietary, names are usually formulated to show the application of the contrast medium to radiography and the specific area of use.

A

Meglumine Iothalamate: 5-Acetamido-2,4,6-triiodo-N-methylisophthalamic Acid Methyl-glucamine Salt (47.1% I)

B

Sodium Iothalamate: 5-Acetamido-2,4,6-triiodo-N-methylisophthalamic Acid Sodium Salt (59.9% I)

III. IOTHALAMIC ACID SALTS

TABLE 1-8. IOTHALAMATE CONTRAST MEDIA FOR ANGIOGRAPHY

Contrast Medium	Percent of Iothalamate Salt MG	Na	Iodine mg./ml.	Source Country-Firm
Angio-Conray	—	80.00	480	Distributors III*
				G. Britain-May & Baker
Angio-Contrix "48"	—	80.00	480	France-Guerbet
Cardio-Conray 400	52.00	26.00	400	G. Britain-May & Baker
Conray	60.00	—	282	U.S.-Mallinckrodt
Conray EV	24.00	36.00	328	Italy-Byk-Gulden
Conray 60	60.00	—	282	Austria-OS
Conray 70	7.10	62.90	410	Austria-OS
Conray 78	52.00	26.00	400	Japan-Daiichi
Conray 80	—	80.00	480	Austria-OS
				W. Germany-Byk-Gulden
Conray 280	60.00	—	282	G. Britain-May & Baker
Conray 300	—	50.00	300	Sweden-Kistner
Conray 400	—	66.80	400	Distributors III*
Conray 420	—	70.00	420	Australia-May & Baker
				G. Britain-May & Baker
Conray 480	—	80.00	480	Australia-May & Baker
				G. Britain-May & Baker
Contrix "28"	60.00	—	280	France-Guerbet
Medio-Contrix "38"	—	64.00	380	France-Guerbet
Neu-Conray FL	24.00	—	113	W. Germany-Byk-Gulden
Sombril(d)	60.00	—	282	Italy-Rovi
Vascoray	52.00	26.00	400	U.S.-Mallinckrodt

* Distributors III: Bulgaria, Czechoslovakia, Ethiopia, Italy, Libya-Bracco; Japan-Daiichi; Sweden-Kistner; U.S.-Mallinckrodt

Each product name is chosen for ease of pronunciation because the chemical names are usually very complex. The product name is frequently modified by a number to show the percent composition of the solution, the milligrams of iodine per milliliter, or the percent of iodine. The product name nearly always indicates a specific preparation, but there are a number of exceptions where the same name has been used for different compositions of matter. The product names collected in Tables 1-6 to 1-9, are based on the publication of Strain,[84] information from manufacturers, and data published in Physician's Desk Reference for Radiology and Nuclear Medicine.[85]

A
Metrizoate Calcium: 3-Acet-N-methylamido-2,4,6-triiodobenzoic Acid Calcium Salt (58.9% I)

B
Metrizoate Magnesium: 3-Acet-N-methylamido-2,4,6-triiodobenzoic Acid Magnesium Salt (59.6% I)

C
Metrizoate Meglumine: 3-Acet-N-methylamido-2,4,6-triiodobenzoic Acid Meglumine Salt (46.4% I)

D
Metrizoate Sodium: 3-Acet-N-methylamido-2,4,6-triiodobenzoic Acid Sodium Salt (58.6% I)

IV. METRIZOIC ACID SALTS
(Isopaque, Metriosil, Ronpacon and Triosil Products)

TABLE 1-9. METRIZOATE CONTRAST MEDIA FOR ANGIOGRAPHY

Contrast Medium	Percent Metrizoate Salt				Iodine mg./ml.	Source Country-Firm
	Ca	Mg	MG	Na		
Isopaque 45% [D]	—	—	—	45.00	260	Distributors IV*
Isopaque 60% [D]	—	—	—	60.00	350	Distributors I
Isopaque 75% [D]	—	—	—	75.00	440	Distributors I
Isopaque 260			—	41.40	260	Distributors I
Isopaque 280 [I]	1.13	—	59.10	—	280	U.S.-Winthrop
Isopaque 300 [I]	1.50	0.50	7.86	43.00	300	U.S.-Winthrop
Isopaque 350	2.80	2.00	—	55.20	350	Distributors I
Isopaque 370 [I]	1.13	—	65.60	10.10	370	U.S.-Winthrop
Isopaque 440	3.50	2.50	—	69.10	440	Distributors I
Isopaque 440 [I]	2.50	0.80	32.00	47.00	440	U.S.-Winthrop
Isopaque Amin 60% [D]	—	—	52.00	8.00	290	Distributors I
Isopaque Amin 280	1.13	—	59.10	—	280	Distributors I
Isopaque Amin 370	1.13	—	65.65	10.10	370	Distributors I
Isopaque Cerebral	1.13	—	59.10	—	280	Distributors I
Isopaque Coronar	1.13	—	65.65	10.10	370	Distributors I
Metriosil '25' [D]	—	—	—	25.00	150	Australia-Glaxo
Metriosil '45' [D]	—	—	—	45.00	260	Australia-Glaxo
Metriosil '60' [D]	—	—	—	60.00	350	Australia-Glaxo
Metriosil '75' [D]	—	—	—	75.00	440	Australia-Glaxo
Ronpacon 280	1.13	—	59.10	—	280	Austria: Cilag Bulgaria: Pharmachim

* Distributors IV: Austria, G. Britain-Glaxo; Belgium, Netherlands, Norway, Sweden-Nyegaard; Denmark-Nycomed; Finland-Medica

TABLE 1-9. METRIZOATE CONTRAST MEDIA FOR ANGIOGRAPHY (*Continued*)

Contrast Medium	Percent Metrizoate Salt				Iodine mg./ml.	Source Country-Firm
	Ca	Mg	MG	Na		
Ronpacon 350	2.80	2.00	—	55.20	350	Czechoslovakia: Chemapol
						Hungary: Medimpex
Ronpacon 370	1.48	1.03	40.00	28.80	370	Poland: Ciech
						Rumania: Chimimport
Ronpacon 440	3.50	2.50	—	69.00	440	Switzerland: Cilag
						W. Germany: Cilag
						Yugoslavia: Agroprogres
Triosil '45'	2.10	1.50	—	41.40	260	Gt. Brit.: Glaxo
Triosil '60'	2.80	2.00	—	55.20	350	Gt. Brit.: Glaxo
Triosil '75'	3.50	2.50	—	69.00	440	Gt. Brit.: Glaxo

Types of Contrast Media

Diatrizoate. The most widely used contrast media for angiography are the solutions of meglumine and sodium salts of diatrizoic acid, given in formulas IA and IB and Table 1-6. Currently, there is considerable interest in comparative evaluation of the toxic effects of these two salts.[86] Evidence has been presented[87] to indicate that a mixture is better than either salt alone, presumably, because the sodium salt enhances the excretion of the diatrizoic acid.[88]

Iodamide. The iodamide contrast media shown in formulas IIA and IIB, and in Table 1-7, have not become available in the United States as yet, and have not been used as widely as the other contrast media. Thus, it is difficult to assess the adverse reactions which are associated with their employment in arteriography and phlebography.

Iothalamate. The iothalamate contrast media, given in formulas IIIA and IIIB and in Table 1-8, have been employed for more than ten years, and are reputedly less neurotoxic than the diatrizoate salts. This is based on their use for visualization of the central nervous system, but adverse reactions are numerous in this application and clearcut claims cannot be made.[89]

A variation of the iothalamate acid molecule has been developed in France but is not yet available in the United States.[90] The new product has a -CO-NH-CH$_2$-CH$_2$-OH grouping at position 3 of the benzene ring in place of the -CO-NH-CH$_3$ grouping of iothalamic acid; it has the generic name of ioxithalamic acid. The contrast media prepared from this acid are offered as Vasobrix 32, a mixture of 41.7 percent ethanolamine ioxithalamate and 20.8 percent meglumine ioxithalamate, with an iodine content of 320 mg./ml.; and as Telebrix 38, a mixture of 51.4 percent meglumine ioxithalamate and 25.6 percent sodium ioxithalamate, with an iodine content of 380 mg./ml.

Metrizoate. The metrizoate contrast media, listed in Table 1-9, were originally offered as meglumine and sodium derivatives, but have been recently altered so that mixtures of calcium, magnesium, meglumine, and sodium salts, shown in formulas IVA-IVD, are employed. Reputedly, these mixtures are more physiologic and produce fewer adverse reactions than the former preparations. The metrizoate media are currently available in the United States on an investigative basis only.

Emergency Treatment of Reactions

Informed consent must be obtained from each patient prior to arteriography or phlebography, especially since the serious complication rate is approximately 1 in 500 angiograms. The angiographer should be responsible for the consent form, and must develop methods of communicating with patients and their relatives.[91]

The angiography suite must be equipped to deal with all cardiovascular emergencies which may arise during the procedure. A DC defibrillator in good working condition should be available at all times. The equipment of the suite should include an emergency cart suitably stocked with ventilatory assisting devices and the following drugs:

Aminophylline 0.5 mg.
Atropine sulfate 0.4 mg.
Diphenhydramine hydrochloride
  (Benadryl)
Calcium chloride
Calcium gluconate
Ephedrine sulfate 50 mg./ml.
Epinephrine (Adrenalin)1:1000
Hydrocortisone sodium succinate
  (Solu-Cortef) 100 mg.
Isoproterenol hydrochloride (Isuprel)
  1:5,000
Lidocaine (Xylocaine) 1%
Metraminol bitartrate (Aramine) 100 mg.
Nalorphine hydrochloride (Nalline)
  5 mg./ml.
Norepinephrine bitartrate (Levophed)
Phenobarbital sodium
Phenylephrine hydrochloride (Neo-
  Synephrine Hydrochloride) 2 mg./ml.
Prochlorperazine edisylate (Compazine)
  5 mg./ml.
Sodium bicarbonate

If resuscitative measures are necessary, the airway must be established, ventilation restored, circulation started, and definitive therapy instituted as quickly as possible. The angiographer must be familiar with all stages of cardiac resuscitation including defibrillation, the indications for epinephrine, isoproterenol, calcium chloride, and lidocaine. If an acute allergic reaction is suspected, epinephrine is probably the single most important drug, and corticosteroid therapy should probably also be given. Epinephrine

should always be ready for use in a loaded syringe fitted with a needle.

All complications cannot be avoided, and it is essential that a plan to deal with complications be ready for immediate use. Barnhard and Barnhard[92] have an excellent summary of the emergency treatment of reactions to contrast media, and their publication should be accessible for rapid reference. They point out that "if reactions to contrast material were common occurrences, radiologists would be skilled in coping with them. Fortunately, such reactions are uncommon, but it is their very infrequency that tends to make the radiologist complacent and ill-prepared to cope with the emergency that will one day come."

A careful history should be taken on each patient undergoing angiography, especially in regard to allergy or specific reaction to iodinated organic contrast media in the past. Contrast agents may cause renal failure in patients with multiple myeloma, and this, as well as other systemic diseases, should be searched for carefully. In pheochromocytomas, the contrast medium may provoke a sudden rise in blood pressure which could prove fatal if not anticipated.

The drugs and ventilatory assist devices should be organized on a "crash cart." This cart should be equipped with oxygen and suction, if not these are piped into the x-ray—surgical facility. A method should be developed to insure continuous inspection and replenishment of all items on the cart. A clear, thin plastic wrap may be employed to cover the cart so that a break in the plastic signals the need for replenishment.

Adverse Reactions to Contrast Media
Adverse reactions to water-soluble contrast media are common. Since the media are very hypertonic and are administered rapidly in large amounts, it is surprising that the adverse reactions are not more common. Arm pain and a metallic taste are experienced by all patients, but fatal and near fatal reactions are the complications of concern.

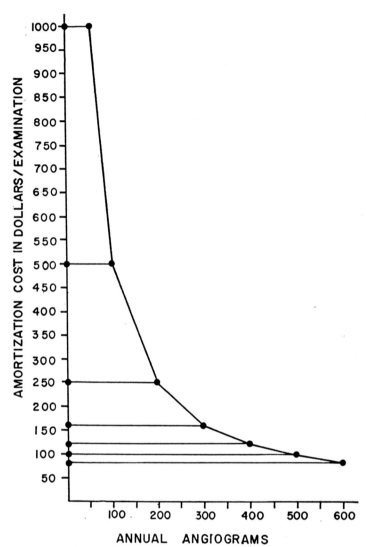

FIG. 1-16. Relationship of annual amortization cost per examination in dollars to the number of examinations, based on an average cost for a well-equipped laboratory of $250,000, and annual amortization of $50,000 over a 5-year period.

The complications from adverse effects seem to be related to the contrast agents, the condition of the patient, and the area of body under study. The media produce renal damage, allergic reactions, CNS disturbances, and cardiovascular changes. The literature on these reactions has been recently summarized by Almén,[93] Ansell,[25] and the Symposium of Contrast Media Toxicity of the Association of University Radiologists.[94] Many other publications could be cited from the world literature. The International Commission of Radiology has a standing Committee on Contrast Media which is presently making a world-wide survey of the incidence and nature of the reactions.

Current views on adverse reactions to the water-soluble agents used in angiography stress interaction with blood protein fractions. Lasser[95] has emphasized that antibody formation does not seem to be involved, but that hypertonicity and radiopaque-protein interactions are the important factors. Kutt and associates[96] have suggested the interference of radiopaques with the normal processes of fibrin and plasma clot formation. Fischer[97] has stressed that hemodynamic reactions are of great importance, as well as techniques of the injections. The tendency to conceal or ignore adverse reactions in the past has greatly hampered realization of the real incidence of untoward effects. There are many oddities to the reactions of contrast media. Lack of severe response to the test dose alone does not insure against a reaction from the diagnostic injection. Some severe reactions may follow as long as a day after the injection.

The Radiographic Facility

The radiographic facility for arteriography and phlebography should be carefully designed, equipped and maintained. The construction, dimensions, and arrangement of this area are of utmost importance in protecting the patient and examiners, and in obtaining the maximum amount of information from each procedure with the least exposure of the patient to contrast medium and radiation. The facility must provide easy traffic flow, and excellent working conditions for the angiographer and his associates. All drugs and instruments needed to deal with emergency situations must be readily available.

Inter-Society Radiology Study Group Report. The report[98] in 1971 of the Inter-Society Radiology Study Group on "Optimal Radiologic Facilities for Examination of the Chest and the Cardiovascular System" emphasizes the need for excellence in cardiovascular diagnosis. The cost of a suitable angiographic suite for a catheterization-angiocardiographic laboratory currently appears to be of the order of $250,000, and this cost must be amortized over a period of a few years because the equipment becomes obsolete so rapidly. Consequently 300 cases annually are recommended as the minimum number, and 450 as the optimum, to maintain the team required for these highly complex procedures and to provide for amortization. The relationship of amortization costs and annual number of examinations performed, based on an average cost of $250,000 for a well-equipped laboratory,

and annual amortization costs of $50,000 over a five-year period, is shown in Fig. 1-16. The facility must be located where the cost of data retrieval will be minimal and the relationship with definitive surgery will be maximal. This will reduce the burden on the patients and the health care system, as well as decrease the potential for complications, which increases with repetitive examinations on the same patient. The other recommendations of the study group are incorporated in this presentation along with the essential facts on radiologic design,[99] and radiation safety.[100-102]

Space Requirements. The x-ray—surgical suite needed for angiography should be located on a broad corridor central to the patients and within the primary radiology department of the institution. The orderly function of this facility is dependent on all the services of the x-ray department. The suite must be large enough to accommodate the basic elements for the arteriography and phlebography procedures. These include the following:

1. A central core consisting of the angiographic table and its associated radiographic x-ray tubes and filming devices.

2. A radiation protected observation area adequate in size for all personnel.

3. Work and storage areas for the equipment and supplies used by all radiographic and surgical personnel.

4. Scrub and gown area for the personnel.

5. Control booth containing x-ray and generator controls.

6. Storage and waiting areas for patients and beds.

7. Space to house the high-voltage transformer.

8. Film processing facilities.

9. Film viewing facilities.

Separate, or sharply demarcated, areas are desirable, but several of these basic elements can be contained in one space. Furthermore, some of the basic requirements can be furnished from the primary radiographic facility.

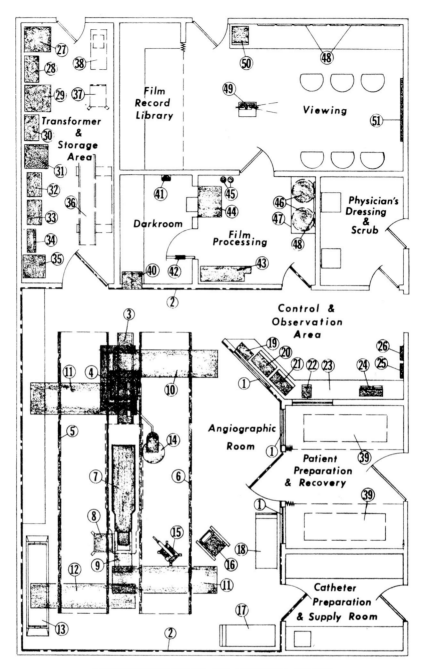

ARCHITECTURAL PLANNING CODE

ANGIOGRAPHIC ROOM
1 Lead glass view window
2 Indicates walls and doors to have lead lining
3 Long film table and cassette changer
4 Recess in ceiling for tube for long film table
5 Ceiling tubemount tracks on 7″ spacer, 23′6″ long
6 Ceiling tubemount tracks, 23′6″ long
7 Floating island table with table top travel indicated
8 Vertical film changer
9 Horizontal film changer
10 Mobile ceiling carriage with amplifier on telescopic column
11 Ceiling tubemount carriage
12 Mobile ceiling carriage with television monitor for procedural observation and physiological monitor
13 Storage area for rotating cradle
14 Surgical light on ceiling tubemount carriage
15 Contrast medium injector
16 Television fluoroscopy monitor

17 Medical monitoring unit
18 Emergency cart

CONTROL AND OBSERVATION AREA
19 Film changer control console
20 Standard control console
21 Grid control console
22 Televised fluoroscopy monitor
23 Shelf for accessory consoles
24 Disc recorder
25 480V. three phase load center
26 120/240V single phase load center

TRANSFORMER AND STORAGE AREA
27 Transformer for standard control generator
28 Power module for standard control generator
29 Transformer for grid control generator
30 Power module for grid control generator
31 Grid capacitor tank
32 Base unit for standard control generator
33 Base unit for grid control generator
34 Film changer control chassis
35 Rack cabinet to contain T.V. chassis, camera control, and brightness stabilizer

36 Storage area for long film table
37 Storage area for vertical film changer
38 Storage area for horizontal film changer

PATIENT PREPARATION AND RECOVERY AREA
39 Patient transport beds

DARKROOM
40 Cassette transfer cabinet
41 Safelight
42 Speaking grille
43 Automatic processor for serial films
44 Automatic processor
45 Water filters

FILM PROCESSING
46 Processor replenisher tanks
47 Removable section of countertop
48 Illuminators for radiographic films

VIEWING AREA
49 Cine film projector
50 Television monitors for procedures and fluoroscopy
51 Viewing screen

A complete angiographic suite with provision for all basic requirements is shown in Figure 1-17. Since the personnel cost is very high for arteriography and phlebography, the greatly increased efficiency and safety of the complete suite repays the expense. Obviously, such a well-equipped area may also be used for other special procedures.

Shell of the Facility. The coordination of several basic elements into one unit may include the central core, the work area, the scrub and gown room, the observation area, and the control booth in one shell. Doors sufficiently wide for easy entrance and turning of hospital beds are essential. The door, or doors, must be well balanced and preferably self-closing for ease of operation. The remaining elements can be housed nearby within the primary radiology department. A space of 700 sq. ft. provides a bare minimum for the grouping of these basic elements.

The entire enclosure, including ceiling and floors, must be constructed of a sufficiently thick radiation barrier to protect personnel outside the room. The exact amounts of this shielding should be determined by the standards established by official government agencies. Usually $\frac{3}{32}''$ of lead, or equivalent,

is sufficient for this enclosure, provided the protective walls extend at least seven feet high. Air conditioning inlets and outlets must be radiation safe and provide adequate air properly conditioned for temperature and humidification. Multiple built-in outlets should be provided around the perimeter of the shell.

Lighting. Abundant overhead lighting must be available for the suite as a whole, and intense beam lighting must be provided in the surgical procedure area. Low level background lighting is desirable for use during fluoroscopy. The general lighting should be controlled by a foot switch available to the angiographer, as well as by conventional wall switches. The suite should be light tight in case film must be loaded within the room in event of malfunction of some part of the system. A red warning light outside the room with a switch in the control booth is essential to indicate that a procedure is in progress, and to prevent inadvertent intrusions into the room at a critical moment.

Control Booth. The control booth serves as a shell within the main shell, and must likewise be constructed of radiation barrier material. The viewing surface of the control booth must be of specially treated lead glass with appropriate built-in voice slots to facilitate communication. The doorway to the control booth must be oriented to the main working area in such a way as to permit rapid flow of traffic between these two locations. Furthermore, this doorway must be located so that radiation does not penetrate the booth. If large enough, the control booth can double as a general protective and observation area.

Structural Details. Great care should be given to the structural details. The floors need not be conductive since explosive anesthetics are not used in the presence of radiographic equipment or other devices capable of producing sparks. The floor should be constructed of a material such as terrazzo, which is easy to clean after each procedure. A floor drain is very helpful in maintaining cleanliness. Oxygen and suction should be

---

Fig. 1-17. The complete angiographic suite must provide facilities for all phases of arteriography and phlebography. The angiographic room itself contains all the primary equipment needed for the radiographic examination and must be large enough for future alteration and expansion. The control and observation room should be sufficiently large to accommodate the angiographic team and several observers. Additional space for patient viewing is available through lead glass windows of the patient preparation and recovery area. Ancillary rooms must be provided for catheter preparation and medical storage; physician's dressing; transformer and equipment storage area; darkroom; film processing; and film viewing. The elongated space shown for transformer and equipment storage provides for better servicing of the transformers and storage of the equipment. An adequate viewing area is most important because it is used so much for clinical evaluation and teaching.

piped into the room at locations convenient to the head of the catheterization table. A clock with a sweep second hand should be located on the wall at the foot of the examination table to serve the needs of the anesthesiologist. An intercom and remote television for monitoring the room are extremely useful adjuncts. The ceiling of the suite should be of sufficient height to permit proper target-film distance for long film angiography, as well as for proper installation of movable tube mounts. Provision should be made for easy access for servicing of all utilities in the examining room. The shell must also contain adequate plumbing services of hot and cold water and venting of the sink.

Electronic Equipment. A vast assortment of cinefluorographic systems, film changers, processors, generators, image intensifiers, tables, and tubes is available for angiography. The state of the art is changing so rapidly that any detailed description of these various elements must of necessity be incomplete and partially obsolete at all times.

Catheterization Table. An "island" type catheterization table is necessary. The top of this table should move freely in the longitudinal and lateral direction. A table which can be raised or lowered is extremely convenient, particularly during the initial insertion of the catheter. The top should be as thin as possible to provide sufficient strength and to give minimal reduction in intensity of the x-ray beam. The tabletop and film changers should be arranged so that patient-film distance is minimized, and so that the table can be easily moved into position over the changers. A Bucky-Potter diaphragm and tray are desirable accessories, as well as a fluoroscopic "spot" film holder. A 90° rotating cradle will allow rapid positioning of the patient during fluoroscopy and filming. The table control handles should be removable so that they can be sterilized, or should have removable sterilizable or disposable covers.

Generators. The radiographic power generator is the heart of the angiography suite.

This generator usually requires three phase 480 v. input, and must be capable of delivering 150 kilovolts at 1,000-2,000 milliamperes. It should be rated at 100 kw. energy capacity, and full power should be available up to 100 kv. Timing is critical and must be in the millisecond range to deliver pulses as brief as one millisecond, or as long as 100 milliseconds. The time required to start the radiation after firing the device should be 4 milliseconds. A three-phase, 100 kw. generator, and a 30 kw., or larger, cine-pulse system are essential for cineangiocardiography.

Generators must be considered from two points of view, serial-film radiography and cine-radiography. In either case, the principal controls which are potentially variable by the operator are kilovoltage (kv.), milliamperage (ma.), and time of exposure. The combination of these three physical factors determines the density and contrast of the angiographic image. The density is primarily a function of the product of ma. $\times$ time, known as mas. In the case of cineangiographic images, the additional feature of automatic density or brightness control is employed.

A basic decision must be made in choosing generators for serial film radiography. Generators are available which allow the operator to individually determine ma. and time separately, or to dial in the desired mas (density). In the latter case, the generator automatically will deliver the highest ma. and shortest time possible for the mas chosen. This insures the most rapid possible exposure and diminishes blurring of the image. Some of these generators also perform this automatic exposure control at the highest kilowattage deliverable by the device, and are known as automatic constant full-power loading, or "iso-watt" devices. There are advantages in each of these basic types of generators which can be considered more fully by the radiologist at the time of design of the angiographic suite. Regardless of the type of generator chosen, it must be three-phase and capable of delivering up to 150 kilovolts at between 1,000-2,000 milliamperes.

X-Ray Tubes and Collimators. The number and kind of radiographic tubes employed in the angiographic facility is determined by the number of imaging devices used. An under the table fluoroscopic tube is needed, and a minimum of 22 inches focal spot—tabletop distance is necessary for satisfactory geometry and minimum skin dosage. An additional tube is required for each serial film changer. The radiographic tubes should be of high capacity with 1.0 mm., or larger, tungsten-rhenium-molybdenum (TRM) anodes capable of rotating at 10,000 rpm. A small focal spot of 0.3 mm., or even smaller, should be available for magnification radiography. Triple-leaf collimation must be used to minimize radiation to patient and technical personnel.

Image Amplification. The choice of image amplifiers varies with the specific functions of the room. Amplifiers are available in 6″, 7″, 9″, and in single or dual mode. The 5″-9″, or 6″-9″, combinations in dual mode are usually used since they are flexible and are preferred for the study of patients with large hearts. The 6″-7″, single mode intensifiers are characterized by high amplification and resolution but are limited in field size, such as for coronary or pediatric angiography. Each amplifier must be calibrated at least every six months. Television display has been a convenience and is developing into a necessity, but optical viewing must be provided as a backup precaution.

Cinefluorography and The Cine Pulsing System. Excellent cinefluorographic detail is provided by using 35 mm. cameras. Generally, reasonable definition can usually be obtained with 16 mm. cameras at lower cost, less patient radiation, and easier viewing and handling than 35 mm. film. It should be emphasized, however, that superior results can only be obtained with 35 mm. equipment. The large size 35 mm. gives optimum detail when used in combination with a small field image intensifier. Normally, the basic apparatus for the majority of the cinefluoro-

graphic needs is provided by a camera film speed of 60 to 80 frames/second and film magazines of 200 to 400 feet. Lenses with focal lengths varying from 50 mm. to 135 mm. and with f stops ranging from 2.0 to 16 are suitable for most purposes. Variable focal lengths may also be employed.

For cinefluorography, a special problem arises in the very rapid repetition of exposures (every 1/60, or even 1/80, of a second), which must be coordinated to occur during the brief interval when the cine-camera shutter is open. A mechanism to provide for these stringent requirements is called the cine-pulse system. Similar to serial film imagery, the energy pulses must be of very brief duration, usually less than 4 milliseconds. The coordination of these pulses with the shutter opening, however, requires either a grid bias applied to the x-ray tube or an electronic valve system using high vacuum tetrode tubes, or the older phase-shifting devices.

The kilovoltage specifications for cine studies is the same as for serial film work. Optimum kv. is usually in the 75-95 kv. range, but may require up to 150 kv. Because of image intensification, however, cine work does not require the very high milliamperage of serial filming. Usually, a cinepulse system supplying up to 200 ma. will suffice for cineangiography, and the capacity should be at least 30 kw.

In cineangiography, the cine pulse system is another special feature incorporated in the generator. This system controls the radiographic exposure and limits this exposure to the period when the camera shutter is open. It also controls and assures proper density for each frame of film. Patient size and thickness of body parts vary as the angiographer studies various organs, or "pans" across a large volume of varying density tissues, such as the chest. Even the opacity of the injected contrast medium changes the overall density of an organ being studied. To compensate for these uncontrollable and sometimes rapidly appearing changes in effective tissue density, the radiographic pulse is modulated by the automatic brightness control device so that the final filmed angiograph is of acceptable and predetermined brightness, or density.

The simplest method of insuring constant film quality is to vary the kilovoltage. A sensor is utilized to determine the exposure of a frame of cine film and, if any adjustments are necessary to bring the next frame into proper exposure range, a motor-driven variable voltage transformer coupled with the sensor then adjusts the kilovoltage to provide the predetermined proper overall exposure. This system has the handicap that unacceptable loss of control occurs if the kilovoltage is allowed to swing to very high levels. Care must be taken to pre-set sufficient milliamperage so as not to drive the kilovoltage too high when filming large density subjects. Three-phase, 30 kw. cine pulsing systems are necessary to provide sufficient energy to avoid this problem.

Milliamperage modulation in principle is similar to kilovoltage modulation in that a sensor determines the need for adjustments in current and a change in milliamperage is then instituted to bring the brightness or density of the frame into proper range. This method obviates the loss of contrast that can occur if kilovoltage modulation is used, assuming that the proper kilovoltage was pre-set by the angiographer. In addition to pre-setting, kilovoltage exposure time can also be determined initially and thus maS is the final variable used to determine brightness. Milliamperage modulation, however, is somewhat slower in response than kilovoltage modulation.

A third method of controlling brightness is achieved by automatically varying exposure time of each frame so that a contrast exposure occurs. This is called pulse width modulation. Kilovoltage and milliamperage are predetermined, and the electronic device varies pulse width by a feed-back system from the frame brightness sensor. The response time is very rapid with this method and phototiming is possible of each frame as it passes through the camera. Pulse width

modulation is very expensive although probably the best method of achieving automatic density control.

Grid and tetrode methods are the two acceptable procedures for cine pulsing, since blurring is minimized by providing exposure time of generally less than 5 milliseconds. The grid method utilizes an x-ray tube fitted with a grid which can control the flow of current in the tube when an appropriate bias voltage is applied. The tetrode method employs a high vacuum switching tube (tetrode) located in the secondary circuit to control the current flow, but short high voltage cables must be used with tetrodes.

To summarize, automatic brightness stabilization systems are of three basic types: (1) kilovoltage modulation; (2) milliamperage modulation; and (3) pulse width modulation. The pulse width modulation is the best of the three methods, and is also the most expensive.

Video System. A video system allows all personnel, as well as the angiographer, to view the fluoroscopic screen. Video recording by tape or disc is invaluable for instantaneous replay of test injections, and for backup during cine filming. A portable system permits usage under diverse radiologic conditions. The system should be operable from within the control booth and should include a high resolution screen, 525-945 lines/inch, visible to all. A remote monitor is helpful for teaching and supervision.

Film Processing. The equipment for processing large film will be determined by the volume of work performed in the angiographic facility. The large films must be handled with great care to prevent creasing or excessive contact with monitors. Preferably, the film processing should be built into the angiographic suite. If this is not possible, the large films can be processed in the equipment of the primary radiologic facilities.

The cine film must likewise be handled with great care. Independent processing facilities for the cine films are extremely desirable, and are essential for superior results. Standard film processing equipment may be used, but at a sacrifice of image quality. Provision must be made for processing all sizes of cine film and for flexibility.

Rapid Film Changers. Rapid film changers are available for film sizes 11″ x 14″, 14″ x 14″, and 14″ x 17″. The large radiographs obtained give optimal resolution of vascular structures and complement the information obtained by cinefluorography. The film changers should provide at least four films per second with automatic numbering and time-marking devices. Higher exposure rates up to 12 frames per second are available and are useful in angiocardiography and/or research, but speeds above 4/sec. are not necessary for most types of angiography. The program selector should operate two changers in biplane mode with electrical synchronization for alternating or synchronous exposures, or in single plane operation in either AP or lateral position. The changers should be designed to provide excellent screen-film contact.

The new improved image intensifiers and reliable spot film cameras give excellent detail comparable to that obtained with large film changers. The cameras employ large film formats, such as the 105 mm. camera, which allow photography of the image tube output phosphor. In addition to convenience of film handling, the repetition rates are more rapid and the radiation dosage to the patient is about one-tenth that required for large film exposure.

Long Film Changers. Changers are also available to move very long films at a slower rate than the rapid film device. A typical changer holds five film cassettes and changes these at the rate of approximately one each 1.5 or 2 seconds. Each cassette contains film covering an area of 14″ x 51″ (3 standard 14″ x 17″ films). This arrangement is extremely helpful because the entire abdomen, thighs, and legs of the average patient can be radiographed after a single injection of contrast medium.

Occasionally, there are problems when long films changers are employed. While this speed of changing films is usually suffi-

cient, there are some patients (frequently normal) whose blood flow is so rapid that visualization of the entire vascular system may not be picked up at this rate. In such cases, a second injection and second series of films may be necessary. Another drawback of this method is that the changing of the long cassettes must be triggered by a hand switch, and it is difficult to achieve uniformity and minimize the interval between exposures.

It is also possible to use conventional rapid film changers with a programmed table top that moves the patient over the film changer as the contrast medium flows through the vascular system. In this system, the exposure time and/or kvP must also change automatically as various thickness body parts are moved into the x-ray field for filming. A special programmer is needed to coordinate table top with film transport motion as the opaque medium flows into the extremities.

Film Viewing. The large films should be viewed immediately after processing. A separate room beyond the hearing range of the patient is extremely desirable. This room should be equipped with a large number of view boxes because so many radiographs must be studied at the same time.

Cine film viewing similarly must be available soon after the examination. Both viewers and projectors may be used, but the projectors are preferable since a larger group can view the results of the angiography at one time. An excellent projector must be used to provide flickerless images, variable speed control, and three projection modes—forward, reverse, and still.

Angiographic Procedures. Vascular catheterization is only the first step in obtaining proper radiographs of the circulatory system. The optimum operation of the radiographic equipment is complex and requires the constant attention of a skilled radiologist. To obtain the greatest amount of information from the available equipment with the least risk to the patient, the angiographer must personally make the injection and select the

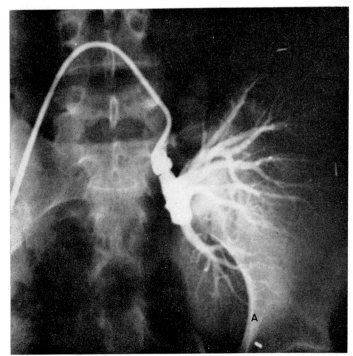

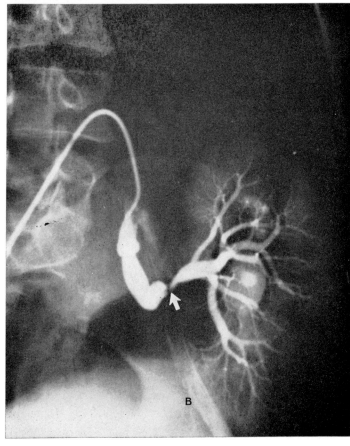

Fig. 1-18. Demonstration of the value of multiple positioning in renal transplant angiography. (*A*) Selective renal angiogram demonstrating anastomosis without evidence of significant stenosis. (*B*) Repeat renal angiogram in the oblique position demonstrates severe stenosis (*arrow*) of the renal artery-internal iliac as a probable cause of marked hypertension.

radiographic techniques. Proper positioning may be decisive in demonstrating the pathology, as shown in Figure 1-18. Fluoroscopy time and milliamperage must be completely controlled and permanently recorded for medical-legal purposes.

Radiation Protection. The radiation hazards to the patient and the examining personnel can be minimized by proper attention to many details. The equipment must be calibrated and checked for stray leakage radiation after installation, and periodically thereafter. The equipment should be checked especially after any maintenance or service procedure which may alter radiation output or shielding. Increased personnel exposure, as indicated by film badge readings, should always be regarded as originating in the equipment. The reports of the National Council on Radiation Protection Measurements[101] should be thoroughly understood, and the radiologist and health physicist in charge of the suite should be informed about all radiation health hazards and techniques for radiation detection. Specific areas for monitoring include the following: the catheterization table area, the observation areas, the control booth, the corridors outside the suite, as well as any areas above and below the angiographic laboratory.

Contrast Medium Injector. An automatic electric injector with built-in safeguards against electrical hazards is required for the injections of contrast medium, especially in selective angiography. The many manual-, gas-, and spring-operated devices cannot match the performance of the electric injectors which should provide the following:

1. Predetermined flow rates of at least 35 ml./sec., preferably 40-50 ml./sec. at body temperature.

2. Syringe capacity up to 100 ml. with built-in protection in the line for excess pressure. Disposable syringes are also available and are preferable.

3. Injection pressures up to 1000 psi, with variable pressure limit devices, and built-in protection for excess pressure.

4. Electrical hazard protection, which should include an audible signal for current leakage as low as 5 ma. and isolation of the contrast syringe from the electrical and mechanical portion of the injector.

5. ECG synchronized injection in certain angiographic techniques; if utilized, the provision should be possible for multiple controlled diastolic injections.

Physiologic Monitors. Physiologic data must be obtained and recorded during many arteriograms or phlebograms. A recording unit with at least four channels for depicting physiologic events is the minimum requirement. An oscilloscope with multiple channels should be available for displaying the electrocardiogram and pressures in full view of the angiographers. Other equipment should be available to determine the following: blood gases, cardiac output, and ergometric data.

Electrical Safety. The increased complexity of electrical equipment in diagnostic procedures has led to a considerable number of arrhythmias and deaths,[103-105] probably far more than have been reported. Ansell[25] described the death of one patient from an electric shock conducted through the x-ray machine from a diathermia apparatus. Whenever two or more pieces of electrical equipment using a common power source are connected to the patient, a hazard may exist if there is a voltage difference between the respective chassis (and the earth). The fluid-filled catheter used in angiography is an additional hazard since it acts as an electrical conductor to the heart, and evidence of shock from this source has been found on ECG tracings during such procedures.

The hazard of electrical shock to patients must be reduced by proper grounding in any facility in which electrical equipment is used. In the catheterization-angiocardiographic laboratory, ground bonding must be provided for both fixed and portable equipment, and must be independent of the electrical

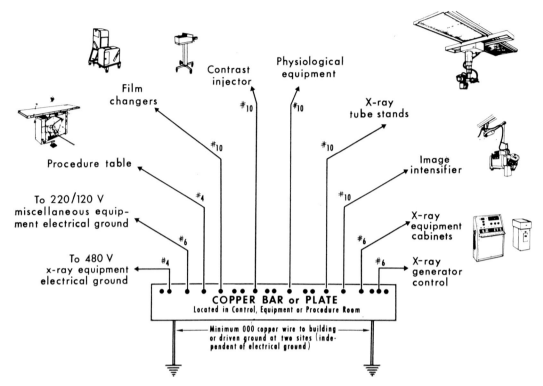

FIG. 1-19. Proper electrical safety system for the catheterization-angiocardiographic laboratory. Extremely small currents transmitted to the heart through the catheter may cause ventricular arrhythmia and death of the patient. Care must be taken to ground all equipment properly to a stable earth ground, independent of the electrical ground. A copper bar or plate may serve as a central grounding terminal for all equipment in the laboratory and should be connected by two independent 000 copper wires to the building ground or to a driven ground; this establishes a stable earth ground. To this plate is grounded all equipment, including, but not limited to, the following types: procedure table, film changers, contrast injector, physiological equipment, x-ray tube stand, image intensifier and its supports, and x-ray equipment cabinet, x-ray generators and transformers, etc. Ground terminals of the electrical service, including both the 120-240 volt and the 480 volt 3 phase lines are grounded on this plate. In some of the United States, an isolation is required of the power lines transformer serving the physiological recording equipment. Manufacturers of acceptable physiological instruments use isolation circuits in their input channels. Pressure transducers require special attention. The object of these measures is to keep the patient and all of his surroundings at ground potential.

ground. The common ground should be connected with special building ground straps, or a driven copper rod. The connections from these grounding sources to a procedure room copper ground plate should not be smaller than 000 copper wire as illustrated in Figure 1-19. The bonding must be appropriately sized to reduce the difference of potential during normal operations to less than five millivolts RMS between any two pieces of equipment within the suite; to handle leakage currents as high as one ampere; and to reduce the potential difference to less than five millivolts between components. The catheterization tabletop and the tube stand should be grounded in a suitable manner by means of a ground strap. All portable equipment must be similarly grounded through an independent ground cord to some other grounded piece of apparatus. Each installation must be checked periodically according to a definite program, and records kept that the bonding standards have been maintained.

Ultrasonic Arteriography. Ultrasonic methods for arteriography have been greatly refined in recent years, but their application seems limited to superficial blood vessels. The method is based on the principle that the frequency of reflected ultrasound from moving blood corpuscles is Doppler shifted from the incident sound.[106] Continuous or pulsed ultrasonic waves are transmitted to the corpuscles from a transducer on the skin overlying the blood vessel under study, and the reflected waves are measured by means of another transducer close to the first. Stenosis of superficial arteries can be detected, but definition is poor.[107]

The risk of tissue damage from ultrasound has been inadequately investigated. The measurements of Taylor and Bond[108] on the production of hemorrhagic injury and paraplegia by ultrasonic radiation of rat spinal cords indicates that damage is produced at the low frequency of 0.5 MHz, but not at frequencies of 5 MHz or higher. In addition, the evidence is conflicting whether ultrasound damages chromosomes.[109]

Radioisotopic Arteriography. The perfection of scintillation cameras during the past 10 years has greatly stimulated the development of radioisotopic arteriography. The procedures are more suitable for screening and for physiological studies than for providing anatomic details comparable to angiography with contrast media.

The scans employing cameras are rapid, and do not require patient preparation. Usually, a saline bolus containing indium-111 or -113M, technetium-99m, or xenon-133, with a radioisotope content ranging up to 20 mCi, is rapidly injected intravenously. Serial scintophotos are made at 2-second intervals with the patient in an upright or reclining position, or both. Tomography may also be carried in special studies. The entire examination is completed within 5 minutes, and the slight pain of venipuncture is the only immediate discomfort experienced by the patient.

The relatively large amount of radiopharmaceutical injected does increase the cost.

There are a number of hidden complications. Precautions must be taken against the radiation hazard to the patient, to the nuclear medicine facility personnel, and to the environment; these hazards have been outlined in NCRP Report 37.[111] Adverse reactions from the radiopharmaceuticals themselves are not common, and are very inadequately reported. Some of these reactions have been summarized by Atkins et al.[112] and Rubis et al.[113] The principal hazards are: improperly prepared radiopharmaceuticals; contamination with long-lived radioisotopes; and poor positioning so that airways are constricted in comatose patients.

Bibliography. In addition to the texts cited, there are many monographs with sections on arteriography and phlebography which also emphasize complications. Other publications that emphasize complications include the following:

Beuren, A. J.: Angiokardiographische Darstellung Kongenitaler Herzfehler: Ein Atlas. New York, De Gruyter, 1966.

Bieniarz, J.: Angiography and Placental Localization. Philadelphia, W. B. Saunders, 1973.

Bunell, I. K.: Selective Renal Angiography. Springfield, Ill., Charles C Thomas, 1968.

Cooley, R. N., and Schreiber, M. H.: Radiology of the Heart and Great Vessels. ed. 2. Baltimore, Williams & Wilkins, 1968.

Curry, J. L., and Howland, W. J.: Arteriography: Principles and Techniques. Philadelphia, W. B. Saunders, 1966.

Djindjian, R.: Angiography of the Spinal Cord. Baltimore, University Park, 1970.

Hanafee, W. N. (ed.): Selective Angiography. *In* Robbins, L. W. (ed.): Golden's Diagnostic Radiology. Baltimore, Williams & Wilkins, 1972.

Nomura, T.: Atlas of Cerebral Angiography. Berlin, Springer-Verlag, 1970.

Plaut, H. F.: Vertebral and Carotid Angiograms in Tentorial Herniations: Including Roentgen Anatomy of the Tentorial Incisure. Springfield, Ill., Charles C Thomas, 1961.

Reuter, S. R., and Redman, H. C.: Gastrointestinal Angiography. Philadelphia, W. B. Saunders, 1972.

Verel, D., and Grainger, R. G.: Cardiac Catheterization and Angiocardiography. Edinburgh, E & S Livingstone, 1969.

Viamonte, M., Jr., and Parks, R. E. (eds.): Progress in Angiography. Springfield, Ill., Charles C Thomas, 1964.

Wackenheim, A., and Braun, J. P.: Angiography of the Mesencephalon: Normal and Pathological Findings. Berlin, Springer-Verlag, 1970.

Weibel, J., and Fields, W. S.: Atlas of Arteriography in Occlusive Cerebral Vascular Disease. Philadelphia, W. B. Saunders, 1972.

Wenz, W., van Kaich, G., Beduhn, G., and Roth, F.-J.: Abdominale Angiographie. Berlin, Springer-Verlag, 1972.

Whitley, J. E., and Whitley, N. O.: Angiography: Principles and Practice. St. Louis, Warren H. Green, 1971.

References

1. Plecha, F. R., and Pories, W. J.: Intraoperative Angiography in the Immediate Assessment of Arterial Reconstruction. Arch. Surg., *105*:902, 1972.
2. Abrams, H. L. (ed.) Angiography. ed. 2, Boston, Little Brown, 1971.
3. Schobinger, R. A., and Ruzicka, F. F.: Vascular Roentgenology. New York, Macmillan, 1964.
4. Szilagyi, D. E., Smith, R. F., Macksood, A. J., and Eyler, W. R: Abdominal aortography. Its values and its hazards. Arch. Surg., *85*:41, 1962.
5. Berberich, J., and Hirsch, S.: Die roentgenographische Darstellung der Arterien und Venen am lebenden Menschen. Klin. Wchnschr., *2*:2226, 1923.
6. Brooks, B.: Intra-arterial injection of sodium iodide. JAMA, *82*:1016, 1924.
7. Moniz, E.: Die cerebrale Arteriographie und Phlebographie. Berlin, Springer, 1940.
8. Seldinger, S. I.: Insertion of catheter by cannula replacement. *In* Schobinger, R. A., and Ruzicka, F. F. (eds.): Vascular Roentgenology, p. 33. New York, Macmillan, 1964.
9. McAfee, J. G.: A survey of complications of abdominal aortography. Radiology, *68*:825, 1957.
10. Beall, Jr., A. C., Morris, Jr., G. E., Garrett, H. E., Henly, W. S., Hallman, G. L., Crawford, E. S., Cooley, D. A., and DeBakey, M. E.: Translumbar aortography: Present indications and techniques. Ann. Int. Med., *60*:843, 1964.
11. Robertson, P. W., Dyson, M. L., and Sutton, P. D.: Renal angiography: A review of 1,750 cases. Clin. Radiol., *20*:401, 1969.
12. Bookstein, J. J., Conn, J., and Reuter, S. R.: Intra-adrenal hemorrhage as a complication of adrenal venography in primary aldosteronism. Radiology, *90*: 778, 1968.
13. Lang, E. K.: A survey of the complications of percutaneous retrograde arteriography: Seldinger technique. Radiology, *81*:257, 1963.
14. Halpern, M.: Percutaneous transfemoral arteriography: An analysis of the complications in 1,000 consecutive cases. Amer. J. Roentgen., *92*:918, 1964.
15. Seidenberg, B., and Hurwitt, E. S.: Retrograde femoral (Seldinger) aortography: Surgical complications in 26 cases. Ann. Surg., *163*:221, 1966.
16. Broadbent, W. H.: Absence of pulsation in both radial arteries, the vessels being full of blood. Trans. Clin. Soc. London, *8*:165, 1875.
17. Fisher, M.: Occlusion of the internal carotid artery. Arch. Neurol. Psychiat., *65*:346, 1951.
18. Loman, J., and Myerson, A.: Visualization of the cerebral vessels by direct intra-carotid injection of thorium dioxide (Thorotrast). Amer. J. Roentgen., *35*: 188, 1936.
19. Turnbull, F.: Cerebral angiography by direct injection of the common carotid artery. Amer. J. Roentgen., *41*:166, 1939.
20. Donald, Jr., D. C., Kesmodel, Jr., K. F., Rollins, Jr., S. L., and Paddison, R. M.: An improved technique for percutaneous cerebral angiography. Arch. Neurol. Psychiat., *65*:508, 1951.
21. Hinck, V. C., and Dotter, C. T.: Appraisal of current techniques for cerebral angiography. Amer. J. Roentgen., *107*:626, 1969.
22. Decker, K.: Clinical Neuroradiology. American edition edited and translated by

Shehadi, W. H., New York, McGraw-Hill, 1966.

23. Allen, J. H., Perara, C., and Potts, D. G.: The relation of arterial trauma to complications of cerebral angiography. Amer. J. Roentgen., *95*:845, 1965.

24. Bergstrom, K., and Lodin, H.: Arteriovenous fistula as a complication of cerebral angiography. Brit. J. Radiol., *39*:263, 1966.

25. Ansell, G.: National survey of radiological complications: Interim report. Clin. Radiol., *19*:175, 1968.

26. Craigmile, T. K.: Carotid angiography. Surg. Clin. N. Amer., *49*:1435, 1969.

27. Chason, J. L., Landers, J. W., and Swanson, R. E.: Cotton fiber embolism. A frequent complication of cerebral angiography. Neurology, *13*:558, 1963.

28. Adams, D. F., Olin, T. B., and Kosek, J.: Cotton fiber embolization during angiography. Radiology, *84*:678, 1965.

29. Bouzarth, W. F., Goldfedder, P., and Shenkin, H. A.: Hypertonic mannitol as a treatment for complications of cerebral arteriography. Amer. J. Roentgen., *104*: 119, 1968.

30. Pearson, H. A., Schiebler, G. L., Krovetz, L. J., Bartley, T. D., and David, J. K.: Sickle-cell anemia associated with tetralogy of Fallot. New Eng. J. Med., *273*: 1079, 1965.

31. Olivecrona, H.: Bericht über die Tagung der Englischen Gesellschaft für Neurochirurgie (Society of British Neurological Surgeons) vom 6, bis 8, Juni 1935 in Stockholm (Offiizieller Bericht). Zbl. Chir., *62*:1903, 1935.

32. Takahashi, K.: Die percutane Arteriographie der Arteria Vertebrales und ihrer Versorgungsgebiete. Arch. f. Psychiat. *111*:373, 1940.

33. Sanders, R. J., and Ramirez, F.: Translumbar aortography. Surg. Clin. N. Amer., *49*:1317, 1969.

34. Lonni, Y. G. W., Matsumoto, K. K., and Lecky, J. W.: Postaortographic cholesterol (atheromatous) embolization. Radiology, *93*:63, 1969.

35. Haney, W. P., and Preston, R. E.: Ocular complications of carotid arteriography in carotid occlusive disease. A report of three cases. Arch. Ophth. *67*:127, 1962.

36. Gudbjerg, C. E., and Christensen, J.: Dissection of the aortic wall in retrograde lumbar aortography. Acta Radiol., *55*: 364, 1961.

37. Coran, A. G., and Tyler, H. B.: Aortic dissection. A complication of translumbar aortography. Amer. J. Surg., *115*: 709, 1968.

38. Margolis, G.: Pathogenesis of contrast media injury: Insights provided by neurotoxicity studies. Invest. Radiol., *5*:392, 1970.

39. Poulias, G. E., and Stergiou, L. E.: Pulmonary infarction and haemothorax as a post trans-lumbar aortography sequel. Brit. J. Radiol., *41*:866, 1968.

40. Candy, J., Grainger, K., and Guyer, P. B.: Aortoduodenal fistula complicating translumbar aortography. Brit. J. Surg., *52*:312, 1965.

41. Killen, D. A., Sewell, R., and Foster, J. H.: Colonic injury resulting from angiographic contrast media. Amer. J. Surg., *114*:904, 1967.

42. Andersen, P. E.: Ischaemic colitis caused by angiography. Clin. Radiol., *20*:414, 1969.

43. Sewell, R. A., Killen, D. A., and Foster, J. H.: Small bowel injury by angiographic contrast medium. Surgery, *64*:459, 1968.

44. Rossi, P., Young, I. S., and Panke, W. F.: Techniques, usefulness, and hazards of arteriography of pheochromocytoma. Review of 99 cases. JAMA, *205*:547, 1968.

45. Caine, M., Kedar, S. S., and Schwartz, A.: Renal angiography by the per-cutaneous non-catheter left brachial technique. Brit. J. Urol., *39*:571, 1967.

46. Carroll, S. E., and Wilkins, W. W.: Two cases of brachial plexus injury following percutaneous arteriograms. Canad. Med. Ass. J., *102*:861, 1970.

47. Armstrong, P. W., and Parker, J. O.: The complications of brachial arteriotomy. J. Thorac. Cardiov. Surg., *61*:424, 1971.

48. Feild, J. R., Lee, L., and McBurney, R. F.: Complications of 1000 brachial arteriograms. J. Neurosurg., *36*:324, 1972.

49. Campion, B. C., Frye, R. L., Pluth, J. R., Fairbairn, II, J. F., and Davis, G. D.: Arterial complications of retrograde brachial arterial catheterization: A prospective study. Mayo Clin. Proc., *46*:589, 1971.

50. Seldinger, S. I.: Catheter replacement of the needle in percutaneous arteriography. Acta Radiol., *39*:368, 1953.

51. Ranniger, K., and Saldino, R. M.: Abdominal angiography. Curr. Probl. Surg., March, 1968.

52. Mortensen, J. D.: Clinical sequelae from arterial needle puncture, cannulation, and incision. Circulation, *35*:1118, 1967.

53. Haut, G., and Amplatz, K.: Complication rates of transfemoral and transaortic catheterization. Surgery, *63*:594, 1968.

54. Takahashi, M., and Kawanami, H.: Femoral catheter techniques in cerebral angiography—an analysis of 422 examinations. Brit. J. Radiol., *43*:771, 1970.

55. Obenchain, T. G., Clark, R., Hanafee, W., and Wilson, G.: Complication rate of selective cerebral angiography in infants and children. Radiology, *95*:669, 1970.

56. Dotter, C. T., Rösch, J., and Bilbao, M. K.: Transluminal extraction of catheter and guide fragments from the heart and great vessels; 29 collected cases. Amer. J. Roentgen., *111*:467, 1971.

57. Curry, J. L.: Recovery of detached intravascular catheter or guide wire fragments. A proposed method. Amer. J. Roentgen., *105*:894, 1969.

58. Sheiner, N. M., Sigman, H., Libman, I., and Palayew, M. J.: An unusual complication of cerebral angiography. Amer. J. Roentgen., *106*:269, 1969.

59. Kocandrle, V., Kittle, C. F., and Petasnick, J.: Percutaneous retrograde abdominal aortography complication. Arch. Surg., *100*:611, 1970.

60. Kirschner, L. P., Twigg, H. L., Conrad, P. W., and Hufnagel, C.: Retrograde catheter aortography in dissecting aortic aneurysms. Am. J. Roentgen., *102*:349, 1968.

61. Shuford, W. H., Sybers, R. G., and Weens, H. S.: Problems in the aortographic diagnosis of dissecting aneurysm of the aorta. New Eng. J. Med., *280*:225, 1969.

62. Harrington, J. T., Sommers, S. C., and Kassirer, J. P.: Atheromatous emboli with progressive renal failure. Renal arteriography as the probable inciting factor. Ann. Int. Med., *68*:152, 1968.

63. Nawar, T., Cadotte, M., LeFebvre, R., Rojo-Ortega, J. M., and Genest, J.: Widespread atheromatous emboli following abdominal aortography. Canad. Med. Ass. J., *100*:1005, 1969.

64. Moore, C. H., Wolma, F. J., Brown, R. W., and Derrick, J. R.: Complications of cardiovascular radiology. A review of 1,204 cases. Amer. J. Surg., *120*:591, 1970.

65. Hall, K. V.: Editorial. Ugeskrift f. Laeg., *134*:13, 1972.

66. Siegelman, S. S., Caplan, L. H., and Annes, G. P.: Complications of catheter angiography. Study with oscillometry and "pullout" angiograms. Radiology, *91*:251, 1968.

67. Pollard, J. J., and Nebesar, R. A.: Abdominal angiography. New Eng. J. Med., *279*:1035, 1968.

68. DeWeese, J. A., and Rogoff, S. M.: Clinical uses of functional ascending phlebography of the lower extremity. Angiol., *9*:268, 1958.

69. DeWeese, J. A., and Rogoff, S. M.: Phlebographic patterns of acute deep venous thrombosis of the leg. Surgery, *53*:99, 1963.

70. Göthlin, J.: The comparative frequency of extravasal injection at phlebography with steel and plastic cannula. Clin. Radiol., *23*:183, 1972.

71. Sanders, R. J., and Glaser, J. L.: Clinical uses of venography. Angiology, *20*:388, 1969.

72. Lea Thomas, M.: Gangrene following peripheral phlebography of the legs. Brit. J. Radiol., *43*:528, 1970.

73. Schobinger, R. A.: Intra-osseous Venography. New York, Grune and Stratton, 1960.

74. Wegner, G. P., Flaherty, T. T., and Crummy, A. B.: Intraosseous lower extremity venography. Arch. Surg., *98*:105, 1969.

75. Sanders, R. J., Ramirez, F., and Kortz, A. B.: Venography. Surg. Clin. N. Amer., *49*:1445, 1969.

76. Lea Thomas, M.: Phlebography. Arch. Surg., *104*:145, 1972.

77. Ferris, E. J., Hipona, F. A., Kahn, P. C., Philipps, E., and Shapiro, J. H.: Venography of the Inferior Vena Cava and Its Branches. Baltimore, Williams & Wilkins, 1969.

78. Bayliss, R. I. S., Edwards, O. M., and Starer, F.: Complications of adrenal venography. Brit. J. Radiol., *43*:531, 1970.

79. Leger, L.: Phlebographie portale par injection splenique intraparenchymatense. Mem. Acad. chir., *77*:712, 1951.

80. Odman, P.: Percutaneous selective angiography of the coeliac artery. Acta Radiol. (Suppl. 159), 1, 1958.

81. Rösch, J.: Roentgenology of the Spleen and Pancreas. Springfield, Ill., Thomas, 1967.

82. Panke, W. F., Bradley, E. G., Moreno, A. H., Ruzicka, Jr., F. F., and Rousselot,

L. M.: Technique, hazards, and usefulness of percutaneous splenic portography, JAMA, *169*:1032, 1959.

83. Damascelli, B.: Study of the cervical veins by the translingual route in man. Amer. J. Med., *47*:392, 1969.

84. Strain, W. H.: Radiologic diagnostic agents. Med. Radiog. Photog., *40*: Suppl., 1964.

85. Blaufox, M. D., and Freeman, L. D. (ed. consult.): Physicians Desk Reference for Radiology and Nuclear Medicine. Oradell, New Jersey, Medical Economics, 1972.

86. Fischer, H. W., and Redman, H. C.: Comparison of a sodium methylglucamine diatrizoate contrast medium of minimal sodium content with a pure methylglucamine diatrizoate preparation. Invest. Radiol., *6*:115, 1971.

87. Fischer, H. W.: Sodium content of contrast media. Invest. Radiol., *5*:266, 1970.

88. Dacie, J. E., and Fry, I. K.: Comparison of sodium and methylglucamine diatrizoate in high dosage urography. Brit. J. Radiol., *45*:385, 1972.

89. Gonsette, R.: An experimental and clinical assessment of water-soluble contrast medium in neuroradiology. A new medium—Dimer-X. Clin. Radiol., *22*:44, 1971.

90. Gonsette, R., and Andre-Balsiaux, G.: Etude expérimentale et clinique de la tolérance des capillaires cérébraux pour une nouxelle substance de contraste (sels de l'acide ioxitalamique). Acta Radiol., *8*:535, 1969.

91. Alfidi, R. J.: Informed consent. A study of patient reaction. JAMA, *216*:1325, 1971.

92. Barnhard, H. J., and Barnhard, F. M.: The emergency treatment of reactions to contrast media. *In* Abrams, H. L. (ed.): Angiography. ed. 2, vol. 1, pp. 63-74. Boston, Little Brown, 1971.

93. Almén, T.: Toxicity of radiocontrast agents. *In* Knoefel, P. K. (ed.): Radiocontrast Agents. Section 76 of International Encyclopedia of Pharmacology and Therapeutics. vol. 2, pp. 443-550. New York, Pergamon, 1971.

94. Association of University Radiologists: Symposium on contrast media toxicity of the Association of University Radiologists. Invest. Radiol., *5*:373, 1970.

95. Lasser, E. C.: Metabolic basis of contrast material toxicity—status 1971. Amer. J. Roentgen., *113*:415, 1971.

96. Verebely, K., Kutt, H., Torack, R. M., and McDowell, F.: The effects of radioopaque contrast media on the structure and solubility of the fibrin clot. Blood, *33*:468, 1969.

97. Fischer, H. W.: Hemodynamic reactions to angiographic media. Radiology, *91*:66, 1968.

98. Radiology Study Group—Abrams, H. L. (chm.), Adelstein, S. J., Elliott, L. P., Ellis, K., Greenspan, R. H., Judkins, M. P., and Viamonte, M.: Optimal radiologic facilities for examination of the chest and the cardiovascular system. Circulation, *43*:A-135, 1971.

99. Scott, W. G. (ed.): Planning Guide for Radiologic Installations. ed. 2, Baltimore, Williams & Wilkins, 1966.

100. Goodwin, P. N., Quimby, E. H., and Morgan, R. H.: Physical Foundations of Radiology., ed. 4, New York, Harper and Row, 1970.

101. National Council on Radiation Protection and Measurements: Medical x-ray and gamma protection for energies up to 10 MeV; equipment design and use; recommendations. Washington, D.C. (NCRP report no. 33), 1968.

102. National Council on Radiation Protection and Measurements: Medical x-ray and gamma-ray protection for energies up to 10 MeV; structural shielding design and evaluation handbook; recommendations. Washington, D.C. (NCRP report no. 34), 1970.

103. Walter, C. W. (ed.): Electric Hazards in Hospitals. Proceedings of a Workshop. Washington, D.C., National Academy of Science, 1970.

104. Sprawls, P.: Electrocution hazards in x-ray installations. Radiology, *100*:157, 1971.

105. Green, H. L., Hieb, G. E., and Schatz, I. J.: Electronic equipment in critical care areas: status of devices currently in use. Circulation, *43*:A-101, 1971.

106. Wells, P. N. T.: Physical Principles of Ultrasonic Diagnosis. New York, Academic Press, 1969.

107. Fish, P. J., Corrigan, T., Kakkar, V. V., and Nicolaides, A. N.: Arteriography using ultrasound. Lancet, *2*:1269, 1972.

108. Taylor, K. F. W., and Pond, F. B.: A study of the production of haemorrhagic injury and paraplegia in rat spinal cord by pulsed ultrasound of low megaHertz frequencies in the context of the safety for clinical usage. Brit. J. Radiol., *45*:533, 1972.

109. Editorial. Brit. J. Radiol., *45*:319, 1972.
110. NCRP REPORT 37. Precautions in the Management of Patients Who Have Received Therapeutic Amounts of Radionuclides. Washington, D.C., National Council on Radiation Protection and Measurement, 1970.
111. Atkins, H. L., Hauser, W., Richards, P., and Klopper J.: Adverse reactions to radiopharmaceuticals. J. Nucl. Med., *13*:232, 1972.
112. Rubis, L. J., *et al.*: Extrinsic and intrinsic hazards associated with brain scanning. Neuroradiol., *4*:128, 1972.

Chapter 2 | Complications of

H. Edward Garrett, M.D. | # Abdominal Aortic Surgery

Achievements in vascular surgery during the past two decades led to the development of numerous operative procedures on the abdominal aorta and its major branches. Concomitantly, improvements in anesthesia, graft materials, and in the understanding of altered physiology in the postoperative patient reduced the risk of operation. Evaluation of this experience has provided rather uniform opinion among surgeons regarding choice of procedure, operative technique, complications encountered, and their prevention and treatment.

The majority of operations on the abdominal aorta are performed for correction of aneurysmal or occlusive disease. Although atherosclerosis is the etiology in most instances, other causes such as congenital anomaly, trauma, embolic disease, and certain inflammatory lesions may be encountered. The basic principles of vascular surgery involved in correction of atherosclerotic aneurysm or occlusive disease may be applied successfully in the treatment of other lesions identified at operation.

Complications of abdominal aortic surgery occur less frequently as the experience of the surgeon increases. This type of surgery is highly technical and many complications have their origin at the operating table as a result of technical factors encountered during operation. A standardized operative technique that results in a high level of proficiency will prevent the majority of com-

plications. When complications occur, immediate detection and vigorous treatment offer the patient the best opportunity for a good result. A review of certain technical points of operative procedures which are considered important in the prevention of complications will be undertaken before considering the treatment of specific complications.

Aneurysm of the Abdominal Aorta

The majority of abdominal aortic aneurysms are atherosclerotic in origin and involve a segmental portion of the abdominal aorta. Most aneurysms arise below the origin of the renal arteries. Occasionally, however, one or both renal arteries or accessory renal arteries may arise from the aneurysm without the superior mesenteric artery being involved[1] (Fig. 2-1, D, E). Thoracoabdominal aneurysms typically involve the origins of the celiac, superior mesenteric, and both renal arteries (Fig. 2-1, F). Distally, an aneurysm may extend to the bifurcation of the aorta (Fig. 2-1, A) or involve one or both common iliac arteries (Fig. 2-1, B). Occasionally, the lesion may include both external and internal iliac arteries (Fig. 2-1, C). Fortunately, the majority of abdominal aortic aneurysms arise below the renal arteries and terminate at the bifurcation of the aorta or the common iliac arteries. Relatively normal arterial segments are usually found above and below the lesion allowing segmental excision and graft replacement.

Abdominal aneurysms usually present as an asymptomatic pulsatile mass. They may be tender on palpation and associated with back pain from compression of the spine or cause severe abdominal and back pain associated with rupture. In general, an aneurysm which is symptomatic or tender should raise immediate suspicion of active expansion or rupture. An abdominal aneurysm occasionally ruptures into the duodenum, vena cava, or left renal vein. More commonly, rupture occurs into the retroperitoneal space and may be contained briefly before fatal hemorrhage occurs. The recommended therapy for

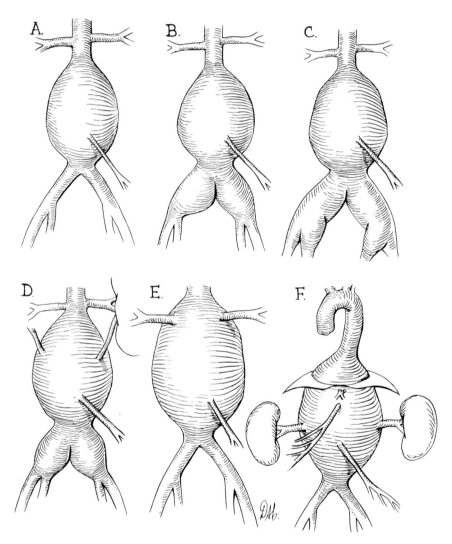

FIG. 2-1. (A) Aneurysm of the distal abdominal aorta; (B) aneurysm of the abdominal aorta and common iliac arteries; (C) aneurysm of abdominal aorta, common, external, and internal iliac arteries; (D) aneurysm of abdominal aorta and common iliac arteries with accessory renal arteries arising from the aneurysm; (E) aneurysm of the abdominal aorta with renal arteries arising from the aneurysm and (F) thoracoabdominal aortic aneurysm with origins of the celiac, superior mesenteric, and renal arteries arising from the aneurysm.

most aneurysms of the abdominal aorta is elective resection with graft replacement. While all ruptured or actively expanding aneurysms should be operated on as true surgical emergencies, consideration should be given to several factors in selecting patients for elective treatment. Size of the aneurysm in relation to the age of the patient has recently been emphasized in several reports. Large aneurysms are far more likely to cause death of the patient by rupture as indicated by the collected figure of at least 70 percent death from rupture of aneurysms 7 cm. in diameter or larger in patients followed without operation. Moreover, the leading cause of death in patients followed without operation is aneurysmal rupture regardless of size. On the other hand, in patients who are 75 years of age or older, whose aneurysms are less than 5 cm. in size and who have significant associated renal, pulmonary, or cardiac disease, consideration should be given to nonoperative management. The incidence of serious complications in this group of patients is significant despite careful operative technique.[2,3,4] With current techniques of vascular surgery, anesthesia, and postoperative care, aneurysms of the abdominal aorta may be successfully managed with low risk to the patient.[5,6,7]

Operative Technique

The patient is placed in the supine position under general endotracheal anesthesia with two indwelling intravenous needles in place in the upper extremities for fluid and blood administration and an indwelling catheter in the bladder attached to a drainage bag. The abdomen and both groins are prepped and draped according to the preference of the surgeon. A vertical midline incision is made from xyphoid to pubis. The peritoneal cavity is explored for associated disease. The omentum and transverse colon are delivered superiorly onto the abdominal wall and the small bowel delivered onto the right abdominal wall. Moist towels are placed over the bowel and large retractors inserted to maintain exposure. The posterior peritoneum is incised between the duodenum and the inferior mesenteric vein from the ligament of Trietz to the pelvis exposing the retroperitoneal space. The periaortic tissue directly overlying the superior portion of the aneurysm is incised until the left renal vein is exposed. This dissection is continued laterally adjacent to the aorta immediately below the renal vein until a finger of the surgeon may be inserted on each side of the aorta providing space for application of the proximal vascular clamp. If necessary, the left renal vein may be encircled with moist umbilical tape and retracted superiorly or inferiorly to provide addition exposure for proximal control of the aorta. The left adrenal vein may be torn during mobilization of the left renal vein and should be sacrificed. The renal arteries are usually exposed if dissection beneath or superior to the left renal vein is required. Transection of the left renal vein with later repair is rarely, if ever, necessary for adequate exposure. Encircling the aorta with umbilical tape proximal to the aneurysm is unnecessary and may be hazardous if a large lumbar artery or vein is torn.

Distal control is obtained by dissecting the tissue over the common iliac arteries anteriorly and laterally to allow placement of vascular clamps. Encircling these arteries is also unnecessary in most instances and may result in injury to the common iliac veins. This is especially true of the right common iliac artery where the left common iliac vein is intimately attached to the posterior surface of the vessel. The ureter must be identified and protected as dissection extends below the bifurcation of the iliac arteries. If the aneurysm extends to the bifurcation of the iliac arteries, distal dissection is less difficult after the aorta is occluded proximally.

Prior to application of vascular occluding clamps near the renal arteries, diuresis is induced by intravenous administration of 12.5 Gm. of mannitol.* If a knitted graft is selected for replacement of the aneurysm,

---

* Merck, Sharp & Dohme.

blood is aspirated from the aorta and pre-clotting accomplished in a small basin. Pre-clotting of the graft should be carefully performed by kneading and stretching the graft so as to work blood into the interstices of the Dacron material over several minutes of deliberate manipulation. Teflon graft material is not recommended because of its tendency to fray at the graft ends and its lesser tendency to hold the neointima which later develops in the graft. Aqueous heparin, 1:1000, approximately 75 units per kilo-

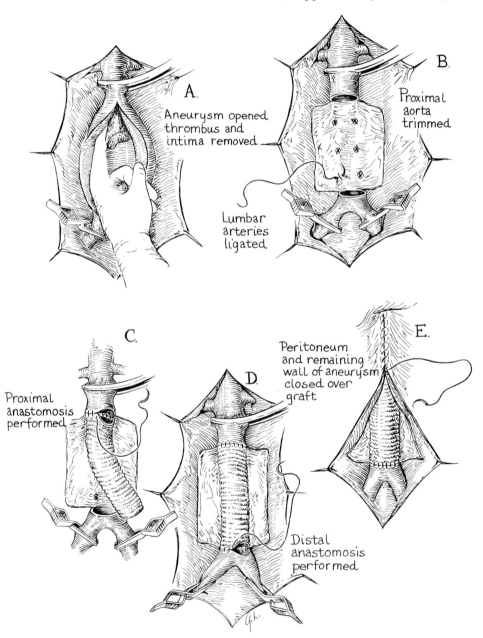

FIG. 2-2. (A) Technique of entering the aneurysm after proximal and distal occlusion; (B) suture of lumbar arteries; (C) proximal anastomosis of Dacron graft; (D) distal anastomosis to bifurcation of aorta, and (E) two-layer retroperitoneal closure over the graft.

gram, is administered intravenously or injected through the aorta proximal to the aneurysm. If heparin is injected through the wall of the aneurysm, thrombus may be dislodged and produce embolic occlusion in the lower extremities.

Occlusion of the aorta and iliac arteries with vascular clamps is accomplished and the aneurysm incised vertically (Fig. 2-2, A). Care is taken to avoid application of vascular clamps on areas of calcified arteriosclerotic plaque formation whenever possible to avoid fracture of this diseased lining which may result in later complications. Blood and atheromatous material is removed by suction and the inferior mesenteric artery and lumbar arteries identified. The inferior mesenteric artery is inspected, however, prior to division. If it is of large size, it should be preserved by control with a vascular clamp and excision of a cuff of aortic tissue for later reimplantation in the aortic graft. The intima is stripped from the ostia of the lumbar and middle sacral arteries and suture ligation accomplished within the lumen of the aneurysm (Fig. 2-2, B). The aorta, proximal to the aneurysm, is incised circumferentially in preparation for proximal anastomosis. Care is taken near the vena cava to obtain a satisfactory cuff of aorta without injuring the cava. The intima within the aneurysm is removed by blunt dissection leaving a fibrous wall to be used later to cover the graft. The graft selected for replacement is then sutured into the cuff of the proximal aorta with a continuous, everting, braided Dacron suture beginning posteriorly and ending anteriorly (Fig. 2-2, C). The choice of graft size, which must be made earlier in the operation before heparinization when using knitted graft material, is made to accommodate the proximal aortic cuff. If a bifurcation graft is to be employed, the distal limbs should be at least 8 mm. in diameter. Any of the Dacron synthetic suture materials may be employed and 3-0 size suture material is generally preferred. Care is taken during the anastomosis to handle the aortic cuff gently to avoid damage to the arterial

wall. The graft is occluded below the suture line and the proximal clamp briefly released to test the suture line. Vascular clamps should be released and reapplied only as often as absolutely necessary to minimize trauma to the vessel wall. Any leaks are repaired prior to proceeding with the distal anastomosis.

If the bifurcation of the aorta is not involved by aneurysmal dilatation, a tube graft replacement may be accomplished with the distal anastomosis performed at the bifurcation using similar continuous suture technique (Fig. 2-2, D). If the aneurysm extends into the common iliac arteries, a bifurcation graft is required with the distal end-to-end anastomosis performed to the common iliac arteries below the lesion. The iliac arteries involved by aneurysm are incised anteriorly until a satisfactory vessel for anastomosis is identified. Circumferential incision of the iliac artery is performed in preparation for the distal anastomosis. The intima of the diseased artery is stripped, leaving a fibrous wall of adventitia. The limb of the graft is cut to an appropriate length and sutured end-to-end with continuous braided Dacron vascular suture. Prior to completion of the suture line, flushing proximally and distally is performed to remove clots and any atheromatous material released by application of vascular clamps. If back flow from a distal vessel is not observed, passage of a Fogarty catheter should be undertaken at this time to recover thrombus or embolized material. On completion of the first distal suture line in a bifurcation graft, blood flow can be restored to that extremity by application of a vascular clamp tangentially at the origin of the remaining limb. This clamp should be carefully applied flush with the graft bifurcation at the origin of the remaining limb to prevent an area of stasis in a blood-filled Dacron graft which may lead to thrombus formation.

Declamping shock is associated with hypovolemia and acidosis and should be prevented. Prior communication between the surgeon and anesthesiologist should always precede release of the proximal clamp allowing for complete blood volume replacement and continuous blood pressure monitoring. If occlusion time has been prolonged, intravenous administration of sodium bicarbonate immediately prior to clamp release should be strongly considered. Many anesthesiologists are now in the practice of monitoring blood gases and pH during such operations, and this offers excellent additional protection to the patient during this maneuver. Distal clamps should be released first allowing the graft to fill and air to be expressed from the lumen. The proximal clamp is then released gradually and the patient briefly observed. Intermittent reapplication of the proximal clamp is seldom necessary and may result in thrombus formation within the prosthesis. Static blood within a Dacron prosthesis has a strong tendency to form thrombus in a very brief period of time. The second distal anastomosis in a bifurcation graft is then accomplished, along with proximal and distal flushing and clamp release, in a similar fashion.

The retroperitoneal area is irrigated thoroughly with an antibiotic solution and inspected for bleeding. Suture lines and lumbar arteries are visualized again and any bleeding controlled with additional sutures. If additional suturing of the posterior aspect of the proximal anastomosis is required at this time and exposure is difficult, the graft may be divided in its midportion and then rapidly repaired after the proximal aortic bleeding point has been controlled. Other bleeding points may be controlled by electrocoagulation. The remaining wall of the aneurysm, including available periaortic tissue, is then sutured over the aortic suture line and graft with continuous chromic catgut (Fig. 2-2, E). Finally the posterior peritoneum is approximated by a second suture line of continuous catgut. This should be accomplished with care so as to definitely interpose adequate tissue between the adjacent duodenum and the aortic graft, especially in the region of the proximal anastomosis where this may be most difficult. Prior planning at the time of retroperitoneal incision so as to leave a flap of retroperitoneal tissue adjacent to the duodenum for later use in closure is usually possible. The inferior

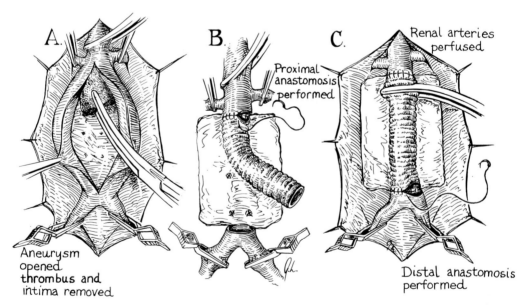

FIG. 2-3. (A) Occlusion of aorta above renal arteries and renal artery occlusion before entering the aneurysm; (B) proximal anastomosis accomplished below the renal arteries, and (C) perfusion of renal arteries before completing distal anastomosis.

mesenteric vein should be protected during retroperitoneal closure by careful placement of sutures in the left lateral retroperitoneal tissues.

The pelvis is aspirated free of blood and fluid and the bowel replaced in anatomical position. Wound closure is accomplished according to the preference of the surgeon. Retention sutures are unnecessary if heavy, interrupted nonabsorbable sutures are used to approximate the linea alba. The vascular status of the lower extremities is inspected and compared to the preoperative state. Should embolic occlusion be suspected, appropriate diagnostic and therapeutic measures are undertaken immediately. If reocclusion of the graft or a limb of the graft is necessary to treat an acute distal occlusion, the occluded portion of the graft must be emptied of blood to avoid thrombosis. If passage of a Fogarty catheter is required, this may be accomplished through a short, transverse incision in the anterior surface of the graft at an appropriate site which can be easily repaired. Exposure of the femoral bifurcation may be useful for extraction of emboli. Following operation, the patient is observed closely for 48-72 hours in a setting with continuous nursing care. Particular attention is directed to blood volume, renal function, and pulmonary function. Early complications are usually evident during this time.

Abdominal Aneurysm Involving Renal Arteries

Occasional aneurysms of the abdominal aorta arise immediately below the ostia of the renal arteries or above the renal arteries, but do not involve the superior mesenteric artery. These lesions are more difficult to manage at operation due to the proximity of the renal arteries and the possibility of producing renal insufficiency.

Aneurysms arising at the ostia of the renal arteries may be managed operatively by proximal occlusion of the aorta above the renal arteries (Fig. 2-3, A). The left renal vein is mobilized and periaortic tissue cleared

above the vein but below the origin of the superior mesenteric artery. The renal arteries are identified and protected during application of the proximal vascular clamp. Renal artery occlusion of a diuresing kidney is well tolerated for periods of up to 30 minutes. This allows ample time to enter the aneurysm, dissect a cuff of aorta below the renal arteries for the proximal anastomosis, and complete the anastomosis (Fig. 2-3, B). The graft is then occluded below the renal arteries and the proximal clamp removed, restoring blood flow to the kidneys (Fig. 2-3, C). The remainder of the operation is completed in standard fashion according to the distal extent of the lesion.

Aneurysms arising above the renal arteries but below the superior mesenteric artery require replacement of each renal artery with a graft. After complete dissection demonstrates the proximal and distal extent of the lesion, an appropriate graft is selected, and prosthetic limbs for each renal artery are sutured to the aortic graft prior to aortic clamping. Diuresis is induced, pre-clotting of the graft accomplished, heparin administered, and vascular clamps applied to the aorta below the superior mesenteric artery and at some point below the renal arteries (Fig. 2-4, A). Both renal arteries are occluded with vascular clamps and the lesion entered. The renal arteries are transacted and prepared for anastomosis (Fig. 2-4, B). The aortic prosthesis with renal branches is sutured proximally to the aorta (Fig. 2-4, C) and one renal anastomosis accomplished thereafter (Fig. 2-4, D). The aortic graft is then occluded below the first renal branch and the proximal clamp removed, restoring circulation to this kidney (Fig. 2-4, E). The second renal branch is sutured promptly and opened, restoring blood flow to the second kidney (Fig. 2-4, F). Then the remaining aneurysm is removed, lumbar and inferior mesenteric branches controlled, and the distal anastomosis accomplished. Renal insufficiency is usually prevented if blood flow to the kidneys is restored within 30-45 minutes after renal artery occlusion.

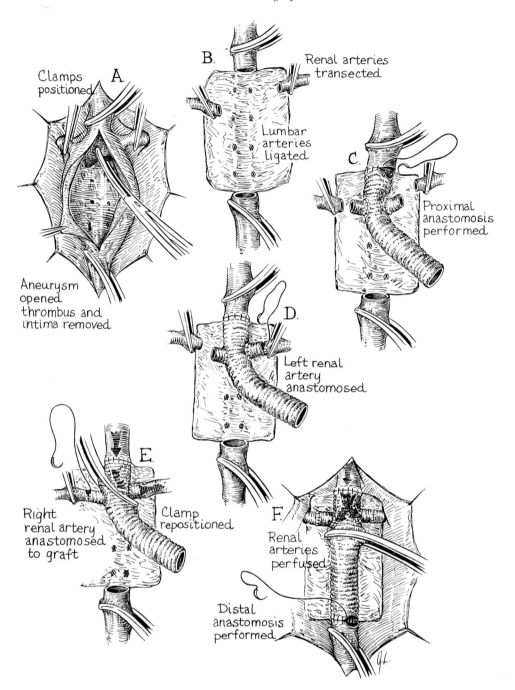

FIG. 2-4. Operative technique employed in resection with graft replacement of abdominal aortic aneurysm involving renal arteries. (A) Entering the aneurysm after occlusion of the aorta above the renal arteries, occlusion of renal arteries and aorta below the lesion; (B) preparation of aorta and renal arteries for anastomosis and ligation of lumbar arteries; (C) proximal anastomosis to aorta performed; (D) one renal anastomosis accomplished; (E) second renal anastomosis performed after opening first renal artery; (F) distal aortic anastomosis accomplished after opening both renal arteries.

Accessory renal arteries occasionally arise from an aneurysm of the abdominal aorta[1] (Fig. 2-5, A). Sacrifice of accessory renal arteries may produce acute renovascular hypertension; therefore, reimplantation into the aortic prosthesis is recommended. These accessory renal arteries are usually small, but may be detached from the aneurysm with a cuff of aortic wall sufficient to suture to the prosthesis without difficulty (Fig. 2-5,

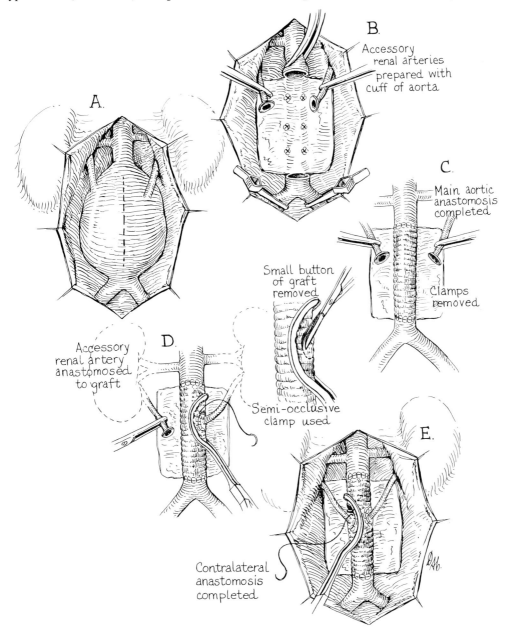

FIG. 2-5. Technique of resection of aneurysm of abdominal aorta with re-anastomosis of accessory renal arteries to Dacron graft. (A) Accessory renal arteries arising from aneurysm; (B) aneurysm resected with cuff of aorta preserved on accessory renal arteries; (C) Dacron graft inserted to restore vascular continuity; (D) partial exclusion of graft with accessory renal artery sutured end-to-side to aortic graft; (E) second accessory renal artery anastomosis accomplished.

B). Partial occlusion of the aortic graft and excision of a small segment of the prosthesis allows reanastomosis without increasing the ischemic time of the lower extremities (Fig. 2-5, C, D, E).

Thoracoabdominal Aneurysm

Thoracoabdominal aneurysm involves primarily the upper abdominal aorta, but usually extends proximally through the diaphragm to involve a portion of the descending thoracic aorta and distally to the bifurcation of the aorta or beyond into the common iliac arteries. These aneurysms are among the most challenging forms of the disease because of their extensive nature involving both body cavities, their difficult anatomical accessibility, and because the major visceral arteries, the celiac, superior mesenteric, and renal arteries, arise from this segment of the aorta.

There are two major considerations in extirpation of aneurysms of this type, both of which are derived from the location and extensive nature of the lesion. The first is concerned with proper anatomic exposure of the aneurysm and a normal segment of aorta above and below the lesion. The second and more significant consideration is concerned with the potential ischemic damage to such vital organs as the kidneys, liver and gastrointestinal tract during temporary arrest of circulation for resection of the aneurysm. Although considerable variation in the tolerance of different organs to ischemia exists, there are definite limits of tolerance that will permit survival. The use of a permanent shunt around the lesion and the performance of the procedure in a manner to reduce the period of circulatory arrest to well within the limits of tolerance has allowed the successful resection of these extensive aneurysms.[7]

Operative Technique

The patient is placed in the supine position with the left side elevated and the left arm suspended from an overhead support. The peritoneal cavity is entered first through a vertical midline incision and a thorough ex-

ploration conducted to determine the extent of the aneurysm and any additional pathology. The distal abdominal aorta is exposed below the aneurysm and a woven Dacron tube graft attached end-to-side by partial exclusion technique. If the aneurysm extends to the bifurcation of the aorta, the limbs of a bifurcation graft are attached by end-to-side anastomosis to both common iliac arteries. Following completion of the distal anastomosis, the graft is occluded at its origin restoring blood flow to the extremities.

The left pleural cavity is entered through an anteriolateral incision in the seventh interspace and the descending thoracic aorta proximal to the aneurysm is exposed. The Dacron tube graft previously attached to the distal abdominal aorta is tunneled in the left retroperitoneal gutter through a hole made in the diaphragm near the aortic hiatus. The graft is cut to an appropriate length and attached to the descending thoracic aorta by end-to-side anastomosis employing a partial exclusion clamp (Fig. 2-5, A). Following completion of this anastomosis, blood flow is routed through the thoracoabdominal bypass graft by occluding the thoracic aorta distal to the anastomosis and removing the occluding clamps from the graft. Woven Dacron tube grafts of appropriate size are attached to the thoracoabdominal graft by end-to-side anastomosis employing a partial excluding clamp (Fig. 2-6, B). Branches for the renal arteries are first attached and each renal artery replaced with end-to-end anastomosis to the proper graft. Subsequently the superior mesenteric and celiac arteries are replaced by similar technique (Fig. 2-6, C). The ischemic time is restricted to that period required to perform an end-to-end anastomosis and rarely exceeds 15 minutes. This period of ischemia is well tolerated by the visceral organs under normothermic conditions.

Following completion of restoration of circulation to the renal, superior mesenteric, and celiac arteries, the aneurysm is entered, lumbar arteries controlled, and the bed over-sewn with continuous chromic catgut. The ends of the thoracic and abdominal aorta are oversewn with nonabsorbable sutures and the posterior peritoneum closed (Fig. 2-6,

D). The abdominal and thoracic incisions are approximated in standard manner.

An alternative method of exposure of the upper abdominal aorta useful in resection of thoracoabdominal aneurysm requires reflec-

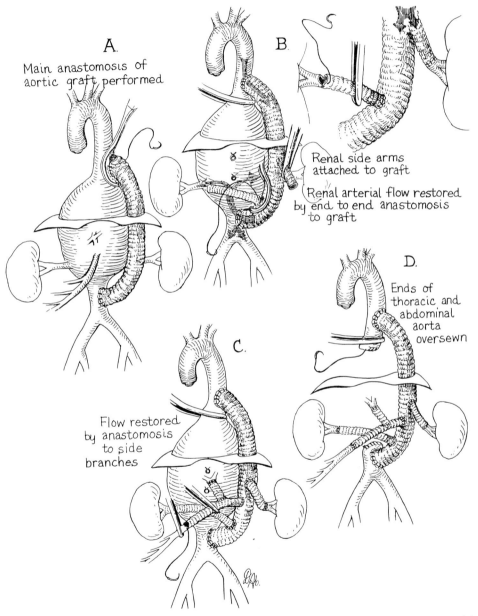

FIG. 2-6. Technique of resection of thoracoabdominal aneurysm and replacement with graft. (A) Dacron bypass inserted around lesion; (B) Dacron tubes for replacement of renal, celiac, superior mesenteric arteries sutured to functioning bypass; (C) anasto-mosis of Dacron limbs to visceral arteries accomplished; (D) aneurysm entered, lumbar arteries suture ligated, and aneurysm wall oversewn; proximal and distal ends of aorta closed.

tion of the left colon, spleen, and stomach medially providing satisfactory visualization of the aorta and major visceral branches.[8]

Ruptured Abdominal Aneurysm

An abdominal aneurysm may rupture into the retroperitoneal space and be contained for several hours before fatal hemorrhage occurs. This condition constitutes a surgical emergency and immediate operation is essential if the patient is to be salvaged. Any delay for administration of blood and restoration of normal blood pressure may increase the retroperitoneal hemorrhage.

The patient is transported to the operating room immediately while blood for transfusion is prepared. Large indwelling catheters are placed in the upper extremities for rapid infusion of blood and fluid. The abdomen and both groins are prepped and draped before induction of anesthesia. As soon as blood is available, rapid infusion is started, induction of anesthesia accomplished, and a midline incision performed. Coordination of restoration of blood volume in large amounts immediately prior to anesthesia is an important feature of the management of such patients as this is one of the most critical periods of their operative management. Proximal and distal control of the aneurysm is obtained while adequate blood replacement is accomplished. Once the operative procedure begins, rapid control of the aneurysm is essential. The single most important determinant of survival of patients with ruptured aortic aneurysms is reducing to a minimum the time between rupture and application of controlling clamps to contain hemorrhage. It may be necessary to occlude the aorta at the diaphragmatic hiatus or immediately above the renal arteries until satisfactory exposure allows placement of a vascular clamp below the renal arteries. If the retroperitoneal hematoma is large and proximal exposure below the renal arteries is uncertain, temporary application of a large, slightly curved aortic clamp by digital dissection at the diaphragmatic hiatus should be considered without hesitation. Resection and graft replacement is then accomplished

as previously described. The retroperitoneal hematoma should be evacuated and the colon inspected before closure. Colon ischemia is more common following resection of ruptured abdominal aortic aneurysms than elective ones because of disruption of the mesocolon by the retroperitoneal hematoma.

Erosion of Duodenum by Aneurysm

Large abdominal aneurysms may become densely adherent to the terminal duodenum and proximal jejunum near the ligament of Trietz. Eventual erosion of the bowel may occur and rupture of the aneurysm into the duodenum with associated massive gastrointestinal hemorrhage results.[9] Bleeding may often be intermittent allowing diagnosis and appropriate operative therapy. Technically these aneurysms present some difficulty in obtaining proximal control which must be achieved before entering the fistula. Occlusion of the aorta above the renal arteries is frequently necessary until the aneurysm is entered, the bowel dissected free from the aneurysm wall, and the aorta below the renal arteries exposed allowing occlusion at this level. The bowel is then repaired by standard technique and graft replacement of the aneurysm accomplished. The fistulous opening into the bowel should be carefully debrided to insure that normal tissue is available for secure closure. Irrigation with antibiotic solution and interposition of viable tissue between aortic suture line and duodenum are important in prevention of infection and recurrent aortoduodenal fistula. If aneurysm wall and periaortic tissue are not available to accomplish this separation, an omental pedicle graft based on the gastroepiploic artery may be utilized.

Aortocaval Fistula

Erosion of the inferior vena cava due to rupture of an aortic aneurysm into the vena cava is occasionally encountered.[10] This lesion may be suspected if evidence of a large arteriovenous fistula or inferior vena caval obstruction is evident. The fistula should not be dissected until control of the aneurysm is achieved with vascular occluding clamps. The aneurysm is then entered and the caval communication controlled with manual pressure. Repair by continuous suture from within the lumen of the aneurysm is then accomplished. Resection and graft replacement of the aneurysm may then proceed in standard fashion.

Dissecting Aneurysm of Abdominal Aorta

The most common form of dissecting aneurysm of the abdominal aorta begins in the thoracic aorta immediately above the aortic valve or distal to the left subclavian artery. An intimal tear results in dissection within the medial layer of the aortic wall producing a double lumen. Re-entry through another intimal defect may occur in the abdominal aorta or iliac arteries. Variation in the point of re-entry of flow into the true lumen and variation in amount and extent of compression of the true lumen may result in distal occlusion of major visceral branches or acute ischemia in the extremities. When the dissection continues into the abdominal aorta, the thin wall of the aorta may progressively dilate under the force of systolic blood pressure producing a fusiform aneurysm. Dissection of the aorta may begin in the abdominal aorta on rare occasions by the same pathologic process. If progressive dilatation of the abdominal aorta occurs, resection with graft replacement is indicated. The operative techniques previously described are employed according to the extent of the aneurysmal disease.

Other anatomical variations occasionally encountered at operation for abdominal aortic aneurysm include horseshoe kidney,[11] double vena cava,[12] and retroaortic left renal vein.[13,14] The variations may not be suspected before operation and present technical difficulties at surgery. Fortunately, such anomalies are rare.

Aorto-Iliac Occlusive Disease

Atherosclerotic occlusive disease is segmental in nature and usually involves the origin or bifurcation of arteries. The disease frequently involves the distal abdominal aorta and common iliac arteries leaving relatively uninvolved distal segments at the level of the external iliac or common femoral arteries. Complete occlusion of the abdominal aorta as originally described by Leriche is manifested clinically by impotence, claudication of the lower extremities, and absent femoral pulses. The development of improved angiography, including safe contrast media, has allowed the recognition of varying degrees of occlusive disease of the abdominal aorta. Some disagreement has existed in the literature regarding the significance of the arteriographic appearance of the distal aorta and proximal iliac arteries. While it is true that arteriograms taken in the anterior-posterior plane may occasionally appear less distinctly abnormal than clinical signs would indicate, indications for operation should never be based wholly on arteriographic appearances alone. If proper consideration is given to the patient's symptoms and to appropriate physical findings, the arteriogram should only serve to confirm clinical impressions and to help in planning the operation. The principles of operative correction are basically the same whether complete or incomplete occlusion of the abdominal aorta and iliac arteries exists.

The operative mortality for aorto-iliac reconstructive operative procedures varies generally between 3 and 6 percent, so the procedure is not one to be casually undertaken. Since the operative mortality of femoropopliteal level reconstruction is approximately 1 percent, the decision as to whether or not arterial reconstruction in any particular patient requires treatment at the aortic level is a critical one. This is especially true when there is coexisting femoropopliteal level thrombosis and partial occlusion at the iliac level. Patients who have significant symptoms, diminished femoral pulses and definite arteriographic findings should be considered candidates for aorto-iliac reconstruction. Failure to appreciate significant proximal disease has led to early failure of femoropopliteal procedures. Furthermore, most patients with coexisting lesions at both levels will obtain a satisfactory result with aorto-iliac reconstruction alone without femoropopliteal repair.[15]

The choice of operation for aorto-iliac occlusive disease depends upon the experience of the surgeon, the extent and nature of the disease, and the results of previous experience. Aorto-iliac endarterectomy or aortofemoral bypass with prosthetic graft are the common operations performed. Endarterectomy requires judgment, experi-

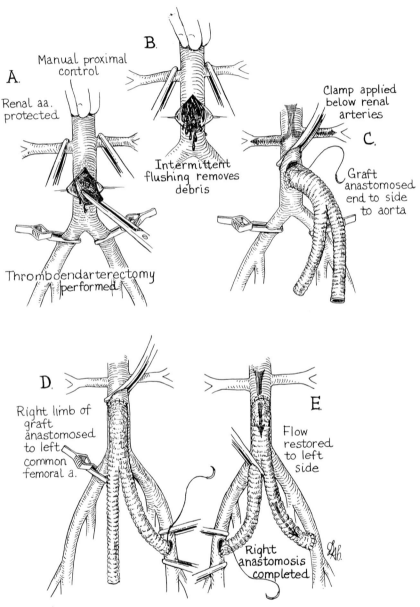

FIG. 2-7. Technique of thrombectomy of abdominal aorta. (A) Aorta and renal arteries occluded, vertical arteriotomy performed while manual proximal control of aorta maintained, thrombectomy performed; (B) intermittent flushing removes debris; (C) aorta clamped below renal arteries and proximal anastomosis performed; (D) one limb of graft anastomosed below occlusive lesion; (E) second limb of graft anastomosed below occlusive lesion after restoring flow through first limb.

ence, and demonstration of satisfactory technical skill. Aortofemoral bypass also requires a smiliar degree of experience, but is less likely to result in complications. Follow-up studies reveal little difference in results with these procedures when performed in selected cases by experienced surgeons.[16,17,18,19]

Complete occlusion of the abdominal aorta begins at the bifurcation of the aorta and extends proximally to the level of the inferior mesenteric artery or the renal arteries. Distally the occlusive process may involve the common iliac arteries leaving the external iliac arteries relatively free of disease. The segmental nature of this disease allows complete correction by several operative techniques including resection with graft replacement, endarterectomy, and bypass with a graft. Thus, normal circulation may be restored distal to the occlusive process.

The technique which allows restoration of circulation with minimum operative trauma is the bypass graft from the abdominal aorta to the external iliac or common femoral arteries, depending on the distal extent of the disease.[20] When the occlusion extends to the ostia of the renal arteries, extreme care is required in removing the thrombus to prevent damage to the renal arteries or emboli to the kidneys. Exposure of the renal arteries and temporary clamp occlusion during intraluminal manipulation of the upper infrarenal aorta may be necessary.

Operative Technique

The abdominal aorta and iliac arteries are exposed through a vertical midline incision. When complete occlusion of the abdominal aorta is present, the proximal portion of the occlusive process is removed by thrombectomy through a vertical arteriotomy below the renal arteries or by transection of the aorta below the renal arteries (Fig. 2-7, A). The proper plane of dissection is entered and thrombectomy accomplished. During this part of the procedure, control of the aorta is obtained with the hand of the surgeon (Fig. 2-7, B). Both renal arteries are occluded

with vascular clamps to prevent emboli. When proximal aortic blood flow is obtained, the renal arteries are opened and the aortic occlusion clamp placed below the renal arteries (Fig. 2-7, C). A Dacron bifurcation graft is sutured either end-to-side or end-to-end to the aorta, depending upon the technique of thrombectomy (Fig. 2-7, D). The distal anastomoses are performed to the external iliac or common femoral arteries as required (Fig. 2-7, E).

The choice of prosthetic graft in any particular operation is not a critical matter. In general, knitted grafts are easier to sew and manipulate, but require pre-clotting before anticoagulants are administered. Woven grafts are preferred when heparin has already been given or when control of blood loss is especially critical. Fixation of pseudo-intima is stronger when knitted grafts are used, but distal emboli from detached pseudointima must be extremely rare from either type of graft.

The choice of suture material is important when sewing prosthetic grafts. Since healing of graft and arterial suture lines does not occur, the future integrity of the anastomosis depends entirely on the suture material. Braided Dacron sutures should be employed in graft anastomoses. Silk and ordinary monofilament sutures are associated with development of false aneurysm and should not be used. Some surgeons prefer specially made monofilament suture material for thoracic aorta anastomoses (see Chap. 6).

Extraperitoneal Approach to the Abdominal Aorta

The employment of an extraperitoneal approach to the aorta, whether for aneurysmorrhaphy or for repair of occlusive disease, has been reported.[21,22] This method is a specialized technique which affords more limited exposure of the vessels. It is not recommended for those inexperienced in its use. There are advantages and disadvantages to this approach. Among the disadvantages, in addition to prohibiting opportunity for abdominal exploration are difficulty of operating on large or high aortic lesions, division of more collateral vessels, and greater difficulty of retraction to accomplish exposure. Among the advantages claimed for the technique are a lower incidence of ileus, atelectasis, wound dehiscence, and greater patient comfort. However, abdominal aortic surgery expeditiously performed through a midline transperitoneal approach with technical precision and meticulous attention to detail postoperatively should result in an extremely low incidence of such complications.

Complications of Abdominal Aortic Surgery

Complications of abdominal aortic surgery may be encountered at operation, occur early in the postoperative period, or develop months or even years after operation. The complications may be discussed from the standpoint of prevention and treatment. Operations for both aneurysmal and occlusive disease have common technical factors, and complications are similar, irrespective of the original lesion.

Operative Complications

On entering the peritoneal cavity, adhesions from previous operations may be encountered. Occasionally, injury to bowel is produced during lysis of adhesions. If small bowel proximal to the distal ileum is entered, primary repair is performed and the proposed vascular operation completed. If colon or distal ileum is injured, repair is accomplished and the vascular operation postponed to avoid the chance of a contaminated field predisposing to an infected prosthesis. Similarly, if an abscess is identified on exploring the peritoneal cavity such as perforated diverticulum, or suppurative cholecystitis, the vascular surgery should be delayed.

Unsuspected intraperitoneal disease or known associated intraperitoneal lesions may be identified during exploration requiring a decision regarding operative priority. In general, nonsuppurative lesions may be treated following completion of the retro-peritoneal aortic surgery without increased risk to the patient. However, suppurative lesions and malignancy are best treated primarily with the elective vascular procedure postponed. Any additional procedure that increases the risk of graft infection, e.g., incidental appendectomy, should be avoided.

During exposure of the aorta and iliac arteries, injury to the vena cava or iliac veins occasionally occurs. Careful dissection during exposure will prevent this complication. The avoidance of unnecessary circumferential dissection for the placement of tapes about the arteries will reduce the incidence of venous injury. The amount of hemorrhage from a major venous laceration can be of fatal proportions and should be dealt with under the best available circumstances by establishing optimal exposure, insuring adequate assistance, and by maneuvers which will not further aggravate the situation.

Ureteral injury is rare, but may occur if the ureters are adherent to a large aneurysm. If the aneurysm is not completely dissected free from surrounding structures, ureteral and vena caval injury will be prevented. If ureteral injury occurs, competent urologic assistance for repair is recommended. Injury to the small bowel mesentery, pancreas, spleen, and superior mesenteric artery may be produced by retractors and excessive retraction should be avoided.

Complications from the aortofemoral tunnel are rare if certain precautions are observed. The tunnel should be made by blunt dissection immediately anterior to the iliac and femoral arteries. The index fingers of the surgeon construct the tunnel satisfactorily; then the graft may be delivered into the groin incision with a sponge forceps. Avoiding the placement of the tunnel medial to the host external iliac and femoral arterial vessels will decrease the chance of lymphatic injury and lymphocele formation in the groin wound. The deep iliac circumflex vein passes over the external iliac artery immediately above the inguinal ligament and may be injured during construction of the tunnel. This vein should be exposed and protected or divided between clamps and ligated prior to constructing the tunnel and passing the graft through the tunnel. Hemorrhage along the tunnel is unusual, but if present should be exposed and controlled. Care should be taken in passing the graft limb to prevent twisting or kinking and to avoid improperly increased or reduced tension of the graft. The proper amount of tension of the graft lies within fairly narrow limits. If the graft is too tight, the anastomosis will be likely to bleed and a false aneurysm may result. If too little tension is permitted, a redundant graft may have poor flow characteristics and will be more likely to erode through adjacent viscera. Injury to the ureter is prevented if the tunnel is constructed by blunt dissection; late ureteral compression from a functioning graft is very rare. The tunnel is made posterior to the ureter and allows normal ureteral function. Obstruction of the ureter has been observed on occasions when the graft limb has been passed anterior to the ureter.[23,24] If malposition of the graft is detected, immediate correction is required to prevent late complications.

Thrombosis in distal arterial segments of the lower extremities may occur during aortic occlusion. Systemic or regional heparin, approximately 75 units per kilogram, is usually preventive providing aortic occlusion does not exceed one hour. Additional heparin is advised when aortic occlusion is prolonged. This complication is more likely to occur when associated occlusive disease of the lower extremities is present. The vascular status of the lower extremities should be compared to the preoperative state as soon as the operation is completed as discussed in Chapter 16. If lower extremity ischemia is detected, appropriate operative diagnostic arteriography and therapy should be employed immediately.

Embolic occlusion of one or more lower extremity arteries is not uncommon, particularly when soft atheromatous material is present in the aorta at the site of application of vascular occluding clamps. Vigorous flushing both antegrade and retrograde prior to removal of clamps usually releases this material and prevents distal emboli. However, in spite of every precaution, an occasional complication of this type occurs and must be treated promptly. Usually this will require passage of an arterial embolectomy catheter as described in Chapter 4. The application of a vascular clamp near the renal arteries may dislodge atheromatous material and produce renal emboli. If this material is visualized through the arteriotomy at the clamp site, aortic occlusion above the renal arteries briefly is recommended. This allows inspection of the aorta and renal ostia and removal of potential embolic material.

Hemostasis following retroperitoneal vascular surgery is extremely important. Careful inspection of suture lines, lumbar arteries, and meticulous control of small bleeding points along the aneurysm wall by electrocoagulation prevents postoperative hematoma and reduces the risk of infection. Irrigation of the retroperitoneal area with antibiotic solutions is advocated by many vascular surgeons in an attempt to reduce the danger of infection.

Inspection of the bowel prior to closure should be practiced routinely. If the color of both small and large bowel is normal and peristalsis is present on palpation, subsequent ischemia is unlikely. If the colon appears of questionable viability, consideration should be given to re-exploration within a 24-hour period to assess the appearance of the bowel. The superior mesenteric artery should be palpated for thrills and the presence of a vigorous pulse.[25] Ligation of the inferior mesenteric artery during abdominal aneurysmectomy is generally well tolerated providing one hypogastric artery is patent. However, if a large inferior mesenteric artery is encountered, suggesting collateral circulation through it, this artery should be reim-

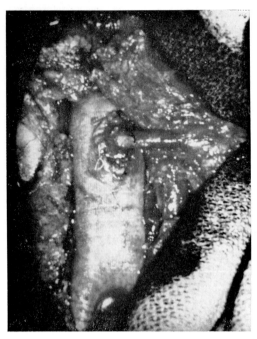

FIG. 2-8. Inferior mesenteric artery reimplanted into Dacron graft.

planted into the aortic graft, thereby possibly avoiding colon ischemia (Fig. 2-8).

Neurologic complications following infra-renal abdominal aortic aneurysm resection are rare, but have been observed.[26,27,28] Cauda equina dysfunction and paraplegia on the basis of spinal cord ischemia may result if arterial circulation to the lower cord or cauda equina is derived from the lower lumbar arteries that are routinely ligated during aneurysm resection. Although this complication is unpredictable, every effort should be made to preserve lumbar branches near the proximal anastomosis. Neurologic complications following thoracoabdominal aortic resection are more common and reimplantation of large lumbar arteries has been advocated. Femoral nerve compression from retractors used to expose the external iliac artery has been observed. Symptoms are usually transient, but may be prevented by proper use of retractors.

Postoperative Complications
Early Postoperative Complications
Hemorrhage may be suspected if vital signs are unstable, urine output reduced, and

tender flanks palpated. If blood administration temporarily corrects hypotension and oliguria and these signs recur, hemorrhage is likely. A central venous pressure monitor is helpful in management of fluid and blood replacement. When hemorrhage is suspected, immediate re-exploration is recommended with inspection of suture lines, lumbar arteries, and the spleen, which is occasionally injured by retractors. Lumbar sympathectomy occasionally produces injury of small blood vessels that produce postoperative bleeding. Evacuation of hematoma is essential to avoid possible retroperitoneal infection. The evacuation of a hematoma by itself will occasionally act to stop bleeding, particularly from small, oozing vessels. This may be due to removal of a local source of activated plasmin from the hematoma, causing local fibrinolysis. A careful search should be made to locate a bleeding point during a time when the patient's blood pressure is in the normal range.

Renal insufficiency following abdominal aortic surgery is not uncommon. Transient oliguria occurs frequently during the first 48 hours as a result of increased output of antidiuretic hormone and the stress response to operation. Osmotic diuretics may be helpful during this period. Severe oliguria or anuria suggests renal vascular insufficiency or renal tubular damage from incompatible blood transfusion or underlying renal disease. There is a growing feeling in many centers that vigorous administration of one of the newer diuretics such as furosemide or ethacrynic acid given early when oliguria is first apparent may prevent the development of the full syndrome of acute renal tubular necrosis. Determination of urine sodium concentration and a comparison of urine and serum osmolalities will help distinguish states that are due to prerenal factors and those associated with increased antidiuretic hormone secretion from those due to tubular necrosis or loss of vascular integrity.[29] Such tests require experienced interpretation when diuretics have been given, and, when possible, urine samples should be obtained prior to their administration. Determination of the renal vascular status by radioisotope renogram or arteriography is essential before relying on return of renal function. Consultation from a nephrologist is very helpful in diagnosis, management, and hemodialysis, if necessary. If renal vascular insufficiency is detected, immediate exploration and revascularization of renal arteries or removal of renal emboli are required.

Thrombosis of arterial prostheses or endarterectomy segments occurs occasionally in the early postoperative period. This complication is almost always entirely technical and requires immediate re-exploration and correction. Because such early failures are technical in nature in the vast majority of cases, an attempt should be made to identify a technical imperfection and to achieve correction so as to prevent recurrence of the early failure. The presence of restored pulses which were absent preoperatively should be established after the original operation to aid in early postoperative assessment along with less objective features of skin temperature, color and distal capillary flow. Further discussion of this topic can be found in Chapter 16.

Intestinal obstruction from adhesions may occur within seven to ten days after operation and generally requires lysis of adhesions. Long tube intestinal decompression rarely corrects the problem, whereas operative intervention usually prevents recurrence. Upper gastrointestinal bleeding from duodenal ulcer, stress ulcer, or gastritis may occur as after any major surgical procedure. Conservative therapy with iced saline gavage often is successful, but if blood replacement above six units is required, re-exploration is advised. Pancreatitis, perforated duodenal ulcer, acute cholecystitis, and other serious intra-abdominal lesions may present in the early postoperative period and require exploration for diagnosis and therapy.[30]

Ischemia of the bowel occurs occasionally after abdominal aortic surgery.[25] Small bowel ischemia may result from injury to the superior mesenteric artery from retractors or vascular clamps placed above the renal arteries or as a result of emboli from the aorta.

The superior mesenteric artery should be inspected at operation to detect unsuspected disease that might precipitate a serious postoperative complication. If superior mesenteric insufficiency is suspected in the postoperative period, immediate arteriography and operation, when indicated, are required. Once gangrene of the bowel occurs, little is accomplished by massive resection. If localized bowel necrosis is present, resection may be life saving.

Colon ischemia is not uncommon following sacrifice of the inferior mesenteric artery. Collateral blood supply from the superior mesenteric and internal iliac arteries is usually adequate if the marginal artery arcades in the sigmoid mesocolon are intact. Any sacrifice of collateral in addition to the inferior mesenteric artery will increase the frequency of colon ischemia. Symptoms may present as diarrhea, bloody mucous rectal discharge, persistent ileus, abdominal pain and tenderness, and alternating constipation and diarrhea.[31,32] The majority of these complaints usually subside, but occasionally colon ischemia progresses to perforation with peritonitis. This complication requires emergency colectomy and colostomy. Careful observation of the postoperative patient is necessary to detect impending colon ischemia or infarction. Sigmoidoscopy and biopsy may be diagnostic in suspected cases. Immediate treatment with antibiotics, steroids and low-residue diet is usually successful, but severe cases require operative intervention. Late stricture of the colon may occur from ischemia and require elective operation for diagnosis and therapy.

Chylous ascites following resection of an abdominal aortic aneurysm is rarely observed.[33] Treatment is conservative initially with re-exploration and suture of the chylous fistula reserved for the patient with a protracted nutritional problem.

Late Postoperative Complications

Late graft thrombosis is encountered when progression of atherosclerotic disease impairs runoff in bypass grafts employed for treatment of occlusive lesions. Progression of disease may occur in endarterectomy segments or distal to bypass grafts and produce thrombosis. Operation is required to restore circulation and each situation is approached following repeat arteriography and estimation of runoff or available patent distal arterial segments. Late thrombosis of one or both limbs of an aortofemoral bypass graft is occasionally encountered. If both limbs are occluded, complete replacement of the graft is required. A single limb thrombosis of an aortofemoral graft may be approached successfully through the groin.[34] Progression of proximal or distal arteriosclerotic disease or false aneurysm is the usual etiology of the thrombosis.

Endarterectomy of the profunda femoris artery distal to its origin almost always provides a satisfactory vessel for restoration of blood flow. The thrombosed graft limb may be opened with arterial strippers if care is taken to prevent injury to the aorta and to

prevent emboli from entering the contralateral open limb of the graft. Manual occlusion by external compression of the patent graft limb in the opposite groin will usually prevent embolic material from entering that limb. Once proximal and distal flow are obtained, a short segment of graft may be interposed between the open limb and the profunda femoris artery. Other thrombosed grafts within the retroperitoneal space, e.g. aortorenal, aortoiliac, aortomesenteric, must be replaced with a new graft providing runoff into an open arterial segment.

False aneurysms occur at suture lines as a result of disruption of suture material employed for the vascular anastomosis or disruption of the arterial wall into which the sutures are placed.[35] Predisposing factors to the development of false aneurysm include silk or monofilament sutures used for prosthetic graft anastomosis, excess graft tension or motion, and suturing grafts to thin arterial

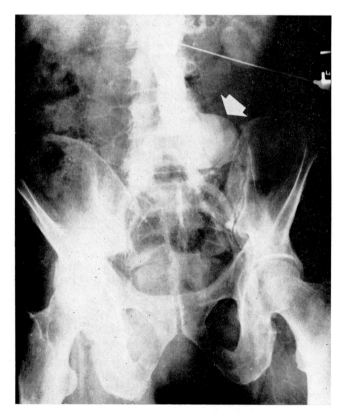

FIG. 2-9. Translumbar aortogram demonstrating a large false aneurysm (arrow) arising at the proximal anastomosis of an aortofemoral bypass graft. The graft had been sutured with silk, and the anastomosis disrupted 8 years postoperatively.

segments in which endarterectomy has been performed. Since Dacron grafts are not ever fully incorporated into the host vessel at the line of anastomosis, permanent suture material is required for support. Silk is not a permanent suture material and therefore should not be employed for suturing prosthetic grafts.

Infection at graft suture lines also produces false aneurysms. When infection is encountered, prosthetic material must be removed, the artery suture ligated or oversewn with wire or synthetic suture material, and circulation restored by bypass technique through clean tissue into a distal arterial segment. False aneurysm occurring from causes other than infection may be approached directly and repaired by resection and graft replacement.

Aortoenteric fistula is a rare, late complication of aortic surgery that requires prompt diagnosis and therapy.[36,37,38,39,40,41] The proximity of the distal duodenum and proximal jejunum at the ligament of Trietz to the infrarenal segment of aorta predisposes to this complication. If the bowel, either duodenum, jejunum or ileum, is allowed to come in contact with the arterial prosthesis, adherence and eventual erosion occurs with contamination of the graft and blood stream. When erosion occurs at the level of the vascular suture line, hemorrhage into the bowel from the aorta occurs. Hemorrhage may present as intermittent, severe upper gastrointestinal bleeding that ceases spontaneously only to recur actively. Eventual exanguination occurs if prompt therapy is not instituted.

Therapy consists of resection of the prosthesis, suture closure of the aorta and distal anastomosis, and suture closure of the bowel. Drainage and antibiotic irrigations locally, as well as systemic antibiotic therapy, are helpful. If distal ischemia results from removal of the graft as is frequently the case, restoration of circulation by extra-abdominal bypass is required. Patients with aortoenteric fistula may present with septicemia without hemorrhage if bowel erosion occurs

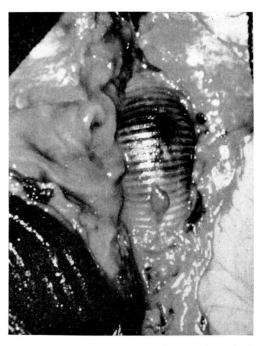

FIG. 2-10. Dacron graft showing erosion of adjacent duodenum. Angulation of graft anteriorly is a predisposing factor in this complication.

at a site away from the vascular suture line.[42] A predisposing factor to this complication is the placement of a graft too long for the aortic defect that bows anteriorly and is difficult to cover adequately with viable periaortic tissue (Fig. 2-10). En bloc resection of bowel and prosthesis with insertion of a new prosthesis has been advocated as an alternative method of therapy.[43] Aortoenteric fistula is a preventable complication if viable tissue such as periaortic fat is sutured over the prosthesis and suture line before closing the posterior peritoneum. If insufficient tissue is available, a free or pedical omental graft may be interposed between arterial prosthesis and bowel.

Sexual dysfunction following aortic surgery is not uncommon, particularly in the male. Impairment of erection and abnormalities of ejaculation have been described in approximately one-third to one-half of male patients who have undergone aortic surgery,[44] although these symptoms are already present to some degree in many of the males in the age group that presents for aortic surgery. Concomitant lumbar sympathectomy appears to increase the frequency of erection problems. Occasional patients have described improvement in one or both these sexual functions following an aortic operation. In the younger, sexually active male, every effort is made to avoid resection of the aortic bifurcation or extensive dissection around the bifurcation. Disruption of nerve pathways in this area appears to increase sexual dysfunction. Lumbar sympathectomy also is usually avoided, when possible, in the younger male.

Infection following aortic vascular surgery is a rare but extremely serious complication. Administration of broad spectrum antibiotics before and after operation,[45] local antibiotics in irrigation solutions,[46] careful hemostasis, and meticulous sterile technique are strongly advocated. Vascular surgery must be performed in "clean" operating rooms where potentially infected cases are not scheduled. In addition, frequent bacteriologic surveys of instruments, ventilation systems and operating fields should be conducted. Traffic of unnecessary personnel in the operating room during the procedure should be eliminated. Thorough skin preparation is very important. Graft material and irrigation solutions should not be permitted to lie exposed to room air for prolonged periods during the procedure. Since the development of infection following insertion of an arterial prosthesis carries a high risk of either fatal outcome or loss of limb, maximum effort toward prevention of infection is mandatory.

Graft infection rarely presents as an early complication unless wound infection overlying a graft occurs. A wound problem must be managed aggressively to prevent underlying infection of a graft. Groin incisions are more commonly involved and should be inspected daily for possible infection. Local hematoma, stitch abscess, lymphocele, and inflammation of skin must be treated promptly by appropriate measures. A small hematoma or lymphocele may be treated

expectantly in many cases. Needle aspiration is usually ineffective and may result in infection. Stitch abscess requires prompt suture removal and continuous warm compresses. If the wound infection involves the graft, open surgical drainage, installation of continuous, appropriate antibiotic solution through a sump suction system followed by delayed secondary closure in several days is often successful in preventing a permanent graft infection. Successful management of an early infection depends upon prompt recognition and, once recognized, upon willingness of the surgeon to accept the necessity for active treatment as outlined. Late graft infections in the groin are rarely successfully managed by this technique and usually require removal of the graft.

Late retroperitoneal graft infection usually presents as a false aneurysm, septicemia, aortoenteric fistula, or localized abscess. Once the prosthesis is involved by infection, removal of the graft and drainage is required.[47] The major problem is protection of the distal circulation from severe ischemia following removal of the graft. Several methods have been employed successfully. Construction of axillary-femoral bypass grafts[48,49] or bypass graft from descending thoracic aorta to one or both femoral arteries is generally recommended.

Late infection in the groin involving prosthetic graft usually presents as hemorrhage, draining sinus, or false aneurysm. Excision of the graft with ligation of the femoral artery is required. A sinogram may be helpful in identifying the extent of the local infection. Preservation of the distal circulation may be accomplished by bypass through the obturator foramen, axillary artery to superficial femoral artery bypass or femoral to superficial femoral artery bypass. In spite of every therapeutic effort, the results of treatment of infected grafts remain poor and reinforce the premise that prevention of graft infection is the primary objective in management of this serious complication.

References

1. Hardy, J. D.: Preservation of accessory arterial supply in abdominal aneurysm resection. Surg. Gynec. Obstet., *123*:1, 317, 1966.
2. Bernstein, E. F., Fisher, J. C., and Varco, R. L.: Is excision the optimum treatment for all abdominal aortic aneurysms? Surgery, *61*:83, 1967.
3. Steinberg, I., and Tobier, N.: Study of 200 consecutive patients with abdominal aneurysms diagnosed by intravenous arteriography: comparative longevity with and without aneurysmectomy. Circulation, *35*: 530, 1967.
4. Szilagyi, D. E., Smith, R. F., DeRusso, F. J., Elliot, J. P., and Sherrin, F. W.: Contribution of abdominal aortic aneurysmectomy to prolongation of life. Ann. Surg., *164*:678, 1966.
5. DeBakey, M. E., Crawford, E. S., Cooley, D. A., and Morris, G. C.: Aneurysm of the abdominal aorta: analysis of results of graft replacement therapy one to eleven years after operation. Ann. Surg., *160*:622, 1964.
6. May, A. G., DeWeese, J. A., Frank, I., Mahoney, E. B., and Rob, C. G.: Surgical treatment of abdominal aortic aneurysms. Surgery, *63*:711, 1968.
7. DeBakey, M. E., Crawford, E. S., Garrett, H. E., Beall, A. C., Jr., and Howell, J. F.: Surgical considerations in the treatment of aneurysms of the thoraco-abdominal aorta. Ann. Surg., *162*:650-662, 1965.
8. Elkins, R. C., DeMeester, T. R., and Brawley, R. K.: Surgical exposure of the upper abdominal aorta and its branches. Surgery, *70*:622-627, 1971.
9. Garrett, H. E., Howell, J. F., and DeBakey, M. E.: Primary aortoduodenal fistula: Case report. Cardiov. Res. Cent. Bull., *3*:96-100, 1965.
10. Beall, A. C., Jr., Cooley, D. A., Morris, G. C., Jr., and DeBakey, M. E.: Perforation of arteriosclerotic aneurysms into inferior vena cava. Arch. Surg., *86*:809-818, 1963.
11. Davis, J. T., Jr., Hardin, W. J., Hardy, J. D., and Neely, W. A.: Abdominal aneurysm and horseshoe kidney. Southern Med. J., *64*:75-77, 1971.
12. Dupont, J.-R.: Isolated left-sided vena cava and abdominal aortic aneurysm. Arch. Surg., *102*:211-212, 1971.
13. Thomas, T. V.: Surgical implications of retroaortic left renal vein. Arch. Surg., *100*: 738, 1970.
14. Yashar, J. J., Hallman, G. L., and Cooley, D. A.: Fistula between aneurysm of aorta and left renal vein: a case report. Arch. Surg., *99*:546-8, 1969.
15. Crawford, E. S., DeBakey, M. E., Morris, G. C., Jr., and Garrett, H. E.: Evaluation of late failures after reconstructive operations for occlusive lesions of the aorta and iliac, femoral and popliteal arteries. Surgery, *47*:79, 1960.
16. Thomas, T. V.: Role of thromboendarterectomy and bypass graft in occlusive vascular disorders. Surgery, *66*:965-8, 1969.
17. Minken, S. L., DeWeese, J. A., Southgate, W. A., Mahoney, E. B., and Rob, C. G.: Aortoiliac reconstruction for atherosclerotic occlusive disease. Surg. Gynec. Obstet., *126*:1056-60, 1968.
18. Moore, W. S., Cafferata, H. T., Hall, A. D., and Blaisdell, F. W.: In defense of grafts across the inguinal ligament: An evaluation of early and late results of aorto-femoral bypass grafts. Ann. Surg., *168*:207-14, 1968.
19. Duncan, W. C., Linton, R. R., and Darling, R. C.: Aortoiliofemoral atherosclerotic occlusive disease: Comparative results of endarterectomy and Dacron bypass grafts. Surgery, *70*:974, 1971.
20. Garrett, H. E., Crawford, E. W., Howell, J. F., and DeBakey, M. E.: Surgical considerations in the treatment of aorto-iliac occlusive disease. Surg. Clin. N. Amer., *46*:949-961, 1966.
21. Rob, C. G.: Extraperitoneal approach to the abdominal aorta. Surgery, *53*:87, 1963.
22. Stipa, S., and Shaw, R. S.: Aortoiliac reconstruction through a retroperitoneal approach. J. Cardiov. Surg., *9*:224, 1968.
23. Thomford, N. R., and Dorfman, L. F.: Ureteral obstruction caused by an aortofemoral bypass prosthesis. Amer. J. Surg., *115*:394-6, 1968.
24. Dorfman, L. E., and Thomford, N. R.: Unusual ureteral injury following aorto iliac bypass graft. Case report. J. Urol., *101*: 25-7, 1969.
25. Williams, L. F., Jr., Kim, R. M., Tompkins, W., and Byrne, J. J.: Aortoiliac steal— A cause of intestinal ischemia. New Eng. J. Med., *278*:777-8, 1968.
26. Edmondson, H. T., and Gindin, R. A.: Paraplegia as a complication of abdominal aortic resection. Amer. Surg., *36*:383-6, 1970.
27. Zuber, W. F., Gaspar, M. R., and Rothschild, P. D.: The anterior spinal artery syn-

drome—A complication of abdominal aortic surgery: Report of five cases and review of the literature. Ann. Surg., *172*:909-15, 1970.

28. Skillman, J. J., Zervas, N. T., Weintraub, R. M., and Mayman, C. I.: Paraplegia after resection of aneurysms of the abdominal aorta. New Eng. J. Med., *281*:422-5, 1969.

29. Jones, L. W., and Weil, M. H.: Water, creatinine and sodium excretion following circulatory shock with renal failure. Amer. J. Med., *51*:314, 1971.

30. Orr, N. W., and Ware, C. C.: Some gastrointestinal complications of abdominal aneurysm surgery. Proc. Roy. Soc. Med., *61*: 342-3, 1968.

31. McBurney, R. P., Howard, H., Bicks, R. O., and Bale, G. F.: Ischemia and gangrene of the colon following abdominal aortic resection. Amer. Surg., *36*:205-9, 1970.

32. Montessori, G., and Liepa, E. V.: Ischemic colitis. Canad. Med. Asso. J., *102*:377-80, 1970.

33. Bradham, R. R., Gregorie, H. B., and Wilson, R.: Chylous ascites following resection of an abdominal aortic aneurysm. Amer. Surg., *36*:238-40, 1970.

34. Lyons, J. H., Jr., and Weismann, R. E.: Surgical management of late closure of aortofemoral reconstruction grafts. New Eng. J. Med., *278*:1035-7, 1968.

35. Sawyers, J. L., Jacobs, K., and Sutton, J. P.: Peripheral anastomotic aneurysms. Development following arterial reconstruction with prosthetic grafts. Arch. Surg., *95*: 802-9, 1967.

36. Garrett, H. E., Beall, A. C., Jordan, G. L., and DeBakey, M. E.: Surgical considerations of massive gastrointestinal trace hemorrhage caused by aortoduodenal fistula. Amer. J. Surg., *105*:6-12, 1963.

37. Shucksmith, H. S.: Duodenal, sigmoid, and ureteric fistulas resulting from aorto-iliac grafts or endarterectomy. Brit. J. Surg., *55*:402-3, 1968.

38. Tyson, R. R., Maier, W. P., and Dipietrantonio, S.: Iliac-appendiceal fistula following Dacron aortic graft. Amer. Surg., *35*: 241-3, 1969.

39. Eadie, D. G., and Pollock, D. J.: A complicated aortoduodenal fistula. Brit. J. Surg., *55*:314-7, 1968.

40. Sheil, G. R., Reeve, T. S., Little, J. M., Coupland, G. A., and Loewenthal, J.: Aorto-intestinal fistulas following operations on the abdominal aorta and iliac arteries. Brit. J. Surg., *56*:840-3, 1969.

41. Donovan, T. J., and Bucknam, C. A.: Aorto-enteric fistula. Arch. Surg., *95*:810-20, 1967.

42. Dass, R.: Small bowel erosion after aortic replacement by synthetic graft. Amer. J. Surg., *116*:460-2, 1968.

43. Najafi, H., Javid, H., Dye, W. S., Hunter, J. A., and Julian, O. C.: Management of infected arterial implants. Surgery, *65*:539-47, 1969.

44. May, A. G., DeWeese, J. A., and Rob, C. G.: Changes in sexual function following operation on the abdominal aorta. Surgery, *65*:41-7, 1969.

45. Moore, W. S., Rosson, C. T., Hall, A. D., and Thomas, A. N.: Transient bacteremia. A cause of infection in prosthetic vascular grafts. Amer. J. Surg., *117*:342-3, 1969.

46. Digiglia, J. W., Leonard, G. L., and Ochsner, J. L.: Local irrigation with an antibiotic solution in the prevention of infection in vascular prostheses. Surgery, *67*:836-40, 1970.

47. Diethrich, E. B., Noon, G. P., Liddicoat, J. E., and DeBakey, M. E.: Treatment of infected aortofemoral arterial prosthesis. Surgery, *68*:1044-52, 1970.

48. Blaisdell, F. W., and Hall, A. D.: Axillofemoral artery bypass for lower extremity ischemia. Surgery, *54*:563, 1963.

49. Mannick, J. A., Williams, L. E., and Nabseth, D. C.: The late results of axillofemoral grafts. Surgery, *68*:1038-43, 1970.

Chapter 3 | Complications of

James A. DeWeese, M.D.

Arterial Reconstruction Distal to the Inguinal Ligament

Prevention of Complications

Most complications are preventable. However, despite all precautions, some complications occur frequently enough that one must be satisfied to decrease the complication rate while attempting to prevent them entirely. There are several areas in management of patients undergoing arterial reconstruction distal to the inguinal ligament where the physician's action can prevent complications or decrease their rate of occurrence. These areas include: selection of the patient for operation, preoperative preparation, and conduct of the operation.

Selection of Patients for Operation

The reconstruction of arteries distal to the inguinal ligament may be necessary because of the presence of aneurysms or following injuries. However, the most frequent reason for operation is symptomatic atherosclerotic and thrombotic occlusion of the leg vessels. These symptoms consist of claudication, or rest pain, or gangrene. The occlusions are best delineated by angiograms. They most frequently occur in the distal superficial femoral artery at the site where it passes beneath the adductor magnus tendon to become the popliteal artery. Occlusions may remain localized there, but more frequently progress proximally or distally. Occlusions less frequently occur at the origin of the superficial femoral artery or at the origin of

the three terminal branches of the popliteal artery. These three popliteal artery terminal branches are called the "run-off" available for arterial reconstruction although there are collateral vessels as well. If none or only one of these three major branches is patent, the run-off is poor, and if two or three are patent, the run-off is good. The length of reconstruction required may be short if the lesion is localized to the region of the adductor magnus tendon, to the superficial femoral artery, or to the popliteal artery. A long reconstruction is required if there is occlusion of both the superficial femoral artery and the proximal or entire popliteal artery. These factors taken together are major influences on patient selection.

The thrombosis rate of femoropopliteal arterial reconstructions, in our experience, has been most consistently influenced by the length of the reconstruction, the arterial run-off, and the presence or absence of diabetes. A group of 157 saphenous vein bypass grafts were followed one month to eight and one-half years.[1] There was a thrombosis rate of 31 percent for short grafts and 51 percent for long grafts. With a good run-off 35 percent of the grafts thrombosed, and with a poor run-off 49 percent of the grafts thrombosed. The thrombosis rate was 37 percent for nondiabetics and 42 percent for diabetics. Long grafts, poor run-off, and diabetes signaled a poor prognosis. The incidence of the poor prognostic signs pro-

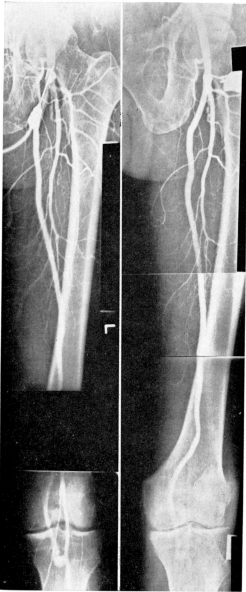

FIG. 3-1. Arteriograms of long autogenous venous bypass graft from the common femoral artery to the popliteal artery below the level of the knee. The arteriogram on the left was obtained five years after the operation and the arteriogram on the right ten years after the original procedure.

gressively increased with the severity of the patient's symptoms from claudication, to rest pain, to gangrene. It is not surprising that the thrombosis rate is closely dependent upon the indication for operation.[2] We were able to follow 56 venous bypass grafts closely for five years.[3] The thrombosis rate in patients with claudication was 27 percent, but was 50 percent in those with rest pain and 56 percent in those with gangrene.

It is obvious that the thrombosis rate could be kept quite low if one accepted for operation only those patients with claudication who were not diabetics, who required only short reconstructions, and whose arteriogram showed a good run-off. Such a restricted selection of patients, however, would result in the amputation of many limbs that might be preserved by an arterial reconstruction. Long reconstructions may remain patent for extended periods of time, and arterial reconstructions may have long-term success even though the arteriogram indicated that the run-off is poor.[4] These facts are well illustrated in Figures 3-1, 3-2, and 3-3.

Preoperative Preparation

Appropriate antibiotics should be administered prophylactically before, during, and after operation.

Infection is one of the most serious of complications that may occur following an arterial reconstruction. It may be responsible for early hemorrhage from anastomotic suture lines, and infection adjacent to a graft may be responsible for thrombosis of the reconstruction. Infections associated with synthetic grafts are responsible for recurrent perigraft abscesses and late bleeding from anastomoses. In a randomized double blind study by Moore, Rasson, and Hall,[5] cephalothin (Keflin) or a placebo was administered intramuscularly the evening before operation, intravenously during operation, and intramuscularly following insertion of Dacron grafts into dogs. A suspension of *Staphylococcus aureus* was injected intravenously immediately following insertion of the graft. The grafts were removed three weeks later and 24 percent of the treated grafts as opposed to 72 percent of the untreated grafts were infected. Although it is not our practice to use antibiotics locally,

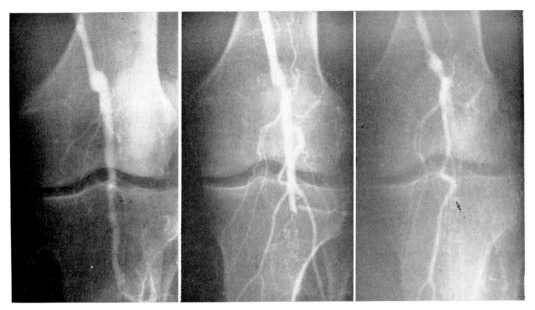

Fig. 3-2. Arteriograms of distal end of femoropopliteal autogenous venous bypass graft. Arteriogram on the left is one week after operation. Only one of the distal vessels is patent, as was also true before operation. The middle arteriogram was obtained six months after operation. The one vessel run-off was then occluded. The arteriogram on the right was obtained seven and one-half years after operation, and the only run-off was through superior geniculate and sural branches. The graft remained patent until the patient's death 14 years and 10 months after operation.[19] (DeWeese, J. A., et al.: Ann. Surg., *163*:205, 1966)

Richardson, *et al.* have presented evidence that soaking grafts in cephalothin or cephaloridine (Loridine) can decrease the incidence and severity of perigraft infections.[6] Darling, Linton, and Razzuk did not observe any suggestive evidence of deep wound sepsis in 294 patients who received penicillin and streptomycin preoperatively and postoperatively.[7]

Conduct of the Operation

The following section is an outline of steps in performance of different types of arterial reconstruction in the leg emphasizing prevention of complications.

Draping of the leg includes coverage of all exposed skin with one of the adhesive-backed plastics. All efforts must be made to prevent infection. Since multiple incisions may be necessary, and the operation may take some time, protection of wounds from skin contaminants is important.

Skin incisions are made directly over the artery or vein being exposed, with the following exception. When the proximal popliteal artery and the greater saphenous vein are both being exposed the incision should be placed parallel to and midway between the two vessels. Otherwise the saphenous vein is removed through multiple short incisions made directly over the vein.

Extensive incisions, particularly when they result in undermining, may cause skin sloughs and superficial wound infections.[7] These complications have occurred in as many as 29 percent of the incisions when care has not been taken to avoid extensive dissection.[8] It is our impression that thrombosis of vein grafts one to three months after their insertion occurs more frequently in the presence of these superficial wound problems.

Mobilization. The arteries are mobilized without excessive traction. All branches are preserved and controlled.

We have observed thrombosis of vessels

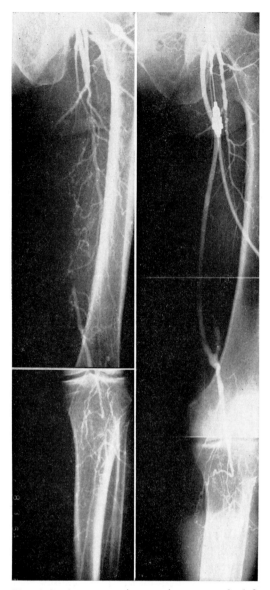

FIG. 3-3. A preoperative arteriogram on the left demonstrates a long occlusion of the femoral artery and also a complete occlusion of the distal popliteal artery. There is reconstruction of the distal arteries of the lower leg through collaterals. The arteriogram on the right was obtained five years after the graft was implanted from the common femoral artery to the proximal popliteal artery. The vein graft remains widely patent despite the distal poor run-off.[3] (DeWeese, J. A., and Rob, C. G.: Ann. Surg., *174*:346, 1971)

which have been encircled with tapes and retracted vigorously during their mobilization. In extensively calcified vessels cracking of the intima is usually incriminated as the cause of such thrombosis. However, occlusion of vessels by traction may also produce stasis and contribute to thrombosis in more pliable vessels. It is important to have control of all posterior branches before occluding a segment of an artery or unnecessary blood loss occurs, and bleeding unnecessarily complicates the performance of anastomosis.

Heparin sodium is administered intravenously in doses of 5,000 to 7,500 units prior to the occlusion of any major artery. Protamine sulfate in doses of 50 to 75 mg. is administered later after all clamps are removed.

Occlusion. Arteries may be occluded for short periods of time without resultant thrombosis. However, proximal or distal thrombosis occurs frequently enough that, in our opinion, the use of anticoagulants is mandatory during the period of arterial clamping. Heparin introduced locally soon produces a systemic effect and has no advantage over the intravenous route.[9]

Soft-walled and thin arteries are occluded with any one of the standard vascular clamps. Vessels with circumferential calcification are occluded only with a tape over an intraluminal occluding catheter. The catheter is introduced through the arteriotomy for the anastomosis and withdrawn just before the anastomosis is completed. If a vessel appears indented or if an intraoperative arteriogram demonstrates an arterial occlusion at the site where a clamp was applied, a Fogarty intraluminal balloon catheter can be used to dilate the vessel.

Arterial thrombosis secondary to vascular clamps is probably much more common than is generally appreciated. The thrombosis may be secondary to permanent narrowing of a nonelastic vessel or to the cracking of the intima producing an intimal flap. In other instances the clamp can dislodge atheromatous material which can embolize and obstruct distal vessels as reported by Dickson, Strandness and Bell.[10] Thrombosis can be recognized and corrected if an operative arteriogram is obtained immediately following arterial reconstruction. Other measures relating to immediate detection of untoward results are discussed in Chapter 16. If not corrected in the operating room the occlusion may be responsible for a suboptimal result and be recognized by a late arteriogram as reported by Darling and Linton.[11] Figure 3-4 is an example of this preventable type of problem.

Venous Bypass Graft. 1. A vein of suitable length is carefully removed from the leg or arm. During removal the branches are ligated 1 mm. from the vein. The vein is then distended with saline and any remaining holes are closed with fine sutures using horizontal mattress stitches.

The saphenous vein is almost always of suitable size and length for even a long femoropopliteal bypass graft. It should have an external diameter of at least 4 mm. Darling, *et al.* believed that veins less than 4 mm. in diameter were often contributing factors to early graft thrombosis.[7] Baddely, *et al.* obtained a significantly better patency rate if the grafts were greater than 5 mm. in diameter.[12] Ray, *et al.* reported a failure rate of 24.4 percent when the grafts were 3 to 4 mm. in diameter, 14.9 percent when they were 5 to 6 mm. in diameter and 0 percent when they were 7 mm. in diameter.[13] The vein may still be acceptable if it is duplicated for a short distance.[14] If the vein is too small or absent the cephalic vein may be acceptable as suggested by Kakkar.[15] Awe and Krippaehne have also successfully used the superficial femoral vein.[16] Turcotte, Dent and Fry were able to distend a small vein over a five-week period by using it as an arteriovenous fistula between the common femoral artery and the distal saphenous vein several days prior to anastomosing the distal end to the popliteal artery.[17] The proximal anastomosis can always be somewhat enlarged by suturing a patch graft of vein to the arteriotomy in the femoral artery, and then performing an end-to-side anastomosis between vein and patch graft as described by Linton.[18]

If the grafts are not long enough it is advisable to perform a proximal endarterectomy and use the vein graft across the knee

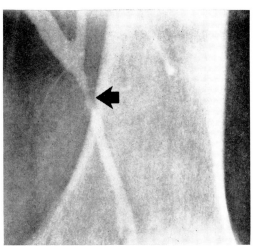

FIG. 3-4. Arteriogram obtained one year following a successful venous bypass graft demonstrating a stenosis, probably secondary to a clamp injury, just distal to the anastomosis. An endarterectomy and patch graft successfully corrected the defect.[54] (DeWeese, J. A., *et al.*: Surgery, *59*:28, 1965)

joint.[18,19] Composite grafts of prosthetics to vein or vein to vein have not been satisfactory. Dale observed thrombosis of 13 of 16 Teflon to vein composite grafts within nine months.[20] Darling, Linton and Razzuk reported occlusion 3 to 39 months after operation in 10 of 29 vein grafts fashioned by multiple end-to-end anastomoses. The occlusion was thought to be secondary to stenosis at the site of venovenous anastomosis. Such a stenosis was demonstrated arteriographically in one patient 20 months following operation.[7]

The vein is removed with care. Ligation of branches too far from the vein may leave small bulges in the graft, but this is probably better than ligating branches too close to the vein. This results in the surrounding adventitia being gathered by the ligature and constriction of the graft.[8] Excessive traction on the vein during its removal causes tears at the junction of the branches and the vein wall. Great care must be taken in suturing these rents with horizontal mattress sutures to avoid constriction of the vein.

2. A hollow bored tunneler is passed between two incisions taking care to pass beneath the sartorious muscle in the thigh

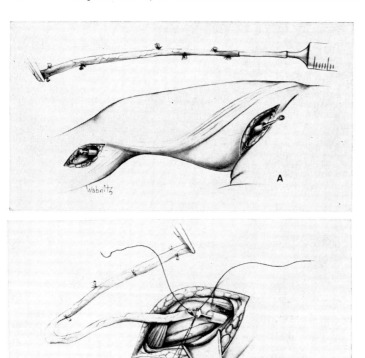

FIG. 3-5. Venous bypass graft. (A) Passage of tunneler in subsartorial plane and orientation of vein; (B) attaching the vein to the metal plate; (C) removing the tunneler.[78] (Rob, C. G., and DeWeese, J. A.: Surgery, *62*:393, 1967)

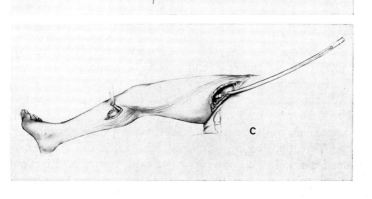

and between the two heads of the gastrocnemius muscle behind the knee. The vein is distended with saline during which time any twist is corrected. An end of the vein is then sutured to the flattened end of the metal rod maintaining proper orientation. The metal rod with the attached vein is pulled through the tunneler. The tunneler is then extracted over the metal rod, the vein detached, and a straight clamp applied to the end of the vein with assurance that the graft is not twisted. Twisting was observed as a cause of early graft failure prior to the use of the tunneler described. It is obviously very important that the vein be reversed prior to tunneling between the incisions. The venous valves are oriented to maintain blood flow toward the heart. The vein must, therefore, be reversed when used in the arterial system where blood flow is away from the heart. Figures 3-5 a, b and c illustrate these steps.

The vein is buried beneath the muscles,

Fig. 3-6. Venous bypass graft. (A) Enlarging the ends of the vein by a "T" incision to form a "cobra" mouth anastomosis; (B) arteriotomy and placing of stay sutures; (C) position of graft and excision of clamped edges; (D) direction of the running stitch at the proximal and distal anastomoses using a double-armed suture.[74] (Rob, C. G., and Smith, J. A.: Surgery Annual 1971, Meredith, New York, 1971, p. 353 (Modified)

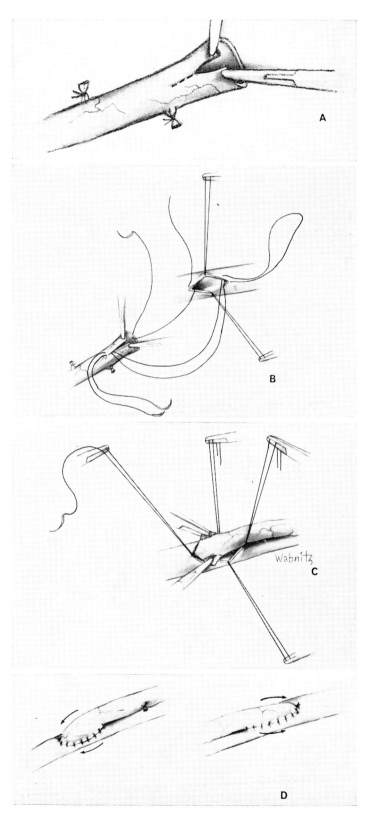

away from the subcutaneous tunnel through which the saphenous vein was removed. It is thus protected if a superficial wound infection should occur.

3. An arteriotomy is made which is twice as long as the diameter of the vein graft. Traction stay sutures are placed on either side of the mid-lateral part of the arteriotomy to avoid the use of forceps to grasp the arterial wall. If the vein is large the end is cut obliquely. If the vein is small its end is enlarged by placing two small clamps adjacent to one another or the proposed bottom edge of the vein and making a longitudinal incision between the clamps for a distance twice the diameter of the vein. Excess adventitia is removed. Proximal and distal stay sutures are placed and tied. The edges of the vein that were clamped are cut off prior to completion of the anastomosis. A continuous everting simple stitch is run down both sides from the double-ended inner stay suture to the end suture. Figure 3-6 a, b, c and d illustrate these steps.

The importance of a meticulous technique in preventing thrombosis of a vein graft cannot be overemphasized. Trauma to the intima of either the vein or artery with clamps or forceps must be avoided. Adventitia pulled within the lumen can initiate clotting, and so all stitches must cause eversion of the edges of the vessels. Sutures can catch the opposite wall of vessels, literally sewing shut the anastomosis. This mistake can best be avoided by beginning both running stitches in the same direction down each side from the inner stay suture as described. Care must be taken not to allow the trailing ends of stitches to pull the adventitia, since this can narrow the size of the anastomosis.

4. Nonreversed venous bypass grafts are performed by mobilizing the proximal and distal ends of the saphenous vein, rupturing the venous valves by passage of catheter or vein strippers through the vein, and then anastomosing the ends of the vein to the appropriate vessels. Significant branches of the vein resulting in arteriovenous fistulae

are identified by palpable thrills, audible bruits, or visible shunts on an arteriogram. Small incisions can be made over these branches for their ligation.

Barner's and our early experiences with nonreversed vein grafts were discouraging. The strippers were occasionally passed through the vein wall, and there were troublesome appearances of arteriovenous fistulae even after leaving the operating room. There was a high incidence of early and then late thrombosis, presumably secondary to incompletely ruptured valves.[21,22] On the other hand, Connolly and Stenner report a greater success, for those interested in learning the method.[23]

Graft Material. Bypass grafts may be performed with other materials including plastic grafts of Dacron, heterografts or venous allografts. The same attention to detail, particularly in regard to twisting of the graft and performance of the anastomosis is just as important as when autogenous veins are being used. The long-term results of prosthetic graft materials below the inguinal ligament have been generally discouraging. The relative merit of alternative graft materials is discussed under the section on late thrombosis elsewhere in this chapter.

Thromboendarterectomy. A longitudinal incision is made at the site of the severest disease and a plane of dissection in the outer media is established. The inner core is divided between two sutures. A Cannon stripper is passed proximally to the thinnest part of the arterial wall above the stenosis, and the core carefully incised through a longitudinal arteriotomy. If the vessel becomes quite thin distally, the stripper is passed carefully to that point where it is incised with a transverse arteriotomy. To prevent subintimal dissection, the posterior cut end of the intima and media is sutured to the adventitia with mattress sutures tied on the outside of the vessel. The arteriotomy is closed with a continuous stitch including all layers of the distal vessel to the adventitia proximally.

FIG. 3-7. Thromboendarterectomy.
(A) Arterial incisions; (B) mobilization of core using Cannon loop;
(C) removal of core; (D) closure
distal arteriotomy.[24] (DeWeese, J.
A.: Surg. Gynec. Obstet., *119*:851,
1964)

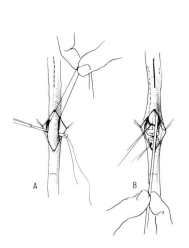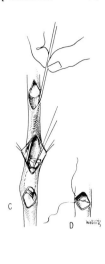

Figures 3-7 a, b, c and d illustrate these
steps. If the vessel is still thickwalled distally, the endarterectomy is ended in the
middle of the arteriotomy, the distal intima
is tacked to the adventitia with a mattress
stitch. A venous patch graft is then applied
to assure an adequate sized outflow.

Early thrombosis following an endarterectomy may be secondary to strands of remaining media, intimal flaps at the end of
the endarterectomy, or constriction of the
vessel by faulty suture lines. A meticulous
technique is necessary if early thrombosis is
to be avoided.

Arteriogram. After completion of any
arterial reconstruction and before the
wounds are closed, an arteriogram should be
performed which visualizes the length of the
reconstruction and the run-off into the
lower leg.

Reliable objective evidence of the status
of the arterial reconstruction and its run-off
should be obtained in the operating room.
Backflow is an unreliable measure of distal
run-off in our experience. Pulsation of the
graft is also unreliable and may actually be
increased by distal obstruction. Digital plethysmography is reported by Dickson, Strandness and Bell[10] to provide a reliable means of
screening for possible occlusion. Angiography
is performed if plethysmography does not record any improvement over the preoperative
measurement. Angiograms are still the most
reliable means of determining patency and
identifying the site of any residual obstruction, which can then be corrected. Constrictions at the site of anastomoses can be
corrected with patch grafts. Constrictions
secondary to clamping of atherosclerotic vessels can be dilated with Fogarty balloon catheters. Emboli can be removed. The only
time that arteriograms are not performed is
when there are strong pedal pulses felt
which were not present prior to the operation. Chapter 16 contains additional discussion of these points.

Lumbar sympathectomies are performed
at the time of their arterial reconstruction on
patients with severe ischemia and poor runoff. Mannick, Jackson and Benjamin have
demonstrated increased blood flow following
sympathectomy in low flow arterial reconstructions.[25] The decrease in peripheral resistance and increased flow occurring after
sympathectomy may maintain patency of
some reconstructions that would otherwise
fail.

Anticoagulants or dextran are not routinely administered postoperatively. Although these materials may decrease the
incidence of thrombotic complications, they
may also increase the risk of other complications. We observed a 9 percent incidence
of significant wound hematomata in the first

100 patients on whom venous bypass grafts or endarterectomies were performed.[26] These all occurred in patients receiving systemic heparinization following operation. Subsequent wound infections, anastomotic bleeding, and/or thrombosis made amputation necessary in five patients.

Rheomacrodex (10%) in saline or 5 percent glucose in water was administered as a continuous infusion of 1,000 ml. per 24 hours for 5 days following arterial reconstruction by Foster, Killen, Jolly and Kirtley.[27] They observed only a 10 percent incidence of thrombosis in the early postoperative period. No wound hematomata occurred but four patients developed pulmonary edema, two of whom died. We have observed wound hematomata following dextran and reserve its cautious use to patients who have required thrombectomy following thrombosis of their reconstruction in the early postoperative period. Further discussion of these measures is contained in Chapter 17.

Identification and Treatment of Complications

The complications which may occur in the early postoperative period include thrombosis, hemorrhage, edema, infection and lymphorrhea. False aneurysms may be identified in the hospital but are more frequently diagnosed later. True aneurysms and atherosclerosis are late complications.

Early Thrombosis

At the end of the operation some objective evidence of patency of the arterial reconstruction is selected for following every two hours for the first 24 hours. In most patients pedal pulses are strong and can be used to assess postoperative status. In patients with poor run-off, the graft pulse or oscillometric readings may be monitored. These extremities should be explored immediately if there is a disappearance of objective evidence of patency anytime in the postoperative period.

Incisions are made at both ends of the graft for removal of thrombi and for careful inspection of the anastomoses from within the lumen of the vessels. Fogarty balloon catheters are passed proximally and distally and through the graft or endarterectomized vessel. Grafts are carefully inspected for twisting, kinking or mechanical obstruction. Any identifiable constrictions are corrected with patch grafts or endarterectomies. Arteriograms are obtained which visualize the entire reconstruction and its run-off into the lower leg. If no mechanical reason for thrombosis is identified dextran is cautiously administered intravenously in 1,000 ml. amounts per 24-hour period for five days. However, it should be emphasized that most early failures will provide a mechanical explanation for thrombosis if it is carefully sought.

Hemorrhage

Hemorrhage was a common complication following the routine use of heparin and dextran. The bleeding was usually diffuse from many small vessels and was not significantly affected by re-exploration, in our experience. Residual hematomas complicated by infection or chronic seroma were common.

Hemorrhage is now a rare complication since these drugs are no longer given routinely, and as soon as it is recognized the wounds should be explored. In the early postoperative period, bleeding has most frequently been from branches of venous bypass grafts which were either not tied or inadequately tied. Anastomotic bleeding has also been observed, but is uncommon. These complications can be quickly remedied with additional sutures. An unusual spontaneous necrosis of a venous bypass graft causing hemorrhage ten days following the operation was observed by Friedman, Cerruit and Amadea.[28] False aneurysms can form and rupture during the patient's hospital stay, but are usually recognized after the patient has been discharged. Hemorrhage may occur in the presence of infection at any time. The management of false aneurysms and infection will be discussed in later sections.

Edema

Edema is frequently observed following an arterial reconstruction. Connolly and Stemmer stated[23] that, "The majority of our femoropopliteal bypass graft patients had postoperative ankle edema which persisted on an average of 3 months." Ray, *et al.* stated[13] that swelling was "quite common," and Downs and Sinha observed edema following 29 of 117 femoropopliteal arterial reconstructions.[29] Husni carefully followed a group of 137 patients following lower extremity arterial reconstructions.[30] All patients with patent reconstructions developed some edema as diagnosed by an increased circumference of the ankle of at least 0.5 cm. in the first few days. The edema disappeared if the reconstruction failed. In some patients the edema became more marked with ambulation. In eight of these patients acute deep venous thrombosis was diagnosed by phlebograms. In several other patients phlebograms and/or venous pressure studies were normal indicating the edema was not related to venous abnormality. They concluded that the mild edema was due to hyperemia and that the more marked edema not due to venous thrombosis was due to hydrostatic pressure accompanying a patent reconstruction with filtration at the capillary end incident to an overstretched precapillary arterial tree.

We also have frequently observed such edema and only rarely have found it to be secondary to deep venous thrombosis. Significant edema has been observed more frequently in patients with wound complications, particularly infection. Vaughan, Slavotinek and Jepson have documented lymphatic abnormalities by lymphangiography in patients after arterial reconstruction.[31] Therefore, it seems that this is lymphedema secondary to destruction of lymphatics by incisions or infection as opposed to increased formation of lymph fluid as postulated by others. This theory is also supported by the observation that the edema becomes persistent and rubbery in consistency. It can be at least partially controlled by elevation of the foot of the bed at night, elevation of the leg above heart level when possible during the day, and the use of strong elastic support, such as Jobst pressure gradient stockings. Further discussion of leg swelling and arterial reconstruction is contained in Chapter 11.

Infection

Infection is the most dreaded of complications occurring after any arterial reconstruction. Fortunately it is also a rare complication occurring in less than 5 percent of arterial reconstructions of the lower extremity.[1,32] Uncontrolled infection in the region of suture lines of patent reconstructions almost invariably results in massive hemorrhage as so well emphasized by Shaw and Baue.[33] This phenomenon has been observed in anastomoses between an artery and vein, homografts or plastic prosthetics. It apparently is related to necrosis of tissue around sutures and not to any effect of infection on plastic grafts or sutures themselves. We have had the dubious privilege of observing a silk suture line in the midportion of an exposed, infected, patent, Dacron graft in the groin for a period of nine months without a single episode of bleeding. Sepsis also causes thrombosis of the graft, particularly venous grafts. In some instances the initial bleed is not massive but remains confined by surrounding tissues. The clotted blood is then compressed by flow of blood through the defect in the suture line. In other words, a false aneurysm develops which almost invariably ruptures at some later date. Sepsis does not usually progress up and down a patent synthetic graft, but may result in recurrent abscesses or chronic draining sinuses for as long as the foreign material is present. Sepsis does progress in thrombosed grafts to cause bacteremia or involvement of suture lines and subsequent hemorrhage.

Aggressive debridement of infected wounds, bathing of grafts in topical antibiotics, and administration of appropriate systemic antibiotics has resulted in long-term salvage of some infected reconstructions.

This type of healing has most frequently been observed in venous grafts as reported by Szilagyi, Ray and Darling.[7,8,13] Najafi, *et al.* reported healing of an infected wound with a Dacron graft replacing the common carotid artery by this local technique.[34] Mundth, *et al.* observed healing of an infected popliteal wound with an iliopopliteal graft exposed.[35] Some experimental studies suggest that the local antibiotics method of management may be even safer in patients with plastic grafts. Massive hemorrhage occurred less frequently when plastic grafts were used in infected wounds than when homografts were inserted by Foster, Berrins and Scott, or when vein grafts were implanted by Bricker, Beall and DeBakey.[36,37] It is our experience that attempts at local management of the infected graft has resulted only in massive hemorrhage or thrombosis of the graft. This more conservative approach should be reserved only for those wounds where suture lines are not exposed, where bleeding has not occurred, and where one of the following methods of management is not possible.

Wylie reported the successful use of an iliac artery autograft for bridging arterial defects in three infected wounds where the autograft was left exposed and healing occurred over it.[38] The method of management which we have preferred was clearly defined by Shaw and Baue in 1963.[33] (1) The reconstruction is defunctionalized by ligations of the involved artery proximal and distal to the area of infection through clean incisions. (2) The ligated artery is bypassed with a suitable graft through clean, distant, noninfected planes. This may involve tunneling of grafts from the iliac vessels through the obturator foramen, and adductor muscles to the distally patent femoral or popliteal artery.[39] If necessary the grafts can be brought down the lateral thigh and anastomosed to the popliteal artery through a lateral approach as described by Danese and Singer.[40] (3) All foreign material, particularly plastic grafts, is removed from the infected area. In some instances the ligation

of vessels and removal of grafts may precede the new bypass graft. In others the bypass graft may be done first. The success of this approach to the problems of infected grafts has been well documented in reports from Fry and Lindenauer, Con, Hardy, Chavez and Fain, and Stipa and Wheelock.[41,42,43]

Lymphorrhea

An occasional patient will develop drainage of a slightly cloudy, watery, fluid from the femoral incision. Initially a diagnosis of seroma is usually made. When drainage becomes profuse and persistent one knows that he is dealing with lymphorrea, apparently secondary to divided lymphatics in the groin wound.

Treatment of this annoying complication is directed toward decreasing lymphatic flow to allow the lymphatics to heal. The patients are placed on bed rest with elevation of the legs to well above heart level in order to decrease capillary hydrostatic pressure. The patient is kept in this position until the wound dressings remain dry, often as long as one week. Then, with tight elastic stockings on, he is allowed to walk, but not to sit. Prophylactic antibiotics are administered.

Aneurysms

Aneurysms occurring after arterial reconstruction may be false aneurysms developing as a result of anastomotic leaks or true aneurysms secondary to degenerative weakness of the wall of the reconstructed vessel or bypass graft.

False aneurysms. False aneurysms are a fairly common complication of arterial reconstruction. Stoney, Albo and Wylie reported a 23.7 percent incidence of false aneurysms in 135 anastomoses of Dacron grafts ending or beginning in the femoral or popliteal arteries.[44] Szilagyi reported a 5 percent incidence in 420 femoral or popliteal anastomoses.[45] Rosenberg, *et al.* observed an 8 percent incidence in 48 femoropopliteal anastomoses using modified bovine carotid arteries.[46] Darling and his colleagues observed less than a 1 percent incidence of false aneurysm in 590 femoral and popliteal artery anastomoses performed with autogenous veins.[7] The femoral site as opposed to aortic, iliac, or popliteal sites is where most false aneurysms occur,[47] and they may occur in the presence of thrombosed as well as patent grafts.[48]

There are several possible causes of false aneurysm including infection and deterioration of the artery, suture material or graft at the site of the anastomosis. Also implicated are shearing forces occurring when rigid grafts are anastomosed in an end-to-side manner across movable joints. Infection is a common cause and cultures should be obtained at the time of repair. Weakening of the arterial wall from atherosclerosis theoretically could contribute, but atherosclerosis is not more prevalent at the femoral than at other sites. The performance of local endarterectomies does not increase the incidence of false aneurysms.[44] The use of silk sutures has been incriminated as the cause of most false aneurysms, particularly when rigid synthetic grafts are used.[49]

We were slow to accept this theory because the first three false aneurysms we observed occurred following the use of synthetic suture material. One occurred at a proximal aortic suture line. Another occurred at the distal end of a femoropopliteal Dacron bypass graft. The third occurred in the distal end of a femoropopliteal venous bypass graft. The distal anastomosis was performed with silk, but an incision had been made in the graft for passage of a Fogarty catheter and this was closed with a plastic suture. At the time of the operation for a rupture of the false aneurysm the incision in the artery was open. Plastic sutures could not be found but the silk suture line was intact. Staphylococcus aureus coagulase-positive was cultured from the wall of the aneurysm. Since then we have observed several noninfected false aneurysms where the silk sutures had deteriorated. We now use plastic nonabsorbable sutures for all arterial anastomoses.

Deterioration of the graft material could,

theoretically, contribute to aneurysm formation since degeneration and/or atherosclerosis has been observed in vein grafts, homografts and heterografts. However, the incidence of false aneurysms is not nearly as high with those materials as it is when plastic grafts are used. The increased frequency of false aneurysms when rigid plastic grafts are used adds credence to the theory that shearing forces are responsible for the late dehiscence of suture lines and formation of false aneurysms.

False aneurysms were first recognized within two months of operation in 12 patients and within eight months in 20 of 26 patients with false aneurysms reported by Spratt, Moran and Baird.[47] Occasionally the aneurysm presented several years postoperatively.

False aneurysms secondary to infection should be handled in the aggressive fashion previously described. The artery should be ligated proximally and distally through clean incisions, the graft should be removed and, if possible, a new bypass graft should be inserted through clean planes. Noninfected aneurysms may be handled in a more conservative fashion. Occasionally it is possible to merely resuture or place a patch graft over the site of disruption. More frequently it is necessary to resect the aneurysm and perform a new anastomosis after sewing a new graft end-to-end to the original graft to increase its length.

True aneurysms. The appearance of an aneurysm at the site of an anastomosis does not necessarily mean the aneurysm must be a false aneurysm or even associated with a graft. We have observed two common femoral aneurysms develop in the host artery above the proximal end of femoropopliteal bypass grafts. The suture lines were quite intact and the dilatation involved only the artery. Sawyer, Jacobs and Sutton have observed five similar cases.[50]

Aneurysms may also develop in the graft itself adjacent to the anastomosis. Aneurysmal degeneration of nylon grafts secondary to the marked loss of tensile strength of

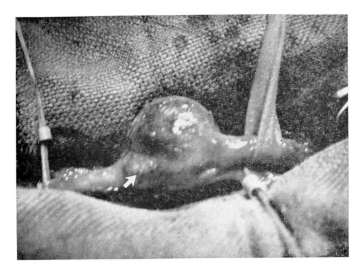

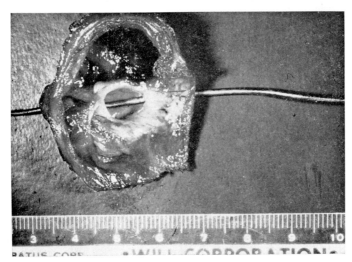

FIG. 3-8. Crimped nylon graft anastomosed to common femoral artery. (A) Aneurysmal dilatation of the end of the graft. Note the black silk (arrow) at the intact suture line. (B) The aneurysm is opened. Fragmented nylon fibers were identified throughout the wall of the aneurysm indicating that it was a true aneurysm.

the material with the first 12 months of implantation was frequently observed.[51,52] We observed four true aneurysms at the distal end of aortofemoral bypass grafts of crimped nylon as illustrated in Figure 3-8.

Aneurysms may also develop in the body of grafts of certain materials. Thirty-five arterial homografts used as femoropopliteal reconstructions were closely followed by Barner, *et al*.[53] Aneursymal degeneration was observed in six (46%) of the 13 grafts patent for more than one year. All of the three grafts patent longer than five years became aneurysmal, as the example in Figure 3-9 shows. Aneurysmal dilatation

has also been observed in at least one modified bovine carotid artery heterograft. Aneurysms have been observed at the ends of two venous bypass grafts one of which is shown in Figure 3-10.[54] A third one was suspected but at operation proved to be an aneurysm of the common femoral artery. Another venous bypass graft, shown in Figure 3-11, was observed to be diffusely aneurysmal five years postoperatively, presumably secondary to atherosclerosis. Venous patch grafts used following thromboendarterectomies have also become aneurysmal 29, 39 and 49 months postoperatively. This occurred in only 4 of 450 or less than one percent of such opera-

FIG. 3-9. Postoperative arteriograms of femoropopliteal arterial homograft. (*Left*) The graft appeared normal 14 months postoperatively. (*Center*) Irregular dilatation was observed 71 months after operation. (*Right*) 79 months after the original procedure there was extensive aneurysmal dilatation.[53] (Barner, H. B., *et al.*: JAMA, *196*:631, 1966)

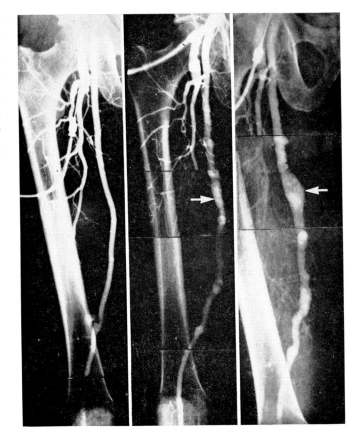

tions performed by Steenart, Troost and Kuypers.[55]

Atherosclerosis

Experimental and clinical evidence indicates that atherosclerotic changes rarely occur in plastic grafts.[52] Some changes have been observed in heterografts.[46] Some experimental studies suggest that autogenous venous grafts are more susceptible to atherosclerosis than arteries.[56] Studies of Penn, *et al.* indicate that the vein is resistant to atherosclerosis.[57] We have observed atherosclerotic changes in three venous grafts. The first was observed within five years after operation in a man whose serum cholesterol levels were consistently greater than 400 mg./100 ml.[58] The second was observed on an arteriogram 11½ years following operation, shown in Figure 3-12, and proved to be atherosclerotic on biopsy at a subsequent operation.

An arteriogram on the same extremity only six years after operation appeared normal. Neither the second or third patient demonstrated abnormal serum lipid studies. Gryska has experimentally demonstrated the susceptibility of thromboendarterectomized arteries to atherosclerosis.[59] Serial arteriograms have also demonstrated the progression of atherosclerosis in arteries on which thromboendarterectomies were performed, examples of which appear in Figures 3-13 and 3-14.

Late Thrombosis

Early thrombosis of arterial reconstructions is almost always related to the arteries selected for reconstruction, and technical mishaps.[60] These failures are preventable if meticulous care is used in the management of the patient in the preoperative, and operative periods as previously described. Throm-

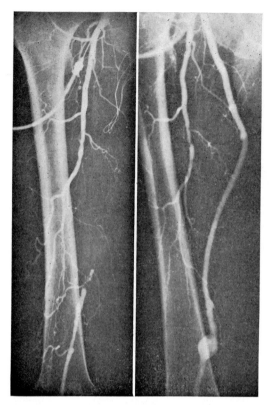

FIG. 3-10. (*Left*) Preoperative arteriogram demonstrating thrombosis of the femoral artery. (*Right*) Arteriogram of patent venous bypass graft from the common femoral to popliteal artery above the level of the knee six and one-half years after operation. An aneurysm of the distal end of the graft is present. The graft remains clinically patent without rupture of the aneurysm 14 years after operation.[54] (DeWeese, J. A., *et al.*: Surgery, *59*:28, 1966)

bosis of an arterial reconstruction after discharge from the hospital is more frequently related to either progression of the underlying disease or complications related to the type of reconstruction and the materials used.

New atherosclerotic occlusive disease may appear proximal or distal to the reconstruction. Morton, Ehrenfeld and Wylie performed late arteriograms on 45 extremities on which endarterectomies were performed and demonstrated progression of distal occlusive lesions in the popliteal artery and its branches.[61] Kirkpatrick and Miller demonstrated experimentally that a critical stenosis

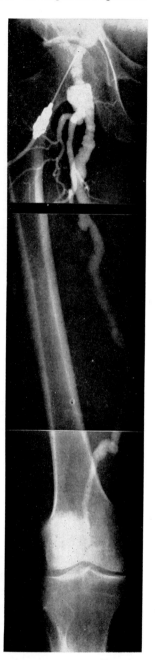

FIG. 3-11. Arteriogram of femoropopliteal venous bypass graft five years postoperatively demonstrating diffuse irregular aneurysmal dilatations. The graft was inserted into this extremity after the last arteriogram on the same extremity in Fig. 3-9 was obtained showing aneurysmal dilatation of a homograft.[63] (DeWeese, J. A., *In* Dale, W. A.: Management of Arterial Occlusive Disease, Yearbook, Chap. 8, Chicago, 1971)

FIG. 3-12. Femoral arteriograms of venous bypass graft. (*Left*) Six years postoperatively the vein appears normal. (*Right*) Eleven and one-half years after operation the graft is irregularly dilated and tortuous. A subsequent biopsy demonstrated arteriosclerotic changes.

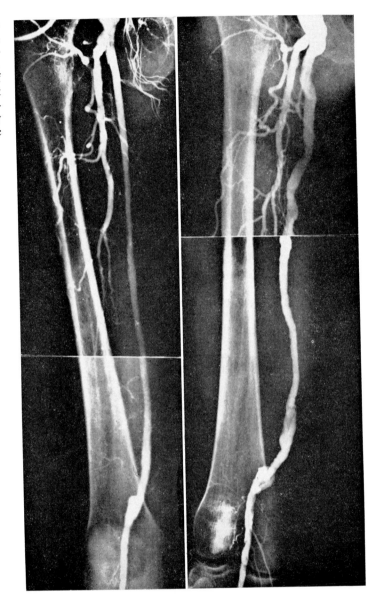

in an artery proximal to a short venous bypass graft caused occlusion of 80 percent of the grafts while a distal stenosis caused thrombosis of 30 percent of the grafts.[62] Szilagyi, Smith, Elliott and Allen followed Dacron graft femoropopliteal reconstructions with serial postoperative arteriograms. They concluded that 63.4 percent of 30 graft thromboses were secondary to progression of disease and 33.3 percent were due to graft failure.[45]

Since progression of disease can be a significant cause of thrombosis it is important that, if possible, the change is recognized and treated prior to occlusion of the reconstruction. Patients are examined every six months and are also asked to return for examination with any change in symptoms. Any decrease in proximal or distal arterial pulsation noted by palpation or recorded by an oscillometer is reason for angiography. A correctible lesion is frequently discovered

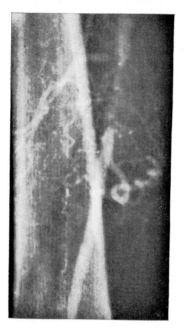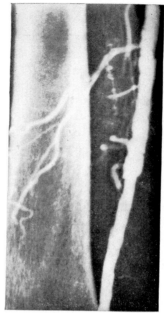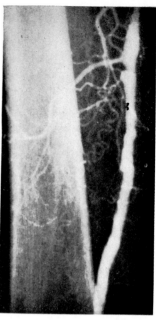

FIG. 3-13. (*Left*) Preoperative arteriogram demonstrates localized arterial occlusion at the level of the adductor magnus tendon. (*Center*) Arteriogram made immediately after thromboendarterectomy was performed shows a slightly dilated vessel. (*Right*) Arteriogram 54 months later demonstrates patent vessel with slight irregularity and narrowing.[63] (DeWeese, J. A., *In* Dale, W. A.: Management of Arterial Occlusive Disease, Yearbook, Chap. 8, Chicago, 1971)

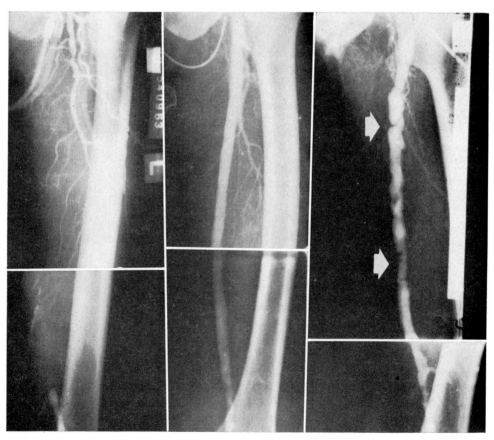

FIG. 3-14. (*Left*) Arteriogram showing femoral artery occlusion. (*Center*) Arteriogram obtained immediately after a long thromboendarterectomy showing smooth-walled vessel. (*Right*) Arteriogram five years later showing irregular-walled vessel with several areas of narrowing.

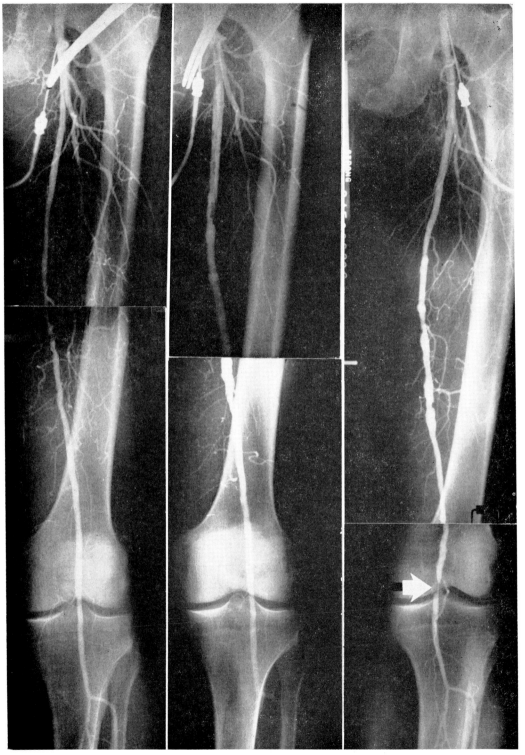

Fig. 3-15. (*Left*) Arteriogram showing atherosclerotic and occluded distal femoral artery. (*Center*) Arteriogram one week after long endarterectomy. (*Right*) Arteriogram 35 months postoperative demonstrating patent femoral artery, but a new stenosis (arrow) of the popliteal artery at knee-joint level.

under these circumstances as shown in Figure 3-15.

Autogenous veins are generally accepted as the best available material for bypass grafts, but even with their use there is a thrombosis rate of approximately 3 percent per year.[7,63] Although some of the occlu-sions are secondary to progression of disease, some occur because of graft failure. Aneu-rysms and arteriosclerosis could also be responsible for some thromboses. In addi-tion, a segmental stenosis of veins either secondary to intimal hyperplasia or valve cusp stenosis has been described.[22,64,65,66]

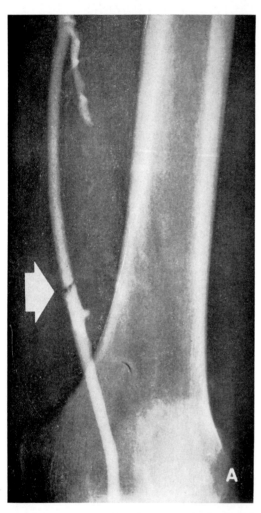

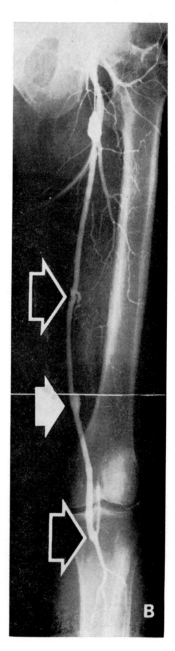

FIG. 3-16. (A) Arteriogram obtained 16 months following venous bypass graft because of recurrence of symptoms of claudication. Localized stenosis was demonstrated in the mid-dle of the graft. Endophlebectomy and venous patch graft were performed.[64] (Breslau, R. C., and DeWeese, J. A.: Ann. Surg. *162*:251, 1965) (B) Arteriogram of same extremity 64 months following the endophlebectomy. The graft (open arrows) is patent with slight dilatation at site of the patch graft (solid arrow).[63] (DeWeese, J. A., *In* Dale, W. A.: Management of Arterial Occlu-sive Disease, Yearbook, Chap. 8, Chicago, 1971)

These lesions appear late, result in new symptoms of arterial insufficiency, cause diminished distal pulses and produce bruits. They cause thrombosis of the graft if untreated. Operative correction by endophlebectomy and application of a venous patch graft, illustrated in Figure 3-16, has resulted in continued patency of grafts for three, six and eight years in three patients in whom we have recognized the complication.

The thrombosis rate for endarterectomies is 6 to 10 percent per year.[63,67] The development of recurrent arterial occlusive lesions in thromboendarterectomies is well demonstrated in Figures 3-13, 3-14 and 3-15. Humphries, Young and McCormack made a detailed pathologic study of 22 specimens of material removed at the time of reoperation for rethrombosis of previously endarterectomized vessels. Seven specimens suggested that the occlusion was secondary to accumulation of thrombi. In 12 specimens atheromatous changes were identified. Despite these complications our thrombosis rate for short thromboendarterectomies was only 4 percent per year.[63] Therefore, we still use the procedure for short occlusive lesions at the level of the adductor tendon when the proximal femoral and distal popliteal vessels appear normal. Edwards recommended application of long venous patch grafts following thromboendarterectomy. These reconstructions became dilated and arteriograms demonstrated slow transit times through the reconstructions.[68] Edwards postulated that slow flow was responsible for gradual thrombosis and later occlusion as is observed in popliteal aneurysms.

The thrombosis rate for knitted Dacron bypass grafts, as determined by the results reported by Szilagyi, would be approximately 9 to 13 percent per year.[45] Arteriographic studies indicated that the possible causes of thrombosis were anastomotic stenosis and intimal thickening possibly related to the slow flow of blood as recognized by the slow transit of dye through the grafts. Crawford, DeBakey, Morris and Garrett felt that kinking or twisting of the grafts might be responsible for some late failures.[69] Autogenous veins and

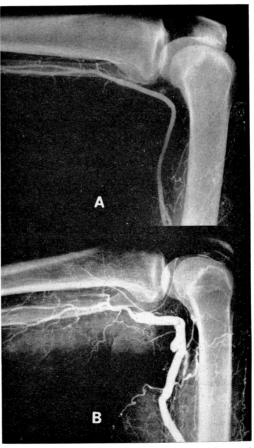

FIG. 3-17. (A) Arteriogram of common femoral to distal popliteal artery bypass graft using the saphenous vein. (B) Arteriogram of similar bypass using a knitted Dacron graft. At the time of angiographic follow-up three years after implantation with knee flexion the autogenous vein graft is flexible, whereas the implanted prosthesis kinks and causes almost complete occlusion of the graft.[11] (Darling, R. C., and Linton, R. R.: New Eng. J. Med., *270*:609, 1964)

small Dacron grafts were used as bypass grafts across a flexion crease in an experimental model by Shirkey, Beall and DeBakey. Fibrin buildup rather than kinking was felt to be responsible for a 36 percent patency rate of Dacron grafts as compared to 93 percent patency of vein grafts.[69] On the other hand, the thrombosis rate of grafts across the knee joint is known to be significantly higher than that for grafts in the thigh.[71] Significant kinking of Dacron grafts can be demonstrated on arteriograms, as shown in Figure 3-17, and may well be re-

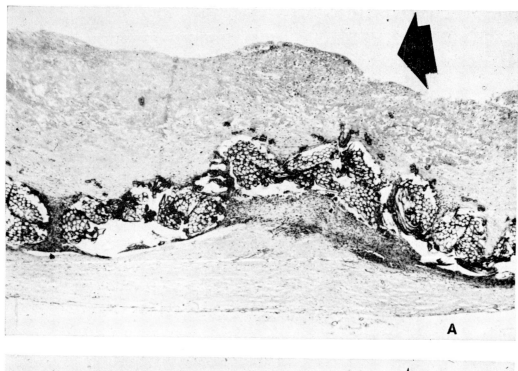

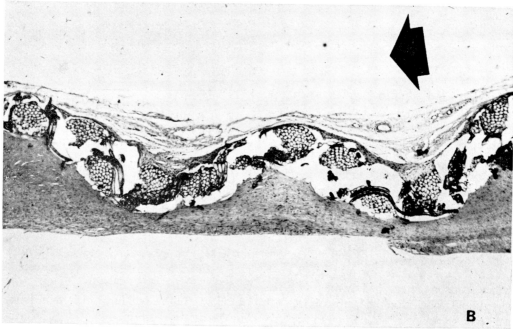

FIG. 3-18. Photomicrographs demonstrating comparative arteriogenesis in plastic fabrics of different construction. (A) Fibrous tissue has grown through the interstices of a knitted Teflon graft resulting in bonding of the inner lining to the outer lining. (B) No fibrous tissue has grown through this woven Teflon graft. Hematoxylin and eosin x 45.[73] (Phillips, C. E., Jr., *et al.*, Arch. Surg., *82*:38, 1961)

lated to late thrombosis.[11] Edwards felt that the inelasticity of all fabric grafts with the resultant kinking made them unacceptable for femoropopliteal reconstructions, particularly if they crossed the knee joint.[72]

Woven grafts have proved unsatisfactory for use in femoropopliteal reconstructions. Small woven grafts of Teflon and Dacron demonstrated significantly higher thrombosis rates than knitted grafts used to bypass the ligated femoral artery of the dog.[73] Fry, *et al.* made histologic studies of thrombosed grafts removed from patients which were very similar to those observed by Phillips, *et al.*[74] The bonding of intima and media, by bridges of fibrous tissue, does not occur in woven grafts. Dissection of the loosely adherent intima can produce occlusion of the grafts (Fig. 3-18).

Heterografts of modified bovine carotid arteries are now available. It is still too early to know what the long-term results of these grafts will be. Rosenberg, *et al.* do indicate that these grafts become rigid and do kink when placed across the knee joint so it is possible that they will share some of the problems of Dacron grafts.[46]

Venous allografts obtained from cadavers or during vein stripping operations have been used as femoropopliteal reconstructions.[75] Ochsner, *et al.* have implanted 22 such veins and followed some of them as long as four years. Fifty percent have thrombosed and one became aneurysmal. It is too early to determine the ultimate use of these grafts.[76]

There are some general rules that we adhere to in the management of patients who thrombose their arterial reconstructions after discharge from the hospital: (1) If an autogenous venous bypass graft does occlude, and the patient is seen within a few days of the thrombosis, the graft is explored. Several grafts have been salvaged at exploration by identifying and correcting new proximal lesions, new distal lesions, or stenoses of the graft or the anastomoses. One graft was successfully salvaged after being thrombosed ten days. (2) Patients with recurrence of

TABLE 3-1. POOR PROGNOSTIC SIGNS RELATED TO INDICATIONS FOR SURGERY

	Long graphs (%)	Poor run-off (%)	Diabetes (%)
Claudication	24	15	15
Rest pain	41	26	21
Gangrene	58	45	43

claudication following thrombosis of a short endarterectomy are restudied. If the patient has an adequate vein and a bypass graft can be done from the common femoral artery to the popliteal artery above the level of the knee, an operation is performed. Otherwise, no reoperations for claudication only are advised. (3) If a patient develops rest pain without gangrene following late thrombosis of an arterial reconstruction, a sympathectomy is performed. (4) Any patient with persistent rest pain following sympathectomy or gangrene is restudied. If an arteriogram demonstrates some patent distal vessels, and leg or arm veins are available, venous bypass grafts are recommended even if the distal anastomosis is to an ankle vessel.[77] Dacron or heterografts would be used only if the anastomosis can be made to the popliteal artery above the level of the knee. (5) Amputations are recommended for persistent rest pain or gangrene in the absence of suitable veins or with extensive occlusive disease of the lower leg.

References

1. Caldwell, R. L., DeWeese, J. A., and Rob, C. G.: Femoropopliteal bypass grafts utilizing autogenous veins. Circulation, *37*:37, 1967.
2. Couch, N. P., Wheeler, H. B., Hyatt, D. F., Crane, C., Edwards, E. A., and Warren, R.: Factors influencing limb survival after femoropopliteal reconstruction. Arch. Surg., *95*:163, 1967.
3. DeWeese, J. A., and Rob, C. G.: Autogenous venous bypass grafts five years later. Ann. Surg., *174*:346, 1971.
4. Mannick, J. A., Jackson, B. T., Coffman, J. D., and Hume, D. M.: Success of bypass vein grafts in patients with isolated popliteal artery segments. Surgery, *61*:17, 1967.

5. Moore, W. S., Rosson, C. T., and Hall, A. D.: Effect of prophylactic antibiotics in preventing bacteremic infection of vascular prostheses. Surgery, *69*:825, 1971.

6. Richardson, R. L., Jr., Pate, J. W., Wolf, A. Y., Ledes, C., and Hopson, W. B., Jr.: The outcome of antibiotic-soaked arterial grafts in guinea pig wounds contaminated with E. coli or S. aureus. J. Thorac. Cardiov., Surg., *59*:635, 1970.

7. Darling, R. C., Linton, R. R., and Razzuk, M. A.: Saphenous vein bypass grafts for femoropopliteal occlusive disease: a reappraisal. Surgery, *61*:31, 1967.

8. Szilagyi, D. E., Smith, R. F., and Elliott, J. P.: Venous autografts in femoropopliteal arterioplasty. Arch. Surg., *89*:113, 1964.

9. Ohlwiler, D. A., and Mahoney, E. B.: Regional heparinization and heparin inactivation by erythrocytes. Surg. Gynec. Obstet., *107*:353, 1958.

10. Dickson, A. H., Strandness, D. E., Jr., and Bell, J. W.: The detection and sequelae of operative accidents complicating reconstructive arterial surgery. Amer. J. Surg., *109*:143, 1965.

11. Darling, R. C., and Linton, R. R.: Management of the late failure of arterial reconstruction of the lower extremities. New England J. Med., *270*:609, 1964.

12. Baddeley, R. M., Ashton, F., Slaney, G., and Barnes, A. D.: Late results of autogenous vein bypass grafts in femoropopliteal arterial occlusion. Brit. Med. J., *1*:653, 1970.

13. Ray, F. S., Lape, C. P., Lutes, C. A., and Dillihunt, R. C.: Femoropopliteal saphenous vein bypass grafts. Amer. J. Surg., *119*:385, 1970.

14. Gaylis, H.: The duplicated saphenous vein in femoropopliteal bypass grafting. Surgery, *67*:277, 1970.

15. Kakkar, V. V.: The cephalic vein as a peripheral vascular graft. Surg. Gynec. Obstet., *138*:551, 1969.

16. Awe, W. C., and Krippaehne, W. W.: Use of the superficial femoral vein for femoropopliteal bypass. Amer. J. Surg., *120*:149, 1970.

17. Turcotte, J. G., Dent, T. L., and Fry, W. J.: Preparation for femoropopliteal bypass. Arch. Surg., *100*:627, 1970.

18. Linton, R. R., and Wilde, W. L.: Modifications in the technique for femoropopliteal saphenous vein bypass autografts. Surgery, *67*:234, 1970.

19. DeWeese, J. A., Barner, H. B., Mahoney, E. B., and Rob, C. G.: Autogenous venous bypass grafts and thromboendarterectomies for atherosclerotic lesions of the femoropopliteal arteries. Ann. Surg., *163*:205, 1966.

20. Dale, W. A., Pridgen, W. R., and Shoulders, H. H., Jr.: Failure of composite (Teflon and vein) grafting in small human arteries. Surgery, *51*:258, 1962.

21. May, A. G., DeWeese, J. A., and Rob, C. G.: Arterialized in situ saphenous vein. Arch. Surg., *91*:743, 1965.

22. Barner, H. B., Judd, D. R., Kaiser, G. C., Willman, V. L., and Hanlon, C. R.: Late failure of arterialized in situ saphenous vein. Arch. Surg., *99*:781, 1969.

23. Connolly, J. E., and Stemmer, E. A.: The nonreversed saphenous vein bypass for femoral-popliteal occlusive disease. Surgery, *68*:602, 1970.

24. DeWeese, J. A.: Transverse distal arteriotomy for femoropopliteal thromboendarterectomy. Surg. Gynec. Obstet., *119*:851, 1964.

25. Mannick, J. A., and Jackson, B. T.: Hemodynamics of arterial surgery in atherosclerotic limbs. Surgery *59*:713, 1966.

26. DeWeese, J. A., Dale, W. A., Mahoney, E. B., and Rob, C. G.: Thromboendarterectomies and autogenous venous bypass grafts distal to the inguinal ligament. Circulation, *29*:171, 1964.

27. Foster, J. H., Killen, D. A., Jolly, P. C., and Kirtley, J. H.: Low molecular weight dextran in vascular surgery: Prevention of early thrombosis following arterial reconstruction in 85 cases. Ann. Surg., *163*:764, 1966.

28. Friedman, S. A., Cerruti, M. M., and Amadeo, B.: Spontaneous necrosis of a functioning saphenous vein graft. Surgery, *66*:1022, 1969.

29. Downs, A. R., and Sinha, B. K.: Assessment of reconstructive procedures for femoropopliteal artery occlusive disease. Canad. Med. Ass. J., *102*:141, 1970.

30. Husni, E. A.: The edema of arterial reconstruction. Circulation, *35*:169, 1967.

31. Vaughan, B. F., Slavotinek, A. H., and Jepson, R. P.: Edema of the lower limb after vascular operations. Surg. Gynec. Obstet., *131*:282, 1970.

32. Vollmar, J., Trede, M., Laubach, K., and Forrest, H.: Principles of reconstructive procedures for chronic femoropopliteal occlusions: Report on 548 operations. Ann. Surg., *168*:215, 1968.

33. Shaw, R. S., and Baue, A. E.: Management of sepsis complicating arterial reconstructive surgery. Surgery, *53*:75, 1963.

34. Najafi, H., Javid, H., Dye, W. S., Hunter, J. A., and Julian, O. C.: Management of

infected arterial implants. Surgery, *65*:539, 1969.

35. Mundth, E. D., Darling, R. C., Alvardo, R. H., Buckley, M. J., Linton, R. R. and Austen, W. G.: Surgical management of the mycotic aneurysms and the complications of infection in vascular reconstructive surgery. Amer. J. Surg., *117*:460, 1969.

36. Foster, J. H., Berzins, T., and Scott, H. W., Jr.: An experimental study of arterial replacement in the presence of bacterial infection. Surg. Gynec. Obstet., *108*:141, 1959.

37. Bricker, D. L., Beall, A. C., Jr., and DeBakey, M. E.: The differential response to infection of autogenous vein versus Dacron arterial prosthesis. Chest, *58*:566, 1970.

38. Wylie, E. J.: Vascular replacement with arterial autografts. Surgery, *57*:14, 1965.

39. Carter, S. C., Cohen, A., and Whelan, T. J.: Clinical experience with management of the infected Dacron graft. Ann. Surg., *158*: 249, 1963.

40. Danese, C. A., and Singer, A.: Lateral approach to the popliteal artery trifurcation. Surgery, *63*:588, 1968.

41. Fry, W. J., and Lindenauer, S. M.: Infection complicating the use of plastic arterial implants. Arch. Surg., *94*:600, 1966.

42. Conn, J. H., Hardy, J. D., Chavez, C. M., and Fain, W. R.: Infected arterial grafts: Experience in 22 cases with emphasis on unusual bacteria and techniques. Ann. Surg., *171*:704, 1970.

43. Stipa, S., and Wheelock, F. C., Jr.: A comparison of femoral artery grafts in diabetic and nondiabetic patients. Amer. J. Surg., *121*:223, 1971.

44. Stoney, R. J., Albo, R. J., and Wylie, E. J.: False aneurysms occurring after arterial grafting operations. Amer. J. Surg., *110*: 153, 1965.

45. Szilagyi, D. E., Smith, R. F., Elliott, J. P., and Allen, H. M.: Long term behavior of a Dacron arterial substitute: Clinical roentgenologic and histologic correlations. Ann. Surg., *162*:453, 1965.

46. Rosenberg, D. M. L., Glass, B. A., Rosenberg, N., Lewis, M. R., and Dale, W. A.: Experiences with modified bovine carotid arteries in arterial surgery. Surgery, *68*: 1064, 1970.

47. Spratt, E. M., Doran, M. L., and Baird, R. J.: False aneurysms in the lower extremity. Surg. Gynec. Obstet., *124*:562, 1967.

48. Sumner, D. S., and Strandness, D. E., Jr.: False aneurysms occurring in association with thrombosed prosthetic grafts. Arch. Surg., *94*:360, 1967.

49. Moore, W. S., and Hall, A. D.: Late suture failure in the pathogenesis of anastomotic false aneurysms. Ann. Surg., *172*:1064, 1970.

50. Sawyers, J. L., Jacobs, J. K., and Sutton, J. P.: Peripheral anastomotic aneurysms. Arch. Surg., *94*:802, 1967.

51. Harrison, J. H.: Synthetic materials as vascular prostheses. Surg. Gynec. Obstet., *108*:433, 1959.

52. Szilagyi, D. E., Pfeifer, J. R., and DeRusso, F. J.: Long term evaluation of plastic arterial substitutes: An experimental study. Surgery, *55*:165, 1964.

53. Barner, H. B., DeWeese, J. A., Dale, W. A., and Mahoney, E. B.: Aneurysmal degeneration of femoropopliteal arterial homografts. JAMA, *196*:631, 1966.

54. DeWeese, J. A., Terry, R., Barner, H. B., and Rob, C. G.: Autogenous venous femoropopliteal bypass grafts. Surgery, *59*:28, 1966.

55. Steenaert, B., Troast, F. A., and Kuypers, P. J.: Aneurysms in autologous venous patches used for arterial reconstruction. J. Cardiov. Surg., *11*:183, 1970.

56. Scott, H. W., Jr., Morgan, C. V., Bolasny, B. L., Lanier, V. C., Younger, R. K., and Butts, W.: Experimental atherosclerosis in autogenous venous grafts. Arch. Surg., *101*:677, 1970.

57. Penn, Israel, Schenk, E., Rob, C. G., DeWeese, J. A., and Schwartz, S. I.: Evaluation of the development of athero-arteriosclerosis in autogenous venous grafts inserted into the peripheral arterial system. Circulation, *31*:192, 1965.

58. Beebe, H. G., Clark, W. F., and DeWeese, J. A.: Atherosclerotic change occurring in an autogenous venous arterial graft. Arch. Surg., *101*:85, 1970.

59. Gryska, P. F.: The development of atheroma in arteries subjected to experimental thromboendarterectomy. Surgery, *45*:655, 1959.

60. DeWeese, J. A.: "Early failures" in arterial reconstruction. Arch. Surg., *85*:901, 1962.

61. Morton, D. L., Ehrenfeld, W. K., and Wylie, E. J.: Significance of outflow obstruction after femoropopliteal endarterectomy. Arch. Surg., *94*:592, 1967.

62. Kirkpatrick, J. R., and Miller, D. R.: Effects of decreased arterial inflow and runoff on vein graft patency. Surgery, *69*:870, 1971.

63. DeWeese, J. A.: Results of thromboendarterectomy vs. venous bypass grafts. *In* Dale, W. A.: Management of Arterial Occlusive Disease; Yearbook, Chap. 8, Chicago, 1971.

64. Breslau, R. C., and DeWeese, J. A.: Successful endophlebectomy of autogenous venous bypass graft. Ann. Surg., *162*:251, 1965.

65. Downs, A. R.: Repair of late vein graft occlusions. Arch. Surg., *103*:639, 1971.

66. McNamara, J. J., Darling, R. C., and Linton, R. R.: Segmental stenosis of saphenous vein autografts. New England J. Med., *277*:290, 1967.

67. Humphries, A. W., Young, J. R., and McCormack, L. J.: Experiences with aortoiliac and femoropopliteal endarterectomy. Surgery, *65*:48, 1969.

68. Edwards, W. S.: Venous patch graft reconstruction of chronic femoral-popliteal occlusions. Surgery, *61*:820, 1967.

69. Crawford, E. S., DeBakey, M. E., Morris, G. C., Jr., and Garrett, E.: Evaluation of late failures after reconstructive operations for occlusive lesions of the aorta and iliac, femoral and popliteal arteries. Surgery, *47*:79, 1960.

70. Shirkey, A. L., Beall, A. C., Jr., and DeBakey, M. E.: The problem of small vessel grafting and the flexion crease. Amer. J. Surg., *106*:558, 1963.

71. Noon, G. P., Heistand, M., Diethrich, E. B., DeBakey, M. E., and Gasior, R. M.: Analysis of 15 years' experience with revascularization of the lower extremity affected by arterial occlusive disease. Presented before the Society for Vascular Surgery, Chicago, Illinois, 1970.

72. Edwards, W. S.: Late occlusion of femoral and popliteal fabric arterial grafts. Surgery, *110*:714, 1960.

73. Phillips, C. E., Jr., DeWeese, J. A., and Campeti, F. L.: Comparison of peripheral arterial grafts. Arch. Surg., *82*:38, 1961.

74. Fry, W. J., DeWeese, M. S., Kraft, R. O., and Ernst, C. B.: Importance of porosity in arterial prostheses. Arch. Surg., *88*:836, 1964.

75. Barner, H. B., DeWeese, J. A., and Schenk, E. A.: Fresh and frozen homologous venous grafts for arterial repair. Angiology, *17*:389, 1966.

76. Ochsner, J. L., DeCamp, P. T., and Leonard, G. L.: Experience with fresh venous allografts as an arterial substitute. Ann. Surg., *173*:933, 1971.

77. Baird, R. J., Tutassaura, H., and Miyagishima, R. T.: Saphenous vein bypass grafts to the arteries of the ankle and foot. Ann. Surg., *172*:1059, 1970.

78. Rob, C. G., and DeWeese, J. A.: Tunneler for arterial bypass grafts. Surgery, *62*:393, 1967.

79. DeWeese, J. A., and Rob, C. G.: The ischemic lower limb—surgical treatment. *In* Surgery Annual 1971. Meredith, New York, 1971, pp. 347.

Chapter 4 | Complications of

Thomas J. Fogarty, M.D.

Arterial Embolectomy

Complications surrounding the management of patients presenting with acute arterial occlusion occurs as a result of underlying cardiac disease, occasions associated with revascularization of ischemic extremities, and technical factors surrounding attempts to unobstruct an acutely occluded artery. The author's experience with such complications is based upon 500 cases of acute arterial occlusion.

Cardiac Pathology

The nature and severity of the underlying cardiovascular pathology influences the clinical course of patients presenting with an acute embolic occlusion more than any other factor. Failure to recognize and appropriately manage cardiac dysfunction can result in serious operative and postoperative complications.

Arteriosclerotic Heart Disease

Reference to Table 4-1 reveals coronary atherosclerosis to be the underlying cause in 78 per cent of the embolic episodes encountered. Sixteen percent of patients embolized following acute myocardial infarction, and in three percent of the patients a ventricular aneurysm was the source of the peripheral embolus.

It should be recognized that the presence of advanced coronary artery pathology puts these patients at risk of sustaining complications associated with chronic and acute myocardial ischemia. Preoperative evaluation of the cardiac status is mandatory, recognizing that recent myocardial infarction, low output states, and worsening heart failure demand intensive care unit monitoring. This evaluation should proceed simultaneously with emergency preparations for surgery. Placement of central venous catheters allows for monitoring of central venous pressure and rapid administration of drugs. This same catheter allows a convenient means of blood sampling and administration of heparin. Cannulation of the internal jugular vein[1] with the Silastic Medi-Cath unit is simple, tolerated for long periods of time, and free of the complications associated with the use of stiff catheters. The mortality and morbidity associated with complications of coronary artery disease can only be decreased by aggressive medical and surgical measures. Some patients who have sustained a peripheral embolus will require direct cardiac surgical procedures also.

Rheumatic Heart Disease

While rheumatic valvular disease is a source of peripheral emboli, it no longer represents the most common cardiac etiology. In general, these patients tend to be younger and present with correctable valvular lesions. Although significant hemodynamic decompensation should be corrected by valvular surgery, it should be recognized that hemodynamic deterioration does not represent the

95

TABLE 4-1. ETIOLOGY OF ARTERIAL
EMBOLUS IN 300 CONSECUTIVE PATIENTS

Atrial Fibrillation	
Arteriosclerotic Heart Disease	183
Rheumatic Heart Disease	48
Acute Myocardial Infarction	50
Arteriosclerotic Plaque	7
Unknown	12
	300

only indication for corrective cardiac surgery. Repeated embolic episodes represent a valid indication for surgical intervention. If valve replacement is required, utilization of the Hancock heterograft has resulted in a statistically significant decreased incidence of emboli when compared to other prosthetic valves.[2] The durability of the gluteraldyhyde-treated tissue valves demands consideration and should be related to the complications associated with long-term anticoagulation necessitated by utilization of plastic prostheses. In this series of patients, on five occasions the presence of a ball valve prosthesis resulted in recurrent emboli requiring replacement of the prosthesis.

Recurrent and Multiple Emboli

The frequency of recurrent arterial emboli in this series has been 17 per cent. When confronted with such patients, serious consideration should be given to elimination of the embolic source, whether it be ventricular aneurysm or left atrial thrombus.

Multiple emboli at initial presentation occurs in approximately 10 per cent of patients. An embolus to vessels supplying an arm or leg represents significantly less challenge from a diagnostic and therapeutic standpoint when compared to visceral and intracranial emboli. The frequency of multiple emboli to critical organs must always be considered in the overall management of the patient. In the presence of abdominal pain, hematuria, or neurological symptoms, arteriographic visualization of vessels supplying the areas of suspected involvement is indicated. The index of suspicion concerning possible presence of emboli to any of these areas must be high. Because of the susceptibility of these organs to ischemia, delay in establishing the diagnosis may result in tissue loss.

**Complications Associated
with Revascularization**

There exists a group of complications that occur as a result of reestablishing blood flow to an extremity that had been severely ischemic. The likelihood of these complications increases with the severity of the ischemia in terms of both volume of tissue and duration of vascular occlusion. The mortality and morbidity encountered under these circumstances can be significantly reduced by anticipation, recognition, and appropriate treatment of the adverse effects of revascularization. We define advanced ischemia as

TABLE 4-2. MEAN VALUES OF BIOCHEMICAL DETERMINATIONS
ON VENOUS EFFLUX OF 10 ISCHEMIC EXTREMITIES
BEFORE AND AFTER RESTORATION OF FLOW

	pH	P_{O_2}	P_{CO_2}	Potassium	Creatine Phosphokinase
Systemic venous blood before embolectomy	7.38	38.2	36.4	4.3	77
Venous blood from ischemic leg before embolectomy	7.31	19.3	45.8	4.7	200
Venous blood from ischemic leg 5 minutes after restoration of flow	6.80	34.8	77.3	7.2	653.4

early rigor and/or complete loss of sensation with some loss of motor movement.

Systemic Complications

Immediately following restoration of arterial continuity in extremities with advanced ischemia, significant alterations in serum electrolytes and systemic acid-base balance may occur.[3] The venous efflux of extremities following restoration of arterial continuity after embolism was studied in ten patients as summarized in Table 4-2. The data clearly indicate that following successful restoration of the circulation there is a sudden return to the heart of acidotic blood with a high potassium content. This metabolic effect, in conjunction with pooling of blood in the dilated vessels of the revascularized extremity, results in hypotension. Adverse effects associated with clamp release, in the form of significant electrocardiographic changes, hypotension, or both, occurred in eight of ten patients studied. The necessity of using buffering agents and antiarrhythmic agents should be anticipated at the time of clamp release. Ideal management should include cardiac monitoring by an anesthesiologist familiar with arrhythmia management; cardiology consultation should be available, too.

Electrolytes must be monitored closely in the postoperative period. The high potassium content noted in Table 4-2 in the venous efflux of the revascularized extremity can have adverse effects on cardiac rhythm and can lead to sudden death. Although elevation in the serum potassium is usually transient, it may persist. Postoperative monitoring of the electrocardiogram and the obtaining of frequent serum potassium values should alert one to the presence of this complication. Monitoring of the creatine phosphokinase level in the postoperative period gives an indication as to the extent of muscle damage which has occurred. In the presence of very advanced muscle necrosis, myoglobinuria may occur. Such an occurrence was responsible for renal failure and death in one patient in the series. Haimovici has reported a similar case.[4]

If embolectomy is to be performed on an extremity with advanced ischemia, prevention of renal complications by a brisk diuresis with the use of furosemide is recommended. Alkalinization of the urine by use of systemic bicarbonate may also be of value in avoiding precipitation of myoglobin in renal tubules.

Stallone and his colleagues have described significant pulmonary complications in those patients who have undergone revascularization in a setting where the extremity was quite ischemic prior to surgery.[5] They felt that these complications were secondary to microembolization of platelet fibrin aggregates, and we would agree that certainly such emboli occur. Whether or not this mechanism is the sole cause of death in a significant number of patients remains to be proven. It has been our experience that the underlying cardiac pathology is so severe that one need not suspect other causes of death.

Local Complications

After successful reestablishment of circulation in an extremity with advanced ischemia, considerable swelling may occur. This may reach such an extent as to embarrass arterial inflow, and reocclusion may result. Capillary damage resulting in fluid exudation into ischemic tissues represents the primary process responsible for this edema. Venous thrombosis, if present, contributes an additional cause of swelling. Failure to recognize and relieve this situation immediately may result in reocclusion of arterial inflow with loss of the extremity. Observation of the extremity in the immediate postoperative hours should be done by an experienced physician. The presence of distal pulses is no reassurance that critical swelling has not already occurred, since disappearance of pulses indicates excessive delay in performing fasciotomy.

Fasciotomy has been required in five percent of our patients who presented with acute embolic occlusions. Initial decompression is carried out through small skin incisions as described by Rosato.[6] If immediate

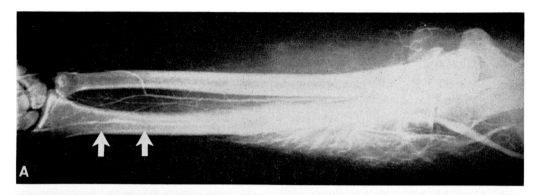

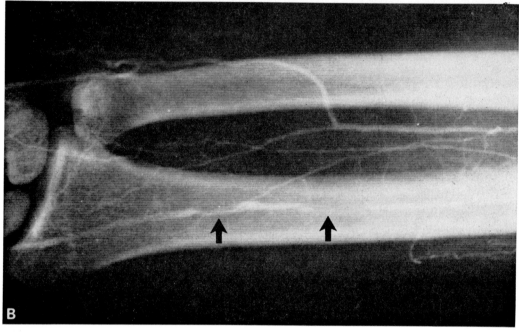

FIG. 4-1. Operative arteriogram showing extensive small vessel occlusions from propagated thrombus after a brachial artery embolus. This patient was a 50-year-old surgeon who delayed 2 weeks after his embolus before seeking attention. (Courtesy H. G. Beebe, M.D.)

improvement is not achieved by the limited fasciotomy, the skin incisions should be extended and the deeper fascial compartments opened wide. Radical decompression requiring fibular resection has not been necessary in our experience. Patman and Thompson[7] have given an excellent review of the techniques of fasciotomy and the indications for its use.

Postrevascularization neuralgia most often occurs with advanced ischemia. If these symptoms persist, sympathectomy in con-

junction with appropriate physical therapy brings relief. Motor deficits may occur in the absence of significant muscle damage. Peroneal nerve involvement with resultant foot drop is the most common neurologic deficit encountered. It has been our experience that these nerve deficits will resolve with time. Consultation with a physical therapist is indicated, and recovery may be slow. Muscle necrosis may occur with the overlying skin remaining viable. The anterior tibial compartment is most often involved, and loss of muscle mass in the gastrocnemius or soleus is less common. Utilization of appropriate orthopedic braces will result in a functional extremity in the majority of cases.

The simultaneous occurrence of major venous occlusion in the presence of advanced ischemia from arterial embolism must be considered. In a series of 300 patients, 8 percent were found to have concomitant major venous obstruction. The majority had advanced ischemia with extensive distal propagation of the clot on the arterial side (Fig. 4-1). If this situation is suspected, the vein is explored before the arterial circulation is reestablished.

Technical Considerations

Certain basic technical concepts should be borne in mind and applied to those patients who have sustained acute arterial occlusions if a successful outcome is to be assured. Possible bilateral disease, either acute or chronic, should be documented prior to surgery. For this reason, the patient is prepared in a manner so that access to both groins, both popliteal spaces, and both tibial arteries can be gained. The preparation ideally extends from the nipple line to both toes, bilaterally. An x-ray casette should be placed beneath the patient in case operative arteriograms should be required.

For lower extremity ischemia, a femoral incision is made regardless of the anatomic location of the embolus. Usually one is able to extract all the embolic and thrombotic material through this femoral arteriotomy. In the event this is not possible, a lower incision can be made. The skin incision is made parallel to the common femoral artery because this allows extension of the incision either superiorly or inferiorly as required. Incisions parallel with the inguinal ligament are more likely to disrupt the numerous lymphatics of the groin and may cause postoperative edema.

It is necessary to dissect and control the common femoral, the superficial femoral, and the deep femoral arteries. The direction of the arteriotomy should be made so as to not compromise the lumen of the artery when it is closed. Generally transverse or tangential incision is preferred. However, the direction of the arteriotomy may be determined by the presence of significant atherosclerotic plaques within the common femoral artery. The arteriotomy, whatever its direction, should be made close enough to the orifices of the superficial femoral and deep femoral arteries so that each of these vessels can be selectively cannulated.

The failure to appreciate the significance of trauma that may be induced by clamping an arteriosclerotic artery can lead to local complications that may extend the length of the operation and, on occasion, lead to failure. Clamps should be placed in relatively soft areas of the artery when this option is available, and the most nontraumatic clamps available should be employed. The occluding silastic vascular pad is a simple and effective means of relatively nontraumatic occlusion (Fig. 4-2). This instrument simultaneously provides an effective vessel tape for traction. The occlusive force can be varied, and the operative field is not cluttered by bulky clamps.

During introduction of the instrument, perforation or dissection may occur. Resistance to passage of the catheter can result in either of these complications if repeated forceful probing is attempted. Appropriate size catheters should be employed. Numbers two, three, and four French catheters should be used for vessels below the popliteal trifurcation and the deep femoral system. Catheters should be introduced without the stylets in place. Further advancement of a catheter is frequently allowed by changing size, bending the tip or simultaneously passing two catheters. If the obstruction appears to occur at the popliteal level, bending the leg at the knee joint will often allow passage. Inability to pass the smaller catheters into the calf vessels is almost always indicative of chronic obstruction. Persistent probing will result in perforation and/or dissection.

Prior to operation for acute ischemia

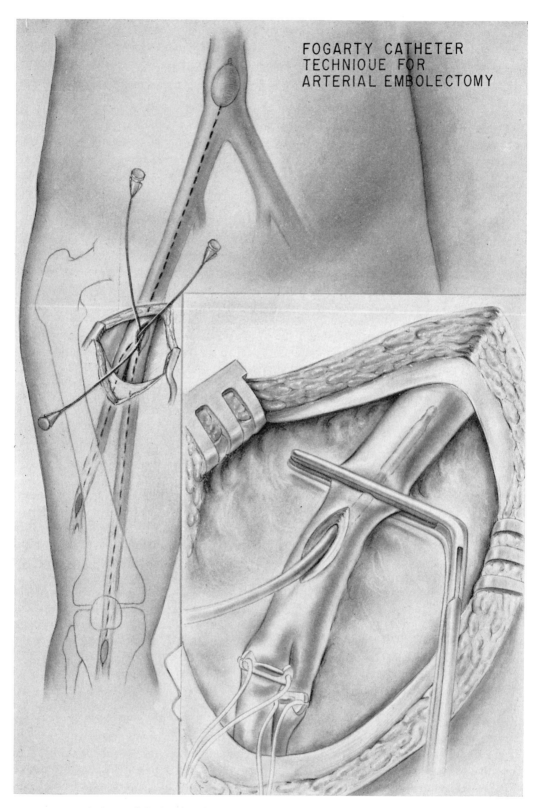

FOGARTY CATHETER
TECHNIQUE FOR
ARTERIAL EMBOLECTOMY

FIG. 4-2. Technique of balloon catheter insertion into proximal and distal vessels at the groin level for arterial embolism to the lower extremities.

thought to be due to an arterial embolus, a history eliciting prior symptoms of chronic arterial insufficiency should be sought. If the patient gives such a history the probability of encountering arteriosclerotic plaques should be borne in mind during passage of the balloon catheter. Arteriosclerotic plaques are frequently present in the absence of such a history, also.

The balloon catheter is designed for extracting emboli and distal thrombotic material. In our experience complications occur when the instrument is applied in other situations. A typical clinical setting is arterial thrombosis as a result of severe atherosclerosis. If the patient is an elderly, poor risk subject with severe ischemia and threatened amputation, one may be tempted to employ the balloon catheter. Although use of the balloon catheter to perform a thrombectomy and blind endarterectomy may be successful, it should be recognized that there is an increase in the incidence of complications when the instrument is employed in this manner.

In the large veins, thrombi are removed by means of venous thrombectomy catheters, and prior to suture closure of the vein, the arterial circulation is reestablished. After removal of the arterial occlusion, the distal arterial system is irrigated with 200 to 300 ml. of a heparinized solution. Then the distal venous clamp is removed to allow any smaller thrombi to be flushed out through this irrigation. The artery is closed first; the vein is flushed again following reestablishment of arterial circulation; and the venotomy is closed last. Venous thrombectomy is discussed further in Chapter 11.

Complications Related to Instrumentation

References in the literature describing clinical experience with the balloon catheter have been uniformly favorable.[8-12] Recognizing the common use of this instrumentation it is surprising to find only infrequent reports describing complications related to its use.[13-17] Undoubtedly, additional complica-

TABLE 4-3. POSSIBLE COMPLICATIONS SECONDARY TO USE OF EMBOLECTOMY CATHETER

Perforation
Dissection
Arterial rupture
Plaque avulsion
Intimal damage
Retention of broken catheter part

tions have occurred but have not been reported.

Despite the fact that the balloon catheter represents a useful tool in the cardiovascular surgeon's armamentarium, it should be recognized that significant complications may be associated with its use. A basic knowledge of vascular pathology and a clear understanding of the mechanism of function of the balloon catheter will aid in decreasing the incidence of complications.

Arterial rupture, plaque avulsion, intimal damage, and retention of broken catheter parts are complications that result from overdistention of the balloon during catheter withdrawal. If the appropriate size catheter is employed, overdistention of the balloon results in balloon rupture prior to vessel damage in the majority of situations. Only minimal traction is required to remove emboli and distally propagated thrombi. In order to judge the appropriate amount of traction being exerted during withdrawal, it is critical that the same surgeon removing the catheter control the balloon volume by manipulation of the syringe during extraction.

The incidence of all complications relating to balloon rupture and catheter tip separation can be significantly reduced if the catheters are not resterilized. Repeated exposure to heat, ethylene oxide, multiple usages, and storage beyond expiration dates are factors that predispose the catheter deterioration. The most significant factors reducing the incidence of complications are familiarity with the use of the catheter and a realization of its limitations.

References

1. Daily, P. O., Griepp, R. B., and Shumway, N. E.: Percutaneous internal jugular vein cannulation. Arch. Surg., *101*:534, 1970.
2. Reis, R. L., *et al.*: Thorac. Cardiovas. Surg., *62*:683, 1971.
3. Fisher, R. D., Fogarty, T. J., and Morrow, A. G.: Clinical and biochemical observations of the effect of transient femoral artery occlusion in man. Surgery, *68*:323, 1970.
4. Haimovici, H.: Arterial embolectomy: A 20 year experience with 163 cases. Surgery, *67*:212, 1970.
5. Stallone, R. J., Blaisdell, F. W., Cafferata, H. T., and Levin, S. M.: Analysis of morbidity and mortality from arterial embolectomy. Surgery, *65*:207, 1969.
6. Rosato, F. E., Barker, C. F., Robert B., and Danielson, G. K.: Subcutaneous fasciotomy. Description of a new technique and instrument. Surgery, *59*:3, 1966.
7. Patman, R. D., and Thompson, J. E.: Fasciotomy in peripheral vascular surgery. Arch. Surg., *101*:663, 1970.
8. Thompson, J. E., *et al.*: Arterial embolectomy: A 20-year experience with 163 cases. Surgery, *67*:212, 1970.
9. Scheinin, T. M., and Inberg, M. V.: Management of peripheral arterial embolism. Acta Chir. Scand., *133*:517, 1967.
10. Buxton, B., and Morris, P.: Arterial embolism of the lower limbs: Experience with the use of the Fogarty embolectomy balloon catheter. Aust. N.Z. J. Surg., *39*:179, 1969.
11. Levy, J. F., Butcher, H. R., Jr.: Arterial emboli: An analysis of 125 patients. Surgery, *68*:968, 1970.
12. Krause, R. J., *et al.*: Further experience with a new embolectomy catheter. Surgery, *59*:81, 1966.
13. Martin, P., King, R. B., and Stephenson, C. B. S.: On arterial embolism of the limbs. Brit. J. Surg. *56*:882, 1969.
14. Cranley, J. J., Krause, R. J., Strasser, E. S., and Hafner, C. D.: A complication with the use of the Fogarty balloon catheter for arterial embolectomy. J. Cardiovasc. Surg., *10*:407, 1969.
15. Rob, C., and Battle, S.: Arteriovenous fistula following the use of the Fogarty balloon catheter. Arch. Surg., *102*:144, 1971.
16. Foster, J. H., Carter, J. W., Graham, C. P., Jr., and Edwards, W. H.: Arterial injuries secondary to the use of the Fogarty catheter. Ann. Surg., *171*:971, 1970.
17. Dainko, E. A.: Complications of the use of the Fogarty balloon catheter. Arch. Surg., *102*:79, 1972.
18. Hogg, E. R., and MacDougall, J. T.: An accident of embolectomy associated with the use of the Fogarty catheter. Surgery, *61*:716, 1967.

Chapter 5 | Complications of Operations for

Norman M. Rich, M.D.

Vascular Trauma, Arteriovenous Fistula and False Aneurysm

Despite the fact that many of the principles and techniques presently included in vascular surgery were recognized at the turn of this century, only in the past 20 years has repair of vascular injuries been accepted and success expected. The overall amputation rate following arterial repair, which is only one method of measuring success or failure, dropped markedly with the general use of repair rather than ligation of arteries after the World War II experience. DeBakey and Simeone analyzed 2,471 cases of acute arterial injuries among American troops, and their report included only 81 arterial repairs.[1] The overall amputation rate following ligation was approximately 49 percent. Hughes reported that this rate decreased to 13 percent following repair of arterial injuries during the Korean conflict.[2] There has been a similar experience in Vietnam with an amputation rate of approximately 13 percent.[3,4] Many civilian series have reported even a lower amputation rate, usually obtained under more ideal conditions.[5-11]

However, the amputation rate is only one method of judging the success or failure of arterial repair. The early complications of injuries to major arteries including hemorrhage, shock, distal ischemia and infection are complications that also can occur following vascular repair (Fig. 5-1). The repair may fail, with viability of an extremity maintained by collateral circulation but the patient may develop symptoms of arterial insufficiency.

Rapid transit and high-velocity missiles continue to contribute to the large numbers of arterial injuries. Despite the fact that the basic principles of arterial surgery are well established, a significant postoperative complication rate exists. This relatively high complication rate remains a disturbing factor which should be lowered by eliminating many avoidable errors in judgment and technique. Nevertheless, it is recognized that a certain number of complications will remain when the surgeon attempts to manage arterial trauma. To obtain the optimum result, a thorough knowledge of the etiology and management of these potential complications is mandatory.

Etiology of the Arterial Injury

The nature of the wounding mechanism can strongly affect the initial outcome of vascular repair and influence the potential development of postoperative complications. For example, recognition of the extent of arterial injury caused by sharp instruments is less difficult compared to high-velocity-missile wounds where massive tissue destruction challenges the surgeon.

Missile Injury. An understanding of the wounding power of missiles is important to the surgeon who treats traumatized patients.[12] Despite the fact that low-velocity

103

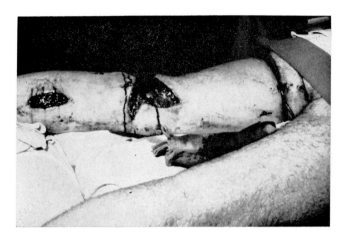

Fig. 5-1. Early complications of injuries to major arteries including infection, hemorrhage from a disrupted vascular repair, shock and distal ischemia can be dramatic. The popliteal artery repair disrupted with resultant severe infection in this patient with infected popliteal fossa and fasciotomy sites. (Rich, N. M., *et al.*: J. Trauma, *10*:359, 1970)

missiles such as the .45 caliber bullet cause minimal surrounding tissue damage (Fig. 5-2), an artery might be injured by being in the direct path of the missile. As in previous wars, many surgeons have been impressed by the massive destructive power of high-velocity missiles used in Vietnam. The contrasting degree in the severity of injury from a high-velocity bullet, such as the M-16, (Fig. 5-3) is most striking when compared to the previously described lower velocity missile wounds. The difference in the wounding power of various missiles is emphasized by the fact that the temporary cavitational effect of a high-velocity missile (Fig. 5-4) can cause thrombosis of an artery by disrupting the intima even though the missile did not actually strike the artery.[13] Recent experimental work evaluating the wounding potential of various missiles has corroborated the clinical findings (Fig. 5-5).[14,15]

In addition to numerous wounds caused by high-velocity bullets, many fragments from artillery, rockets, grenades and booby traps have contributed to high-velocity wounds at close range (Table 5-1). Among 1,000 acute major arterial injuries in Vietnam, fragments were responsible for 60.1 percent, bullets for 34.5 percent and blunt trauma for only 1.1 percent of the total.[4]

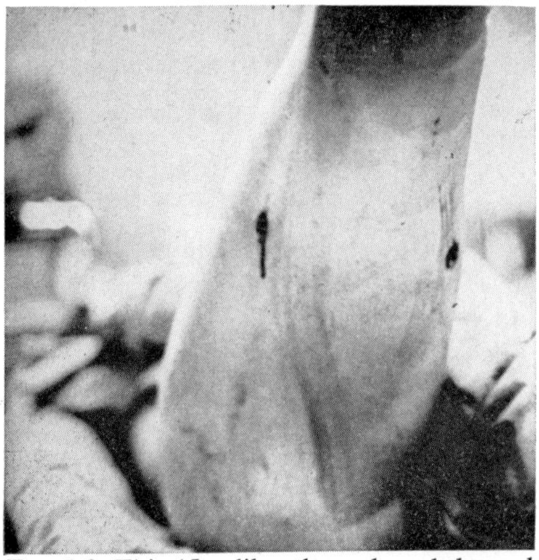

Fig. 5-2. This 45-caliber through-and-through gunshot wound of the posterior thigh is representative of a low velocity missile which causes minimal tissue destruction. (Rich, N. M.: Milit. Surg. *133*:9, 1968)

TABLE 5-1. ETIOLOGY OF 1,000 ACUTE
MAJOR ARTERIAL INJURIES*
INTERIM REPORT
VIETNAM VASCULAR REGISTRY

Wounding Agent		Number	Percent
Fragment		601	60.1
Bullet		345	34.5
Blunt		11	1.1
Punji stick		4	0.4
Miscellaneous		6	0.6
Questionable		33	3.3
	Total	1,000	100.0

* Modified from Rich, N. M., *et al.*, J. Trauma, *10*:359, 1970.

FIG. 5-3 (A). The entrance wound caused by a high velocity M-16 bullet on the lateral aspect of the right forearm is similar in size to the lower velocity 45-caliber entrance and exit wounds, all measuring about 1.5 cm.

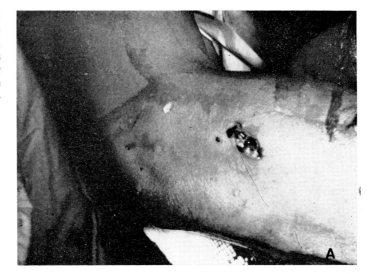

(B). There is a marked contrast, however, in the massive exit wound of the M-16 bullet measuring 8 × 10 cm. on the volar surface of the forearm. (Dimond, F. C., and Rich, N. M.: J. Trauma, 7:619, 1967)

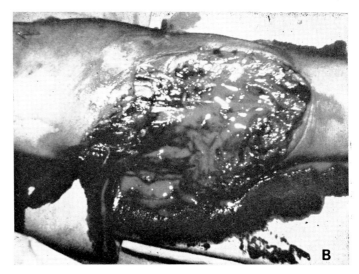

Civilian Missile Injury. Injuries to arteries are more commonly caused by penetrating wounds than by blunt trauma, even in civilian experience. American urban violence has shown a relative increase in gun-shot wounds, including some of high velocity. Perry and co-authors found that gun-shot wounds accounted for the majority of 259 patients in their series in Dallas: 143 cases (Table 5-2).[11] Edged instruments accounted for 92 injuries and blunt trauma for 24 injuries. They emphasized that aggressive acts of violence occurred in the majority of their injuries and only a small number were due

to accident. In another recent large civilian series, Drapanas and co-workers in New Orleans found that penetrating arterial injuries occurred in 90.2 percent, 204 patients, and blunt trauma caused the arterial injury in 9.8 percent, 22 patients, in their 226 patients.[10] Among the penetrating injuries to the major arteries in their series, 56.4 percent were due to low velocity gun-shot wounds and 43.6 percent were due to puncture wounds or lacerations.

Other Injuries. Fractures and dislocations are a common cause of vascular trauma. Frequently, this is a form of blunt trauma

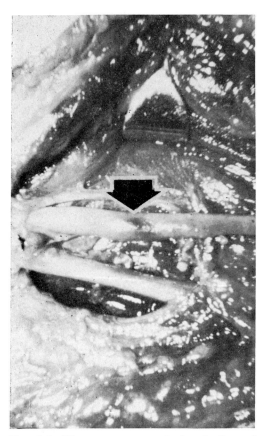

FIG. 5-4. The temporary cavitational effect of a high velocity M-16 bullet caused contusion of this brachial artery (arrow) with the median nerve seen below. The lack of arterial flow beyond the contused segment can be appreciated by the smaller size of the artery distally to the right. (Rich, N. M., *et al.*: Surg. Dig., 1971)

to the vessel; however, sharp spicules of bone can also lacerate arteries. Arterial trauma can be caused by diagnostic procedures such as catheterization for angiographic studies (see Chap. 1). Vascular injuries can be associated with unrelated operative procedures such as excision of a herniated nucleus pulposus resulting in an iliac arteriovenous fistula.

Unique and interesting sources of recorded arterial trauma have included primitive Vietnamese punji sticks responsible for nearly a dozen arterial injuries,[16] transection of the thoracic aorta by an arrow[17] and blunt trauma caused by a surf board resulting in abdominal aortic thrombosis.[18]

Clinical Pathology

The Arterial Lesion

Depending on the nature of the wounding agent, arterial trauma can vary from a single, small, sharp laceration with no adjacent damage to transection with gross and microscopic changes in both the proximal and distal ends. A laterally lacerated vessel, held open by a small portion of the wall, will continue to hemorrhage while completely severed vessels tend to retract and thrombose.

The mechanism of arterial injury following blunt trauma usually consists of fracture of the intimal layer permitting blood to dissect beneath it causing disruption and thrombosis or subintimal hematoma. One of the most common causes of such an injury in civilian practice is posterior dislocation of the knee usually occurring in an automobile accident. The fractured popliteal intima causes thrombosis at the site of injury. At operation the external appearance of the vessel may be quite unimpressive, showing only a small, subadventitial hematoma in many cases.

Occasionally there can be significant perivascular hemorrhage creating a compression stenosis or even thrombosis. Needle penetration of an artery in diagnostic or thera-

TABLE 5-2. CAUSE AND TYPE
OF ARTERIAL INJURY*
CIVILIAN EXPERIENCE IN DALLAS

Wounding Agent		Number	Percent
Gunshot		143	55.2
Edged instruments		92	35.5
Blunt trauma		24	9.3
	Total	259	100.0

Resultant Injury		Number	Percent
Laceration		133	51.4
Transection		99	38.2
Puncture		18	6.9
Contusion		7	2.7
Spasm		2	0.8
	Total	259	100.0

* Modified from Perry, M. O., *et al.*, Ann. Surg., *173*:403, 1971.

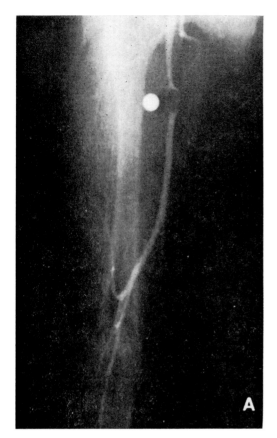

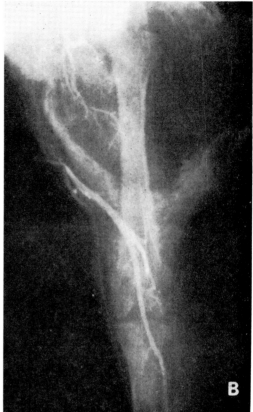

FIG. 5-5 (A). A 16-grain sphere neatly sheared the femoral artery in an experimental model without disrupting the remaining artery at the time of impact.

(B). Moments later the temporary cavitational effect of the high velocity 16-grain sphere travelling at 3,000 feet per second is dramatic. There is stretching, compression and disruption of the femoral artery after the missile has passed. (Amato, J. J., *et al.*: J. Trauma, *11*:412, 1971)

peutic procedures can also elevate a strip of intima in a fashion similar to the disruption of the intima and thrombosis caused by blunt trauma. The most common type of injury to an artery is lateral laceration. In a large civilian series, 133 lateral lacerations represented the most commonly encountered arterial injury as contrasted with transection present in 99 cases (Table 5-2).[11] Also in this series of 259 cases, arterial puncture occurred in 18, contusion in seven and spasm in two. The situation in the military experience in Vietnam has been similar in that laceration and transection were the most common injuries. A study evaluating 100 arterial segments among wounded military personnel showed only four did not involve a significant laceration or transection (Table 5-3).[19]

TABLE 5-3. EXTENT OF ARTERIAL TRAUMA*
VIETNAM PATHOLOGIC STUDY

Degree of Involvement	Number	Percent
Thrombosis	4	4.0
Laceration	23	23.0
Incompletely severed	33	33.0
Transected	40	40.0
Total	100	100.0

* Modified from Rich, N. M., *et al.*, J. Trauma, *9*:279, 1969.

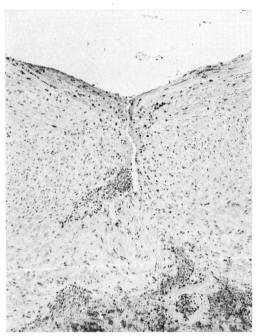

FIG. 5-6. Included in the pathologic study of the Vietnam arterial injuries is this representative photomicrograph of an H&E stained cross section of a popliteal artery (X275) showing partial laceration involving the intima and media. A fibrin plug is present over the site of injury and there is loss of intima. The adventitia shows minimal damage. (Rich, N. M., *et al.*: J. Trauma, *9*:279, 1969)

Considerable controversy has existed in the past 20 years regarding evaluation of the extent of trauma to an artery and its contribution to postoperative complications. Because of the experience and follow-up with patients from the Korean War, it was empirically recommended that 1 cm. of grossly normal appearing artery on either side of the obvious arterial damage should be resected. Others have recommended resecting up to 3 cm. of normal appearing artery, while many surgeons have felt that adequate resection included only the grossly traumatized arterial wall and that sacrifice of normal artery was unwarranted. Because of this controversy, more than 100 arterial segments were obtained in Vietnam for a thorough evaluation including gross and microscopic pathological studies.[19] Microscopic changes in the arterial wall included focal

disruption of the internal elastic membrane, areas of intimal loss, fibrin deposition, infiltration of polymorphonuclear cells into the media, focal disruption of the media and perivascular hemorrhage (Fig. 5-6). Focal areas with these microscopic changes were found more than 1 cm. into what appeared to be grossly normal artery.

The level of arterial injury is an important consideration in determining final results. The potential development of collaterals plays an important role in this determination. The amputation rate following popliteal artery injuries is disproportionately higher than the amputation rate following other extremity injuries. Concomitant injuries to adjacent structures in and adjacent to the popliteal fossa contribute to this problem. Arterial injuries accompanied by fractures are associated with a high amputation rate. Trauma to the aorta carries a higher mortality rate than injuries to major arteries in the extremities because there is usually rapid exsanguination.

Associated injuries are frequently present and often act as major determinants in the eventual outcome of the management of vascular trauma. In the Vietnam experience the severity of the injury secondary to high-velocity missiles has often adversely affected results obtained in arterial repair. Massive soft tissue destruction has created such large tissue defects that it has been difficult at times to find suitable viable tissue to cover the arterial repair. Perry and colleagues found that significant venous injuries occurred in 34 percent of their patients in association with arterial injury. Isolated venous injuries were found in 10.8 percent of their patients with vascular injuries. They also found that major nerve involvement occurred in 18.5 percent. Approximately seven percent of their patients had more than one significant arterial injury. In the military experience in Vietnam, where a greater percentage of high-velocity-missile wounds have been seen, the percentage of associated injuries has been even higher. In a review of 1,000 acute major arterial injuries, asso-

TABLE 5-4. CONCOMITANT INJURIES
ASSOCIATED WITH 1,000 MAJOR
ARTERIAL INJURIES
VIETNAM EXPERIENCE*

Injury	Patients	Percent
Nerve	424	42.4
Vein	377	37.7
Bone	285	28.5

* Modified from Rich, N. M., *et al.,* J. Trauma, *10*:359, 1970.

ciated trauma to nerves occurred in 42.4 percent, venous injuries occurred in 37.7 percent and fractures occurred in 28.5 percent of the patients (Table 5-4).[4]

If the surrounding tissues confine the vascular perforation, either a pulsating hematoma or an arteriovenous fistula may occur. Drapanas and his colleagues reported the management of eight acute arteriovenous fistulas (3.5%) among the 226 patients in their series.[10] If these injuries are not recognized at the time of initial debridement, either a false aneurysm or a chronic arteriovenous fistula will develop.

Clinical Evaluation

A rapid, yet thorough physical examination is most important in evaluating the traumatized patient for possible arterial damage. The obvious arterial injury presents with spurting, bright red blood exiting from a wound or the formation of a rapidly expanding hematoma in the area of injury. Absence of distal pulses, a cool, painful, pale extremity, numbness and loss of voluntary motion of an extremity all herald the possibility of major arterial injury. Location of the wound may immediately suggest the possibility of vascular injury when it is directly overlying the anatomic course of a major vessel. However, it is a common observation that missiles may take widely divergent paths between wounds of entry and exit or come to rest in the body after taking circuitous routes. Therefore, wound location itself is not a reliable criterion for evaluating all vascular injuries.

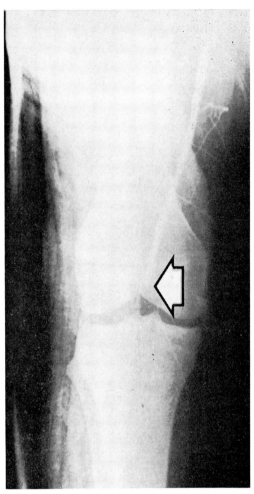

FIG. 5-7. This arteriogram shows the typical appearance of popliteal artery thrombosis after posterior knee dislocation. The foot remained cool, pale and pulseless after the cast had been bivalved. A popliteal artery vein graft replacement restored circulation. (Courtesy of Dr. H. G. Beebe)

In association with a fracture, signs of ischemia should suggest arterial injury until proved otherwise by definitive diagnostic efforts. If a cast has been applied to the affected part, it should be loosened or bivalved immediately. If diminished or absent distal pulses, coldness or pallor persists, an arteriogram should be obtained promptly (Fig. 5-7).

The patient may volunteer that there was bright red, spurting bleeding at the time of wounding which may have stopped spon-

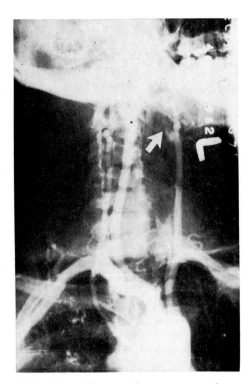

FIG. 5-8. Although there were no signs or symptoms to confirm the clinical suspicion, this arch study demonstrates acute thrombosis of the left internal carotid artery (arrow) following a gunshot wound of the neck.

taneously or with externally applied pressure. Patients, may present with hypotension or in shock resulting from major hemorrhage. Drapanas and co-authors found that 50 percent of their 226 patients were admitted in shock due to blood loss which they defined by systolic pressure of less than 80 mm.[10] They also found that among major arterial injuries in the neck and extremities, active arterial bleeding was present in 13.5 percent of the patients. The absence of shock, however, in no way mitigates against the presence of significant arterial injury.

Distal pulses may be diminished or absent, but these findings can be unreliable. The transmitted pulse wave may proceed easily in an artery which is only partially obstructed and it also may be carried through small areas of soft intraluminal thrombus or beyond injured intimal flaps.

Drapanas[10] and Perry[11] and their colleagues found about 25 percent of patients with injuries to major arteries of extremities had palpable pulses distal to the injury. The converse may also be true. Distal pulses can be absent with no significant arterial trauma; however, one must be extremely careful in making the diagnosis of arterial spasm in the traumatized patient.

Occult Injury. There may be no obvious evidence of ischemia where collateral vessels permit excellent distal perfusion, particularly with subclavian and axillary artery injuries. In some such patients distal pulses may even be detectable because of excellent collateral flow. In one large series of civilian arterial injuries, obvious clinical signs of ischemia distal to the injury were found in only 24.1 percent of the patients with arterial injuries of the extremities.[10] There may be a bruit or a thrill over, or distal to, a site of arterial injury in about 10 percent of cases, as was documented by these same authors. Edema may also be present depending on the time of injury and the extent of associated injuries.

Diagnostic Procedures

In addition to routine studies, special tests can provide valuable information for specific injuries. For example the use of an intravenous pyelogram is helpful in determining renal function where renal artery trauma is questioned. Plain roentgenograms of the abdomen can be helpful in demonstrating a large retroperitoneal hematoma associated with central abdominal vascular trauma.

Although arteriography can be an important part of the evaluation of many patients with suspected arterial injuries in civilian trauma, this examination has frequently been omitted in military experience where the nature of the wound and the limited time frequently make arteriography unnecessary and undesirable prior to operation. Drapanas and colleagues performed arteriography in 30 percent of their patients with major wounds of the extremities or neck, and 94 percent of these arteriograms demonstrated the arterial injury.[10] In two patients arteriography failed to demonstrate an injury, but clinical findings prompted exploration which demonstrated arterial injury. Perry and colleagues also reported two cases where arteriography failed to demonstrate significant arterial injury.[11] Exploration was prompted by anatomical proximity of the wound to a major artery. Arteriography is particularly helpful in patients with blunt trauma and in patients with associated fractures and dislocations. Whenever the diagnosis of arterial spasm is entertained, arteriography can be particularly valuable in determining the patency of the artery. Patients with shotgun wounds of the legs and forearms should also be evaluated thoroughly with a preoperative arteriogram because these injuries often require only superficial debridement and arteriography offers reliable evidence of the presence or absence of significant arterial injury.[11] Arteriograms are also particularly useful in evaluation of penetrating cervical wounds near the base of the skull, and may demonstrate previously undetected injuries to the intracranial arteries (Fig. 5-8).

Although arteriography is not mandatory when obvious clinical signs make arterial injury a certainty such as in posterior knee dislocations presenting with a cadaveric lower leg, the ready availability of this technique in hospitals equipped to care for major trauma should not be overlooked.

Operative Management

Early recognition and prompt repair of vascular injuries are most important in obtaining successful results. Because immediate repair is usually advocated for all acute arterial injuries, development of many delayed complications such as arteriovenous fistulas and false aneurysms can be avoided.

Time Until Repair. An important factor influencing the success of arterial repair is a reduction of the lag time between injury and vascular repair. In the experience in Vietnam, continued reduction in the time from wounding to the operating room, which has been made possible by helicopter evacuation, has favorably affected the results obtained.

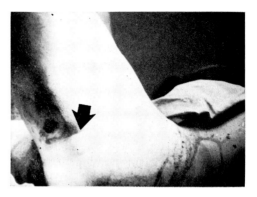

FIG. 5-9. The mark from a soldier's webbed belt (arrow) which had been used as a tourniquet for 16 straight hours is visible high in the proximal thigh. Marked ischemia and cadaveric changes had occurred by the time he was evacuated to a definitive surgical center.

There, 229 vascular patients arrived at the operating room within six hours, with the average time after wound to arrival at the hospital only 90 minutes.[3] Some civilian experience has varied enormously from 18 minutes up to 30 hours.[10] The average delay for civilian injuries to arteries in the extremities and neck was approximately five hours in this study by Drapanas and associates. They found delay was least among survivors of abdominal aortic injuries which averaged only 36 minutes.

Control of Hemorrhage. An immediate problem in arterial trauma involves the control of hemorrhage. This can usually be accomplished by direct external pressure. Tourniquets are usually unnecessary and dangerous because irreversible ischemic changes occur when they are left in place too long (Fig. 5-9). Also hemorrhage can be augmented in venous injury when the improperly used tourniquet allows continued arterial inflow. The temptation to apply hemostats to bleeding wounds in the emergency room should be scrupulously resisted as iatrogenic nerve injury commonly results from such misguided efforts. Also, there might be additional trauma to normal artery when large crushing clamps are applied. Shock is often a prominent feature with arterial trauma and should be rapidly treated with whole blood fluid replacement. There appears to be little justification for use of the pressure suit. It is occasionally necessary to continue resuscitation in the operating room while controlling hemorrhage and stabilizing patient. Intravenous antibiotics in large doses should be started as soon as possible, continued during the operation and in the early postoperative period.

In order to obtain rapid proximal and distal control of injured arteries, adequate exposure is mandatory. This is frequently best obtained through an elective incision. The surgeon should never settle for inadequate exposure by attempting to explore the arterial injury through an entrance or exit wound far removed from the injured artery. This is particularly true in exploring major abdominal vessels surrounded by retroperitoneal hematoma. Proximal and distal control at a site distant from the hematoma should always be established prior to opening the retroperitoneum over the injury and thus releasing the tamponading structures. Failure to observe this has resulted in fatal massive hemorrhage which otherwise might have been avoidable.

Debridement and Thrombectomy. Adequate debridement of the artery is mandatory; but, wide excision of grossly normal appearing adjacent artery does not insure success of the arterial repair.[19] All other devitalized adjacent tissue should also be debrided. Special atraumatic vascular instruments should be utilized. Even these instruments can occasionally injure an artery by creating a break in the intima. Adequate illumination in the operating field, suction apparatus, fine synthetic vascular sutures and meticulous surgical technique have all aided in repairing damaged arteries. The surgeon should never allow the urgency of dealing with trauma to compromise the employment of usual careful vascular techniques.

Residual distal thrombus is a complication which will defeat an attempt to restore arterial flow. Passage of a Fogarty catheter will help insure that there is no distal thrombus even in the presence of what might be con-

sidered good back bleeding. This must be accomplished carefully, however, to avoid additional arterial trauma. Complications with the use of this instrument are described in Chapter 4.

Although somewhat controversial in the trauma patient, anticoagulation may be helpful in preventing distal thrombus formation. Two methods utilized have been systemic heparinization or "distal heparinization" with approximately 3,000 units of dilute heparin solution. Anticoagulation should not be continued in the postoperative period because of the dangers of additional hemorrhage and hematoma formation. Perry and colleagues employed copious amounts of cool, balanced salt solution containing a one to ten dilution of heparin in combined arterial and venous injury.[11] This technique retards intravascular thrombosis by removal of small thrombi and by the anticoagulant effect of the heparin.

Type of Arterial Repair. An ideal repair of the injured artery is end-to-end anastomosis with one suture line. This can frequently be accomplished, particularly in the brachial and superficial femoral arteries without sacrifice of major branches and without tension on the suture line. Perry and co-workers were able to perform an end-to-end anastomosis in 107 of 249 patients with arterial injuries. The severity of the injury determined the type of arterial repair. If there is any suggestion of tension on the anastomosis, however, end-to-end anastomosis should not be employed. In attempting to eliminate tension on the suture line, important collaterals should not be sacrificed to gain additional length. Other maneuvers with potential complications involve marked flexion of joints. If this flexion is maintained for a period of approximately three weeks, considerable rehabilitation problems can occur before the patient will again be able to ambulate. Drapanas and colleagues found that 70 percent of the injuries in their series were repaired by suture or resection and suture with only 16 percent of the repairs requiring vein graft interpositions.[10] Although military experience differs considerably, end-to-end anastomosis was still possible in a significant percentage of repairs.[4] Occasionally, lateral repair with or without an autogenous vein patch graft will be acceptable in large arteries with limited lacerations such as wounds of the aorta.

If repair by suture is not possible, a reversed, hydrostatically dilated, autogenous vein graft is the preferable arterial substitute. Although the greater saphenous vein has been found to be the best arterial substitute, other veins including the cephalic vein have been used on occasion. The majority of veins accompanying major arteries are more thin-walled than the saphenous vein and early dilatation with aneurysmal change may occur under arterial pressure. Autogenous artery grafts, using the splenic artery or hypogastric artery, for example, have occasionally been helpful as arterial substitutes. Plastic prostheses in acute arterial injuries are sometimes necessary, particularly in larger arteries such as the aortoiliac system. However, the danger of infection in placing foreign material in contaminated wounds may have serious complications of life-endangering nature. The use of synthetic graft material whether Dacron, Teflon or bovine heterograft, should only be occasioned by necessity.

Patients who have sustained a popliteal artery blunt injury in association with fracture dislocations of the knee have often been unsuccessfully treated in the past by Fogarty catheter extraction of the thrombus alone. This has occurred in inexperienced hands because of failure to appreciate the significant internal injury to the arterial lining and the deceptively innocent external appearance. Repair of these blunt injuries should include resection of the arterial segment with the intimal fracture and either end-to-end anastomosis or vein graft.

Additional Measures in Repair. If associated abdominal visceral injury has resulted in massive fecal or other contamination, this should be repaired first. Then consideration can be given to extra-anatomical bypass sites such as the axillofemoral grafting or to ancillary techniques to prevent infection. Among

these are copious irrigation including the topical use of antibiotic solutions and the placement of omental pedicle wrapped about the prosthetic graft which has proven useful in preventing experimental graft infection.

Adequate coverage of the arterial repair is mandatory to prevent drying of the artery and to help eliminate the possibility of the development of infection and subsequent disruption with resulting hemorrhage. If necessary, viable muscle can be transferred over the arterial repair unless the soft tissue deficit is so large that there is no adjacent muscle present. Split thickness skin grafts and tissue flaps of various types have also been utilized; however for a variety of reasons, these efforts have only a limited application and are frequently unsuccessful. Occasionally, placement of a vein graft in an extra-anatomic position to the usual arterial course may be necessary. Subcutaneous tissue and skin should routinely be left open for three to six days followed by closure. This will provide a safety factor if the wound becomes infected and delayed primary closure of the wound will not delay wound healing.

Arterial Spasm. If normal distal flow is not obtained immediately, operative arteriography is usually indicated. This will show the status of the vascular repair and also help locate an additional distal arterial injury or distal thrombus. Multiple arterial injuries in the same extremity are recognized more frequently when sought by such careful techniques.

If arterial spasm is thought to be the cause of extremity ischemia, the safest approach is to consider the probability that thrombosis exists rather than spasm when associated with arterial trauma. Arteriography is helpful but often misleading in this regard. It may be possible to relieve spasm by direct application of chemical vasodilators such as topical one percent procaine or lidocaine or intra-arterial papaverine and by mechanical dilatation including use of the Fogarty catheter. However caution must be exercised to insure that there is not an intimal injury or subintimal hematoma. Williams and col-

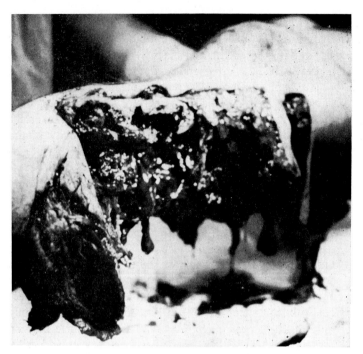

FIG. 5-10. The massive soft tissue injury of the right lower extremity was caused by fragments from a 105 mm. artillery round. In addition to destruction of the popliteal artery, there was also significant osseous loss, nerve deficits and venous insufficiency. (Rich, N. M., *et al.*: Am. J. Surg., *118*: 531, 1969)

leagues have documented some success in applying surgical sympathectomy[20] and the use of sympatholytic drugs has also been reported occasionally to be successful, but obviously has a limited role in the patient with major trauma.

Primary Amputation. The majority of surgical training programs place an appropriate emphasis on management of arterial injuries by repair. Nevertheless, there is considerable variation among surgeons regarding interest and ability in managing these injuries. Preoperative assessment of the degree of tissue involvement and experienced decision making regarding the requirement for primary amputation are important to the ultimate outcome. There is still a place for primary amputation in the very severely injured extremity where massive tissue destruction involves neurovascular, osseous and soft tissue (Fig. 5-10). Although arterial reconstruction may be feasible in this situation, the poor chance of success and the danger of infection must be considered. Occasionally, this decision for a primary amputation may be quite difficult; however, the patient's life must not be lost while attempting to reconstruct an unsalvageable extremity.

Concomitant Venous Injury. When both the major arteries and veins are injured, concomitant venous repair can usually be performed prior to completion of the arterial repair. A more aggressive approach than has been used by many in the past has the possibility of contributing to additional success in the management of vascular trauma, particularly in major venous injuries in the extremities.[21] Failure of limb salvage and amputation of an extremity because of acute venous insufficiency with an associated patent arterial repair has repeatedly been experienced. In general, smaller veins, particularly when accompanied by preserved collaterals, should be ligated as close to functioning branches as possible. Acute venous insufficiency with venous stasis and swelling of the extremity may contribute to the failure of the arterial repair. Numerous patients have been treated in Vietnam with concomitant popliteal or superficial femoral artery and vein injuries. At the time that an amputation was required on the second or third postoperative day, the lower extremity was found to be markedly edematous, bluish in color and cool. The arterial system frequently revealed patency, however, there was essentially no patent venous return.

Pulmonary embolization has been reported following repair of axillary venous injuries in two patients.[22] However, in more recent experience involving hundreds of venous repairs, the incidence of acute thrombophlebitis has been less than in those patients having ligation of their injured vein, and documented pulmonary embolization has not occurred.[21] When major venous injuries, particularly in the lower extremities, are not repaired, the problems of postphlebitic sequelae are increased. In the long term follow-up of patients through the Vietnam Vascular Registry, the problems of stasis changes with edema, pigmentation and ulceration are frequently seen (Fig. 5-11).

Fasciotomy. Following arterial injury of the extremities, fasciotomy is often necessary to maintain tissue viability. Major indications for considering the use of fasciotomy include the presence of swelling in the extremity, a significant delay between the time of wounding and arterial repair, concomitant arterial and venous injuries and massive soft tissue destruction. Numerous reports have emphasized that the anterior compartment of the leg is the most susceptible to changes in tissue pressure producing vascular compression. The posterior compartment may be similarly affected.

An inadequate fasciotomy must be avoided. The extent of the skin and fascial incision is somewhat debatable. Limited incisions for prophylactic fasciotomy can occasionally be useful. However, intact skin and fascia can continue to confine underlying tissues and contribute to compression. With any form of fasciotomy, there is always a possibility of superficial nerve or vessel injury. Particular care should be taken to preserve the peroneal nerve. This is particularly true if a transfibular four-compartment fasciotomy is indicated. Secondary infection can occur in the fasciotomy wound and this can complicate the problem of maintaining

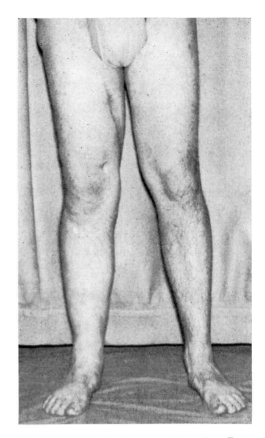

FIG. 5-11. Nearly five years later, the effects of ligation of the right superficial femoral vein are evident. Chronic edema and venous stasis changes are present. The end-to-end anastomosis of the superficial femoral artery which was performed in Vietnam remains patent.

viability of the extremity. This local infection can also contribute to a generalized septicemia.

Although fasciotomy should not be routine, even in the lower extremities, consideration must be given to avoid being "too late with too little." The original injury may make unreliable the usual signs of anterior compartment compression in the leg such as hypesthesia in the web space between the first and second toes or foot drop. The presence of distal pulses felt at the ankle level is not a reliable guide to the absence of leg compartment compression. To delay until they become absent is to delay too long.

TABLE 5-5. PERCENTAGE OF LIMB LOSS RESULTING FROM LIGATION OF DAMAGED MAJOR VESSELS

Injured Artery	*Percentage of Limb Loss*
Subclavian	28.6
Axillary	43.2
Common brachial	55.7
Brachial	25.8
Common iliac	53.8
External iliac	46.7
Common femoral	81.1
Superficial femoral	54.8
Popliteal	72.5

Reported by DeBakey, M. E., and Simeone, F. A. Modified from Hughes, C. W.: Traumatic Lesions of Peripheral Vessels, Thomas, Springfield, 1961.

Fracture Stabilization. Surgeons who elect to stabilize fractures with internal fixation have emphasized that this should be performed prior to repairing the arterial injury. There is a danger of disruption of the arterial repair during manipulation which might be necessary in realignment of the fracture and placement of fixation devices. Considerable controversy remains regarding the use of internal fixation and many feel that immobilization by external fixation is usually adequate.[23] There is general agreement that internal fixation should be avoided in combat zones because potential complications including infection compound an already complex problem.

Arterial Ligation. What might be considered minor arterial trauma such as an injury of the radial artery of the wrist can become a significant arterial injury if the ulnar artery is also traumatized. Also, false aneurysms and arteriovenous fistulas developing in minor arteries can create pressure on nerves and pose a threat to viability of the extremity through potential complications. It is easier to detect and manage minor arterial injuries at the time of initial surgery, whether by repair or ligation, than to operate at a later time on these well-developed complications.

Because of the documentation of the British experience in World War I by Makins and of the American experience in World War II by DeBakey and Simeone, the expected poor results of ligation of major arteries have been well understood. Consideration must be given to the location of the arterial injury as shown in Table 5-5. Loss of extremity viability following ligation of the subclavian or axillary artery is certainly much less likely because of the rich collateral arterial flow of the arm when compared to ligation of the distal popliteal artery where there is considerably less collateral supply. Ligation of the acute arterial injury may occasionally still be indicated in the management of a patient with more immediate life-threatening injuries. Brisbin and colleagues extended this thought on the basis of their experience with secondary disruption of vascular repairs following war wounds in Vietnam to a provocative recommendation that more routine ligation of major arteries be carried out.[24]

Results

Whether in civilian or military experience, the majority of the arterial injuries in patients who survive to reach a definitive surgical center are in the extremities. This has been emphasized by the recent interim statistics from the Vietnam Vascular Registry where only nine percent of the acute major arterial injuries were not in the extremities (Table 5-6).[4]

Repair of arterial injuries by either lateral suture or end-to-end anastomosis has frequently been possible. This was particularly true in the Korean experience (Table 5-7). There has been an increase in the tendency to utilize autogenous vein grafts more frequently in the Vietnam experience where high-velocity missile wounds are common. There has been a similar experience in the civilian community with 84 percent of the arterial repairs in the Dallas series managed by lateral suture or end-to-end anastomosis.[11] In one large civilian series of arterial injuries, Perry and colleagues reviewed the records of 908 patients undergoing operative exploration for vascular injury between 1950

TABLE 5-6. LOCATION OF 1,000 MAJOR
ARTERIAL INJURIES IN VIETNAM*

Location	Artery	Number	Percent
Neck	Carotid	50	5.0
Chest	Innominate	3 }	1.1
	Subclavian	8 }	
Upper Extremity	Axillary	59 }	34.2
	Brachial	283 }	
Abdomen & Pelvis	Abdominal aorta	3	
	Common iliac	9	2.9
	External iliac	17	
Lower Extremity	Common femoral	46	
	Superficial femoral	305	56.8
	Popliteal	217	
	Total	1,000	100.0

* Modified from Rich, N. M., et al., J. Trauma, 10:359, 1970.

and 1968 in Dallas.[10] They documented 508 significant arterial injuries. This meant that approximately one-third of the patients in their series had a vascular exploration without finding major arterial injury. They did emphasize that in many of their operations the vascular exploration was performed at the time of debridement of a significant wound of the extremity and did not constitute the primary indication for operation.

It is also important to emphasize that in 312 patients explored without finding major arterial injuries, there was no mortality and the only significant morbidity was a wound infection rate of about three percent. Identification of an arterial injury does not always result in successful repair. Drapanas and his co-workers found that arterial reconstruction was possible in 83 percent of their 226 patients sustaining arterial trauma.[11]

Although it is difficult to compare the various types of management of arterial repair, the evaluation of the methods of repair used during the Korean War reveal a relatively high failure rate associated with

TABLE 5-7. METHOD OF ARTERIAL REPAIR

Repair	Korean Experience* Arteries	Korean Experience* Percent	Vietnam Experience† Arteries	Vietnam Experience† Percent
Lateral suture	35	13.4	87	9.4
End-to-end anastomosis	145	55.3	377	40.5
Autogenous vein graft	34	13.0	459	49.4
Autogenous artery graft	48	18.3	3	0.3
Prosthesis	0	0.0	4	0.4
Totals	262	100.0	930	100.0

* Modified from Hughes, C. W.: Ann. Surg., 147: 555, 1958.
† Modified from Rich, N. M., et al., J. Trauma, 10:359, 1970.

artery homografts (Table 5-8). Wounds requiring arterial replacement are usually more severe and a higher complication rate might be anticipated. However, attempted end-to-end anastomosis or lateral suture repair under less than ideal conditions will also result in repair failure.

In the management of 1,000 acute major arterial injuries in Vietnam, the complication rate was 30 percent.[4] However, this included a number of complications which were recognized and corrected at the time of the initial procedure. Although thrombosis was the most frequent complication, hemorrhage with or without infection from a disrupted suture line was the most dramatic. Throm-

TABLE 5-8. EVALUATION OF METHODS OF
REPAIR—KOREAN EXPERIENCE*

Method	Treated	Amputated	Percent
Anastomosis	145	13	9.0
Vein graft	34	4	11.8
Artery homograft	48	16	33.3
Transverse suture	35	1	2.9
Conservative care	5	—	—
Release spasm	2	1	50.0
Total	269	35	13.0

* Modified from Hughes, C. W., Ann. Surg., 147: 555, 1958.

TABLE 5-9. VIETNAM AMPUTATION RATE—919 MAJOR ARTERIAL INJURIES*

	Artery	Injuries	Amputation	Percent	
Upper Extremity	Axillary	59	3	5.1	2.0
	Brachial	283	16	5.7	
Abdomen	Common iliac	9	1	11.1	0.1
Lower Extremity	Common femoral	46	7	15.2	
	Superficial femoral	305	37	12.1	11.4
	Popliteal	217	64	29.5	
	Total	919	128		13.5

* Rich, N. M., *et al.*, J. Trauma, *10*:359, 1970.

bosis of the repair or disruption with hemorrhage necessitating major arterial ligation does not necessarily lead to disaster. The important role of collateral circulation has recently been reviewed in the management of vascular injuries seen at Walter Reed General Hospital.[25]

A final measure of success or failure of an arterial repair is the amputation rate. In addition to thrombosis and hemorrhage from a disrupted suture line, massive tissue necrosis, sepsis, venous insufficiency and large osseous defects contribute to the amputation rate. Table 5-9 outlines the Vietnam experience with an overall amputation rate of approximately 13 percent. Injuries to the popliteal artery remain an enigma with a relatively high amputation rate of about 30 percent.[4,26]

Associated injuries usually contribute to the mortality of patients with vascular trauma. It is impressive, nevertheless, that less than two percent of the 1,000 acute major arterial injuries in the interim report from Vietnam ended in death.[4]

The requirement for an additional procedure to correct a complication of the initial arterial repair must be individualized. An attempted end-to-end anastomosis resulting in thrombosis because of tension on the suture line can be corrected at the same time by utilization of a vein graft replacement. Table 5-10 outlines the number and type of operation utilized in an attempt to correct complications after the initial vascular repair both in the immediate and late postoperative

period. However, many patients with complications do not require an additional operation.

In evaluating 57 patients with complications of their initial arterial repair performed in Vietnam who were seen at Walter Reed General Hospital, only 24 patients required additional vascular operations.[27] Thrombosis and stenosis of upper extremity arterial repairs required operative intervention in only 4 of 27 patients (Fig. 5-12). In this group, concomitant nerve deficits frequently remained the limiting factor. In the lower extremity, thrombosis and stenosis of arterial repairs caused significant intermittent claudification in 8 of 13 patients, necessitating additional operative procedures (Fig. 5-13).

Missile embolization in both the arterial and venous circulations has been described. If a bullet is known to reside in the vascular

TABLE 5-10. ADDITIONAL PROCEDURES UTILIZED IN AN ATTEMPT TO CORRECT COMPLICATIONS AFTER INITIAL OPERATIONS IN VIETNAM*

Autogenous Vein Graft	92
Thrombectomy	88
Ligation	35
End-to-End Anastomosis	33
Prosthesis	20
Suture	15
Total	283

* Rich, N. M., *et al.*, J. Trauma, *10*:359, 1970.

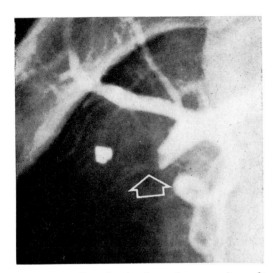

FIG. 5-12. Thrombosis of a saphenous vein graft of the right distal axillary—proximal brachial artery is evident in this arteriogram. Collateral circulation maintained viability of the extremity and the patient remained asymptomatic. (Rich, N. M., *et al.*: Arch. Surg., *100*:646, 1970)

space, it should be extracted at the time of the original operation and vascular repair (Fig. 5-14).

Arteriovenous Fistulas and False Aneurysms

The majority of complications previously discussed in the management of acute vascular trauma also can occur in treating arteriovenous fistulas and false aneurysms. This is particularly true of acute arteriovenous fistulas and acute false aneurysms, pulsating hematomas, treated within hours after initial trauma. However, there are problems of particular concern in management of long-established arteriovenous fistulas and false aneurysms which deserve special mention. These have also been recently reviewed by Fomon and Warren.[28]

These lesions have been particularly notable by their frequent occurrence in battle casualties during the last 100 years. They also occur in civilian life and can be found in some injuries which were initially felt to be very minor. It has been of particular interest in follow-up of approximately 7,500 Vietnam casualties with vascular injuries that

more than 400 arteriovenous fistulas and false aneurysms have been documented. In organization of the Vietnam Vascular Registry in 1966, the initial opinion was that very few arteriovenous fistulas and false aneurysms would be seen. With many well-trained young surgeons, the majority of whom had an excellent background in vascular surgery, who were interested in performing arterial repairs, it seemed that very few vascular injuries would be missed. However, several factors continue to contribute

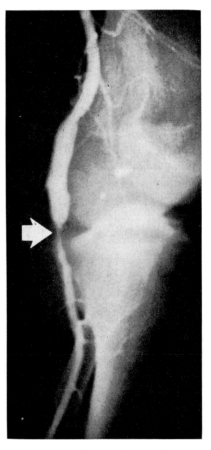

FIG. 5-13. This arteriogram demonstrates marked stenosis of the distal left popliteal artery saphenous vein graft anastomosis. Because the patient had severe claudication, the stenotic area was excised and repaired with good results. (Rich, N. M., *et al.*: Arch. Surg., *100*:646, 1970)

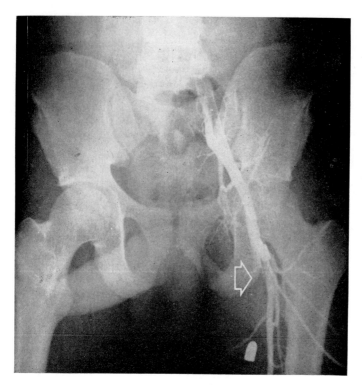

FIG. 5-14. Two days previously this patient had an aortic laceration repaired. Plain films gave the impression that the bullet was in the buttock. Left leg pulses remained normal for two days and then suddenly disappeared. This left femoral arteriogram demonstrates superficial femoral artery thrombosis due to a bullet embolus. Fogarty catheter extraction and thrombectomy was successful. (Courtesy of Dr. H. G. Beebe)

to these vascular lesions which usually have a delayed recognition.

A patient with multiple penetrating injuries, such as an individual hit with 100 or more small fragments from an exploding mortar round, creates a challenging problem for the surgeon. Despite the fact that a general recommendation can be made to explore all arteries and veins that are in proximity to a missile or the path of a missile, it should be obvious that this is not practical in a patient with such a large number of small wounds. Also, some arteriovenous fistulas and false aneurysms might not be immediately apparent. A contusion may exist initially with disruption of a portion of the arterial wall several days later.

In the past 50 years numerous operations have been designed for managing such lesions. The endoaneurysmorrhaphy described by Matas in 1888[29] and the multitude of various methods of ligating portions or all of the components of an arteriovenous fistula have generally been replaced by an effort to repair the majority of the arteries and veins, except in minor vessels where ligation is considered inconsequential.

Historical Note

William Hunter (1757)[30], (1762)[31] provided the first detailed documentation of an abnormal communication between an artery and vein. He noted that pressure over the site of communication or on the proximal artery would eliminate the palpable thrill and venous distention. He also stated that the artery proximal to the site of the communication was enlarged and tortuous. Nicoladoni (1875)[32] demonstrated a slowing of the pulse rate by compression of the artery proximal to the arteriovenous communication. Branham (1890)[33] again demonstrated a slowing of the pulse rate, in his case by direct manual obliteration of a large acquired arteriovenous fistula. Reid (1920)[34] developed an experimental and clinical evaluation which provided evidence of enlargement of the heart in the presence of an arteriovenous fistula. Holman (1937)[35] established and clarified many of the anatomic and hemody-

FIG. 5-15. Types of operation employed for treatment of aneurysms prior to the introduction of Matas' endoaneurysmorraphy in 1888. (Elkin, D. C.: Surg. Gynec. Obstet. *82*:1, 1946)

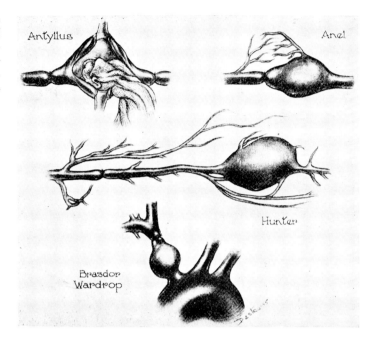

namic changes that occur with both traumatic and congenital arteriovenous fistulas.

False aneurysms have been recognized and treated for a much longer period of time than arteriovenous fistulas. Nearly 2,000 years ago Antyllus devised an operative method which consisted of ligation of the artery above and below the sac followed by evacuation of its contents and application of an astringent or of packing (Fig. 5-15).[29] In Elkin's report on traumatic aneurysms, he reviewed some of the older operative methods of management. He noted that Anel's operation (1710) consisted of ligation of the proximal artery close to the sac. One-half century later John Hunter ligated the superficial femoral artery at a distance from a popliteal artery aneurysm to establish clotting in the aneurysm and at the same time preserve the collateral circulation. Elkin emphasized that the Matas endoaneurysmorrhaphy was based on the same principle of preservation of collateral circulation. Elkin also mentioned that Brasdor and Wardrop independently ligated the artery on the distal side of the sac in an attempt to arrest the circulation through it, but this operation was make-shift at best. All of the described

methods, except for the Matas endoaneurysmorrhaphy, were frequently followed by infection, hemorrhage, gangrene or failure to cure the condition.

Prior to World War II, Matas was the recognized authority on managing traumatic aneurysms. In addition to treating large numbers of aneurysms by his obliterative technique with endoaneurysmorrhaphy, he also advocated reconstruction and restorative procedures. In 1913, Soubbotitch presented the experience of Serbian military surgeons in managing 72 vascular injuries during the Serbo-Turkish and Serbo-Bulgarian Wars and revealed that there were 32 vascular repairs.[36] Matas in discussing Soubbotitch's report emphasized that one of the most notable features was the suture, both circular and lateral repair, and the fact that it had been utilized more frequently in the Balkan conflict than in previous wars.

Prior to World War II, Matas, Reid and Holman were the recognized authorities in the management of arteriovenous fistulas. Other names familiar to those interested in trauma and vascular surgery are Elkin, Freeman and Shumacker because of their experience with World War II casualties and

TABLE 5-11. MAJOR VESSEL INVOLVEMENT FROM A TOTAL OF 215 LESIONS WALTER REED GENERAL HOSPITAL* †

Vessel	Arterio-venous Fistulas	False Aneurysms	Total
Common Carotid	7	2	9
Internal Carotid	3	—	3
Subclavian	6	2	8
Axillary	9	11	20
Brachial	10	9	19
Iliac	3	1	4
Common Femoral	7	1	8
Superficial Femoral	24	7	31
Popliteal	22	10	32
Total	91	43	134

* The majority of these injuries were sustained during the first two years of the Korean War.
† Modified from Hughes, C. W., and Jahnke, E. J., Jr., Ann. Surg., *148*:790, 1958.

Hughes and Jahnke with their Korean War experience. There were 215 arteriovenous fistulas and false aneurysms treated at Walter Reed General Hospital over a seven-year period reported in 1958 by Hughes and Jahnke.[37] More than one-half of the lesions involved major vessels (Table 5-11). Another equally large series of 200 traumatic arteriovenous fistulas was reported from the Surgical Clinic of the University of Heidelberg from 1939 to 1967 by Vollmar and Krumharr (Fig. 5-16).[38] Representative civilian experience can be found in several recent series.[39,40,41,42]

Obliterative surgery for arteriovenous fistulas was routinely used until about 20 years ago and is still applicable for arteriovenous fistulas of noncritical, minor vessels. The acceptable type of obliterative surgery implies quadruple ligation and excision. Ligation of the artery and vein both proximal and distal to the fistula should be followed by removal of the fistula and associated false sac because of the possibility of additional communications which will allow restoration of the fistula.

Quadruple ligation and excision of a fistula of major vessels is undesirable because

arterial insufficiency or gangrene may result. Other methods of managing arteriovenous fistulas such as ligation of the artery only proximal to the lesion, as was once advocated, is contraindicated. Gangrene may result because of retrograde arterial flow through the fistula into the less resistant venous system. If both the artery and the vein are ligated only proximal to the fistula, severe venous stasis will result with massive swelling of the extremity.

Diagnosis

One of the problems associated with arteriovenous fistulas and false aneurysms is in not

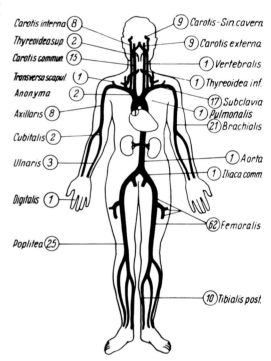

FIG. 5-16. Similar to series of acute arterial injuries, the majority of arteriovenous fistulas and false aneurysms are found in extremity vessels. The above is a representative large series of arteriovenous fistulas with 88.5 percent caused by World War II projectiles; 5.0 percent caused by fractures; 3.5 percent due to stab wounds; 2.0 percent from iatrogenic trauma; and the remaining 1.0 percent from civilian gunshot wounds. (Vollmar, J., and Krumhaar, D., *in* Hiertonn, T., and Rybeck, B.: Traumatic Arterial Lesions, page 102, Forsvarets Forskningsanstalt, Stockholm, 1967)

recognizing the presence of the lesion. A "misdiagnosis" can lead to complications involving other organ systems in addition to the pathophysiologic changes directly related to arteriovenous fistulas.

There is usually a bruit, often with a large area of radiation from the point of maximal intensity, and frequently a thrill associated with these lesions. The nature of the bruit will frequently help differentiate an arteriovenous communication from a false aneurysm. A systolic bruit is associated with false aneurysm, and a continous bruit with arteriovenous fistula. It must be remembered that false aneurysms are frequently found in juxtaposition to an arteriovenous communication (Fig. 5-17).

There may be a palpable mass, particularly associated with false aneurysms, pain on application of pressure, and local warmth and erythema of the overlying skin. There can be a reduction in the quality of the peripheral pulse or even an absence of peripheral pulses if a large false aneurysm compresses the artery. With arteriovenous fistulas of some duration, venous hypertension and stasis occur with an increase in extremity size and development of superficial varicosities. Also, with an arteriovenous fistula of relatively large size which has been present for a number of years, there may be: a palpable, dilated proximal artery, associated cardiac enlargement, an increase in cardiac output, an increase in blood volume and red cell mass, and even signs of cardiac failure.

Other specific signs and symptoms may suggest the possibility of vascular involvement. One soldier developed severe hypertension after an abdominal wound which caused a false aneurysm of the abdominal aorta.[43] Angiograms demonstrated compression of the right renal artery by a large false aneurysm. Angiography can be an invaluable diagnostic aid. It not only assists in delineating the communication, but it also helps in determining the operative approach. It must be remembered that more than one arterial lesion can exist. Such a diagnosis

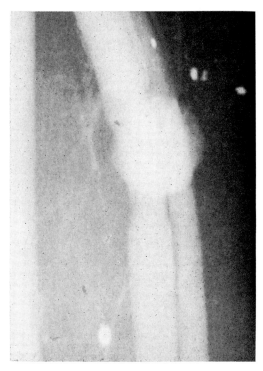

Fig. 5-17. Both an arteriovenous fistula and a false aneurysm might result from vascular trauma. The false aneurysm seen on the above angiogram is in juxtaposition to a superficial femoral arteriovenous fistula.

may be possible only by angiographic demonstration.

Preoperative Complications

The danger of rapid expansion, even perforation, is greater for a false aneurysm than an arteriovenous fistula, because the latter will tend to decompress itself by shunting the blood from the artery to the low pressure venous system. An arteriovenous fistula can be converted into an aneurysm by thrombosis of the fistual or venous component with sudden expansion of the weak sac which will act as a false aneurysm. Rapid expansion of the false aneurysm may compress an adjacent nerve with immediate distal neurologic changes (Fig. 5-18). If the fistula is not decompressed, the neurologic deficits may become permanent. An aneurysmal sac can cause severe nerve damage without further expansion by repeated pulsa-

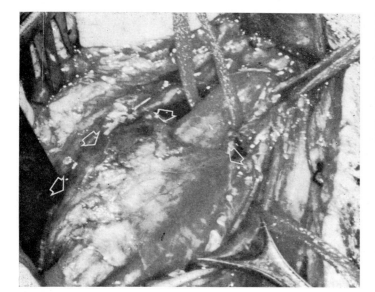

FIG. 5-18. Pressure from a false aneurysm can compress an adjacent nerve. A false aneurysm of the brachial artery has compressed both the median and ulnar nerves with resultant neurologic deficit. The false aneurysm sac overlying the median nerve is outlined by arrows.

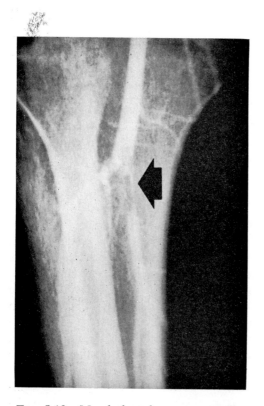

FIG. 5-19. Mural thrombus may embolize from either a false aneurysm or an arteriovenous fistula. On the above angiogram an embolus from a proximal popliteal artery false aneurysm is seen in the distal popliteal and the proximal posterior tibial arteries.

tions which injure adjacent motor nerves or erode bone. Rapid expansion may also compress venous return and cause severe venous stasis and insufficiency. If expansion occurs in a closed compartment, such as the anterior tibial compartment or the popliteal fossa, immediate operative intervention is indicated to prevent loss of muscle viability and probable loss of an extremity.

Infection is always a potential hazard in these lesions. The possibility of erosion and perforation with resulting hemorrhage is increased. Although fairly rare, the complication of bacterial endocarditis and endarteritis associated with arteriovenous fistulas can threaten the patient's life.

Infrequent complications also include thrombosis of the aneurysmal sac which in turn occludes the artery. This may require immediate surgical intervention if the thrombosis involves a critical artery. Both false sacs and arteriovenous fistulas may contain mural thrombi which have produced emboli (Fig. 5-19). In the Vietnam experience, distal emboli have occluded the popliteal and internal carotid arteries.

Another uncommon complication resulting from arteriovenous fistulas is cardac failure. Degeneration of the dilated proximal artery associated with a long-standing arterio-

FIG. 5-20. Proximal and distal control of both the artery and vein are important in successful management of arteriovenous fistulas. It was possible to repair the popliteal vein (open arrow) by lateral suture and the popliteal artery (solid arrow) by an end-to-end anastomosis in correcting the arteriovenous fistula demonstrated above.

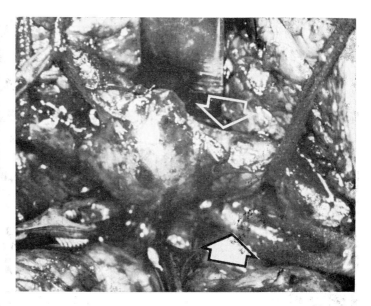

venous fistula has not been reported frequently in the past, but this condition has caused considerable interest in the past ten years.

Surgical Management

Although there have been individual reports of spontaneous closure of small fistulas and inconsequential thrombosis of small false aneurysms, the incidence is still so low that it would be unwise to delay treatment for this. One patient at Walter Reed General Hospital with a distal axillary arteriovenous communication had a spontaneous closure within three weeks following angiographic studies via a catheter placed percutaneously through the transaxillary route. This was only a very small communication.

Arteriovenous fistulas and false aneurysms should be repaired within a short time after recognition. There is no reason to wait six months for the development of collateral circulation as was once advocated. Occasionally it may be necessary to correct an acute arteriovenous fistula as a surgical emergency because of distal arterial ischemia. Also, as previously alluded to, the rapidly expanding false aneurysm or hemorrhage may necessitate immediate surgical intervention.

At the time of surgical correction both proximal and distal control of the involved vessel should be obtained. In the case of false aneurysm, sharp dissection can be carried toward the defect in the arterial wall from both the proximal and distal control sites. This will preserve some of the length of the artery which might have otherwise been lost if an "en block" resection were carried out. Care must be taken in dissecting around the false sac to insure that adjacent nerves are not injured. It may be best to leave part of the sac in place after it has been opened and the thrombus evacuated. The sac should not be used in the arterial repair. It may be possible, nevertheless, after adequate debridement, to close the arterial defect with several interrupted vascular sutures without compromising the lumen. Usually an end-to-end anastomosis after resection of the small area of involvement will accomplish the most satisfactory repair. Occasionally, a vein graft will be needed to restore arterial continuity.

In arteriovenous fistula, particularly when larger vessels are involved, an attempt should be made to repair both the artery and the vein. Again, proximal and distal control, this time of both the artery and the vein should be obtained (Fig. 5-20). When this control is difficult because of the location of

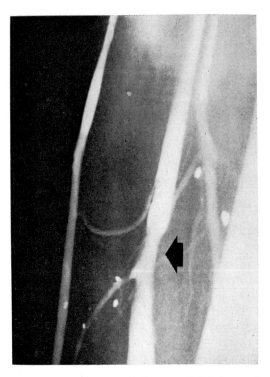

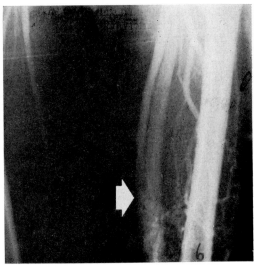

FIG. 5-22. This angiogram corroborated the clinical impression of a left femoral arteriovenous fistula. Additional assistance was provided establishing that the communication involved a muscular branch of the superficial femoral artery (arrow). Note the development of collaterals. Also, note the proximal arterial dilatation in this former soldier who had been wounded in Vietnam five years previous to this study.

FIG. 5-21. Patency of the superficial femoral vein is demonstrated by phlebography approximately one month after lateral repair of the vein in a 20-year-old Vietnam casualty who had multiple fragment wounds with a resultant superficial femoral arteriovenous fistula. (Rich, N. M., Hughes, C. W., and Baugh, J. H.: Ann. Surg., *171*:724, 1970)

TABLE 5-12. METHODS OF MANAGING MAJOR VESSEL LESIONS
WALTER REED GENERAL HOSPITAL EXPERIENCE REPORTED IN 1958*

Vessel	Ligation and Excision	Anasto-mosis	Vein Graft	Artery Graft	Lateral Repair	Division of Fistula	Sponta-neous Closure	Total
Common Carotid	–	6	–	–	–	1	2	9
Internal Carotid	2	–	–	–	–	1	–	3
Subclavian	3	2	–	1	1	1	–	8
Axillary	4	8	2	1	2	–	3	20
Brachial	6	9	1	1	1	1	–	19
Iliac	–	3	–	1	–	–	–	4
Common Femoral	–	3	2	1	–	2	–	8
Superficial Femoral	6	14	9	–	–	2	–	31
Popliteal	9	16	3	1	–	2	1	32
Total	30	61	17	6	4	10	6	134

* Modified from Hughes, C. W., and Jahnke, E. J., Jr., Ann. Surg., *148*:790, 1958.

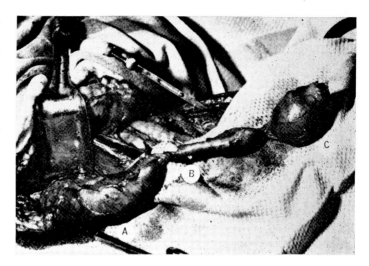

Fig. 5-23. Aneurysmal dilatation of the superficial femoral artery (A), narrowed segment (B) where the artery transversed Hunter's canal and popliteal artery aneurysm (C). This patient had had a closure of an anterior tibial arteriovenous fistula of 21 years' duration and 14 years after the fistula closure multiple aneurysms of the femoropopliteal arteries had developed. (Sako, Y., and Varco, R. L.: Surgery, *67*:40, 1970)

the communication, or if the communication is inadvertently entered during dissection, intraluminal control using a Fogarty balloon catheter may be of great value in preventing exsanguinating hemorrhage. Hemorrhage at the time of dissection is one of the most catastrophic complications associated with difficult arteriovenous fistulas. Once the fistula is divided, a lateral suture repair of the vein is frequently possible and patency maintained. Large veins should be repaired.[44] The artery can be repaired in the manner mentioned above (Fig. 5-21).

The method of managing arteriovenous fistulas and false aneurysms in the large Walter Reed General Hospital series reported in 1958 is outlined in Table 5-12.

Dilatation of the artery proximal to an arteriovenous fistula which has been present for at least several years has been widely recognized (Fig. 5-22). Although the etiology is not completely understood, it is known that the dilatation and aneurysmal changes can continue even after the distal arteriovenous communication has been corrected. Sako and Varco documented four cases in their series of arteriovenous fistulas with progression of these pathologic changes in the artery proximal to the fistula even after the fistula was closed by operative intervention (Fig. 5-23).[42]

Repair of arteriovenous fistulas and false aneurysms for major arteries and some small critical arteries is an established principle. Venous repair should also be carried out in large arteriovenous fistulas. The results should generally be more successful than those in managing acute vascular trauma.

References

1. DeBakey, M. E., and Simeone, F.A.: Battle injuries of the arteries in World War II: An analysis of 2,471 cases. Ann. Surg., *123*: 534, 1946.
2. Hughes, C. W.: Arterial repair during the Korean War. Ann. Surg., *147*:1555, 1958.
3. Rich, N. M., and Hughes, C. W.: Vietnam vascular registry: A preliminary report. Surgery, *65*:218, 1969.
4. Rich, N. M., Baugh, J. H., and Hughes, C. W.: Acute arterial injuries in Vietnam: 1,000 cases. J. Trauma, *10*:359, 1970.
5. Morris, G. C., Beall, A. C., Roof, W. R., and DeBakey, M. E.: Surgical experience with 220 acute arterial injuries in civilian practice. Amer. J. Surg., *99*:775, 1960.
6. Ferguson, I. A., Byrd, W. M., and McAffee, D. K.: Experiences in the management of arterial injuries. Ann. Surg., *153*:980, 1961.
7. Smith, R. F., Szilagyi, D. E., and Pfeifer, J. R.: Arterial trauma. Arch. Surg., *86*: 153, 1963.

8. Treiman, R. L., Doty, D., and Gaspar, M. R.: Acute vascular trauma: A fifteen year study. Amer. J. Surg., *111*:469, 1966.

9. Dillard, B. M., Nelson, D. L., and Norman, H. G.: Review of 85 traumatic arterial injuries. Surgery, *63*:391, 1968.

10. Drapanas, T., Hewitt, R. L., Weichert, R. F., and Smith, A. D.: Civilian vascular injuries: A critical appraisal of three decades of management. Ann. Surg., *172*:351, 1970.

11. Perry, M. O., Thal, E. R., and Shires, F. T.: Management of arterial injuries. Ann. Surg., *173*:403, 1971.

12. Rich, N. M.: Vietnam missile wounds evaluated in 750 patients. Milit. Med., *133*:9, 1968.

13. Rich, N. M., Amato, J. J., and Billy, L. J.: Arterial thrombosis secondary to temporary cavitation. Surg. Digest, 1971.

14. Amato, J. J., Billy, L. J., Gruber, R. P., Lawson, N. S., and Rich, N. M.: Vascular injuries: An experimental study of high and low velocity missile wounds. Arch. Surg., *101*:167-174, 1970.

15. Amato, J. J., Rich, N. M., Billy, L. J., Gruber, R. P., and Lawson, N. S.: High velocity arterial injury. A study of the mechanism of injury. J. Traum., *11*:412-416, 1971.

16. Rich, N. M.: Vascular trauma in Vietnam. J. Cardiov. Surg., *11*:3, 1970.

17. Edmundson, K.: Transfixion of the aorta. Brit. J. Surg., *23*:869, 1936.

18. Ngu, V. A., and Konstam, E. G.: Traumatic dissecting aneurysm of the abdominal aorta. Brit. J. Surg., *52*:981, 1965.

19. Rich, N. M., Manion, W. C., and Hughes, C. W.: Surgical and pathological evaluation of vascular injuries in Vietnam. J. Trauma, 9:279, 1969.

20. Williams, G. D., Crumpler, J. B., and Campbell, G. S.: Effect of sympathectomy on the severely traumatized artery. Arch. Surg., *101*:704, 1970.

21. Rich, N. M., Hughes, C. W., and Baugh, J. H.: Management of venous injuries. Ann. Surg., *171*:724, 1970.

22. Cook, F. W., and Haller, J. A., Jr.: Penetrating injuries of the subclavian vessels with associated venous complications. Ann. Surg., *155*:370, 1962.

23. Rich, N. M., Metz, C. W., Jr., Hutton, J. E., Jr., Baugh, J. H., and Hughes, C. W.: Internal versus external fixation of fractures with concomitant vascular injuries in Vietnam. J. Trauma, *11*:463, 1971.

24. Brisbin, R. L., Geib, P. O., and Eiseman, B.: Secondary disruption of vascular repair following war wounds. Arch. Surg., *99*: 787, 1969.

25. Levin, P. M., Rich, N. M., and Hutton, J. E., Jr.: Collateral circulation in arterial injuries. Arch. Surg., *102*:392, 1971.

26. Rich, N. M., Baugh, J. H., and Hughes, C. W.: Popliteal artery injuries in Vietnam. Amer. J. Surg., *118*:531, 1969.

27. Rich, N. M., Baugh, J. H., and Hughes, C. W.: Significance of complications associated with vascular repairs performed in Vietnam. Arch. Surg., *100*:646, 1970.

28. Fomon, J. J., and Warren, W. D.: Late complications of peripheral arterial injuries. Arch. Surg., *91*:610, 1965.

29. Elkin, D. C.: Traumatic aneurysm, the Matas operation—57 years after. Surg., Gynec. Obst., *82*:1, 1946.

30. Hunter, W.: The history of an aneurysm of the aorta with some remarks on aneurysms in general. Med. Obs. Soc. Phys. (London), *1*:323, 1757.

31. Hunter, W.: Further observations upon a particular species of aneurysm. Med. Obs. Soc. Phys. (London), *2*:390, 1762.

32. Nicoladoni, C.: Phlebarterietasie der rechten obern Extremitat. Arch. Klin. Chir., *18*:252, 1875.

33. Branham, H. A.: Aneurismal varix of the femoral artery and vein following a gunshot wound. Int. J. Surg., *3*:250, 1890.

34. Reid, M. R.: The effect of arteriovenous fistula upon the heart and blood vessels: An experimental and clinical study. Bull. Hopkins Hosp., *31*:43, 1920.

35. Holman, E.: Arteriovenous Aneurysms: Abnormal Communications Between the Arterial and Venous Circulations. New York, Macmillan, 1937.

36. Soubbotitch, V.: Military Experience of Traumatic Aneurysms. At the XVIIth International Congress of Medicine. Section VII, Surgery, Part II, pp. 179, 185, 1913. London, 1914. Oxford Univer. Press.

37. Hughes, C. W., and Jahnke, E. J., Jr.: The surgery of traumatic arteriovenous fistulas and aneurysms: A five year follow-up study of 215 lesions. Ann. Surg., *148*:790, 1958.

38. Vollmar, J., and Krumhaar, D.: *In* Hiertonn, T., and Rybeck, B.: Traumatic Arterial Lesions, p. 102, Stockholm, Forsvarets Forskningsanstalt, 1967.

39. Gomes, N. M. R., and Bernatz, P. E.: Arteriovenous fistulas: A review and ten

year experience at the Mayo Clinic. Mayo Clin. Proc., *45*:81, 1970.

40. Conn, J. H., Hardy, J. D., Chaves, C. M., and Fain, W. R.: Challenging arterial injuries. J. Trauma, *11*:167, 1971.

41. Hunt, T. K., Leeds, F. G., Wanebo, H. J., and Blaisdell, F. W.: Arteriovenous fistulas of major vessels in the abdomen. J. Trauma, *11*:483, 1971.

42. Sako, Y., and Varco, R. L.: Arteriovenous fistulas: Results of management of con- genital and acquired forms, blood flow measurements and observations on proximal arterial degeneration. Surgery, *67*:40, 1970.

43. Rich, N. M., Clarke, J. S., and Baugh, J. H.: Successful repair of a traumatic aneurysm of the abdominal aorta. Surgery, *66*:492, 1969.

44. Rich, N. M., Hughes, C. W., and Baugh, J. H.: Management of venous injuries. Ann. Surg., *171*:724, 1970.

Chapter 6 | Complications of Procedures of

Edward B. Diethrich, M.D. | # The Aortic Arch and the Thoracic Aorta

Among the various areas of the arterial tree with potential for the development of complications, the ascending aorta, aortic arch, and descending thoracic aorta probably rank among the highest, both in severity and complexity. Anatomically, there is potential for injury to many nervous structures passing through the mediastinum in close proximity to the great vessels. The thoracic duct, both pleural cavities containing lungs, bronchi and large veins draining from above and below the diaphragm all increase the risk of complication when dealing with arterial problems in this region. The arterial blood supply to every part of the body originates through the ascending aorta and is distributed either cephalad to the upper extremities and brain or caudad to the subdiaphragmatic structures. Interruption of this arterial supply, even on a temporary basis, may lead to permanent, even lethal complications. Finally, as diagnostic abilities have increased with more satisfactory methods of visualizing arterial problems within the chest, so has the frequency with which the surgical team has intervened for correction of congenital and acquired defects. Thus the opportunity is increased for development of a complication in what may be an already complex situation.

A detailed description of all the potential complications which may arise in treating arterial problems within the chest would be impractical. The principles of management as they relate to the prevention or avoidance of difficulty in treating certain lesions can be applied readily to the majority of situations. For that reason, some specific areas of potential difficulty will be described and at least one method of prevention or treatment of the complication suggested.

Aneurysms of the Aortic Arch

There is probably no more difficult vascular lesion to treat surgically than an aneurysm involving the arch of the aorta. Located directly in the thoroughfare for arterial distribution to all the vital structures of the body, and frequently associated with accompanying problems of tracheal compression and nerve involvement, management of this type of aneurysm has always been associated with a high morbidity and mortality. A large aortic arch aneurysm frequently involves the ascending aorta and may be accompanied by aortic valvular insufficiency. This in itself does not present serious difficulty since resection of the ascending aortic aneurysm and replacement of the aortic valve can be accomplished in the routine manner. It is important to recognize that an extended period of operating time will be required for arch resection and valvular replacement, and while ischemic cardiac arrest may be quite satisfactory for valvular replacement alone,[1] myocardial tissues usually will not tolerate prolonged periods of ischemia necessary for this combined procedure. It is therefore important to establish coronary perfusion

131

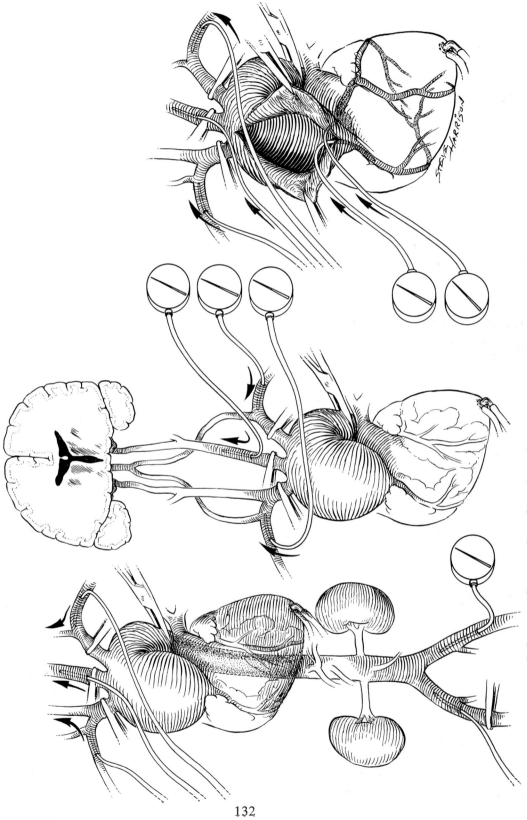

FIG. 6-1. Technique use for resection of aortic arch aneurysms with four vessel cerebral and coronary perfusion. Blood flow and pressure in each of the lines is continually monitored to assure adequate perfusion.

132

throughout the majority of the procedure to avoid irreversible cardiac muscle damage.

Protection of brain tissue from any but the slightest period of ischemia is also essential. Consideration for four-vessel cerebral perfusion has been adopted with this technique. A median sternotomy incision is used for exposure of the heart and great vessels. Even if the aneurysm extends a distance down the descending thoracic aorta, as it frequently may, this incision provides adequate exposure and enhances the view of the vessels originating from the arch.

During opening of the mediastinum, use of the sternal saw has caused inadvertent entry into the ascending portion of an aortic arch aneurysm when the aneurysm rests directly beneath the sternum, or when a previous operation has resulted in close apposition between the vessel and bone. Unless proper precautions are taken under these circumstances, the entire anterior surface of the aorta may be lacerated during opening of the sternum with a resultant exsanguinating hemorrhage. A perfusion technique has been developed which is particularly useful, not only to prevent this particular complication, but also for the routine perfusion during resection and graft replacement involving the entire aortic arch.

A bilateral thoracotomy is also possible, but with this approach there is often difficulty exposing the most cephalad portion of the aneurysm and the innominate and carotid arteries as they traverse into the neck. Following total body heparinization, the superior and inferior venae cavae and one femoral artery are cannulated to establish the basic extracorporeal circuit. The right axillary artery is exposed through a transverse incision in the axillary fold for retrograde perfusion of the right vertebral and right common carotid arteries. The left axillary artery is similarly exposed and cannulated for perfusion of the left vertebral artery. At this point, cardiopulmonary bypass is started, three-vessel cerebral perfusion already having been established. The left common carotid artery is dissected free above the aneu-

rysm and cannulated to complete four-vessel cerebral perfusion. If there is extension of the aneurysm into the left common carotid, this artery can be exposed in the neck through a short, transverse incision.

Using this technique of cerebral perfusion, there is only a brief period of cerebral ischemia during cannulation of the left common carotid artery. It is also possible to begin temporary cardiopulmonary bypass and cerebral perfusion prior to entering the chest by cannulation of the common femoral artery and vein. This is particularly useful when there is a possibility of entering the aneurysm upon opening the sternum or when dealing with a ruptured aneurysm of the ascending aorta or aortic arch where only the tamponading effect of the closed chest is maintaining arterial continuity.

Over-perfusion of the brain during extracorporeal pumping may be as detrimental as supplying insufficient blood. In order to prevent this complication, it is important to monitor both flow and pressure in the lines supplying blood to each of the four cannulas. The complete perfusion circuit with the usual pressure and flow relationships is shown in Figure 6-1.

While this technique obviously does not eliminate all the possible difficulties which can arise in dealing with aneurysms of this magnitude, the serious problem of assuring adequate cerebral perfusion is dealt with. Many of the other technical details are similar to those employed in treating aneurysms anywhere in the arterial tree.

Aneurysms of the Descending Thoracic Aorta

The most frequently encountered aneurysm within the thoracic cavity is located just distal to the left subclavian artery, extending a variable distance toward the diaphragm. Aneurysms in this location may be either the classical atherosclerotic variety or more uncommonly one or another form of dissecting aneurysm. There has been considerable experience treating this latter type of aneurysm with antihypertensive medications since it is most commonly associated with severe hypertension.[2] While the final answer regarding the preferred treatment of dissecting aneurysms has yet to be defined, there is general agreement that if a complication of dissection occurs such as acute aortic insufficiency, occlusion of a major arterial branch of the aorta or rupture of the aneurysm, emergency surgical intervention is required. In addition, if aortography reveals a definite false channel, the follow-up results favor surgical over medical treatment.[3]

Dissecting aneurysms in any location in the thoracic aorta may present several special problems, not the least of which is determination of the precise site of origin of the dissection and its extent. Even with the best angiographic techniques, it may be difficult to establish the origin of the intimal tear and

re-entry point. From the standpoint of operative therapy, this can prove extremely important since in Type I and II dissections, a median sternotomy incision affords the best exposure while for a Type III dissection, a left posterolateral incision is more satisfactory.[11] Clinical findings and physical examination can be helpful especially if sudden aortic insufficiency or cerebral insufficiency symptoms occur. If the initial incision proves to be inadequate to repair the arterial defect, there should be no hesitation to extend or even perform a second incision in order to accomplish removal and graft replacement of the aneurysm (Fig. 6-2).

Regardless of the nature of the lesion, one of the major complications of treating aneurysms of the descending thoracic aorta relates to cross-clamping the aorta and inter-

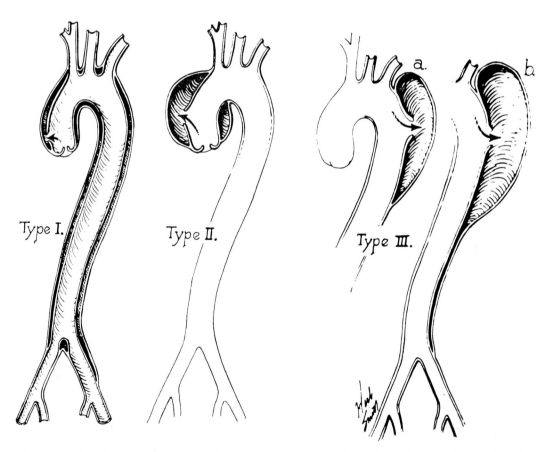

FIG. 6-2. Classification of types of dissecting aneurysms of the aorta. (From DeBakey, M. E., *et al.,* Surgical management of dissecting aneurysms of the aorta. J.T.C.V.S., *49*:130, 1965)

FIG. 6-3. Technique of atriofemoral bypass frequently used for controlling proximal hypertension and perfusion of subdiaphragmatic structures during resection and graft replacement of aneurysms of the descending thoracic aorta.

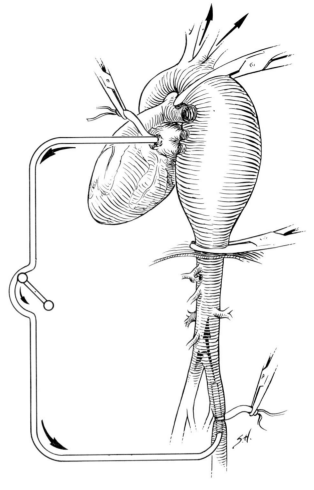

ruption of its blood flow during extirpation and graft replacement of the aneurysm.[4,5,6,7] Since the descending thoracic aorta must be cross-clamped at the level of the left subclavian artery, and under some circumstances proximal to this artery, the available arterial "run off" bed is drastically reduced, thereby resulting in arterial hypertension proximal to the occluding clamp. Cerebral blood pressure is increased, which if not controlled, may precipitate cerebral edema or result in a hemorrhagic cerebral vascular accident. In addition, this increased pressure can produce acute left ventricular strain since the resistance against which the heart must work to expel blood into the ascending aorta is increased. Adequate control of proximal hypertension can prevent both of

these complications. This has been accomplished most satisfactorily in the past using a temporary bypass from the left atrium to the femoral artery.[8] Withdrawal of blood from the atrium not only reduces the volume presented to the left ventricle for each systolic ejection, but it also permits perfusion of the subdiaphragmatic structures beyond the distal occluding clamp (Fig. 6-3).

The use of atriofemoral bypass obviates a second potential complication related to spinal cord and renal ischemia. If a pressure in the abdominal aorta of approximately 70 mm. Hg is maintained, satisfactory perfusion of the structures most sensitive to prolonged lack of blood flow can be accomplished. Urine output during the procedure is maintained at adequate levels and the occurrence

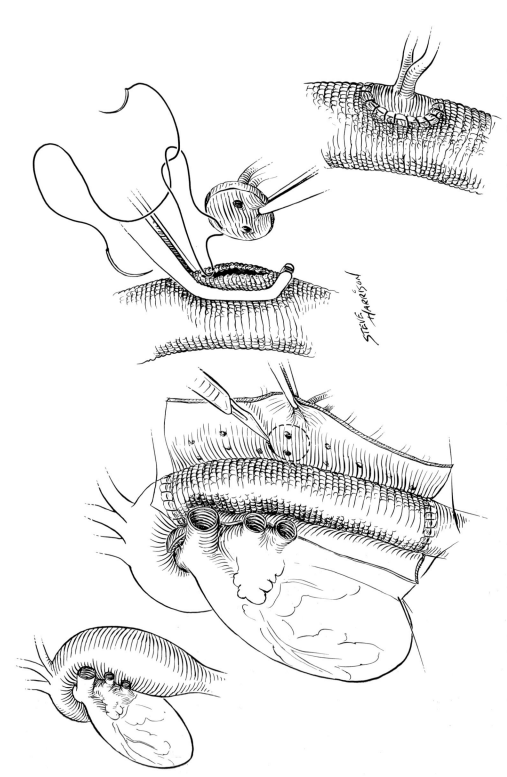

FIG. 6-4. Technique used to preserve intercostal arteries during resection of low aneurysm of the descending thoracic aorta where spinal cord blood supply may be jeopardized. A button of aorta with the intact intercostal artery is preserved and attached to the graft.

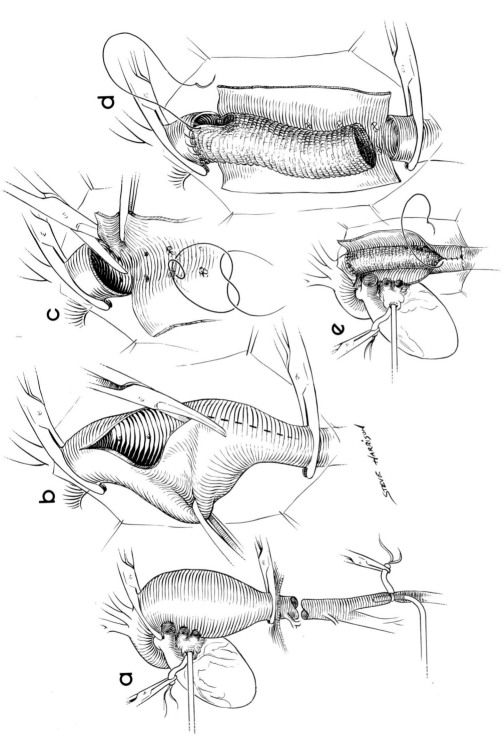

Fig. 6-5. Operative technique used in resection and graft replacement of aneurysms of the descending thoracic aorta. After proximal and distal control, the aneurysm is entered and intercostal arteries are ligated from within the lumen. The Dacron prosthesis is sutured proximally and distally using a continuous suture incorporating a wide margin of aortic cuff. The graft is covered with pleura and the remaining outer layers of the aneurysm to prevent later formation of bronchial or pulmonary communication with the prosthesis or suture line.

of postoperative neurologic deficit secondary to spinal cord ischemia is minimized.

At times, even with adequate atriofemoral bypass, it is necessary to administer a vasodilator drug to further decrease the proximal arterial pressure. This does not adversely affect distal perfusion since the volume of blood delivered by the pump is essentially unchanged. During the performance of these procedures, the anesthesiologist must monitor both proximal and distal arterial pressures continuously since over-perfusion of the subdiaphragmatic structures can result in decreased flow to the cerebral circulation. Intra-arterial catheters are recommended for this monitoring technique.

The use of drugs to lower the arterial pressure has been required more frequently with a recently advocated "no pump" technique.[9] It has been demonstrated that both the spinal cord and kidneys can tolerate brief periods of ischemia without damage. If an aneurysm can be resected with graft replacement in 30 to 40 minutes of occlusion time, the results appear to be comparable to the technique of atriofemoral bypass. It should be emphasized, however, that when prolonged arterial occlusion is anticipated, a method of assuring distal arterial blood supply should be provided if renal and spinal cord damage are to be avoided. For the surgeon who only occasionally deals with aneurysms in this region, use of some form of temporary bypass is recommended since a hurried operation performed under unnecessary time limitations can lead to disastrous results.

Occasionally, spinal cord ischemia occurs resulting in either temporary or permanent neurologic deficit. This is probably related to the direct interruption of the lower intercostal arteries supplying the thoracic segment of the spinal cord. Unfortunately, it is impossible to predict with reliability which intercostal arteries can be ligated, and therefore, it is unlikely that the incidence of this complication can be reduced appreciatively.

Some surgeons have recommended preserving large intercostal arteries encountered in the lower thoracic aorta and re-attaching them to the prosthetic graft. This can be accomplished quite simply by excising a button of tissue around the origin of the intercostal artery (Fig. 6-4). Re-attachment of the cuff of aorta with the intact intercostal artery, while technically easy, unfortunately does not assure that some damage to the spinal cord will not occur since the selection of the appropriate artery for resuturing is arbitrary and the arterial supply to the spinal cord extremely variable.[10] It is probably a worthwhile technique to consider, however, when one or a pair of large intercostal arteries are encountered, especially if the resection demands removal of multiple pairs of intercostal arteries along the entire length of the descending thoracic aorta.

Control of bleeding from inadvertently severed intercostal arteries during resection of descending thoracic aneurysms can be as troublesome as lumbar arterial and venous bleeding during abdominal aneurysmectomy. Therefore, the technique of entry into the aneurysm after proximal and distal control is established, with suture ligation of the intercostal arteries from within the lumen of the aorta is recommended. Each bleeding site is readily identified, the posterior adventitial wall of the aorta is left intact and the anastomoses are performed using a woven Dacron graft with large atraumatic needles taking a generous cuff of aortic wall to assure a strong, bloodless suture line (Fig. 6-5).

Whenever possible, either the outer wall of the aneurysm or the pleura should be sutured over the graft to prevent adhesion between the prosthesis and the lung. When this precaution is not taken, especially at the suture lines, erosion of the lung and bronchus has resulted in fistula formation with hemoptysis and even exsanguination. A woven graft is usually preferable in thoracic aortic procedures since the amount of bleeding through the prosthesis is considerably less than with more porous graft material. If the patient is heparinized, as would be the case for all temporary bypass procedures, use of the woven graft is mandatory.

Probably the greatest single difficulty encountered with operative treatment of dissecting aneurysm pertains to the friable nature of the tissue. Frequently, the entire aortic wall and surrounding tissues are involved with edematous swelling and occasionally subadventitial hemorrhage. Unawareness of this pathologic condition can lead to inadvertent entry into the aortic lumen or tear and laceration of a large intercostal artery. While removal and graft replacement can be accomplished in the manner described for atherosclerotic aneurysms, excessive bleeding at the suture line may be encountered, once again due to the delicate aortic wall. The use of Dacron felt pledgets for reinforcement along the anasto-

motic line significantly reduces the potential for leakage due to tearing of the suture material through the aorta (Fig. 6-6).

Selection of the proper suture material is also important in reducing bleeding at the anastomotic site. Multistranded suture of excessive size tends to tear the friable aorta and increase bleeding through the needle holes. New monofilament sutures currently available in 2-0 and 3-0 sizes provide the required tensile strength and at the same time reduce the chance for tear of the aortic wall. Reinforcing interrupted sutures tied on Dacron felt pledgets should be used wherever the integrity of the suture line is questionable, and especially in posterior areas where accessibility is difficult once the anas-

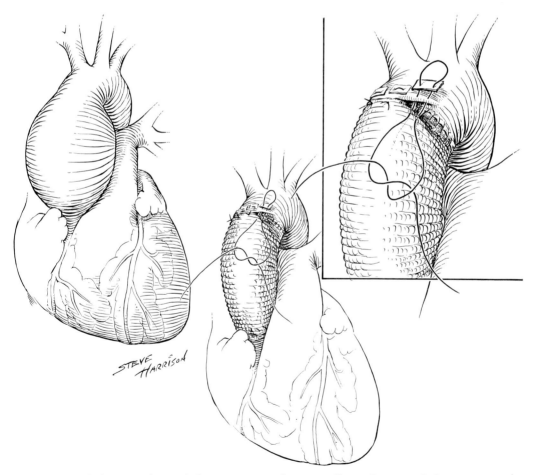

FIG. 6-6. Technique used to reinforce anastomotic suture lines. Dacron pledgets prevent the suture material from tearing the friable aortic tissue.

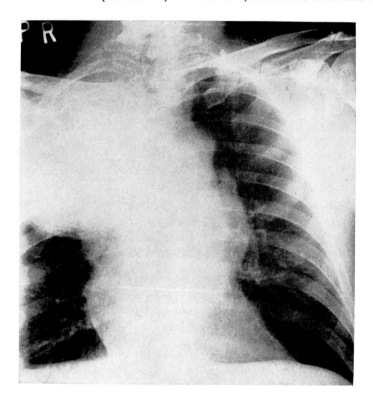

FIG. 6-7. Roentgenograms of the chest showing opacification in the right upper mediastinum thought to be ruptured aneurysm of the ascending aorta. At operation, a ruptured aneurysm of the descending thoracic aorta with bleeding into the right upper chest was encountered.

tomosis has been completed and the occluding clamps removed.

As a general principle, whenever anastomotic bleeding is encountered, the reparative sutures usually can be placed more accurately if the occluding clamp is reapplied. If suturing is attempted in the tense aorta at normal or increased aortic pressures, frequently the size of the leak is increased resulting in more bleeding and further injury to the aorta.

With the increased awareness by physicians of the potential lethality of aneurysms in general, and particularly those aneurysms in the thorax, most patients are referred for surgical treatment prior to rupture. However, when presented with a ruptured thoracic aneurysm, the surgeon faces one of his greatest challenges. The roentgenogram of the chest usually localizes the area of rupture, but occasionally the film can be misleading and create an additional technical complication. This is particularly true if an aneurysm of the descending thoracic aorta ruptures into the right pleural space. If the

presenting opacity on the chest film is in the right upper lung field, the natural conclusion is that an aneurysm of the ascending aorta or aortic arch has ruptured into that area (Fig. 6-7). An aneurysm of the *descending* thoracic aorta, however, can rupture posteriorly across the vertebral column into the *right* pleural space. Previous pleural adhesions can be responsible for the direction of bleeding accounting for a rather confusing problem for the operator. Since both the incision and method of handling aneurysms in these two locations differ, an awareness of this possibility with an effort to make the correct preoperative diagnosis is essential.

Traumatic Injury

Traumatic stab and missile wounds to the neck and chest may involve single or multiple arterial injuries. While some surgeons prefer a conservative approach in these cases, a policy of exploration of all neck and chest wounds assures that no potentially dangerous lesion will produce a sudden or irreversible complication. Delayed hemorrhage when a clot over an injured artery becomes dislodged is thus avoided. A few cases of negative exploration is a small price to pay for the high salvage rate experienced from the more aggressive approach.

Traumatic injury of the thoracic aorta and the major arteries arising from the aortic arch is relatively common, and with the ever-increasing incidence of high velocity deceleration injuries resulting from motor vehicle accidents, the frequency is increasing.[12-21] Rapid deceleration injuries of the thoracic aorta vary from intimal tears to partial or complete transection of the aorta.[22-23] Initially small intimal tears may progress to further subintimal dissection and occlusion of the lumen or subsequent aneurysm formation. Unless the attending physician has

a high index of suspicion, the diagnosis of traumatic transsection of the aorta may be missed. Whenever there is any possibility of this condition suspected on either physical examination or plain roentgenograms of the chest, thoracic aortography should be performed immediately.[34]

Aortography is most helpful in locating the area of aorta laceration or transsection in order to plan accurately the operative approach. In the event of rapid clinical deterioration of the patient, it may be necessary to proceed with operation without the benefit of aortography. Clinical localization with the aid of plan roentgenograms of the chest is possible in most cases since by far the greatest majority of these rapid deceleration injuries to the aorta occur near the

FIG. 6-8. Technique of femoral vein to femoral artery bypass using pump oxygenator for partial cardiopulmonary bypass.

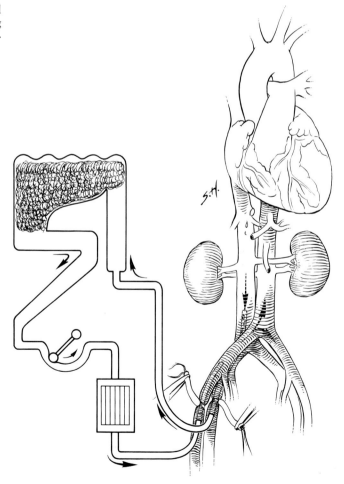

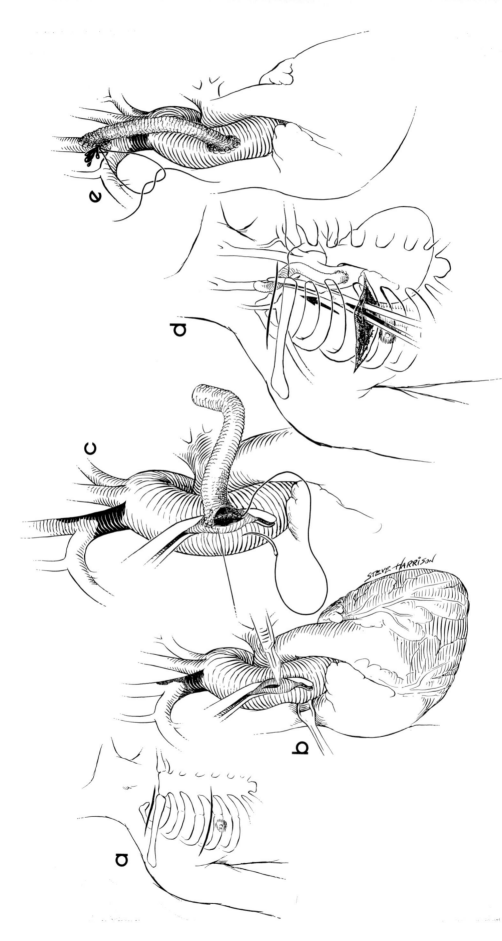

Fig. 6-9. Technique used to bypass obstructive lesions of the great vessels. Graft is anastomosed to the ascending aorta after exposure through a right second or third intercostal incision. Bypass can be taken to any of the cervical vessels. Potential complication of compression in the graft and erosion of the prosthesis is eliminated with this operative approach.

attachment of the ligamentum arteriosum. More than a single injury may be present, however, and the possibility of a second intimal tear should always be considered.

Preparation for extracorporeal support should be made for maintenance of distal circulation during the period of aortic occlusion necessary for isolation and repair of aortic lacerations in the usual location at the attachment of the ligamentum arteriosum. Either left atrial-to-femoral artery bypass without an oxygenator as described for the management of aneurysms of the descending thoracic aorta,[35] or partial cardiopulmonary bypass from the femoral vein to femoral artery with an interposed pump oxygenator is satisfactory (Fig. 6-8).[36] The advantage of this latter technique is the avoidance of left atrial cannulation with its inherent risk of tear and bleeding. It also has the advantage of eliminating further manipulation and tubing within the pericardial sac.

Since the hematoma surrounding an injury in the region often covers most of the proximal descending thoracic aorta, with extension over the pericardium and transverse aortic arch, attempts to obtain proximal aortic control from outside the pericardial sac may result in entry into the mediastinal hematoma. This may release the tamponading effect of the hematoma and result in rapid exsanguination. Exposure from within the pericardial sac allows access to the proximal aorta between the left common carotid and left subclavian arteries without danger of entering the hematoma. Control of the distal aorta should also be well beyond the mediastinal hematoma. The clamp may be moved closer to the site of injury once the hematoma has been evacuated in order to diminish blood loss from intercostal arteries between the area of aortic laceration and the cross-clamped aorta.

A graft usually is necessary for restoration of aortic continuity in cases of complete transsection since the ends are often fragmented and friable even after debridement of the aorta. If a portion of the aortic circumference remains intact, primary repair

may be possible. However, even under these circumstances, use of a strip of Dacron cloth on either side of the anastomosis to buttress the suture line is quite helpful in preventing further tearing and bleeding.

One of the major complications resulting from these injuries is ischemic spinal cord damage probably occurring as a result of compression and occlusion of intercostal arteries by the hematoma.[37] Paralysis resulting from this injury may be temporary, especially if there is not a concomitant direct injury to the cord itself. Unfortunately, in a few cases, paraplegia may be permanent even when operation is performed within a short time after injury. Because of the occasional occurrence of such a complication, an accurate neurologic evaluation of these patients must be recorded at the time of hospital admission.

The Great Vessels Originating from the Aortic Arch

Many of the occlusive lesions of the great vessels originating from the aortic arch can be treated best by extrathoracic procedures such as carotid-subclavian bypass (see Chap. 7). However, if the occlusive lesion involves the origin of the innominate artery, either endarterectomy of the vessel or bypass graft around the obstruction affords a satisfactory opportunity for a good long-term result. Localized endarterectomy of the innominate or the proximal common carotid arteries does present a potential for complication since cerebral circulation must be temporarily suspended during the thromboendarterectomy and repair. A partially occluding clamp can be placed across the origin of the vessel including a portion of the aortic arch, but once again the risk of cerebral ischemia or embolization from a friable intimal plaque poses a potential danger.

These difficulties are alleviated by the use of a Dacron bypass graft from the ascending aorta to beyond the obstructing lesion. Originally, a median sternotomy was the preferred incision for exposing the ascending aorta. A Dacron graft was anastomosed to the ascending aorta over a partially occluding clamp and the distal end of the graft sutured to one or more branches of the arch outside the thoracic cavity. Two difficulties, however, have been discovered using this approach. First, when the sternum is closed pressure on the graft lying between the bone and the aorta can result in decreased blood flow with compromise of the bypass graft. While this is not always the case, since the available retrosternal space is variable, the possibility should be considered when a median sternotomy is used. Second, erosion of the graft, lying in the enclosed space has resulted in false aneurysm formation. There is little tissue available to cover the prosthesis as it originates from the ascending aorta and unlike the locations for prostheses in the descending thoracic aorta or the abdominal aorta where either pleura or peritoneum are available to cover the prosthesis and suture line, the graft lies rather naked in the retrosternal space.

Both of these potential complications can be eliminated if the bypass graft is taken from the right lateral side of the ascending aorta (Fig. 6-9). Exposure for this anastomosis is through a right anterior thoracotomy in either the second or third intercostal space. The incision is carried to the right medial aspect of the sternum although it is not necessary to divide the internal mammary vessels. The lung is then retracted laterally, exposing the ascending aorta covered by the pericardium. An incision is made in the pericardium and extended cephalad for approximately two inches up the ascending aorta. Pericardial retraction sutures can be used to provide better exposure of the ascending aorta which in this location has a natural curvature to the right. A partially occluding clamp is placed on the aorta and the anastomosis performed. The graft then lies to the right of the ascending aorta well below the sternum with sufficient free space in the superior mediastinum. Pericardium and loose pleural connective tissue can be used to cover the anastomosis so that both compression from the sternum and the

possibility of fistula between the suture line and contiguous pulmonary structures are eliminated. The graft is then tunneled into the supraclavicular area beneath the clavicle and the anastomosis performed to the appropriate artery beyond the stenotic lesion. If more than one artery is being bypassed, a second or even third graft can be taken from the primary Dacron graft originating from the ascending aorta. Use of this procedure and its several modifications converts a previously major operative procedure with several inherent opportunities for the development of complications into a relatively low risk procedure with a high assurance of success in terms of relieving the patient's symptoms and avoiding any major postoperative difficulties.

Patent Ductus Arteriosus

Interruption of a patent ductus arteriosus is among the early operations performed by residents in cardiovascular surgery training. This is an appropriate operative procedure to introduce more technically challenging operations since both the potential for and actual incidence of complications are low.[38] A clear understanding of the anatomy is most important in the avoidance of difficulty in dealing with a patent ductus arteriosus since one of the most frequent complications is injury to the recurrent laryngeal nerve. The vagus nerve courses directly over the aorta and at the level of the ductus gives off the recurrent laryngeal branch. This nerve then curves posteriorly and circles behind the ductus. If the operator does not identify the vagus nerve and this recurrent branch, either transsection or crushing by hemostat or occluding clamp may occur. Once the recurrent laryngeal nerve is identified, it is unlikely that injury will occur since the ductus can be encircled easily with a heavy ligature, leaving the nerve to lie posteriorly.

Opening the pericardium allows the pericardial fluid to escape. This is helpful in infants where the heart is large and this fluid may impede lung retraction and adequate exposure of the ductus. In order to obtain full length of the ductus prior to placing the occluding clamps, the fibrous pericardial reflection is cut posterior to the ductus. Dissection in the area posterior to the ductus must be done carefully since in about 15 percent of the cases one or more mediastinal branches of the aorta cross at the ductus level. These small arteries should be identified and ligated before division of the ductus.[39]

It is generally accepted now that the operative treatment of choice for patent ductus arteriosus is division rather than ligation. The hazards of ligating any large vessel in continuity are well recognized. The incidence of either recanalization or incomplete occlusion of a ligated ductus arteriosus is sufficiently high to consider it a second choice procedure except under unusual circumstances. Another important complication which has resulted from ligation is the development of an aneurysm at the site of ligature placement around the ductus.[40-44] If this complication is associated with infection, it represents an extremely serious problem necessitating reoperation, excision of the aneurysm and complete division of the ductus.[45] Initial division of the ductus avoids the potential for these complications.

Several techniques have been described for routine division of the ductus and in the uncomplicated situation with a long, narrow communication between pulmonary artery and aorta, application of two clamps and division is accomplished without incident. If however, the ductus is short and any difficulty in applying the clamps with an acceptable cuff of aorta and pulmonary artery is anticipated, it is wise to incise the ductus a short distance and begin a running mattress suture. As the suturing progresses, the ductus is divided further. In this way, there is always complete control, and hemostasis is assured should the occluding clamp slip.

When the ductus is very short, an alternative technique is useful. First the aorta is occluded both proximal and distal to the ductus. Then a third clamp is applied across the ductus near the pulmonary artery. The ductus is then divided flush with the aorta and the aorta is closed transversely (Fig. 6-10).[49]

In the adult patient with a patent ductus, there is often calcium present in either the aortic wall or ductus itself. Application of occluding clamps across the ductus can cause a fracture of the calcified wall or a tear with resultant hemorrhage. Adequate mobilization of the aorta proximal and distal to the ductus is important under these circumstances, so that if necessary occluding clamps can be placed for temporary decompression in a similar manner as described for a very short ductus.[47] This maneuver avoids clamping the ductus, pulsating at systemic pressures, and provides an opportunity to perform the repair even in the presence of a calcified artery.

Coarctation of the Aorta

Coarctation of the aorta is another congenital defect for which operative therapy can yield a cure in most cases.[48,49] Even infants with heart failure and hypoxemia due to a high-grade obstruction of the coarcted aorta have been operated upon with good results.[50] Occasionally, cardiac failure is observed in a patient in the geriatric age range due to a coarctation missed during earlier life. It is generally agreed now that all patients with coarctation of the thoracic aorta should undergo operative correction since the incidence of intraoperative and postoperative complications is extremely low.

In early infancy, the major complications at the operating table are associated with either a critical state of cardiac competence due to left ventricular failure or the presence of other congenital cardiac anomalies. Patent ductus arteriosus is very common in the early age group, but even if recognized, creates no additional operative hazard. Congenital mitral stenosis, intracardiac shunts and other complex anomalies in the presence of a coarctation present additional hazards since general anesthesia alone with partial collapse of the left lung and possible shift of

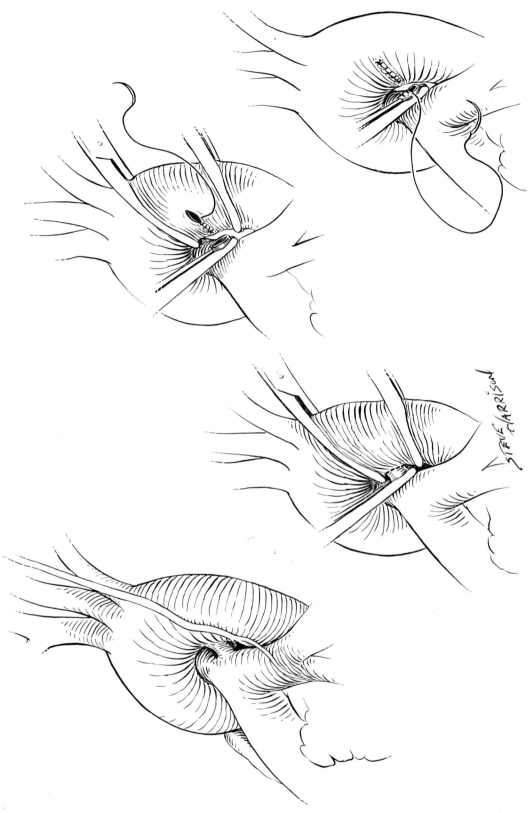

FIG. 6-10. Operative technique used for division of short ductus arteriosus. This technique permits safe division and repair of the pulmonary artery and aorta without compromising either lumen.

146

the mediastinum can cause further cardiac decompensation. Any of these combinations can produce a rather anxious state for both the surgeon and anesthesiologist resulting in a hurried operation which may yield less than the desired long-term results.

A factor known to produce a delayed complication of coarctation surgery, restenosis of the aorta, relates to the amount of constricted tissue which is removed at the time of operation.[51-56] Ideally, effort should be made to excise all the constricted tissue and

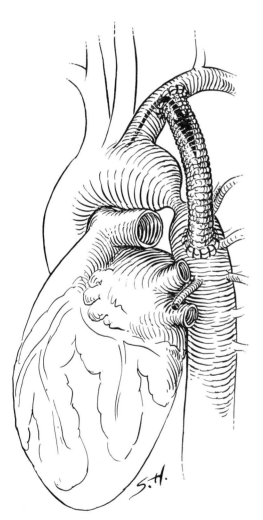

FIG. 6-11. Technique of bypass graft from the left subclavian artery to the descending thoracic aorta used for recurrent coarctation of the aorta or in adult patients where large intercostal arteries may create technical difficulties.

cut back to normal aortic substance on each end. If this is not accomplished, the remaining ends are somewhat thickened and non-elastic. In spite of an adequate early repair, scarred ends of this type at the anastomotic site will not grow normally in subsequent years, and restenosis is the end result.

Many times the failure to excise all the abnormal tissue is the result of the surgeon's concern that there will not be sufficient length to reunite the aortic ends without undue tension. Under most conditions, this should not be a concern in the infant or young child since, with adequate mobilization of the distal and proximal aorta including the left subclavian artery origin, an anastomosis can be performed without tension. As a technical aid during the performance of the anastomosis, the assistants should hold an occluding clamp in each hand, bringing the transsected aortic ends close together until the entire suture line has been completed. If the clamps are allowed to move, the sutures may tear the aortic wall resulting in excessive bleeding.

In an additional effort to prevent restenosis and permit the reconstructed aorta to grow normally, many surgeons now use interrupted sutures for at least the posterior suture line. It is not entirely clear whether this precaution provides better long-term results than anastomosis performed using the continuous technique, but the theoretical advantages seem to justify its use.

Patients who are not operated upon electively in early life for repair of aortic coarctation usually develop one or another manifestation of severe narrowing of the thoracic aorta. Systemic hypertension above the coarctation is the most commonly encountered complication which may appear as early as late adolescence. If the usual signs of coarctation including decreased pulses in the lower extremities, rib notching on roentgenograms of the chest, a characteristic systolic murmur and evidence of increased periscapular collateral channels are not recognized, hypertension may be misdiagnosed and the patient treated for an erroneous cause of it. Unfortunately, the end result of failure to recognize the true cause of the hypertension may result in left ventricular decompensation. Another, but less frequently observed consequence of this misdiagnosis is intermittent claudication of the lower extremities.

Persons in the early twenties or late teens may have typical symptoms of intermittent claudication due to coarctation of the aorta. Both systemic hypertension and intermittent claudication are reversible with correction of the coarctation. There are, however, a significant number of patients who have persistent hypertension for a period following operation. The exact nature of this phenomenon is not entirely understood, but it may be related to a "high set" of the baroreceptors below the coarcted level of the aorta.[57-60] After a period of time, these baroreceptors become readjusted to the new pressure level and the hypertension disappears.

Other postoperative visceral manifestations have been reported following repair of the coarcted aorta.[61-64] Intestinal symptoms and abdominal pain may well be due to changes in the vessel walls of the arterioles below the coarctation in combination with a complex relationship of reflexes from the baroreceptor area and an increase in norepinephrine levels.

This mesenteric arteritis may present typical signs of advanced intestinal ischemia. Often this syndrome is accompanied by severe hypertension even though the coarctation has been removed.[65] Treatment with antihypertensive agents, usually reserpine is best, is often effective. With control of the idiopathic hypertension, abdominal symptoms may subside. If improvement with these measures and nasogastric decompression is not prompt, exploration of the abdomen to rule out or treat bowel infarction has been undertaken. There is no known prophylaxis of this condition, but fortunately its occurrence is rare.

In both the adult patient with coarctation and the patient who requires reoperation for either stenotic or occluded primary repair,[66]

consideration should be given to the use of a bypass graft from the left subclavian artery to the aorta beyond the coarctation. In both of these circumstances it may be technically difficult to resect the coarctation due to scar tissue and extremely large intercostal arteries. In order to avoid this complication, a partially occluding clamp is placed on the left subclavian artery just beyond its origin. A woven graft is then anastomosed side-to-side to the subclavian artery proximally and to the aorta beyond the coarctation over a similarly placed partially occluding clamp on the descending thoracic aorta (Fig. 6-11). This type of bypass restores circulation and from a technical standpoint provides a highly satisfactory method of dealing with an otherwise potentially complicated problem.

References

1. Cooley, D. A., et al.: Surgical management of aneurysms of the ascending aorta. Surg. Clin. N. Amer., 46:1033-44, 1966.
2. Wheat, M. W., Jr., et al.: Dissecting aneurysms of the aorta: Present status of drug versus surgical therapy. Progr. Cardiovas. Dis., 11:198-210, 1968.
3. McFarland, James, and Willerson, J., et al.: The medical treatment of dissecting aortic aneurysms. J. Med., 286:115-19, 1972.
4. Cole, P. T., and Gutelius, J. R., Jr.: Neurologic complication of operations on the descending thoracic aorta. Canad. J. Surg., 12:435-43, 1969.
5. Cooley, D. A.: Complications of procedures on the thoracic aorta, In: Complications of Surgery and Their Management. Artz, C. P., and Hardy, J. D. Eds. Philadelphia, Saunders, 1960, p. 511.
6. Edwards, R. H., and Killen, D. A.: Prevention of spinal cord ischemia incident to extensive mobilization of the thoracic aorta from the posterior parieties. Surg. Forum, 15:285, 1964.
7. Cole, P. T., and Gutelius, J. R., Jr.: Paraplegia resulting from use of the subclavian artery as a shunt source during resection of the descending thoracic aorta. Ann. Surg., 169:293-4, 1969.
8. Cooley, D. A., DeBakey, M. E., and Morris, G. C., Jr.: Controlled extracorporeal circulation in surgical treatment of aortic aneurysm. Ann. Surg., 146:473, 1957.

9. Crawford, E. S., Fenstermacher, J. M., *et al.*: Reappraisal of adjuncts to avoid ischemia in the treatment of thoracic aortic aneurysms. Surg., *67*:182-96, 1970.

10. Bolton, B.: The blood supply of the human spinal cord. J. Neurol. Psychiat., *2*:137, 1939.

11. DeBakey, M. E., and Henly, W. S., *et al.*: Surgical management of dissecting aneurysms of the aorta. J. Thorac. Cardiovas. Surg., *49*:130-147, 1965.

12. Beall, A. C., Jr., Arbegast, N. R., *et al.*: Complete transection of the thoracic aorta due to rapid deceleration, report of successful repair in two cases. Amer. J. Surg., *114*:769-73, 1967.

13. Strassmann, G.: Traumatic rupture of the aorta. Amer. Heart J., *33*:508-515, 1947.

14. Parmley, L. F., Mattingly, T. W., *et al.*: Non-penetrating traumatic injury of the aorta. Circulation, *17*:1086-1101, 1958.

15. Greendyke, R. M.: Traumatic rupture of aorta: Special reference to automobile accidents. JAMA, *195*:527-530, 1966.

16. Spencer, F. C., *et al.*: A report of 15 patients with traumatic rupture of the thoracic aorta. J. Thorac. Cardiov. Surg., *41*:1-22, 1961.

17. Eiseman, B., and Rainer, W. G.: Clinical management of post-traumatic rupture of the thoracic aorta. J. Thorac. Surg., *35*: 347-358, 1958.

18. Ellis, F.: Surgical repair of a traumatic rupture of the thoracic aorta. Brit. J. Surg., *46*:495-499, 1958-59.

19. Passaro, E., Jr., and Pace, W. C.: Traumatic rupture of the aorta. Surgery, *46*: 787-791, 1959.

20. Fleischaker, R. J., Mazur, J. H., and Baisch, B. F.: Surgical treatment of acute traumatic rupture of the thoracic aorta. J. Thorac. Cardiov. Surg., *47*:289-297, 1959.

21. Stoney, R. J., Roe, B. B., and Reddington, J. V.: Rupture of the thoracic aorta due to closed-chest trauma. Arch. Surg., *89*:840-847, 1964.

22. Slaney, G., Ashton, F., and Abrams, L. D.: Traumatic rupture of the aorta. Brit. J. Surg., *53*:361-364, 1966.

23. Dobell, A. R., MacNaughton, E. A., and Crutchlow, E. F.: Successful early treatment of subadventitial rupture of the thoracic aorta. New Eng. J. Med., *270*:410-412, 1964.

24. McKnight, J. T., Meyer, J. A., and Neville, J. F., Jr.: Nonpenetrating traumatic rupture of the thoracic aorta. Ann. Surg., *160*: 1069-1072, 1964.

25. Jahnke, E. J., Jr., Fisher, G. W., and Jones, R. C.: Acute traumatic rupture of the thoracic aorta: Report of six consecutive cases of successful early repair. J. Thorac. Cardiov. Surg., *48*:63-77, 1964.

26. Cammack, K., *et al.*: Deceleration injuries of the thoracic aorta. Arch. Surg., *79*:244-251, 1959.

27. Bromley, L. L., Hobbs, J. T., and Robinson, R. E.: Early repair of traumatic rupture of the thoracic aorta. Brit. Med. J., *2*:17-19, 1965.

28. DeMuth, W., Roe, H., and Hobbie, W.: Immediate repair of traumatic rupture of the thoracic aorta. Arch. Surg., *91*:602-603, 1965.

29. Lawrence, M. S., and Ehrenhaft, J. S.: Trauma to the thoracic aorta. J. Iowa Med. Soc., *55*:637-643, 1965.

30. Mulder, D. G., and Grollman, J. H., Jr.: Traumatic disruption of the thoracic aorta: Diagnostic and surgical considerations. Amer. J. Surg., *118*:311-6, 1969.

31. Baker, N. H., Ewy Hg.: Surgical significance of extraluminal aortic perfusion after acute thoracic aortic dissection. Amer. Surg., *35*:688-90, 1969.

32. Rittenhouse, E. A., Dillard, D. H., and Winterscheid, *et al.*: Traumatic rupture of the thoracic aorta—A review of the literature and a report of five cases with attention to special problems in early surgical management. Ann. Surg., *170*:87-100, 1969.

33. Beall, A. C., Jr., and Arbegast, N. R., *et al.*: Aortic laceration due to rapid deceleration. Arch. Surg., *98*:595-601, 1969.

34. Blake, H. A., Inmon, T. W., and Spencer, F. C.: Emergency use of antegrade aortography in diagnosis of acute aortic rupture. Ann. Surg., *152*:954-956, 1960.

35. Bloodwell, R. D., Hallman, G. L., and Cooley, D. A.: Partial cardiopulmonary bypass for pericardiectomy and resection of descending thoracic aortic aneurysms. Ann. Thorac. Surg., *1*:46-56, 1968.

36. Neville, W. E., *et al.*: Resection of the descending thoracic aorta with femoral vein to femoral artery oxygenation perfusion. J. Thorac. Cardiov. Surg., *56*:39, 1968.

37. Herendeen, T. L., and King, H.: Transient anuria and paraplegia following traumatic rupture of the thoracic aorta. J. Thorac. Cardiov. Surg., *56*:599-602, 1968.

38. Jones, J. C.: Twenty-five years' experience with the surgery of patent ductus arteriosus. J. Thorac. Cardiov. Surg., *50*:149, 1965.

39. ———: Complications of the surgery of patent ductus arteriosus. J. Thorac. Surg., 16:305, 1947.
40. Payne, R. F., and Jordan, S. C.: Postoperative aneurysms following ligation of the patent ductus arteriosus. Brit. J. Radiol., 41:858-861, 1968.
41. Rosenkrantz, J. G., and Kelminson, L. L., et al.: False aneurysm after ligation of a patent ductus arteriosus. Ann. Thorac. Surg., 3:353-357, 1967.
42. Hallman, G. L., and Cooley, D. A.: False aortic aneurysm following division and suture of a patent ductus arteriosus: Successful excision with hypothermia. J. Cardiov. Surg., 5:23, 1964.
43. Kerwin, A. J., and Jaffe, F. A.: Postoperative aneurysm of the ductus arteriosus. Amer. J. Cardiol., 3:397, 1959.
44. Ross, R. S., Feder, F. P., and Spencer, F. C.: Aneurysms of the previously ligated patent ductus arteriosus. Circulation, 23:350, 1961.
45. Schieppati, E., Viola, A. R., and Leyro-Diaz, R. M.: Postoperative infected aneurysm of patent ductus arteriosus. Dis. Chest, 46:503, 1964.
46. Jones, J. C.: Twenty-five years' experience with the surgery of patent ductus arteriosus. J. Thorac. Cardiov. Surg., 50:149, 1965.
47. Morrow, A. G., and Clark, W. D.: Closure of the calcified patent ductus. J. Thorac. Cardiov. Surg., 51:534, 1966.
48. Gross, R. E.: Surgery for coarctation of the aorta in infants. Amer. J. Cardiov., 25:507-508, 1970.
49. Crafoord, C., Ejrup, B., and Gladnikoff, H.: Coarctation of the aorta. Thorac. Surg., 2:121, 1947.
50. McNamara, D. G.: Prevention of infant deaths from cogenital heart disease. Pediat. Clin. N. Amer., 10:127, 1963.
51. Hartman, A. F., Jr., Goldring, D., and Hernandez, A., et al.: Recurrent coarctation of the aorta after successful repair in infancy. Amer. J. Cardiol., 25:405-410, 1970.
52. Parson, C. G., and Astley, R.: Recurrence of aortic coarctation after operation in childhood. Brit. Med. J., 1:573, 1966.
53. Mulder, D. G., and Linde, L. M.: Recurrent coarctation of the aorta in infancy. Amer. Surg., 25:908, 1959.
54. Khoury, G. H., and Hawes, C. R.: Recurrent coarctation of the aorta in infancy and childhood. J. Pediat., 72:801, 1968.
55. Stansel, H. C., Jr., and Newbold, R.: Recurrent coarctation of the aorta. Ann. Thorac. Surg., 11:380-384, 1971.
56. Ibarra-Perex, C., Castaneda, A. R., and Varco, R. L., et al.: Recoarctation of the aorta: Nineteen year clinical experience. Amer. J. Cardiol., 23:778-84, 1969.
57. Sealy, W. C.: Coarctation of the aorta and hypertension. Ann. Thorac. Surg., 3:15-28, 1967.
58. Harris, J., Sealy, W. C., and DeMaria, W.: Renal dynamics and hypertension in aortic coarctation. Amer. J. Med. Sci., 9:734, 1950.
59. Kirkendall, W. M., Culbertson, J. W., and Eckstein, J. W.: Renal hemodynamics in patients with coarctation of the aorta. J. Lab. Clin. Med., 53:6, 1959.
60. Sealy, W. C., Harris, J. S., and Young, W. G., Jr., et al.: Paradoxical hypertension following resection of coarctation of the aorta. Surgery, 42:135, 1957.
61. Benson, W. R., and Sealy, W. C.: Arterial necrosis following resection of coarctation of the aorta. J. Lab. Invest., 5:359, 1956.
62. Lober, P. H., and Lillehei, C. W.: Necrotizing panarteritis following repair of coarctation of aorta. Surgery, 35:950, 1954.
63. Mays, E. T., and Sergeant, C. K.: Postcoarctectomy syndrome. Arch. Surg., 91:59, 1965.
64. Trummer, M. J., and Mannix, E. P., Jr.: Abdominal pain and necrotizing mesenteric arteritis following resection of coarctation of the aorta. J. Thorac. Cardiov. Surg., 45:198, 1963.
65. Tawes, R. L., Bull, J. C., and Roe, B. B.: Hypertension and abdominal pain after resection of aortic coarctation. Ann. Surg., 171:409, 1970.
66. Berroya, R. B., Aleman, J., and Mannix, E. P., Jr.: A long-term failure of prosthetic graft in coarctation. J. Cardiov. Surg., 11:329-332, 1970.

Chapter 7 | Complications of

Charles G. Rob, M.D.,
and Hugh G. Beebe, M.D.

Extracranial Cerebrovascular Procedures

The extracranial cerebral arteries may be defined as the innominate, common carotid, subclavian, internal carotid, vertebral and external carotid arteries when the ipsilateral internal carotid artery is occluded. Operations upon the innominate, left common carotid and left subclavian arteries as they arise from the aortic arch have been discussed in Chapter 6 and will be only briefly referred to here. Arterial reconstruction of the extracranial cerebral arteries is usually performed for occlusive arterial disease or atherosclerosis and this accounts for fully 95 percent of such procedures. Other indications include: tortuous or kinked arteries, aneurysms, arteriovenous fistulas, arterial injuries, various forms of arteritis, congenital abnormalities, carotid body tumors, arterial emboli, and the occasional involvement by a malignant tumor.

The development of operations for occlusive disease of the extracranial cerebral arteries dates from the realization by Ramsey Hunt,[1] Hutchinson and Yates[2] and others that many strokes were due to occlusions of the extracranial as opposed to the intracranial cerebral arteries. The true frequency of these lesions was not fully known until the introduction of cerebral angiography[3] and percutaneous catheter angiography.[4] This was followed by reports of operations for the correction of occlusive lesions of the carotid arteries by Eastcott, Pickering and Rob[5] and by Rob and Wheeler.[6]

Radiographic Evaluation

Whenever possible, arch aortography with visualization of all of the major extracranial vessels should be obtained. Variation in the intracranial collateral anatomy suggests that the blood supply of the brain be regarded as a single, total entity with variable contributions by the carotid and vertebral-basilar systems. Some patients with isolated internal carotid artery stenosis and an otherwise normal extracranial arterial supply may have serious and disabling symptoms, while other patients may be observed radiographically to have completely occluded one or more major vessels without significant symptoms at all.

This variability of clinical symptoms is a reflection of collateral pathway differences, and shows that a single anatomic lesion does not have identical neurologic implications for all patients. A variety of techniques has been described for obtaining contrast visualization of the cerebral vessels in the neck including bilateral direct common carotid artery injections coupled with direct puncture subclavian injection, retrograde pressure injection from the brachial artery and limited studies involving only unilateral carotid injection. The desirability of arch aortography, however, is demonstrated by the fact that approximately two thirds of

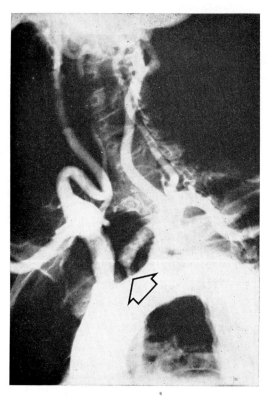

Fig. 7-1. This arch aortogram of a 56-year-old woman with transient episodes of dizziness demonstrates marked tortuosity of the right common carotid artery and stenosis of the left common carotid artery at its origin (arrow). The left carotid stenosis was repaired by endarterectomy through a cervical approach. She has remained asymptomatic postoperatively without anything being done on the right side.

patients will present with multiple lesions in surgically accessible sites.[7]

Moreover, arch aortography permits some degree of physiologic evaluation of flow. The importance of this is illustrated by the relatively late description of the subclavian steal syndrome which was understood only when total and sequential radiographic demonstration of the extracranial blood supply became available. Another example of the importance of evaluating the total cerebral arterial supply as a unit is supported by recent evidence suggesting the importance of internal carotid artery stenosis in association with a subclavian steal phenomenon which may be insufficient to result in clinical symptoms by itself. Planning the conduct of a reconstructive operation or series of operations can be done with greatest safety for the patient when the entire arterial tree is defined. Moreover, approximately 12 percent of patients with significant occlusive disease of at least one carotid artery will present without classic symptoms.[8] Therefore, arteriographic visualization of isolated, single vessels should be avoided in favor of more complete study whenever possible.

The complications of arteriography are discussed in Chapter 1. However, it should be mentioned here that complications of arteriography, or any other investigative procedure, cannot be considered separately from the results of surgical treatment. So long as the complications of arteriography are few and the yield from this study of candidates for operation is made high by appropriate selection of patients for x-ray investigation, surgical results will not be adversely affected. If on the other hand, radiographic complications were high and arteriography indiscriminately employed yielding a low percentage of operative candidates, then surgical results would have to overcome a handicap of the morbidity of the x-ray examination. With properly selected patients, and careful arteriography the incidence of significant radiologic complications should be less than 1 percent, and the postoperative improvement in surgical patients should be approximately 90 percent.

The interval between the arteriogram of the extracranial cerebral arteries and the operation is of importance. We always allow at least one full day between these procedures unless an emergency situation develops. And if the arteriogram is followed by transient worsening of the cerebral function a longer interval is recommended. In this connection we prefer to have an interval of several days between the operation and the last transient ischemic attack and of at least two weeks between the onset of a complete stroke and the operation.

Patient Selection

A critical understanding of the natural history of cerebrovascular disease is necessary for proper selection of patients for operation. To a large degree the incidence of complications and the risk of mortality following operation for carotid artery disease can be controlled by appropriate patient selection.[9] The great majority of patients with carotid arterial lesions will have typical symptoms of transient ischemic attacks consisting of difficulty with speech, ipsilateral eye symptoms, contralateral motor and sensory symptoms or various combinations of these. When such symptoms are brief, intermittent, self-resolving and leave no significant residual, these patients may be properly classified as symptomatic with transient ischemic attacks. Assessment of the degree of stenosis is difficult to make from radiographic studies, but may be estimated from biplaner views. No degree of stenosis can be accurately calculated from single plane radiographs. It should be remembered that symptoms of transient cerebral ischemia are more likely to be due to microembolization from an ulcerated atheromatous lesion of the proximal internal carotid artery than to the degree of narrowing by the plaque itself.[10,11,12]

There should be a clear distinction made between patients with transient ischemic attacks and patients who have so-called progressing strokes or completed strokes. A progressing stroke is one in which a minor residual deficit persists after an ischemic attack and is observed subsequently to be worsening neurologically over a short period of time. A completed stroke is one in which a major neurologic deficit has developed and remains fixed for a long period of time or permanently. This is important because the early results of operation for patients with progressive and completed strokes are in marked contrast to the early results of operation for patients with transient ischemic attacks.

There is wide disagreement of opinion over whether or not patients with asymptomatic carotid bruits should be treated surgically. Although the immediate postoperative status of such patients is excellent, the argument in favor of this treatment should rest on demonstration that such patients sustain a lower incidence of strokes at a later time in their follow-up. Because of the variable nature of cerebrovascular disease, this remains an unsettled issue presently. The reported incidence of mortality due to stroke following major vascular reconstructive surgery for noncerebrovascular lesions is sufficiently high that consideration should be given to prophylactic carotid endarterectomy in patients with asymptomatic bruits who are candidates for a major operation elsewhere. A more liberal approach to the patient with an asymptomatic bruit has been advocated by some, who consider that operation may be advised in patients with asymptomatic bruits unless they are extremely poor risk, elderly patients with generalized, serious disease.[13] It has been pointed out, however, that if carotid surgery is advised for such asymptomatic patients, it is mandatory that operative morbidity and mortality must be exceedingly low.

Patients with complete occlusion of the internal carotid artery are often seen after having sustained a major frank stroke and thus are not ordinarily considered candidates for a reconstructive procedure. In other patients with complete occlusion who have not suffered a permanent residual the lesion may be approached surgically but with less than 50 percent likelihood of restoring patency. Carotid reconstruction is best performed at the stage of arterial stenosis. Once the internal carotid artery has thrombosed the whole situation changes. The thrombus rapidly extends up through the carotid canal to the first branch which is the ophthalmic artery. This thrombus soon becomes adherent to the arterial wall in the carotid canal and complete removal becomes impossible often in less than 24 hours. More than a third of patients with complete occlusion will show significant neurologic improvement without operation.[8,13] Therefore, surgical attack of complete occlusions has a limited role.

The diagnosis between carotid arterial stenosis and internal carotid thrombosis is usually made by an arteriogram, but sometimes a doubt exists. Under these circumstances exploration of the carotid bifurcation is justified and if the blood in the distal internal carotid artery is fluid and a good retrograde flow is obtained then an arterial reconstruction procedure should be performed.

The so-called "kinked" carotid artery may be identified on arteriography by its markedly tortuous appearance. Despite the striking radiographic features and experimental evidence of diminished flow[14] such vessels are seldom the cause of symptomatic disease and usually do not require operative treatment. If a clear history of positional precipitation of symptoms can be obtained and reproduced on examination, treatment reasonably can be advised. These ectatic vessels are apt to be abnormally thin and friable and deserve careful handling if operated upon.

Fibromuscular hyperplasia of the carotid arteries has been treated surgically by some using the technique of dilitation of the artery,[15] patch graft or other measures.[16]

Some authors have advocated external carotid artery endarterectomy when significant stenosis of this vessel is associated with ipsilateral internal carotid artery total occlusion.[17] The rationale for this procedure rests on improvement in extracranial collateral supply to the brain. The variable nature of cerebral collaterals and the natural history after carotid occlusion make the results of such treatment difficult to evaluate.[18]

During the past 17 years changes in surgical technique and in anesthesia have improved the results, but the most important changes have been in the indications for performing these operations and in the selection of patients for this form of surgery.[12] The main indications for surgery in patients with atherosclerosis of the extracranial cerebral arteries are now considered to be:

1. Transient ischemic attacks or incipient strokes due to stenosis of the extracranial cerebral arteries.

2. Asymptomatic but significant stenosis of the common or internal carotid arteries.

3. Embolic obstruction of the extracranial cerebral arteries.

4. Patients with completed strokes due to a correctable lesion of the extracranial cerebral arteries, if surgery is performed very early (within two or three hours) or late (after at least two weeks).

5. The aortic arch syndrome.

Operation is not recommended for patients with acute progressing strokes, nor for the majority of patients with acute completed strokes.

Technique of Internal Carotid Artery Endarterectomy

We perform this operation under general anesthesia and take great care to maintain a satisfactory cardiac output and a blood pressure at least equal to the preoperative level during the period that the carotid artery is clamped. In the past we performed these operations under general anesthesia with whole-body cooling, with hypercarbia and under local anesthesia with monitoring of the cerebral function during the procedure in attempts to protect the brain during the period of carotid artery clamping, but we have abandoned these techniques as unnecessary and unhelpful.

The patient is positioned supine on the operating table and the anesthesiologist positioned laterally opposite the operative side so as to afford easy access by the assistant to a small operating field. The head is turned away from the side of operation with care not to overdo this in elderly patients with cervical osteoarthritis. Attention should also be paid to insuring adequate protection of the cornea of the eye from abrasion as the face will be covered with surgical drapes during the operation. This can be done by the installation of ophthalmic jelly beneath the eyelid or by lightly taping the eyelid shut or preferably, by doing both.

The incision is centered upon the carotid bifurcation and follows the transverse skin

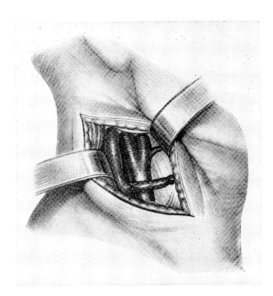

FIG. 7-2. Exposure of the carotid artery bifurcation. (Rob, C. G., and DeWeese, J. A.: Occlusions of the internal carotid and vertebral arteries. *In* Rob, C. G. (ed.): Operative Surgery, vol. 3. London, Butterworth, 1968)

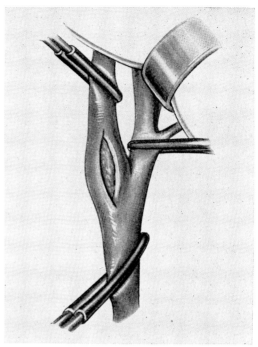

FIG. 7-3. The carotid artery incision. (Rob and DeWeese, *op. cit.*)

folds of the neck. This produces a better scar than an incision parallel to the anterior border of the sternomastoid muscle. It is important not to carry the incision too far back because the great auricular nerve may be divided producing anesthesia of the ear. After division of the facial vein the bifurcation of the common carotid artery is exposed and mobilized. At this point we divide the carotid sinus nerve and take great care to preserve the hypoglossal and vagus nerves. The hypoglossal nerve (cranial nerve XII) should be identified crossing the carotid arteries high in the neck just beneath the digastric muscle. This nerve should be carefully protected as a common cause of unnecessary postoperative morbidity is palsy of this nerve resulting in ipsilateral tongue deviation. This is seldom due to inadvertent division of the nerve, but rather to direct and excessive retraction on it, especially when the bifurcation of the carotid artery is high in the neck.

Attention should be paid to monitoring of the patient's blood pressure at frequent intervals throughout the operation, and this is especially useful during the time when the carotid bulb and carotid sinus nerve are being manipulated. Hypotension should be guarded against by both surgeon and anesthesiologist. If any significant drop in blood pressure is encountered, the anesthesiologist should infuse appropriate amounts of a premixed, immediately available solution containing a pressor drug. If the carotid sinus nerve, easily identified lying in the angle between the internal and external branches, is promptly divided before manipulation of the carotid bifurcation, hypotension and bradycardia will be infrequent. Care should be taken while dissecting in this region to avoid excessive manipulation of the carotid bifurcation and the proximal internal carotid artery so as not to dislodge embolic material from an ulcerated atherosclerotic plaque. When sufficient lengths of the vessels have been exposed and encircled with umbilical tape, the patient is given 7500 to 10,000 units of systemic, intravenous aqueous heparin.

Occluding vascular clamps are applied and a longitudinal incision is made beginning

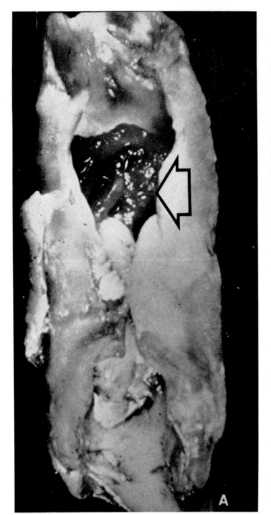 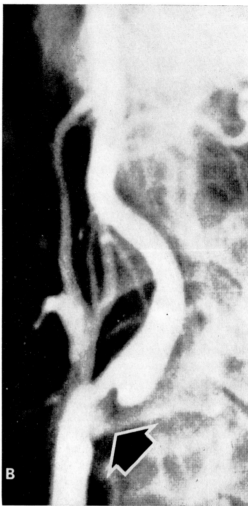

FIG. 7-4 (A). This carotid arteriogram demonstrates the typical appearance of a ulcerated atheromatous lesion. Great care should be taken not to manipulate this region during dissection of the vessels prior to clamping so as to avoid possible embolism. (B) Gross specimen of the lesion shown in the arteriogram in (A). Fibrinous and atheromatous debris can be seen within the core of the vessel which has been removed.

on the last portion of the common carotid artery and extending up the internal carotid artery to beyond the upper limit of the main atheromatous plaque. Some surgeons make an initial incision in the arterial wall only through the adventitia and outer media to enable placement of stay sutures and partial performance of the thromboendarterectomy before the vessel is occluded by clamps. This will decrease the amount of occlusion time but increase the risk of embolization of debris from the atheromatous plaque. Such a technique should be considered with caution in patients whose arteriogram or retinal findings suggest the presence of an ulcerated plaque. During the time when the carotid is clamped, the systemic blood pressure is kept approximately 20 mm. Hg above the patient's normal level recorded on the ward unless there is pre-existing significant hypertension. The strict avoidance of any hypotension during this period of the operation is

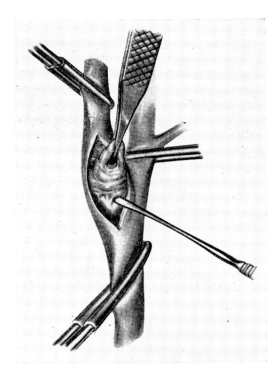

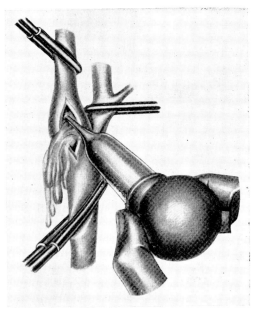

FIG. 7-6. Careful irrigation and meticulous removal of all debris. (Rob and DeWeese, *op. cit.*)

FIG. 7-5. Discussion of the atheromatous plaque. The proper plane of cleavage within the vessel wall must be obtained. This can often be identified by a distinct color change between the internal and external elastic laminae. (Rob and DeWeese, *op. cit.*)

of great importance as shown by Max, *et al.*[19]

Although many techniques have been suggested for assessing the necessity for an indwelling arterial shunt, a good and simple method is to permit a brief amount of back bleeding from the distal internal carotid artery to assess both the pressure of this flow and the color of the back bleeding. When back bleeding is of good character as judged by these criteria, the operation may be safely continued without employment of an indwelling arterial shunt. If back flow is of a questionable nature, such a shunt should be employed and should always be available for use prior to commencing this portion of the operation. Some authors have routinely employed an indwelling arterial shunt during the period of carotid artery clamping.[13] This is not a secure protection against the development of postoperative neurologic sequelae,

however, and in most cases is not necessary.[8,20,21]

It is important to remove completely the distal end of the atheromatous plaque so that the intima just distal to the thromboendarterectomy is normal or nearly so. Fortunately the plaque of atheroma usually ends within 4 cm. of the carotid bifurcation and just distal to the carotid bulb. Complete removal of the plaque prevents rethrombosis and possible distal dissection. With complete removal it is not necessary to suture the intima to the arterial wall except at the ends of the line of closure of the longitudinal arteriotomy incision.

No aspect of this operation is more important than meticulous removal of all atheromatous debris, leaving a smooth lumen free from any loose tags of medial tissue. Irrigation of the vessel should be routinely accomplished to remove even the smallest fragments of material. Other portions of the body subjected to arterial reconstruction may be tolerant of tiny embolism, but the brain is not. Compulsive attention to detail in accomplishing a technically perfect endarterectomy is of signal importance in this region

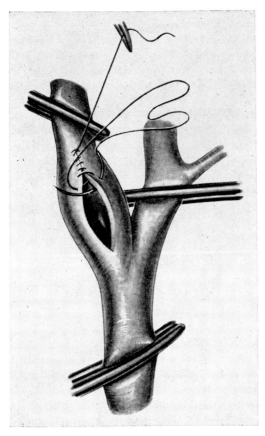

FIG. 7-7. Closure of the artery without a patch graft by careful suture technique. (Rob and DeWeese, *op. cit.*)

and will help prevent postoperative complications. If the atheromatous disease extends into the external carotid artery, this should be removed also.

Closure of the arteriotomy is accomplished with a running suture of carefully placed 5/0 silk on a fine atraumatic needle. In most cases a satisfactory closure can be achieved by simple, direct arterial suture without employment of a patch graft. The arterial clamps can now be removed and at this point the anesthesiologist counteracts the heparin with intravenous protamine sulfate. The surgeon now applies light pressure with a gauze sponge until hemostasis is complete. The wound is closed in layers and a soft Penrose drain is routinely employed. This drain is removed at the end of 24 hours and seldom drains a significant amount of material

during this time. Its purpose is prophylactic to decompress the visceral space of the neck if early postoperative hemorrhage should occur. A light, noncircumferential dressing is employed to permit easy postoperative observation of the neck.

Prevention of Complications by Preoperative Care

The important thing here is careful case selection. It must be stressed that these patients usually have generalized atherosclerosis. The operation can only have a regional effect, and so the local and regional manifestations of this generalized disease must predominate if surgery is to succeed. Fortunately this is often the case, but the usual reason for a poor result is still failure to appreciate this obvious fact. Too often a patient with very severe diffuse generalized atherosclerosis is subjected to an arterial reconstruction procedure and develops an arterial thrombosis at another site. The state of the coronary arteries is of special importance. If there is any question, a cardiologist should see the patient before operation.

Many of these patients are hypertensive or suffer from diabetes mellitus. The diabetes must be controlled before, during and after operation. In patients with arterial hypertension we do not advise reduction of the blood pressure before operation because a fall of blood pressure may be disastrous in a patient with severe carotid stenosis. Once the stenosis has been corrected, arterial hypertension should be treated.

The long-term management of the patient's primary problem, atherosclerosis, can begin before operation. If possible, the patient should stop smoking, and advice should be given on a diet and exercise. Some patients, depending on the opinion of their internist, will be taking clofibrate, aspirin, anticoagulants, vasodilators, vitamin E or other drugs in an attempt to control the atherosclerosis or the associated thrombosis. These may be continued but anticoagulants should be stopped three days before operation and started afterwards if necessary.

TABLE 7-1. TECHNIQUE OF OPERATION
FOR OCCLUSIVE DISEASE OF THE
CAROTID BIFURCATION
(1009 Patients; 192 Bilateral Operations)

Thromboendarterectomy	1168
Venous Patch	12
Prosthetic Patch	8
Resection and End-to-end Anastomosis	8
Vein Graft Replacement or Bypass	5

Postoperative Complications

We have performed a reconstruction of the bifurcation of the common carotid artery for occlusive disease on 1201 occasions. As Table 7-1 shows, this consists of thromboendarterectomy with or without patch graft angioplasty on 1188 occasions or another operation on only 13 other patients. The complications of these procedures will now be considered.

Worsening of Cerebral Function

As with most surgical operations, the incidence of complications drops with increasing experience of the surgeon, and this has been so with the reconstruction of the carotid arteries. The most important and potentially most disastrous complication is worsening of cerebral function as a direct result of the procedure. Such worsening is usually transient, but may be permanent and may even result in the death of the patient. The hospital mortality in our hands has been 27 of 1009 patients. But 19 of these patients died before 1960 after operations for progressing or acute completed strokes which we no longer consider to be indications for this form of surgery.

At one time it was thought that worsening of cerebral function in the immediate postoperative period was due to clamping of the carotid artery during operation. We now think that this is not the most common cause, and that worsening which may follow operation is usually due to embolization. Such emboli may be dislodged during mobilization of the artery before it has been clamped, during insertion of a shunt, or at the conclusion of the procedure when the clamps are opened and a loose fragment left in the vessel at the operation site becomes an embolus. The important thing is to prevent this complication by meticulous surgery and a full realization of the importance of emboli as a cause of postoperative worsening in these patients.

The other causes of worsening of cerebral function are ischemia during the period of carotid arterial occlusion and thrombosis of either an intracranial artery or the internal carotid artery at the site of operation. Worsening due to cerebral ischemia during the period of carotid artery clamping may be prevented by using an indwelling shunt. We do not use such a shunt in every case, but use it whenever there is evidence of reduced retrograde flow from the internal carotid artery after the common carotid artery has been clamped and in every patient with a history of a recent acute stroke. Retrograde flow is estimated by temporary removal of the clamp on the internal carotid artery after this vessel has been opened. If retrograde flow is fast and red, then a shunt is not inserted. If it is slow and cyanosed, or if there is any doubt, then we use an indwelling shunt. The reason why we do not use a shunt in every patient is that emboli may be dislodged when the shunt is inserted or re-

TABLE 7-2. EARLY RESULTS OF RECONSTRUCTION
OF THE CAROTID ARTERIES IN 1009 PATIENTS

Type of Stroke	No. of Patients	Good Flow Established	Asymptomatic	Objectively Better	No Change	Died
Transient	761	744	492	187	74	8
Progressing	74	35	15	15	32	12
Completed	174	92	42	76	49	7

moved. In our opinion the risk of this is sufficiently high to make the use of a shunt in every case undesirable.

Thrombosis at the site of thromboendarterectomy is rare and probably due to the excellent outflow artery in most patients. The usual cause when this complication occurs is inadequate removal of the distal portion of the atheromatous plaque. Thrombosis of an intracranial artery may develop in a previously diseased artery during the period of reduced flow when the common carotid artery is clamped. The use of an indwelling shunt in patients with known disease of the ipsilateral intracranial cerebral arteries appears to prevent this complication.

The treatment of worsening cerebral function commencing immediately or very soon after operation consists first of establishing the cause. Ophthalmodynamometry, if positive, will establish a diagnosis of internal carotid thrombosis at the site of the operation. The treatment is urgent reoperation to correct the imperfections of the first procedure. For patients without clear evidence of carotid artery thrombosis, the treatment we recommend is administration of clinical dextran intravenously unless there is evidence of cardiac decompensation, the maintenance of satisfactory cardiac output, blood pressure, oxygenation and hematocrit. Both early and long-term use of physiotherapy and speech therapy are recommended if necessary. Severe neurologic deficits will require measures to maintain a satisfactory airway such as tracheal suction or occasionally a tracheostomy. Antibiotics may be required for pulmonary infections.

Reports of attempts to treat acute postoperative carotid thrombosis by means of cervical sympathetic block have appeared in the literature. Such nonoperative methods are unlikely to prevent serious neurologic sequelae and cannot be recommended.[22]

Wound Hematoma

Hemorrhage occurring immediately postoperatively in a carotid wound is usually either from the arterial suture line or from the divided facial vein. During cough with its accompanying strenuous Valsalva maneuver, cervical venous pressures may exceed systemic arterial pressures. We recommend the drainage of the wound for the first 24 hours in every patient, and as a result hematomas and seromas have been rare. This complication can lead to severe respiratory obstruction or may be followed by a wound infection. As a result we recommend urgent reexploration of the wound if a hematoma develops. The blood clot should be evacuated and a search made for the bleeding point. Again we recommend drainage of the wound after this second procedure, and it is wise to give a course of prophylactic antibiotic therapy if it has been necessary to reopen the wound.

Damage to the Adjacent Nerves

It is important to avoid damage to the hypoglossal nerve during the initial dissection. The retraction of this nerve, if required, must be both careful and gentle if either temporary or permanent paralysis is to be avoided. It is also wise to place the incision behind and below the line of the inframandibular branch of the facial nerve and in front of the great auricular nerve to prevent weakness of the corner of the mouth or anesthesia of the ear which may follow injury to these nerves. The carotid sinus nerves are divided, and we have not encountered complications from either the unilateral or bilateral division of these nerves. Hypotension and bradycardia may occur during mobilization of the carotid bifurcation before division of these nerves.

The superior laryngeal nerve is important also. It is rarely seen during operation and is rarely divided, but it is often temporarily damaged by retraction. This results in anesthesia of the entrance to the larynx. This is not a serious problem when unilateral, but it can be disastrous if bilateral. This is one of the reasons why we do not perform bilateral carotid arterial reconstruction procedures under the same anesthetic. We recommend an interval of at least four days between the two operations when bilateral reconstruction is required.

A Technically Poor Operation

Our standard procedure is thromboendarterectomy with a simple closure. A patch graft is rarely used. Technical defects include an incomplete thromboendarterectomy, particularly at the distal end of the atheromatous plaque, which may result in postoperative thrombosis or late recurrence of symptoms due to re-stenosis. As already described, we recommend urgent operation for early postoperative thrombosis.

Sometimes thromboendarterectomy has so damaged the arterial wall that a patch graft or even complete arterial replacement is required to restore continuity. This is our main indication for patch graft angioplasty at this location. In our opinion, patch grafts are not required to increase the lumen of the carotid arteries. The lumen at the carotid bulb is larger than the lumen of the internal carotid artery, and an adequate thromboendarterectomy leaves a good lumen with the most narrow point just distal to the suture line in the internal carotid artery. If a patch graft is used the narrowest point is still at the same place in the internal carotid artery just distal to the patch. The frequent association of false aneurysm formation with the use of Dacron patch material in this vessel suggests the use of a venous patch to prevent this complication,[23,24,25] if angioplasty is required.

As Table 7-1 shows, we have used a patch in only 20 or 1.66 percent of 1201 operations for carotid stenosis. Twelve of these have been venous patches and eight Dacron patches. When a thromboendarterectomy is not possible, we restore continuity by an end-to-end anastomosis. Eight patients or 0.66 percent had this operation, and in five patients or 0.4 percent an arterial substitute was used to restore continuity.

Postoperative Hypertension

At least 10 percent of our patients had a significant rise of systolic and diastolic blood pressure very soon after operation. This usually developed in the recovery room and reached a level of 300 mm. Hg or more in several patients. At first this caused considerable alarm, and we treated some of these patients with hypotensive agents. However, none of these patients suffered any ill effects, and in every case the blood pressure returned to the preoperative level in a few days without special treatment.

Other groups have recommended control of hypertension by the use of dilute intravenous solutions of trimethaphan (Arfonad). If such hypotensive agents are employed, continuous arterial blood pressure monitoring by an indwelling catheter is recommended. Postoperative *hypo*tension is more likely to cause serious complications than is *hyper*tension. A fall of the blood pressure and of the pulse rate was noted in 60 percent of our patients during mobilization and dissection of the carotid bifurcation. However, these returned to normal very soon after the carotid sinus nerve was divided. It is our opinion that this hypotension and bradycardia may cause worsening of the cerebral status unless rapidly corrected. These patients have a stenosis of the internal carotid artery and reduction of cardiac output will produce its worth effects distal to such a lesion. For this reason we divide the carotid sinus nerve as early as possible in the operation, usually before the carotid arteries have been fully mobilized. And as stated earlier, we have not seen ill effects follow bilateral division of the carotid sinus nerves. Presumably other baroreceptor nerves arising from the aortic arch and elsewhere take on their function.

Bilateral carotid endarterectomy results in loss of carotid body function and the usual compensatory responses to hypoxia according to Wade and his associates.[26] Treatment for bilateral lesions should not be withheld for such reason, however, as this is not accompanied by clinically significant changes. Hickey and others have attempted to preserve carotid body function after bilateral carotid endarterectomy without success.[27] But, response to hypoxia was improved spontaneously after seven months.

Fifty-four percent of our patients were hypertensive at the time of preoperative examination.[8] The association of renovascular hypertension with occlusive disease of the extracranial cerebral arteries is of interest. When a patient has evidence of both occlusive disease of the extracranial cerebral arteries and hypertension, and if the patient is below 65 years of age and in good general health, we recommend arteriography of both the extracranial and renal arteries through the same Seldinger catheter positioned appropriately for each study. To date we have demonstrated a renovascular cause for hypertension in 10 percent of patients who have had this combined study. In these patients we correct the extracranial occlusive lesion first, and then about four days later operate upon the renal artery stenosis.

Wound Infection and False Aneurysm

Wound infection is almost unheard of, and late infection of an arterial suture line in the carotid artery has been seldom reported except in some cases of false aneurysm occurring in association with a Dacron patch graft. This type of patch graft material has a notorious reputation in comparison with autogenous veins, and chronic low-grade infection may be related to this observation.

Ehrenfeld and Hays have discussed the management of false aneurysms occurring after carotid surgery in four patients of whom two were infected.[28] Successful repair was accomplished.

Attempts to restore flow in the completely occluded carotid artery using manipulation of the intracranial portion of the vessel by means of the Fogarty catheter have resulted in carotid-cavernous sinus fistula.[29,30]

Postoperative Fits and Seizures

At one time we thought these were connected with postoperative hypertension, but now feel there is no connection and other causes must be looked for. This is a rare complication and has occurred in only four of our patients. One was found to have a meningioma which had not been diagnosed before the operation on this patient's carotid stenosis. In one patient no cause was found and the fits stopped after about two weeks, and two patients had an associated subclavian steal syndrome which was also operated upon. It is possible that hyperemia and edema in a previously ischemic zone may be the cause of this problem, or the cause may be a small intracerebral hematoma. Fortunately, in both these patients the fits subsided after a few weeks and have not recurred.

Rationale Against Surgery for Acute Stroke Patients

In 1957 we wrote[6] that it was better to operate at the stage of arterial stenosis in patients who were suffering from transient ischemic attacks and in 1972[31] we still consider this to be the correct policy. The reasons include the high incidence of worsening after operations on patients with progressing and acute completed strokes. This worsening is observed both in the immediate postoperative period and later due to delayed intracranial hemorrhage in some of those patients with a successful revascularization operation.[32,33,34]

The fact is that it is extremely difficult to arrange to operate early on patients with acute completed strokes. We now believe that operation should begin within two or three hours of onset of the stroke if it is to be effective in most patients. Unless the stroke is diagnosed in the recovery room after another surgical procedure, it is rarely possible to schedule operation as quickly as this even if an early diagnosis has been made. Even under these optimum conditions it is difficult to be certain that the progress of the patient is any better after a successful arterial reconstruction procedure than it would have been with good conservative care. It is well known that complete recovery often follows a major stroke which has been treated conservatively. We are therefore opposed to operation in the great majority of these patients.

Late Recurrence of Symptoms

These may be due to extension of disease to other arteries, a recurrence at the site of operation or to a completely new lesion that has developed. If late recurrence develops, an arteriogram is an important investigation. Ophthalmodynamometry may also give valuable information. Fortunately recurrence at the site of the original operation is rare and has occurred in only 11 of our patients or 0.9 percent of the operations. The reason for this is probably the extraordinarily well-localized lesion at the carotid bifurcation and the very nearly normal arterial wall immediately distal to the site of operation. A thromboendarterectomy leaves no disease in the immediate outflow artery in nearly every patient. The treatment of a recurrent stenosis is re-operation when possible.

Reconstruction of the Vertebral and Subclavian Arteries

Patient Selection

Many patients have atherosclerosis of both the internal carotid and vertebral arteries. In these patients it has been our policy to restore a normal lumen to the internal carotid arteries first and only operate upon the vertebral stenosis if symptoms persist after carotid reconstruction. The result of this policy has been that we have reconstructed about ten times as many internal carotid as vertebral arteries.[35]

The patient with vertebral artery disease has characteristic symptoms, but they are more variable than the characteristic symptoms of carotid artery disease. Dizziness, vertigo, tinnitus, syncope, blurring of vision, diplopia, hemianopsia, dysarthria, motor and sensory loss and dysesthesia particularly about the face are all symptoms encountered in patients with vertebral artery disease. It is also true that many of these same symptoms may be associated with carotid artery stenosis.

A variety of lesions may produce vertebral artery stenosis. Characteristically it is less common than carotid artery stenosis and results from a short atheromatous plaque at the origin of the vessel from the subclavian artery. The vertebral artery may also be narrowed by a fascial band in the neck, by an osseous spur impingeing on the artery during its course through the vertebral boney canal or after spinal trauma.[36]

Technique of Vertebral Reconstruction

The origin of the vertebral artery from the subclavian artery is the usual site of the lesion. The vertebral artery origin and adjacent subclavian artery can be exposed adequately by a supraclavicular approach. This is particularly true in elderly individuals because the subclavian artery tends to rise above the clavicle as the vessels leaving the aortic arch elongate and unfold with age. An incision is made above the medial end of the clavicle and the sternum. The sternomastoid muscle is divided to expose the carotid sheath. The common carotid artery is identified and mobilized. The lateral margin of the common carotid artery is then followed proximally until the subclavian artery is identified. This vessel is then isolated and the vertebral artery identified. It is important to note that the anterior scalene muscle has not been divided. Two structures must be specially identified and avoided; the recurrent laryngeal nerve on the right side of the neck and the thoracic duct on the left side.

Injury to adjacent venous structures during operation may cause significant bleeding and be difficult to control. The danger of air embolism should be born in mind. In general, more is to be gained by packing for five minutes by the clock to permit venous bleeding to cease than by an immediate attempt to repair the vein. If a real problem with the proximal subclavian or innominate vein develops, claviculectomy will measurably aid exposure.

About 3 cm. of both the subclavian and vertebral arteries are now fully mobilized and the vertebral artery followed until it enters the osseous canal. The vessels are then clamped and the origin of the vertebral artery opened by a curved incision which begins on the subclavian artery and passes up the vertebral artery. A thromboendar-

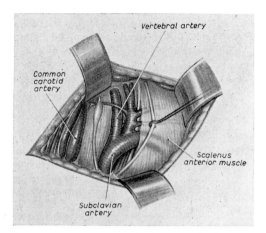

FIG. 7-8. Exposure of the vertebral artery through a cervical approach. The thromboendarectomy is then performed in the way already described. (Rob and DeWeese, *op. cit.*)

terectomy is then performed and the arterial incision closed with a venous patch graft to enlarge the lumen obtained from the external jugular or lesser saphenous vein. We believe that a patch graft angioplasty is necessary to achieve a good result here and use it in every operation at this site.

The integrity of the pleura should be checked prior to closure as the cupula of the thorax lies within the operative field. If the pleural space has been opened, the wound is closed with a catheter in place under suction which is removed after closure of the skin. A soft Penrose drain is left in the wound for 24 hours if the pleura is intact.

Postoperative Complications

The complications of vertebral reconstruction are similar to those already listed for the carotid procedure but with two differences. The first is anatomic. The right recurrent laryngeal nerve can easily be injured as it crosses the right subclavian artery. An exact dissection is necessary. This insures an anatomically intact nerve but even so paralysis may follow. Fortunately, this is usually transient if the nerve is anatomically intact. On the left side, the thoracic duct may be injured. If unrecognized this can result in a lymph fistula. The important thing is to ligate the duct if it is damaged.

The lesion is recognized by discharge of lymph into the wound. Ligation of the thoracic duct at this point is not followed by any problems because there are alternate pathways for the lymph.

The most important difference between internal carotid and vertebral arterial reconstruction is the much higher incidence of rethrombosis after the vertebral procedure. The reasons for this include the smaller size of the vertebral artery and the fact that the disease is not so well localized in the vertebral as in the internal carotid artery. Atheromatous disease often remains in the wall of the vertebral artery just distal to the operated lesion. The higher incidence of rethrombosis after vertebral reconstruction is one of the main reasons why we often recommend reconstruction of only the internal carotid artery in patients with involvement of both arterial systems. Respiratory embarrassment may be observed postoperatively from causes other than recurrent laryngeal nerve injury. The phrenic nerve may be palsied even though carefully preserved, resulting in diminished tidal volume. This can be recognized by physical signs or by inspiratory chest roentgenograms. Usually such patients will be asymptomatic at rest and only dyspneic on exertion. Unnoticed pleural injury causing pneumothorax with or without a pulmonary air leak may be a cause of early postoperative distress.[37] Unless a fluid accumulation accompanies it, such pneumothoraces can be managed without treatment or by simple needle aspiration.

Occasionally chylothorax or hemothorax will be seen postoperatively and will require tube drainage. Horner's syndrome and neck or arm pain from brachial plexus neuralgia can be prevented by avoiding excessive retraction on adjacent structures by deep instruments.

Thrombosis of the Subclavian Arteries and the Steal Syndromes

There are three major steal syndromes in the extracranial cerebral arterial circulation: the subclavian steal, the innominate steal and the carotid steal. The subclavian steal syndrome is the most frequent, both the innominate and carotid steal syndromes being rare, and still a controversial lesion. Although some experimental work has questioned the significance of retrograde vertebral artery flow in terms of its effect on overall cerebral perfusion,[38] the fact remains that symptomatic patients are seen whose postoperative improvement can only be attributed to change in vertebral artery blood flow. However, many patients with cerebral ischemic symptoms and a radiographically apparent subclavian steal syndrome will have an associated stenosis of either the internal or common carotid vessels.

Generally patients who are symptomatic from subclavian steal syndrome manifest symptoms of vertebrobasilar insufficiency, primarily vertigo, transient blindness and syncopal episodes. When these are accompanied by blood pressure differential between the two arms of 20 mm. Hg or greater and a typical radiographic appearance, treatment is indicated.[39]

In patients who do not have a blood pressure differential between the arms, another explanation for the cause of their symptoms should be sought such as cerebellar neoplasm which may present with a similar history. Occasional patients may be seen with bilateral subclavian steal who therefore do not have a blood pressure differential, but such patients will be extremely symptomatic. Failure to appreciate the significance of a contralateral subclavian stenosis may result in prompt recurrence of symptoms postoperatively.[40]

A false appearance simulating subclavian steal radiographically may result from certain catheter placement locations within the aortic arch causing the subclavian artery to appear as if it is filling late by retrograde flow when in fact it is not.[41] This appearance will not be deceiving if blood pressure differences between the arms are sought in every patient thought to have subclavian steal syndrome.

Choice of Operation

The ideal to aim at is the restoration of a normal arterial flow to both the upper limb and the brain. This, however, is not always required. Although the pathophysiology is identical in both the right and left-sided subclavian steal syndrome, the anatomic differences between the two sides influence the selection of operative procedure. Left-sided subclavian steal syndrome is somewhat more common than right-sided in most series, but the difference is not marked.

Among the procedures employed are: subclavian endarterectomy, carotid-subclavian bypass graft, subclavian-subclavian bypass graft and ipsilateral vertebral artery ligation.

Subclavian artery endarterectomy can be safely and easily approached through a supraclavicular cervical incision for right-sided lesions and has been employed as the procedure of choice. However, left subclavian artery endarterectomy requires a transthoracic approach with attendant greater morbidity and mortality. This has stimulated interest in extrathoracic methods of treatment.[42] We believe that treatment of this lesion should be different on each side of the neck. On the right a thromboendarterectomy of the occluded first part of the right subclavian artery can be performed through the incision already described for exposure of the vertebral artery. Through this incision it is also possible to perform a thromboendarterectomy of the innominate artery. In more than 80 patients we have never found it necessary in a patient with occlusive arterial disease to enlarge this simple cervical incision even by a sternal split. A curved arterial clamp is placed around the adjacent aortic arch to occlude the origin of the innominate artery and the thromboendarterectomy procedure performed in the usual way. A thromboendarterectomy of either an occluded first part of the right subclavian artery or of the innominate artery restores normal blood flow to the right upper limb and the right extracranial cerebral arteries.

On the left side the situation is different.

It is difficult and often impossible to expose the origin of the left subclavian at the aortic arch through a cervical incision. This means that a thoracotomy is often required to perform a thromboendarterectomy of the first part of the left subclavian artery. This is rarely justified because two lesser procedures produce satisfactory results. These are a bypass from the left common carotid artery to the second or third parts of the left subclavian artery or a simple ligature of the left vertebral artery in patients with a left subclavian steal syndrome.[43]

Carotid-subclavian bypass graft represents an alternative approach, applicable to either side, which is especially useful for left-sided lesions because only supraclavicular exposure is required.[44] A theoretical concern that such an anastomosis would deprive the carotid artery of blood flow has been expressed in experimental studies by Barner[45] and by others.[46] Clinical experience with its use has proved satisfactory, however, when appropriate precautions are taken to insure that patients with proximal common carotid artery lesions are excluded. The existence of a lesion in the proximal common carotid artery which is apparent on arteriography should constitute an absolute contraindication to carotid-subclavian bypass regardless of whether a pressure gradient can be demonstrated or not.

The advantages of the bypass procedure are that it increases the blood flow to the left arm and slightly increases the blood flow to the brain. The bypass may reduce the left internal carotid flow, but reverses the vertebral flow resulting in an overall increase of cerebral flow. The main disadvantage of this procedure is that there is a slight, but definite incidence of cerebral embolus during the first ten days after the operation. Presumably small emboli are common after bypass procedures. When these pass into the limbs the only ill effect is a short episode of cramplike pain or local necrosis of a small area of skin, but the same embolus can produce a serious deficit if it lodges in a branch of the middle cerebral artery.

The carotid anastomosis should be performed using a partially occluding clamp permitting continuous perfusion. Care should be taken in construction of this anastomosis particularly at the inferior aspect. Indentation of the common carotid artery by a right Dacron graft has been suspected as a possible cause of technical malfunction by resulting in proximal carotid stenosis. This consideration plus the location of the graft in a region of high motility suggests the use of autogenous vein as the graft material of choice for this procedure.

We believe that a left common carotid to subclavian bypass should be used if the patient has ischemic symptoms in the left upper limb or if the patient is left handed. For other patients the simple procedure of left vertebral artery ligation increases cerebral blood flow by abolishing retrograde flow in the left vertebral artery.[47] The slight further reduction of arterial flow to the left arm is not a problem in right-handed people.[39] It is also important to stress that many patients with cerebral symptoms and a subclavian steal syndrome have in association a stenosis of one or both internal carotid arteries. The surgical correction of this carotid arterial lesion is usually of greater therapeutic benefit than is the relief of the subclavian steal syndrome.

Subclavian-subclavian bypass graft employed by Rush and his colleagues has proved a useful measure in their hands.[48] The added difficulty of a more extensive operation and the requirement of crossing the anterior neck with a vascular graft make this approach seem less appealing than carotid-subclavian graft.

Carotid Body Tumors, Aneurysms and Other Lesions

Injuries to the carotid arteries should be repaired. Arterial aneurysms which often involve the carotid bifurcation are best treated by resection and an end-to-end anastomosis between the common and internal carotid arteries after the external carotid artery has been divided between ligatures to provide greater mobility. Sometimes a vein graft replacement is required.

Arteriovenous fistulas in this region are now rare. In the days of direct puncture vertebral arteriography an arteriovenous fistula between the vertebral artery and vein was quite a frequent complication of this procedure. This was located in the vertebral canal and was best treated either by quadruple ligature or repair of the vertebral artery with ligation of the vertebral vein. The postoperative complications of these operations do not differ from those already described, but carotid body tumors present special problems.

Carotid body tumors are usually very vascular lesions with an easily heard systolic and diastolic bruit over the tumor. If this bruit is not present the lesion is almost certainly a mass of enlarged lymph nodes. Sometimes true carotid body tumors are silent with no bruit, but this is rare. When in doubt an arteriogram helps to make the diagnosis.

The incision to expose a carotid body tumor is the same as that for reconstruction of the internal carotid artery, but after that the procedures differ. The first step is to isolate the common carotid proximally. The next, and an important step, is to isolate the internal carotid artery distal to the tumor. This must precede division of the branches of the external carotid artery. The reason is that if the external carotid branches are divided first there is a tendency to rotate the tumor so much that clot forms in the twisted internal carotid artery. Later this becomes dislodged with production of a cerebral embolus. Once the internal carotid artery has been isolated distally it can be observed and this rotation prevented. During this part of the operation it is important to identify and preserve the hypoglossal nerve and at the same time to make sure that the patient does not have an associated tumor of the glomus jugulare.

The tumor is now mobilized and the branches of the external carotid artery are divided between ligatures as they leave the tumor. These tumors are very vascular and

if the capsule is injured brisk bleeding occurs which can usually be controlled by pressure. The anesthesiologist now gives the patient heparin and then common and internal carotid arteries are clamped and the tumor divided from end to end in the line of the common and internal carotid arteries. This is most easily performed by entering the adventitia of the common carotid artery proximal to the tumor and then peeling the divided tumor off the arteries in this plane. This will leave a defect at the point of origin of the external carotid artery which is closed with sutures. The clamps are then removed, protamine sulfate given, and when hemostasis is satisfactory the wound is closed with drainage. Using this technique shunts are not required.

It has been our experience that most carotid body tumors are benign. The histologic picture is one of possible malignancy, but of 34 personal cases only one metastasized and in this case metastases were slow growing and had been present for years in the adjacent cervical nodes before they and the tumor were excised. Fear of malignancy is not really an indication for excising these tumors. Unless the surgeon is confident that he can perform the procedure without producing a cerebral deficit, it is better to observe these lesions.

The patients a surgeon operates upon with occlusive disease of the extracranial cerebral arteries are usually suffering from transient ischemic attacks or have a significant but asymptomatic arterial stenosis. In the case of asymptomatic patients and patients with transient ischemic attacks the operation is essentially a prophylactic procedure designed to prevent future and possibly catastrophic strokes. These patients often have no deficit before the operation. The surgeon's technique must therefore be meticulous and every precaution taken to prevent complications, particularly those which lead to a cerebral deficit. As has been stated on many occasions, it is impossible to improve the symptoms of an asymptomatic patient.

References

1. Hunt, J. R.: The role of the carotid arteries in the causation of vascular lesions of the brain, with remarks on certain features of symptomatology. Amer. J. Med. Sci., *147*: 704, 1914.

2. Hutchinson, E. C., and Yates, P. O.: Carotico-vertebral stenosis. Lancet, *1*:2, 1957.

3. Moniz, E.: L'Encephalographie arterille son importance daus la localizarion des tumeurs cerebralis. Rex. Neurol., *2*:72, 1927.

4. Seldinger, S. I.: Catheter replacement of the needle in percutaneous arteriography. Acta Radiol. Stockl., *39*:368, 1953.

5. Eastcott, H. H. G., Pickering, G. W., and Rob, C. G.: Reconstruction of the internal carotid artery. Lancet, *2*:994, 1954.

6. Rob, C. G., and Wheeler, H. B.: Thrombosis of internal carotid artery treated by arterial surgery. Brit. Med. J., *2*:264, 1957.

7. Hass, W. K., Fields, W. S., North, R. R., Kricheff, I. I., Chase, N. E., and Bauer, R. B.: Joint study of extracranial arterial occlusion. JAMA, *203*:159, 1968.

8. DeWeese, J. A., Rob, C. G., Satran, R., Norris, F. H., Lipchik, E. O., Zehl, D. N., and Long, J. M.: Surgical treatment for occlusive disease of the carotid artery. Ann. Surg., *168*:85, 1968.

9. Rob, C. G.: Operation for acute completed stroke due to thrombosis of the internal carotid artery. Surgery, *65*:862, 1969.

10. Ehrenfeld, W. K., Hoyt, W. F., and Wylie, E. J.: Embolization and transient blindness from carotid atheroma. Arch. Surg., *93*: 787, 1966.

11. Moore, W. S., *et al.*: Ulcerated atheroma of the carotid artery. A cause of transient cerebral ischemia. Amer. Jour. Surg., *116*: 237, 1968.

12. Rob, C. G.: The surgical treatment of occlusive disease of the extracranial cerebral arteries. *In* Dale, W. A.: Management of Arterial Occlusive Disease. pp. 345-51, Chicago, Year Book, 1971.

13. Thompson, J. E., Austin, D. J., and Patman, R. D.: Carotid endarterectomy for cerebrovascular insufficiency. Ann. Surg., *172*: 663, 1970.

14. Derrik, J. R.: Circulatory dynamics in kinking of the carotid artery. Surgery, *58*:381, 1965.

15. Morris, G. C., Lechter, A., and DeBakey, M. E.: Surgical treatment of fibromuscular disease of the carotid arteries. Arch. Surg., *96*:636, 1968.

16. Perry, M. O.: Fibromuscular disease of the carotid artery. Surg. Gynec. Obst., *134*:57, 1972.

17. Diethrich, E. B., Liddicoat, J. E., McCutchen, J. J., and DeBakey, M. E.: Surgical significance of the external carotid artery in the treatment of cerebrovascular insufficiency. J. Cardiov. Surg., *3*:213, 1968.

18. Fields, W. S., Bruetman, M. E., and Weibel, J.: Collateral circulation of the brain. Mono. Surg. Sci., *2*:183, 1967.

19. Max, T. C., Muyshondt, E., Schwartz, S. I., and Rob, C. G.: Studies of carotid blood flow in unilateral occlusion. Arch. Surg., *86*:65, 1963.

20. Bloodwell, R. D., Hallman, G. L., Keats, A. S., and Cooley, D. A.: Carotid endarterectomy with a shunt. Arch. Surg., *96*:644, 1968.

21. Wylie, E. J., and Ehrenfeld, W. K.: *In* Extracranial Occlusive Cerebrovascular Disease. pp. 191-2, W. B. Saunders, Philadelphia, 1970.

22. Gilligan, B. S., and Stirling, G. R.: Cervical sympathetic block in the treatment of acute hemiplegia following carotid endarterectomy. Med. J. Aust., *2*:1022, 1967.

23. Raskind, R., and Doria, A.: Wound complications following carotid endarterectomy —Report of two cases. Vasc. Surg., *1*:127, 1967.

24. Vellar, I. D.: Aneurysm of the internal carotid artery following endarterectomy for carotid stenosis. Med. J. Aust., *2*:803, 1969.

25. Ahliquist, R. E., Jr.: False aneurysms complicating synthetic arterial reconstruction. Am. Surg., *36*:627, 1970.

26. Wade, J. G., Larson, C. P., Jr., Hickey, R. F., *et al.*: Effect of carotid endarterectomy on carotid chemoreceptor and baroreceptor function in man. New Eng. J. Med., *282*:823, 1970.

27. Hickey, R. F., Ehrenfeld, W. K., Hamilton, F. N., and Larson, C. P., Jr.: Bilateral carotid endarterectomy with attempted preservation of carotid body function. Ann. Surg., *175*:268, 1972.

28. Ehrenfeld, W. K., and Hays, R. J.: False aneurysms after carotid endarterectomy. Arch. Surg., *104*:288, 1972.

29. Davie, J. C., and Richardson, R.: Distal internal carotid thromboendarterectomy using a Fogarty catheter in total occlusion. J. Neurosurg., *27*:171, 1967.

30. Barker, W. F., Stern, W. E., Krayenbuhl, H., and Senning, A.: Carotid endarterectomy complicated by carotid cavernous sinus fistula. Ann. Surg., *167*:568, 1968.

31. Rob, C. G.: The origin and development of surgery for occlusive disease of the carotid arteries. Rev. Surg., *29*:1, 1972.

32. Gonzalez, L. L., and Lewis, C. M.: Cerebral hemorrhage following successful endarterectomy of the internal carotid artery. Surg. Gynec. Obst., *122*:773, 1966.

33. Bland, J. E., Chapman, R. D., and Wylie, E. J.: Neurological complications of carotid artery surgery. Ann. Surg., *171*:459, 1970.

34. Brentman, M. E., Fields, W. S., Crawford, E. S., and DeBakey, M. E.: Cerebral hemorrhage in carotid artery surgery. Arch. Neurol., *9*:458, 1963.

35. Rob, C. G.: Obliterative disease of the extracranial cerebral arteries—surgical treatment. *In* Stroke Symposium. Stockholm, Nordiska Bokhandelns Forlag, 1967, pp. 267-75.

36. Bell, H. S.: Basilar artery insufficiency due to atlanto-occipital instability. Amer. Surg., *35*:695, 1969.

37. Wheeler, H. B.: Surgical treatment of subclavian artery occlusions. New Eng. J. Med., *276*:711, 1967.

38. Eklof, B., and Schwartz, S. I.: Effects of subclavian steal and compromised cephalic blood flow on cerebral circulation. Surgery, *68*:431, 1970.

39. Resnicoff, S. A., DeWeese, J. A., and Rob, C. G.: Surgical treatment of the subclavian steal syndrome. Circulation 41, Supplement *2*:147, 1970.

40. McDowell, H. A., Jr.: Surgical correction of vertebral steal followed by contralateral retrograde vertebral flow. Ann. Surg., *168*: 154, 1968.

41. Pineda, A.: True and false subclavian steal syndromes. Arch. Surg., *92*:258, 1966.

42. Blaisdell, W. F., Clauss, R. H., Gailbraith, J. G., Imparato, A. M., and Wylie, E. J.: Joint study of extracranial arterial occlusion. IV. A review of surgical considerations. JAMA, *209*:1889, 1969.

43. Rob, C. G.: Technique of surgical therapy. *In* Siekert, R. G., and Whisnat, J. P.: Princeton Conference on Cerebrovascular Disease; New York, Grune & Stratton, 1961, p. 110.

44. Diethrich, E. B., Garrett, H. E., Ameriso, J., Crawford, E. S., El-Bayar, M., and DeBakey, M. E.: Occlusive disease of the common carotid and subclavian arteries treated by carotid-subclavian bypass: Analysis of 125 cases. Amer. J. Surg., *114*:800, 1967.

45. Barner, H. B., Rittenhouse, E. A., and Willman, V. L.: Carotid-subclavian bypass for "subclavian steal syndrome". J. Thor. Cardiov. Surg., *55*:773, 1968.

46. Lord, R. S., and Ehrenfeld, W. K.: Carotid-subclavian bypass—A hemodynamic study. Surgery, *66*:521, 1969.

47. Yum, K. Y., and Myers, R. N.: Vertebral artery ligation. *In* Management of the Subclavian Steal Syndrome. Arch. Surg., *98*: 199, 1968.

48. Finkelstein, N. M., Byer, A., and Rush, B. F., Jr.: Subclavian-subclavian bypass for the subclavian steal syndrome. Surgery, *71*:142, 1972.

Chapter 8 | Complications of

Visceral Arterial Procedures

Complications Associated with the Operative Treatment of Renovascular Hypertension[*]

John H. Foster, M.D., and Richard H. Dean, M.D.

The successful operative management of the patient with renovascular hypertension (RVH) requires meticulous attention to detail. Although renal revascularization has the attendant complications associated with any major vascular procedure, the added insult of the side effects of hypertension and the drugs used to treat hypertension increase the propensity for complications during the perioperative period.

In a recent review of our experience with the operative management of 122 patients with renovascular hypertension,[1] over 60 per cent had evidence of associated left ventricular hypertrophy, overt heart disease, or cerebrovascular disease. These disorders added to the fluid and electrolyte aberrations associated with hypertension and renal dysfunction combine to form a very precarious pre- and postoperative state. Many of the complications described in this chapter may be averted and the remainder minimized by a systematic approach to the patient and attention to the multiple details of evaluation and management.

Patient Selection and Errors in Diagnosis

Historically the surgical treatment of renovascular hypertension has undergone wide fluctuations in its acceptance. Following the experimental work of Goldblatt,[2] later corroboration by Page and Corcoran,[3] many centers performed nephrectomy based on the indications of a small kidney demonstrated by intravenous pyelography and concomitant hypertension. This proved to be no panacea. Reports such as Smith,[4] in 1956, which showed only a 26 per cent cure of hypertension, dampened the earlier enthusiasm for the surgical treatment of hypertension. In the mid 1950's aortography came into widespread use. In this era many patients with hypertension and renal artery stenosis, demonstrated arteriographically, had operative treatment. However, less than 50 per cent were benefited. Only in the past decade has sufficient knowledge of the pathophysiology of renovascular hypertension allowed a renewed interest in the applicability of operative management. The establishment of meaningful studies of split renal function (by Howard, et al.[5] and by Stamey, et al.[6]) and of a reliable assay of plasma renin has made possible surgical treatment for those

* Supported in part by: NIH Grant #5 P17 HL 14192, Specialized Center of Research in Hypertension and NIH Grant #5 M01 RR 00095, Clinical Research Center.

patients with renal artery stenosis who have renovascular hypertension.

Controversy has continued in some centers regarding intensive evaluation of certain groups of patients for the presence of renovascular hypertension. Chamberlain[7] feels that liberal use of arteriography is too high a price to pay for recognition of the occasional patient who may have renovascular hypertension. Sixteen per cent of the patients studied by our group have proven to have RVH. Ours is admittedly a selected series, and the true incidence of RVH in the hypertensive population is unknown. From our experience it seems very likely that at least 5 per cent of the hypertensive population has renovascular hypertension. It has been variously estimated that 30 to 60 million people in the United States have hypertension, thus by our estimate, 1.5 to 3 million people have RVH.

Shapiro advocates investigating only those patients with "positive" rapid-sequence intravenous pyelograms and recommends operative treatment only to patients under 50 to 55 years old with contralateral good renal function.[8] In our 122 patients with RVH the rapid-sequence intravenous pyelogram gave a false-negative result in 31 per cent of the patients. Fifty-two of the patients were over 50 years of age, and 85 per cent of them were either cured or improved following operative treatment. The operative mortality (10 per cent) was higher in these older patients, but this mortality occurred primarily in patients who had simultaneous operative treatment of extrarenal vascular lesions such as abdominal aortic aneurysm or aortic occlusive disease. Four of the seven operative deaths occurred in such patients.

Over the past 12 years all patients admitted for evaluation of hypertension at the Vanderbilt University Hospital have undergone a general evaluation that includes the measures listed below. If a significant lesion is found on arteriography, the patient is then submitted to differential renal vein renin assay and split renal function studies (Howard and Stamey Tests). Using this protocol, 1,070 patients have undergone evaluation (Table 8-1). Forty-three per cent, or 460 patients, were found to have renal artery lesions, and 176 patients, or 39 per cent of the patients with renal artery stenosis, were found to have renovascular hypertension by our criteria for establishing the diagnosis (i.e., positive split renal function studies and/or renal venous renin assays).

We have used liberal criteria for a "positive" test in interpreting the results of the split renal function studies: (1) Consistent discrepancies in all three samples; (2) Howard Test—25 per cent reduction in urine volume and 15 per cent increase in creatinine concentration from the involved kidney as compared with the contralateral side; and (3) Stamey Test—25 per cent increase in PAH concentration and 25 per cent reduction in urine volume when comparing the side with renal artery stenosis to the uninvolved side. The renal vein renin assay was considered "positive" if the ratio of renin activity from the involved to the uninvolved kidney ratio is 1.5 or greater. Of our 122 patients, 101 underwent Howard

TABLE 8-1. RESULTS OF EVALUATION OF 1,070 HYPERTENSIVE PATIENTS

	Renal Arteriogram	Renovascular Hypertension*	
Normal	610 (57%)	—	} 16%
Renal artery stenosis due to:			
Atherosclerosis	297 } (43%)	114 } 39%**	
Fibromuscular dysplasia	163	62	

* Positive functional tests—split renal function studies or renal venous renin assays.
** 122 of these patients have had operative treatment and a minimum follow up of at least 12 months.

and Stamey Tests, and 99 had renal vein renin assay prior to operation. Using the above criteria, 97 per cent of the patients with unilateral lesions had a positive Howard or Stamey Test and 80 per cent had a positive renin assay. When these tests are combined, all patients with unilateral lesions had either a positive Howard Test, a positive Stamey Test or a positive renal vein renin assay.

A most difficult problem is the patient with severe bilateral renal artery lesions. In most instances the functional studies did lateralize to one side and thereby indicated the primary cause of the hypertension. There were 39 patients with bilateral renal artery stenosis and resultant RVH. Twenty-eight had lateralizing split renal function studies or renal vein renin assays by the above criteria. In patients with severe hypertension and marked bilateral lesions without lateralizing functional studies, we have adopted the policy of reconstructing only one side initially. If hypertension persists, split renal function studies and renal vein renin assay are repeated. Occasionally, however, we have done bilateral renal artery reconstruction in patients with severe stenoses and bilateral elevated renal vein renin assays. However, we have serious reservations about simultaneous bilateral renal artery recon-

GENERAL EVALUATION OF PATIENT WITH HYPERTENSION

History and Physical Examination

Hemogram, SMA 12, Urinalysis, Urine Culture, Serum Kx3, Electrocardiogram and Chest X-Ray, Analysis of 24-Hour Urine Collection for:

Creatinine clearance, Electrolytes, Catecholamines, VMA, and 17OH Steroids and Ketosteroids

Rapid Sequence Intravenous Pyelogram

Renal Arteriography

struction as will be noted subsequently in this chapter.

Occasionally a patient will present with RVH and severe extrarenal vascular lesions. The abdominal aortogram of such a patient is seen in Figure 8-1. This patient had celiac artery occlusion, superior mesenteric artery stenosis, aortic occlusion, occlusion of one renal artery, and greater than 90 per cent stenosis of the other renal artery. He had abdominal angina; his hypertension was uncontrollable; and his lower extremities were of borderline viability. As a life-saving procedure, we have undertaken operative correction of both the renal and extrarenal lesions in such patients. Of 16 patients in

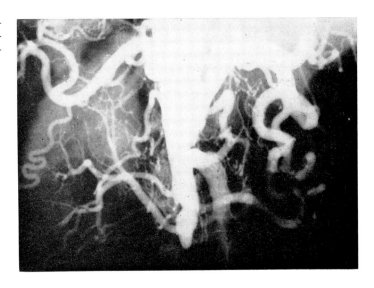

FIG. 8-1. Anteroposterior aortogram showing severe bilateral renal and extrarenal vascular lesions.

this extreme category, 12 are living, relatively well and their hypertension improved or cured (Fig. 8-2).

Considerations in Preoperative Evaluation and Management

Many patients present with severely elevated diastolic pressures ranging from 140 to 160 mm. Hg. In this group of patients, the first priority of management is control of hypertension. The subjection of patients with uncontrolled hypertension to the multiple diagnostic procedures may have catastrophic consequences. Only after an adequate period of treatment with antihypertensive medications are these patients submitted to an evaluation for the presence of a curable lesion.

Rapid Sequence Excretory Pyelogram

Many physicians still rely on the rapid sequence intravenous pyelogram alone to screen patients for the presence of significant renal arterial lesions and resultant hypertension. The findings suggestive of the presence of RVH are: (1) Unilateral delay in calyceal appearance time; (2) Difference in renal length of 1.5 cm or more as compared to the contralateral kidney; (3) Hypercon-

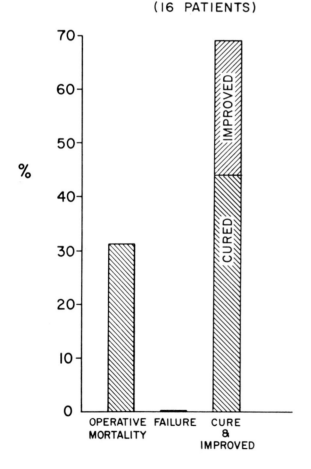

RESULTS OF COMBINED OPERATIONS

SIMULTANEOUS OPERATIVE TREATMENT OF
RENAL AND EXTRA RENAL VASCULAR LESIONS
(16 PATIENTS)

Fig. 8-2. Early results of simultaneous treatment of renal and extrarenal lesions in 16 patients.

centration of the contrast medium on late films; (4) Ureteral notching secondary to increased size and tortuosity of the ureteral artery; and (5) Defect in the renal silhouette suggestive of segmental renal infarction. In 122 proven cases of RVH only 69 per cent in our experience had a "positive" IVP using the above criteria (Fig. 8-3).

Although we do not believe the rapid sequence intravenous pyelogram should be used as the sole screening test for the detection of renovascular hypertension, it is valuable in the evaluation of associated lesions of the genitourinary tract. Furthermore, if positive preoperatively, it is a simple examination which gives valuable information in postoperative assessment of the revascularization. A normal postoperative pyelogram is very reassuring. Allergic reactions are the only important complication secondary to intravenous pyelography. Most are associated with urticaria and wheezing and are readily controlled by the administration of intravenous antihistamine preparations. The rare instance of hypotension and sudden death from anaphylactic shock has been recorded by Pendergrass[9] to occur once per 120,000 injections, but it has never occurred in our experience.

Renal Arteriography

There continues to be controversy over the use of aortography and renal arteriography in the routine screening of hypertensive individuals. Some feel it should be reserved for select groups of patients. We do not share this conservative view and proceed with arteriography in any patient who would be a candidate for renal artery revascularization if a lesion were found, irrespective of intravenous pyelogram results, age, or duration of known hypertension.

In our institution, renal arteriography is performed via the percutaneous retrograde femoral route. When known disease of this vessel precludes its use, the transaxillary approach is utilized. Of 1,423 renal arteriograms in 1,070 patients with hypertension, no deaths have occurred, and complications attended the procedure in only 10 patients (0.7 per cent). In a larger survey conducted by Lang[10] involving 11,402 retrograde percutaneous aortograms, there were only seven deaths (.06 per cent) and 81 (0.7 per cent)

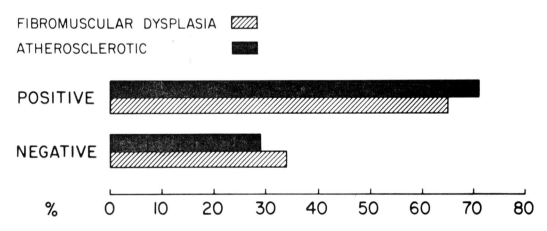

FIG. 8-3. Interpretation of preoperative rapid sequence pyelogram in 122 patients with proven renovascular hypertension.

serious complications. Errors in interpretation of renal arteriography can occur when the renal artery is examined only in the anteroposterior projection. Some lesions situated near the orifice of the renal artery can be masked in the A-P plane. They can be masked in the distal renal artery, also. Oblique projections are required to demonstrate such lesions (Fig. 8-4) and should be used in all examinations.

Although allergic phenomena occur with arteriography, reactions are less common than with intravenous pyelography. In instances of previous allergy to intravenous pyelography, we prepare to treat an allergic reaction following aortography but rarely have to do so. This is commonly thought to be due to the fact that serious reactions to injections of contrast media are related to the high concentration of the drug reaching the lungs following intravenous injection. Intraarterial injections rarely cause a problem.

Renal toxicity of contrast media has long been recognized.[11] Although the true incidence of transient renal damage from contrast media is unknown, it is probably much more frequent than is commonly recognized. Severe toxicity is accompanied by albuminuria, hematuria, oliguria, and azotemia. The specific etiology of this toxicity is uncertain, but it is probably related to the amount and concentration of the contrast media perfus-

ing the kidney. The time of exposure of the kidneys to the medium is also important[12] and severe toxicity is more likely in patients with diffuse parenchymal disease. Because of the real possibility of renal toxicity, we routinely obtain pre- and postarteriographic blood urea nitrogen levels. Occasionally the post study value will be elevated. Since the injury is usually transient, further evaluation and operation are delayed until renal function has returned to the prearteriogram level. This problem is treated more extensively Chapter 1.

Although extremely rare, red blood cell agglutination[13] and hemolytic phenomena sometimes occur following abdominal aortography. For this reason, we also routinely recheck serum hemoglobin and hematocrit levels following arteriography.

Another rare complication of the injection of contrast media is hypotension. It is usually mild, transient, and often goes undocumented. Its significance is usually clouded by the use of premedications and psychosomatic reactions consequent to arteriography. A much more hazardous problem however is the precipitation of a hypertensive crisis in patients with unsuspected pheochromocytoma as the etiology of the hypertension. Because of this remote possibility, we assay urinary catecholamines and/or vanillyl mandelic acid levels prior to this examination in

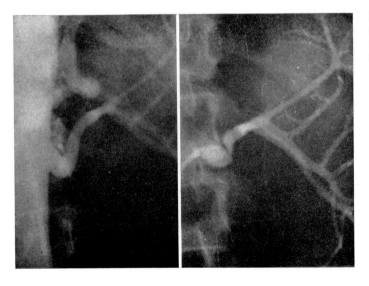

Fig. 8-4. Anteroposterior and oblique renal arteriogram showing stenosis only in the oblique projection.

patients with any sign or symptom suggestive of the condition.

Technical complications of percutaneous retrograde aortography and renal arteriography include femoral artery thrombosis, plaque dislodgement and embolism, subintimal dissection, false aneurysm, and aortic perforation by the guide wire or catheter. Femoral thrombosis is the most common serious complication encountered and can usually be recognized at the time of arteriography. Although distinction must be made between this and severe arterial spasm, if improvement is not prompt following the institution of heparin anticoagulation, one should proceed to exploration and thrombectomy. Finally, hematoma formation at the site of arterial puncture is the most common complication and is much more likely in hypertensive patients. For this reason, manual pressure should be applied to the puncture site for at least fifteen minutes following completion of arteriography. This is then followed for the ensuing 12 hours with frequent blood pressure determination and observation for local bleeding.

Renal Venous Renin Assays

Transfemoral venous catheterization of the renal veins is a relatively innocuous test. In over 500 selective renal vein renin assays during the past seven years only one major complication was encountered. This patient had femoral vein thrombosis with subsequent pulmonary embolism but recovered completely and subsequently had successful bilateral renal artery revascularization. Other complications such as renal vein thrombosis or perforation are, at most, rare with this procedure and have not occurred in our experience.

Split Renal Function Studies

Since the establishment of reliable assays for renin, some centers question the need for the concomitant use of split renal function studies in the evaluation of renal arterial lesions.[14,15,16] These investigators feel that the risk of complications coupled with the

inaccuracies of the studies limit their usefulness, and they employ renal vein renin determinations alone. In contrast, others feel as we do, that valuable diagnostic and management insight can be obtained by the use of both studies.[17] We have found split renal function tests especially helpful in evaluating the viability of severely ischemic kidneys and the likelihood of salvage in these instances. In unilateral renal artery stenosis they are useful in evaluating renal function in the contralateral kidney. Furthermore, in our experience, about 10 per cent of patients with unilateral RVH who have been cured following operative treatment had nonlateralizing renin results and lateralizing split renal function studies. An equal number of different patients had negative split renal function studies and positive renin ratios.

Serious complications associated with split renal function studies include subsequent urinary tract infection, bacteremia, ureteral edema and obstruction with resultant oliguria or anuria, and azotemia. In Dahl's series[18] of 271 studies, serious complications occurred in only 5 per cent, while minor complaints of headache, suprapubic pain, flank pain, nausea, and dysuria were seen in 39 per cent. Rhamy, et al.[19] have reviewed the complications attendant to 1,633 studies performed in the recent Cooperative Study of Renal Vascular Hypertension. Major complications were uncommon, occurring in 3.1 per cent, and minor complications occurred in 32.8 per cent. A significant increase in problems was also seen when large ureteral catheters were employed (greater than #7 French). Technically unsatisfactory tests were less common with regional anesthesia (12 per cent) than local (15 per cent) or general anesthesia (29 per cent). We routinely obtain pre- and postexamination blood urea nitrogen levels and urine cultures. In those patients with preexisting urinary tract infections, the study is withheld until a successful course of appropriate antibiotics has sterilized the urine. Likewise, in the rare case of *induced* azotemia or urinary tract infection, operation is delayed until the patient has fully recovered.

In our experience with over 500 studies in 439 patients, serious complications of urinary infection or azotemia were encountered in nine patients. Each patient recovered fully, so there was no lasting damage. Flank pain is a very common complaint, and analgesics are frequently required for 12 to 18 hours after examination. Liberal fluid intake minimizes this complication.

Other Preoperative Considerations

Several other considerations are important in patients to be submitted to operative management of renovascular hypertension. Since most of these patients will have been taking antihypertensive medications, and because of the inherent impairment of renal function, fluid and electrolyte imbalances are often present. To alleviate untoward effects of hypokalemia, close evaluation of serum electrolytes is necessary. Likewise, concomitant heart disease and congestive failure may be present secondary to prolonged uncontrolled hypertension. In these cases preoperative digitalization is often required. During the postoperative period we rely heavily on daily body weight in regulating fluid therapy. Preoperative body weight is recorded using the same scales to be used in the postoperative period.

Occasionally patients who present for surgical correction of renovascular hypertension have significant cerebrovascular disease. We recommend arteriographic study of the cerebrovascular tree in all patients with a past history of cerebrovascular disease and in any patient with a carotid bruit. We agree with Javid[20] that significant obstructive carotid lesions should be corrected prior to any other major operative procedure. This is especially appropriate in the patient who is to undergo correction of RVH. Since perfusion pressure may be significantly reduced postoperatively and the possibility of episodes of relative hypotension during the operative period is great, the likelihood of stroke is greater in these patients. Therefore,

if significant carotid artery lesions are found, they are corrected prior to any renovascular operation. We have done this for 20 patients (five bilaterally) who subsequently had renal artery surgery. There were no postoperative central nervous system problems in any of these patients.

The preoperative management of antihypertensive medications is occasionally a problem. Drugs such as guanethidine and reserpine should be stopped at least 2 weeks before surgery. For those patients with severe diastolic pressures in excess of 120 in whom continued medications are required, alphamethyldopa is preferred because it does not deplete nerve endplates stores of epinephrine and norepinephrine and its effects are of relatively short duration. Ordinarily it can be discontinued 24 hours prior to operation, but in over 40 cases in which it was continued until the time of operation, no untoward effects were seen. It is most important for the anesthesiologist to know what medications the patient has been taking so he can take steps to avoid intra- or postoperative hypotension.

Blood volume determinations should be performed preoperatively in all patients. In our experience, 27 per cent of patients undergoing operative treatment had significant deficits in red blood cell mass or plasma volume. In these 33 patients, deficits in total blood volume ranged up to 1,740 cc. (see Table 8-2). Any patient with a blood volume deficit of 500 cc. or greater should have this replaced in the 24 hours prior to operation to avoid hypotensive episodes in the intra- and postoperative periods. Early in our experience we encountered serious post-

TABLE 8-2. PREOPERATIVE BLOOD VOLUME DEFICITS IN 33 PATIENTS

Deficit	Mean (ml.)	Range (ml.)
Blood Volume	997	504-1740
Red Blood Cell	560	90- 984
Plasma Volume	438	45-1140

operative thrombotic complications which were directly attributable to unrecognized blood volume deficits. We delay restoration of any blood volume deficit until the day prior to operation in order to avoid aggravation of the patient's hypertension by volume expansion.

Finally, the benefits of preoperative instruction in pulmonary toilet and introduction to assistive pulmonary devices is obvious. As in any other major abdominal procedure, the propensity for atelectasis and retained pulmonary secretions in the immediate postoperative period can be minimized by instruction in the correct use of these measures.

Intraoperative Considerations

Certain general considerations are of note in the intraoperative management of patients undergoing renal revascularization. If the patient has been on drugs such as reserpine or guanethidine preoperatively it will take 10 to 14 days after cessation of these drugs for the effects to be cleared. As mentioned above, they should be discontinued or replaced by Alphamethyldopa 2 weeks prior to operation. Rarely, operation may be required while the effects of reserpine or guanethidine are still present. The possibility of profound vasomotor collapse is real in this setting, and preventive measures should be readily available. Because the stores of epinephrine and norepinephrine are severely depleted, we recommend the use of a neosynephrine infusion, because its action is not dependent on the release of endogenous epinephrine and norepinephrine.

Patients with RVH frequently have impairment of both renal and cardiac function. Renal ischemia during revascularization causes further impairment, at least temporarily, of renal function. Because of this, intravenous fluids must be administered very judiciously. If appropriate steps are taken to replenish preoperative blood volume deficits and if intraoperative blood loss is recorded accurately and appropriately replaced, large fluid loads are not required and should

not be given. Continuous monitoring of central venous pressure and urine output are helpful in assessing fluid balance and avoiding overload in these patients with secondary myocardial disease and renal impairment. Fluid overload is frequently the cause of congestive failure, pulmonary edema, and further aggravation of the hypertension in these patients. Conversely, inadequate blood replacement and resultant hypotension is also poorly tolerated, especially when concomitant coronary or cerebrovascular disease is present.

In all revascularization procedures, we routinely use systemic anticoagulation, 5,000 units heparin is administered intravenously prior to application of occluding vascular clamps. If bleeding is excessive following completion of all anastomoses, this can be counteracted with protamine, but this is rarely necessary with present-day suture techniques. Mannitol is administered both prior to and during the period of renal artery occlusion. Its osmotic diuretic effect and its possible direct effect on the arteriolar walls of the kidney to provide some vasodilatation combine to give significant protection against acute tubular necrosis. There are many different declamping routines following aortic cross-clamping. Aortic occlusion time is usually very short (10 to 15 min.) during the construction of an aortorenal bypass. When this is the case, administration of sodium bicarbonate is not required. If occlusion time is long, as in transaortic bilateral renal endarterectomy or concomitant aorto-iliac grafting, $NaHCO_3$ is given immediately prior to aortic clamp release. Cautious administration of a fluid load is also used if occlusion time has been long. When this is necessary, we prefer an osmotically active colloid solution of whole blood over simple electrolyte solutions.

Complications Associated with Specific Operations

A wide variety of operations have been employed for revascularization of the renal artery. Table 8-3 depicts the variety of procedures employed in our experience with 122 patients over the past 11 years. Since splenorenal shunts and the resection of lesions with reimplantation of the renal artery are rarely used now, they will not be discussed in this chapter. Saphenous vein aortorenal bypass has been the mode of revascularization most frequently employed (55 per cent). Dacron aortorenal bypass was employed in 23 per cent, while thromboendarterectomy (both transrenal and transaortic) was used in 19 per cent and autogenous hypogastric arterial graft used in only three patients (3 per cent).

Although the use of an autogenous saphenous vein introduces the possible complication of thigh hematoma in the heparinized patient, this can be averted by exact hemostasis at the time of vein procurement. We also routinely use a Hemo-Vac drain in the thigh incision. We have had one patient who required formal drainage of a large groin hematoma. There was no late morbidity associated with this complication. Because of the theoretical advantage of using autogenous artery for arterial bypasses, some authors have advocated the use of an autog-

enous hypogastric artery for the graft.[21,22] We have very limited experience with this technique. If it is used, one should have careful ateriographic visualization of the vascular supply to the bowel preoperatively. Occasionally patients will have occlusive lesions of the celiac, superior mesenteric, and/or inferior mesenteric artery. In this setting the sacrifice of the hypogastric may lead to abdominal angina and possible bowel infarction. Ordinarily the hypogastric artery is not an important source of arterial blood supply to the intestines. However, such a phenomenon occurred in one of our three patients who had an aortorenal bypass utilizing the hypogastric artery. This seven-year-old boy had RVH with concomitant multivessel involvement of his celiac, superior mesenteric, and inferior mesenteric arteries with fibrodysplastic disease. Subsequent aortosuperior mesenteric artery bypass relieved his symptoms of severe intestinal angina. The hypogastric artery in older patients may contain significant atheromatous disease that necessitates thromboendarterectomy prior to its use as a bypass graft. Whether these grafts will prove to be superior to saphenous vein grafts will only be

TABLE 8-3. PRIMARY OPERATIVE PROCEDURES

| Procedure | Renal Artery Lesion | | |
	Fibromuscular Dysplasia	Atherosclerosis	Total
VEIN BYPASS GRAFTS			
Single Aortorenal	22	25	47
Bilateral Aortorenal	3	5	8
DACRON BYPASS GRAFTS			
Single Aortorenal	1	10	11
Bilateral Aortorenal	1	7	8
THROMBOENDARTERECTOMY			
Single	3	13	16
Bilateral		3	3
NEPHRECTOMY	11	15	26
OTHER			
Autogenous Arterial Bypass	3	—	3
	44	78	122

Fig. 8-5. Graphic demonstration of intimal flap at suture line and the preferred method of management.

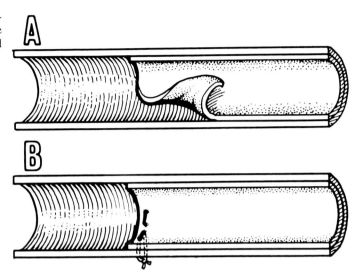

determined by long-term follow-up studies. There is accumulating evidence that saphenous vein grafts sometimes develop aneurysmal changes.[23]

Errors of Technique

Intimal Flap Creation Revascularization of atherosclerotic lesions of the renal arteries often entails thromboendarterectomy to some extent. When the lesion is at the orifice of the renal artery, this can often be performed by a transaortic approach. If the lesion is more distal or if the endarterectomy is performed in conjunction with an aortorenal bypass, it is approached through a renal arteriotomy. In either instance the possibility of creating an intimal flap exists (Fig. 8-5). The intimal flap must be either trimmed

away or meticulously tacked down with fine interrupted mattress sutures, preferably with the use of magnifying loops. With transrenal thromboendarterectomy the distal intima is easily visualized and appropriately handled. With the transaortic approach, visualization may be more difficult. In this case an "on the table" arteriogram, as recommended by Wylie and Stoney,[21] should be done at the end of this procedure. If an intimal flap is found, it must be corrected.

Renal Artery Injury In performing end-to-side anastomoses, it is easy to injure the renal artery. If the surgeon injudiciously performing arteriotomy inserts the scalpel too deeply, he can easily lacerate the opposite wall of the vessel (Fig. 8-6). A #11 scalpel blade should be used to make a very

Fig. 8-6. Schematic representation of incorrect (*A*) and correct (*B*) method of performing arteriotomy.

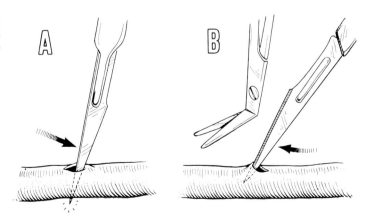

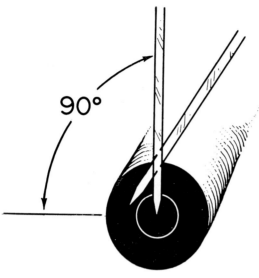

FIG. 8-7. Sketch illustrating hazard of angulation of scalpel from a 90-degree angle with the vessel lumen during arteriotomy.

small arteriotomy which is then extended with right angle scissors. Likewise, by inadvertent angulation of the scalpel from a 90-degree angle with the plane of the lumen, it is possible to miss the lumen completely or enter the vessel lateral to the ideal entrance point (Fig. 8-7).

Graft Misalignment and Anastomotic Stenosis Several errors in technique can lead to anastomotic stenosis and bypass thrombosis.

Early in our experience, we used a running simple suture from each vertex of the anastomosis. This can result in a purse-string effect if too much tension is held on the suture while making the anastomosis. Furthermore, any artery that is cross-clamped undergoes a relative state of collapse. Arterial pressure is no longer distending the vessel. An anastomosis made in the collapsed state will have a purse-string effect when the vessel is again distended by arterial pressure. To avert these problems, we use four interruption points in the anastomosis (Fig. 8-8) and distention of the arteriotomy by traction on the four sutures. The use of operating loop magnification also helps with the exact placement of the sutures in performing these anastomoses.

Malan[24] has stated that when the angle between the direction of flow in the aorta and a graft or between the graft and the distal renal artery exceeds 90°, turbulence at the anastomotic site is increased and thrombosis is more likely to ensue. (Fig. 8-9 attempts to depict the hemodynamic consequences of various anastomotic angles in accordance with this concept.) If this concept is correct, end to end anastomosis between the graft (Fig. 8-10) and the renal artery would be advantageous, and, by the same token, suprarenal aortic implantation

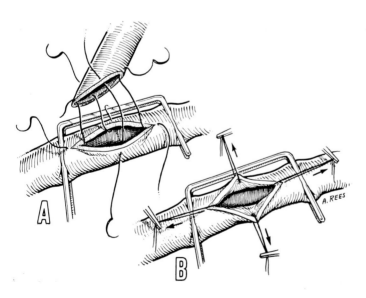

FIG. 8-8. Illustrative demonstration of correct method of employing "traction sutures" and interrupted suture line.

FIG. 8-9. Drawings depicting the correct and turbulence-producing incorrect angles of aortic and renal artery-vein anastomoses.

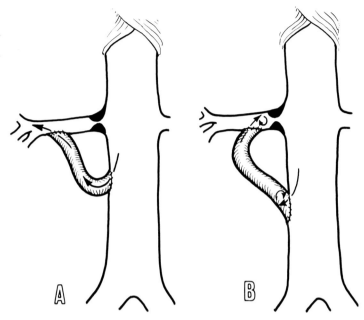

of the graft would also have merit although it would make the operation more difficult. Wylie and Fry[21,26] and their associates prefer an end-to-end anastomosis between the graft and the renal artery. Fry's group observes that following end to side anastomosis between the graft and the renal artery, the renal artery proximal to the anastomosis usually thromboses. They believe such thrombus may propagate distally and occlude the anastomosis. More concrete follow-up data, including follow-up arteriographic studies, will be necessary to evaluate these theoretical concepts. Constriction of anastomotic sites can also occur by using inordinately deep bites of vein graft in the

FIG. 8-10. Illustration of two types of end-to-end renal artery graft anastomoses.

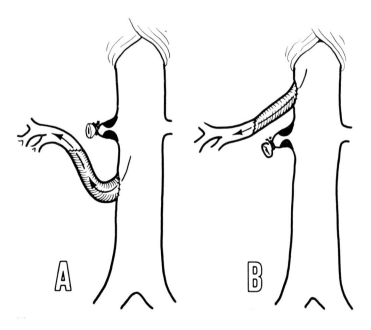

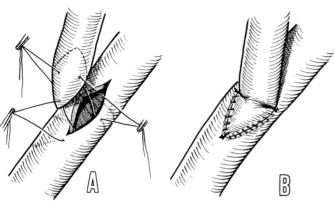

FIG. 8-11. Demonstration of stenosis producing effects of "deep-bites" in vein at the anastomotic heel.

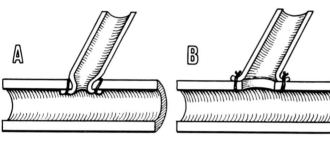

FIG. 8-12. Representation of stenosis-producing "intima-to-intima" running anastomosis and nonstenotic interrupted "intima-to-adventitia" aortic anastomosis.

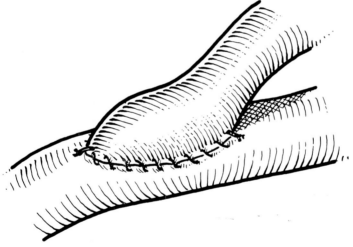

FIG. 8-13. Illustrative drawing of desired "cobra-hood" effect of vein anastomosis.

mid-portion of the anastomosis (Fig. 8-11). This results in a band-like constriction which narrows the diameter of the vein at that point.

Another cause of anastomotic stenosis is found in the older patient with an aortic wall thickened by atherosclerosis. A running suture interrupted at each end of the anastomosis will draw a graft down into the aortic orifice and cause some degree of narrowing (Fig. 8-12). The percentage of narrowing increases directly in proportion to the thickness of the aortic wall and inversely with diameter of the anastomosis. If the saphenous vein used is 4 mm. or less in diameter, this effect can be quite significant. It can be completely avoided by the use of an everting horizontal mattress suture line resulting in the so-called cobra hood anastomosis (Fig. 8-13). An objection may be raised to this

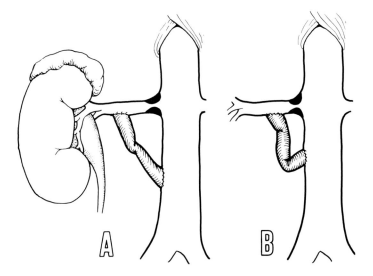

FIG. 8-14. Representation of the most frequent points of kinking in redundant grafts.

procedure in that it does not produce an intima-to-intima anastomosis. The intima of the vein is approximated to the aortic adventitia. The importance of this objection is questionable. A synthetic prosthesis has no intima, and in the atherosclerotic aorta intimal approximation is often difficult or impossible.

Other factors of importance in aortorenal bypass grafting are graft length and orientation. Grafts that are too long may kink. The common site and causes of graft kinking are shown in Figure 8-14. A number of factors can contribute to kinking: placement of the aortic anastomosis; caudal traction of the renal artery during the anastomosis and cephalad retraction when completed; grafts that are too long or too short; and twisting of the graft along its horizontal axis. End-to-end anastomosis between the renal artery and the graft will eliminate most of the problems but may introduce others by decreasing the diameter of the anastomosis. If there is a kink or some other misalignment in the graft at the completion of the anastomosis, it must be redone. Attempts to reorient the course of the graft with anchoring sutures or pyloroplasty-type procedures have resulted in graft thrombosis in our experience. One or both anastomoses must be taken down and redone. A helpful maneuver in orienting the graft is shown in Figure

8-15. A cannula is fixed in the aortic end of the graft with a ligature. The graft is distended with saline and oriented in a proper course between the renal artery and aorta. This technique is also useful in checking for

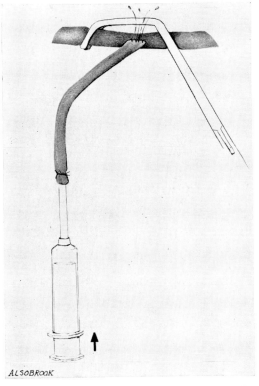

ALSOBROOK

FIG. 8-15. Method of vein orientation by distention with saline-filled syringe and cannula.

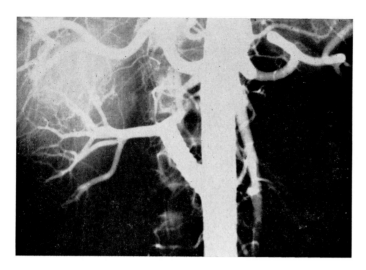

FIG. 8-16. Aortogram showing patent Dacron aortorenal bypass 2 years after operation.

leakage points in the renal arterial anastomosis and checking for presence of adventitial bands which may compromise the lumen of the graft.

The anatomy and course of the renal artery varies from patient to patient. The operative procedure employed for revascularization must be varied accordingly. In some cases an end-to-end anastomosis is the

BLOOD REPLACEMENT REQUIRED DURING SAPHENOUS VEIN AORTO-RENAL BYPASS

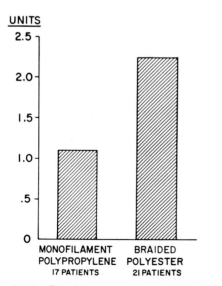

FIG. 8-17. Graphic comparison of blood replacement required during aortorenal saphenous vein bypass when using braided polyester and monofilament polypropylene suture material.

only solution. In some situations a Dacron prosthesis, which has a little more rigidity and less propensity to kink, will work better than a saphenous vein. Long-term results with Dacron grafts that are successful initially are as good as those with saphenous vein in our experience. Others have made similar observations.[25] Another factor in graft failure is the use of a saphenous vein that is too small in diameter. The vein is spatulated widely in an attempt to increase the size of the anastomosis, but this in turn creates angulation problems at the site of origin of the graft. In such a situation a Dacron graft of appropriate size will allow a 90-degree angle of origin of the graft from the renal artery (Fig. 8-16) and a successful anastomosis.

Finally, Fry[26] has evaluated the problem of suture line scarring and anastomotic contracture. He recommends spatulation of the saphenous vein to three times the diameter of the renal artery to avoid this cause of late operative failure.

Anastomotic Bleeding In our experience with braided polyester suture material in performing saphenous vein aortorenal bypasses, hemorrhage from the suture line routinely resulted in the need for blood transfusion and reversal of the heparin with protamine. For the past 2 years we have used a monofilament polypropylene suture (Prolene) and have seen minimal anastomotic leakage and have not had to give protamine. A review of 38 comparable procedures shows over twice as much blood replacement was required when the braided polyester suture was used (Fig. 8-17). Under the microscope the braided suture appears quite porous; it has an irregular, serrated surface when compared to the smooth monofilament polypropylene. When the braided polyester is pulled through an artery or vein, a sawing effect results which enlarges the hole created by the needle. We think this is the cause of more suture line bleeding with the braided polyester suture.

Intrarenal Complications   The most paradoxical of all complications in renal revascularization is acute tubular necrosis and renal failure. The true incidence of its occurrence is not known. However, clinically unrecognized minor renal damage secondary to temporary occlusion of the renal artery during the operation is much more common than had been recognized previously. Since most operations involve a unilateral reconstruction with a relatively normal contralateral kidney, even major degrees of acute tubular necrosis are not reflected in serum creatinine or blood urea nitrogen levels. The good kidney takes over until the injured kidney has recovered. For the past 7 months we have been doing triple isotope renograms serially beginning on the first postoperative day. This study has routinely shown normal renal blood flow but poor tubular function for 1 to 3 weeks. Renal transplantation experience has shown that if the vascular tree of the donor kidney is washed out and cooled with an acellular perfusate, tubular necrosis is minimized. We have recently used 500 ml. of a hypothermic saline solution (1° to 2° C) to wash out and cool the kidney. This is accomplished by inserting a cannula into the renal artery at the site of the arteriotomy (Fig. 8-18). A 14-gauge needle is placed into the renal vein with proximal occlusion to collect the perfusate and prevent it from entering the systemic circulation. Following this, the cannula is removed and the revascularization is performed. The core tempera-

ture of the kidney is reduced to about 15° C by this maneuver. Serial postoperative renograms show normal or near normal tubular function in these recent cases. The reader is admonished to remember that our experience with this technique is limited to 12 patients; there have been no complications attendant to the procedure, but further study and observation will be required to establish its merit.

Complications Inherent in Any Vascular Procedure   Aside from operative considerations peculiar to renal artery surgery, there are several complications associated with any vascular procedure on the abdominal aorta and its branches. Thrombosis of the renal artery or aorta distal to the point of cross-clamping is usually averted by systemic heparinization. In the unusual case when this does occur, immediate thrombectomy should be performed with Fogarty catheters of appropriate size. In patients with atheromatous disease of the abdominal aorta, distal embolization owing to plaque dislodgement at the time of cross-clamping is a real danger. Since the groin and the thighs are prepped and included in the operative field for saphenous vein procurement, distal pulses and lower leg color can be assessed during

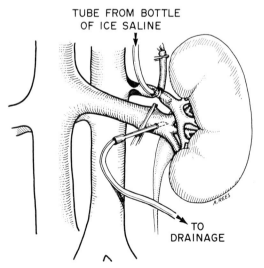

TUBE FROM BOTTLE
OF ICE SALINE

TO
DRAINAGE

FIG. 8-18. Technique of cannulation and core cooling of kidney through arteriotomy prior to graft anastomosis.

the operation. Femoral embolectomy can be performed if there is evidence of distal thrombosis or embolization. Ureteral injury and ureteral fistulae are possible with any abdominal vascular procedure and have been reported as the result of aortorenal bypass procedure.[27] We have not had such an injury in over 200 renal artery revascularizations. Nevertheless, depending on the site of injury, either direct reconstruction or renal autotransplantation with ureteroneocystostomy have been used successfuly in reported cases.[28]

Postoperative Considerations

The routine management of patients following renal revascularization includes the usual therapeutic maneuvers appropriate for any major abdominal operation. Patients are kept on nasogastric suction for 3 to 5 days postoperatively. Central venous pressure is routinely monitored. Serum and urinary electrolytes are determined until the patient is stable and on a regular diet. As stated earlier, body weight is determined daily; we consider it very important in regulating fluid balance. Hourly urine output and monitoring of central venous pressure are valuable in determining the patient's state of hydration. During the convalescent period a rapid sequence IVP and renogram are obtained to evaluate both the success of the operation and renal function. If the preoperative rapid-sequence IVP was positive and the postoperative examination normal, the revascularization is considered to be successful. If, however, the postoperative study is still positive or if renal function has deteriorated, an arteriogram is obtained.

Early Postoperative Complications

Two problems may present in the immediate postoperative period. Hypovolemia and resultant hypotension may occur from inadequate blood replacement during the procedure or from postoperative blood loss. We have had one instance of anastomotic disruption that required reoperation. Certainly the successful outcome of such a catastrophic event is dependent on astute diagnostic acumen. Severe hypertension in the first few postoperative hours may be from any one of several causes. Prior to our renewed attention to intraoperative temperature control, postoperative total body hypothermia with resultant vasoconstriction and severe hypertension was disturbingly common. When this has occurred we have administered Thorazine to counteract peripheral vasoconstriction while we warmed the patient. Fluid overload during operation may also result in hypertension immediately postoperatively. This is most easily controlled by accurate blood and fluid replacement intraoperatively. Occasionally diuretics are required to correct overexpansion of the blood volume. Finally, severe hypertension not produced by the above errors may occur immediately. When the above conditions have been ruled out or if no response occurs after initiating treatment for vasoconstriction, antihypertensive medications should be instituted. Control has usually been obtained by the intravenous use of 500 mg. of alphamethyldopa every 4 to 6 hours. Many patients may remain hypertensive for days, weeks, or even months following successful revascularization. If antihypertensive medications are necessary during the postoperative course, they are continued following discharge and then gradually withdrawn over a period of weeks or months, depending on the degree of blood pressure rehabilitation. Over 50 per cent of the patients who were eventually classified as cured were discharged from the hospital on antihypertensive drugs.

Clinically significant acute tubular necrosis and subsequent renal failure has occurred in four cases (3 per cent) in our experience. With the use of daily serum and urine electrolytes, blood urea nitrogen, creatinine, and hourly urine output recordings, this can be demonstrated early in its course and appropriate treatment can be initiated. Renal hemodialysis has afforded a successful means of managing the more severe cases with uncontrollable hyperkalemia and azotemia. Two of the four patients made a full recov-

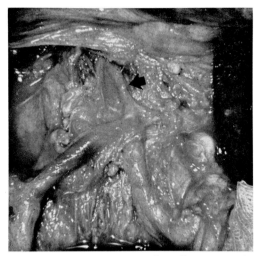 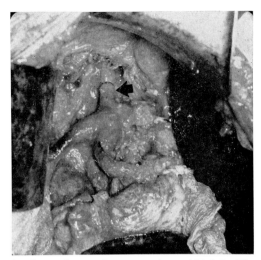

FIG. 8-22. (*Left*) A stenotic celiac artery (*arrow*) after release of compression. (*Right*) The change in diameter after dilatation can be seen (*arrow*).

through an arteriotomy in the splenic artery, thus avoiding a suture line in the celiac axis proper. Care should be taken in manipulation of the celiac artery origin, as this vessel is frequently thin-walled and may be torn.

If celiac isolation is required, Wylie and Stoney[3] have preferred complete aortic occlusion by widely spaced clamps, rather than partial occlusion which we have employed. Unless the occlusion time can be kept brief,

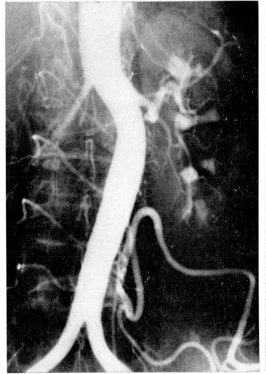 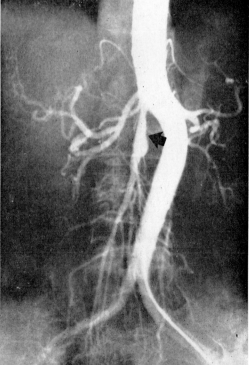

FIG. 8-23. (*Left*) Preoperative arteriogram showing scant flow in celiac and superior mesenteric distribution with large inferior mesenteric artery. Contrast this with vessel's appearance following endarterectomy and venous patch grafting (*Right*).

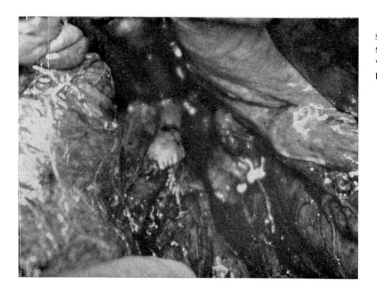

FIG. 8-24. Patch graft in superior mesenteric artery shown in Figure 8-23. The vessel was exposed through the gastrohepatic ligament.

complete aortic occlusion at this level invites renal ischemic complications.

Wylie and Stoney have also advised caution in positioning a superior mesenteric

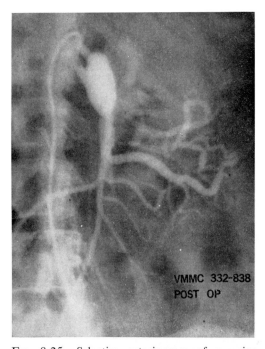

VMMC 332-838
POST OP

FIG. 8-25. Selective arteriogram of superior mesenteric artery obtained 19 months postoperatively, showing dilated ovarian venous patch graft. The patient continues to do well and is being observed.

artery bypass graft, since the acute angle between the aorta and this vessel may result in kinking of the graft.[3] Reimplantations or endarterectomy with venous patch grafting offer alternatives (Figs. 8-23, 8-24). For bypass grafting, Dacron prostheses have shown an excellent long-term patency. Care should be taken to close the posterior peritoneum securely to prevent graft erosion into adjacent bowel. We have preferred reconstructive procedures utilizing repair of the involved artery and have grafted or reimplanted the vessel in only three of 31 cases of either celiac or superior mesenteric disease. Figure 8-25 illustrates a late complication of venous patch grafting of the superior mesenteric artery using ovarian vein. We no longer regard this as a satisfactory venous grafting material.

The routine use of pressure and flow measurements (Fig. 8-26) adds greatly to the understanding of patients with visceral ischemia and will help determine the adequacy of arterial reconstruction. As pointed out by Rob,[4] patients with reduced hepatic blood flow may tolerate poorly the rapid transfusion of acid citrate dextrose treated blood. Diminished liver metabolism, perhaps aggravated by hypothermia, may result in citrate intoxication under these circumstances.

Acute Ischemia

Problems in Diagnosis

Patients with acute embolic or thrombotic occlusion of a major mesenteric artery characteristically have prompt onset of severe abdominal pain, which is usually out of proportion to physical findings depending on the duration of occlusion when the patient is seen. The progression from pain to hyperperistalsis, to ileus and distention, to bleeding, and eventually to peritonitis has been well described by Williams.[5] Usually mesenteric infarction is considered in the diagnosis, especially when there is evidence of cardiac arrhythmia, past myocardial infarction, or other evidence of arteriosclerosis.

The problem in diagnosis lies in distinguishing such patients from those with so-called nonocclusive mesenteric ischemia. Many consider this a nonoperative lesion,[6] and recommend such measures as Dextran, epidural or splanchnic block, heparinization, and cardiac support. Fogarty and Fletcher have pointed out patients with nonocclusive mesenteric ischemia frequently have severe congestive heart failure, digitalis intoxication, and hemoconcentration.[7] The results in these patients are uniformly disappointing, as illustrated by Ottinger and Austen's report of 100 per cent mortality in 67 patients.[8]

Technical Considerations

Superior Mesenteric Artery

Since most of these emboli will lodge distally beyond the origin of the vessel, exposure beyond its ostium is satisfactory for embolus extraction. If the embolus appears to have lodged at the origin of the superior mesenteric artery, preexisting arteriosclerotic narrowing should be suspected. Failure to correct this at the time of embolectomy may result in postoperative thrombosis.

Although a thoracoabdominal approach has been advocated by some authors, we have found laparotomy alone to be satisfactory in all 18 patients who underwent elective or emergency surgery on the superior mesenteric artery. Ottinger and Austen pointed

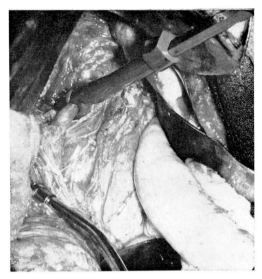

FIG. 8-26. Electromagnetic flowmeter probe positioned on the common hepatic artery. Reversal of flow can occasionally be demonstrated by this technique.

out[8] the added morbidity of such an approach should prohibit its use in emergency circumstances.

Postoperative Complications

A variety of experimental studies have been directed at investigation of the biochemical, acid-base, and toxic abnormalities of intestinal revascularization. Hyperkalemia and acidosis were documented in dogs by Robertson, et al.[9] after an average of 2 hours of superior mesenteric artery occlusion was released. Williams and his colleagues[10] showed evidence of a myocardial depressant factor using a dog plasma fraction and rat muscle.

Wilson and Ebert questioned the validity of this concept after they were unable to demonstrate myocardial depression in unanesthetized dogs with a 6-hour superior mesenteric artery occlusion.[11] Hashimoto and Thal[12] thought that phenoxybenzamine treatment protected dogs against decreases in cardiac output after superior mesenteric arterial occlusion release. Others have felt that hemodynamic events such as sequestration of fluid alone was a sufficient explanation for shock in experimental dogs without invoking toxic product absorption.[13]

Although it is generally true that salvage of patients with acute mesenteric ischemia is difficult, there is little documentation of the same biochemical postoperative abnormalities occurring in humans. Indeed, studies such as that of Bergen, Haid, and Conn[14] have shown an encouraging absence of the problems of hyperkalemia, acidosis, and large, "third space" fluid shifts. Nine of 11 patients with acute bowel ischemia from thrombosis or embolus were successfully revascularized; six were followed up. No evidence of severe acidosis, massive hyperkalemia, or toxic product absorption was noted.

Until the significance of experimental observations becomes known in the clinical setting, postoperative observation for such changes should be carefully pursued, including measurement of central venous pressure, arterial blood gases and serum electrolytes at frequent intervals in the early postoperative period. Some of these patients may have very little margin between too much and too little fluid administration, and we have seen one death after mesenteric arterial surgery from refractory pulmonary edema following overzealous intravenous fluid replacement.

Cardiac arrhythmia has been shown to decrease superior mesenteric artery blood velocity, and correction of arrhythmias may improve diastolic flow through areas of recent reconstruction or in treatment of "nonocclusive" mesenteric ischemia.[15] Digitalis preparations, often used for treatment of atrial arrhythmias, may decrease mesenteric blood flow themselves, however.[16] Control of arrhythmia by electrical cardioversion might be considered more rational in such patients.

Occasional patients may develop late bleeding from eventual slough of gangrenous mucosa without full thickness bowel involvement. Strictures of localized segments, particularly in the left colon, may be transient or permanent after ischemic injury. The assessment of bowel viability may be impossible at the time of original operation, and clinical signs are not reliable indices of bowel viability after revascularization. Therefore, the "second look" concept has been widely advocated following surgery for acute mesenteric ischemia. While some have recommended reoperation to assess bowel viability at 24 to 48 hours, Williams has preferred a period of 6 to 8 hours so that repair of rethrombosis of the reconstructed vessel may still be usefully undertaken if required.[5] Unless the surgeon is confronted with frankly gangrenous bowel in a late situation, greater conservation of intestine may be expected by delayed resection at a second look procedure. Often striking improvement will have occurred that makes resection unnecessary. Routine use of antibiotics has been practiced by most, since the integrity of the bowel membrane is jeopardized.

References

1. Szilagyi, D. E., Rian, R. L., Elliott, J. P., and Smith, R. F.: The celiac artery compression syndrome: Does it exist? Surgery, 72:849, 1972.
2. Stanley, J. C., and Fry, W. J.: Median arcuate ligament syndrome. Arch. Surg., 103:252, 1971.
3. Wylie, E. J., and Stoney, R. J.: Management of visceral arterial occlusions. In Dale, A. W. (ed.): Management of Arterial Occlusive Disease. Chicago, Year Book Medical Publishers, 1971.
4. Rob, C.: Surgical diseases of the celiac and mesenteric arteries. Arch. Surg., 93:21, 1966.
5. Williams, L. F.: Progress in gastroenterology: Vascular insufficiency of the intestines. Gastroenterology, 61:757, 1971.
6. Bergen, J. J., Dry, L., Conn, J., and Trippel, O. H.: Intestinal ischemic syndromes. Ann. Surg., 169:120, 1969.
7. Fogarty, T. J., and Fletcher, W. S.: Genesis of nonocclusive mesenteric ischemia. Amer. J. Surg., 111:130, 1966.
8. Ottinger, L. W., and Austen, W. G.: A study of 136 patients with mesenteric infarction. Surg., Gynec., Obstet., 124:251, 1967.
9. Robertson, G. S., Lyall, A. D., and Macrae, J. G. C.: Acid-base disturbances in mesenteric occlusion. Surg., Gynec., Obstet., 128:15, 1969.

10. Williams, L. F., Goldberg, A. H., Polansky, B. J., and Byrne, J. J.: Surgery, *66*:138, 1969.

11. Wilson, J. M., and Ebert, P. A.: Hemodynamic effects of superior mesenteric artery occlusion: A comparison in anesthetized and unanesthetized dogs. Ann. Surg., *175*: 214, 1972.

12. Hashimoto, E., and Thal, A. P.: The lung lesion produced by materials released from the superior mesenteric vein after superior mesenteric arterial occlusion. Jap. Circ. J. *35*:1071, 1971.

13. Chiu, C. J., Scott, H. J., and Gurd, E. N.: Volume deficit versus toxic absorption: A study of canine shock after mesenteric arterial occlusion. Ann. Surg., *175*:479, 1972.

14. Bergen, J. J., Haid, S. P., and Conn, J.: Systemic effects of intestinal revascularization. Amer. J. Surg., *117*:235, 1969.

15. Benchimol, A., Desser, K. B., and Gartlan, J. L.: Superior mesenteric artery blood velocity in man during cardiac arrhythmias. Gastroenterology, *62*:950, 1972.

16. Shanbour, L. L., *et al.*: Effects of Ouabain on splanchnic hemodynamics in the rhesus monkey. Amer. Heart J., *81*:511, 1972.

Chapter 9 | Complications of

J. Cuthbert Owens, M.D. | # Sympathectomy

Most surgeons agree that operations performed on the sympathetic nervous system do not involve a diseased or injured structure. Therefore it has been concluded that each procedure is relatively safe and simple and results in fewer complications than most surgical procedures.[1,2,3] Excluding technical misadventures, however, studies do not support this casual concept. Often the complication is not recognized as being directly related to the procedure, and sometimes the patient's postoperative complaint is accepted as an inevitable sequela. Technical complications plus those that are unexpected and difficult to understand result in much confusion, controversy, and disagreement among surgeons regarding not only indications for sympathectomy but also the results. Although new approaches to vascular disorders have proved worthwhile, sympathectomy may offer much to patients who have been screened properly.

Complications of sympathectomy may be divided into three categories: (1) technical errors, (2) unexpected complications due to the surgeon's poor judgment or inadequate knowledge of the physiology of the underlying disease process, and (3) complications peculiar to ablation of the sympathetic nervous system.

The sequelae of the several types of sympathectomy may be more clearly understood if the history of each procedure is reviewed.

History

Since sympathectomy was introduced as a treatment for neurological and vascular disorders at the end of the 19th century it has had a turbulent though colorful history.

1896–1921. The fluctuations of the popularity of sympathectomy began in 1896 when Jennesco advocated periarterial sympathectomy as a means of therapy for epilepsy, glaucoma, and migraine.[4] Three years later, Jaboulay utilized it to treat ulceration of the feet.[5] The popularity of the procedure was short-lived owing to the fact that results were neither predictable nor lasting. Leriche, who was a student of Jaboulay, reintroduced periarterial sympathectomy and for two decades advocated its use in vascular disease and in painful conditions of the extremities.[6-9] Leriche erroneously believed that the sympathetic fibers reached the periphery of the extremity along the course of the arterial adventitial network. Kramer and Todd, in 1914, correctly described the pathway of the sympathetic fibers to the extremity via the peripheral nerves.[10] These studies were later confirmed by Woollard and Norrish, and periarterial sympathectomy was generally replaced by ganglionectomy.[11]

1921–1940. Interestingly, Jennesco, who first advocated the use of periarterial sympathectomy, was one of the first to recommend a *stellate ganglionectomy* for Raynaud's disease in 1921.[12] During the same year,

Brüing[13] suggested its use because it had a more lasting periphereal vascular effect than periarterial sympathectomy. However, the procedure did not achieve expected results in certain patients, and the vasomotor tone almost invariably returned.[14]

Kuntz, in 1927, was the first to explain the reason for the unpredicable results following a stellate ganglionectomy and its short-lived effect on vascular tone.[15] He described direct connections between the second and third thoracic (dorsal) ganglia to the first intercostal nerve which bypassed the stellate ganglion and reached the extremity via the peripheral nerves. Following this report surgeons extended the stellate ganglionectomy procedure to include the second thoracic ganglion, namely a *cervicothoracic* or *cervicodorsal sympathectomy*.[16,17] Again vascular tone returned, though not so soon as after stellate ganglionectomy or periarterial sympathectomy.[17-21]

Complications developed when the stellate ganglion was included with the ablation of the upper thoracic sympathetic ganglia, and clinicians recognized that an adequate sympathectomy could be accomplished by an *upper thoracic sympathectomy* in which the upper thoracic ganglia are sectioned up to the lower portion of the stellate ganglion just below the entrance of the preganglionic fibers of the first thoracic ganglion.[22, 23] In some patients, however, an adequate sympathectomy was not obtained until the stellate ganglion was removed.[24-26]

In 1923 Royle and Hunter, experimenting on goats, concluded that the sympathetic component of a dual innervation of striated muscle was responsible for its spastic tone.[27-31] Royle therefore performed *lumbar sympathetic ramisections* on patients with spastic paralysis.[32-34] Adson performed the same procedure but with disappointing results.[35] However, he confirmed Royle's observation that after lumbar sympathetic ramisection and division of the sympathetic trunk, the skin of the toes of the ipsilateral side became warm and dry.[17,36,37] Although sympathectomy for spastic paralysis failed

to stand the test of time, the procedure began to be used to improve the peripheral circulation.[14] However, within a few years enthusiasm waned when it became apparent that the gratifying vasodilation noted immediately postoperatively was not maintained as well several days after denervation. Further it was noted that sympathectomy for the upper extremity had a briefer effect than that performed for the lower extremity, and ultimate results were closely related to the nature of the underlying disease.[38] These disappointing observations caused clinicians to lose interest in surgery on the sympathetic nervous system.

1940–1950. There was a hiatus of approximately 10 years before surgery on the sympathetic nervous system again became a common operative procedure, not only for peripheral vascular diseases[39] but for hypertension[40,41] and a seemingly endless number of disorders including angina,[42,43] burns, frostbite,[44,45] megacolon,[46] pancreatitis,[47,48] hyperhidrosis,[49] causalgia,[50,51] and numerous other maladies.[39,52,53] Two procedures had been added, a *thoracolumbar sympathectomy* for hypertension and a *splanchnicectomy* for abdominal visceral disorders. During sympathectomy's third return to popularity, surgeons again began to express widely divergent opinions about the precise value of the procedure.

Again the primary objections to sympathectomy were that certain patients failed to achieve expected results and that the beneficial effects were short-lived.

During the first half of this century no surgeon advocated the use of sympathetic denervation more than Leriche. He constantly searched for some means to completely ablate the effects of the sympathetic nervous system on a part by performing periarterial sympathectomy, arterectomy, ganglionectomy, and even sympathectomy combined with subtotal adrenalectomy.[54-56]

1950–Present. In spite of the inadequacies of the operation,[23,57-59] the procedures continued to be performed, and a trend developed not only to extend the number of ganglia removed but also to utilize several operative approaches. The list of complications increased to include some of the most unexpected and interesting postoperative problems in the field of surgery. Furthermore, clinical investigators were even more confused as to the benefits derived by the patient when published physiologic studies were found to vary, especially studies which involved peripheral vascular disorders.[21,59-65] With the advent of ganglion blockers and reconstructive vascular surgery, sympathectomy, particularly as a treatment for occlusive arterial disease, was reappraised.[21,66-69]

Selection of Patients

There are four primary indications for a sympathectomy: (1) to relieve vasospasm, (2) to aid in the development of small collateral channels, (3) to obviate causalgia or causalgic type pain, and (4) to eliminate hyperhidrosis. Proper selection of patients who can benefits from a sympathectomy for any of these indications would be easier if an accurate prediction of the results could be made preoperatively by means of some test. However, no test is infallible, and since there are no fixed rules for selecting patients for operation, this goal cannot be consistently maintained.[66,70,71] Generally patients who have a favorable response to preoperative testing will do well after sympathectomy.[72] Estimates of accurate preoperative predictability of benefit vary from 90 per cent to 50 per cent.[73]

De Takets stated: Sympathectomy for occlusive vascular disease has had a hard time. . . . The operation has suffered criticism through its wholesale use and its abuse in being applied to conditions which, either through poor diagnosis or poor understanding of physiology, could never be hoped to be aided by such surgery. . . . It is obvious that sympathectomy will fail to improve circulation, abolish rest pain, or save a part from amputation (1) when there is no capability for the vascular bed to dilate, (2) when there is insufficient collateral circulation because the extent of the main trunk obstruction is too great, and (3) when the lesion actually is not circulatory in origin in the first place and thus an increase in circulation has nothing to do with the therapeutic needs.[69]

Before there can be a discussion of the methods used for selecting patients for sympathectomy and what can be expected from the procedure, there must be some comment on its limitations.

Limitations

Complications result from sympathectomy when its limitations are not clearly understood and its indications are not properly applied. It is essential that the clinician have a sound knowledge of the anatomy of the sympathetic nervous system and its variables and also of the pathophysiology of the disorder for which the procedure is being considered.

The dissimilarities and variables of diseases and disorders in sympathectomy patients are great. Technically the operation may seem to be relatively simple. However, it is difficult to perform correctly;[74,75] it is impossible to prevent the return of sympathetic tone,[76-81] and any analysis of clinical results should have subjective statements proved or disproved objectively.[59,61]

Relief Pain

Sympathectomy relieves only one type of pain, namely, causalgia or causalgia-type pain, which is superficial.[51,61,66,74,82] Deep pain of somatic root origin is not affected by medical or surgical sympathetic denervation. In visceral pain patterns such as those in chronic pancreatitis[47,48,83] and angina pectoris due to myocardial ischemia,[42,43,84] sympathectomy has been used with some success. However, the neurologic pathways followed by such painful stimuli and the vasomotor function of the sympathetic nervous system, especially as it applies to the coronary vessels, are not completely understood.[85] Fewer sympathectomies are being performed today for visceral pain than in the past. Yet from increased experience with external painful states, it is our belief that a similar dual pain pattern may exist in visceral organs, and results of sympathectomy for pain may be comparable to those reported on other areas of the body.

Lasting Effects

Sympathectomy performed in vasospastic and occlusive arterial disease has been challenged frequently as to the lasting effect and the limitations of the procedure.[23,57-59,85] Ironically, causalgia-type pain, which has a dramatic response to sympathectomy, has the highest incidence of complications, since it may produce bizarre and unexpected pain syndromes postoperatively.[86]

The failure of a sympathectomy to have a lasting effect in vasospastic disorders such as Raynaud's phenomenon is well documented, especially for the upper extremity.[87-90] In scleroderma and other diseases where Raynaud's phenomenon is secondary, a sympathectomy may produce dramatic benefit in the early postoperative period, but the ultimate result is frequently so poor that the procedure is generally considered to be of little value.[91-93] In primary Raynaud's disease sympathectomy is usually done only when skin necrosis or pain is a prominent complaint.[87] Here the lasting effect of the operation is subject to the problem of return of sympathetic tone.

A discouraging complication which may follow a sympathectomy is the return of sympathetic tone. The cause of this remains obscure although several theories have been proposed, such as the establishment of "intrinsic tone" and increased sensitivity to circulating catecholamines or some other hormone; pathways which may remain following sympathectomy; and "regeneration" of sympathetic fibers.[61,76-81,93-95] Studies conducted by Parks et al. in a sympathectomized patient[80] and the benefits derived by the use of reserpine in the treatment of Raynaud's phenomenon[96,97] lead to the belief that any sympathetic fibers that may remain after surgery have little to do with the return of tone postoperatively. It has been suggested that "changes in the catecholamine content of the tissue and increasing sensitivity to both these and circulatory amines may be closely related to the phenomenon."[80,98] These observations help to explain some of the confusion regarding return of sympathetic tone following sympathectomy and also point out the limitations of sympathectic ablative surgery in certain patients where supplemental therapy may be required to accomplish the desired response.

In chronic obliterative arterial disease, the decreased arterial flow to the distal part may result in complete sympathetic denervation in the small peripheral vessels, which therefore develop a paralytic vasodilatation or chronic hyperemia identified as "dependent rubor" with loss of sensation in the distal skin.[86] In patients with this finding, ischemia has become so advanced that pregangrenous changes are present and sympathectomy is not indicated unless causalgia-type pain can be demonstrated proximal to the area of sensory loss. No improvement in circulation should be expected in this setting. Interestingly, patients with "dependent rubor" who are operated on for relief of pain have a return of sympathetic tone manifested by the same pain on approximately the sixth postoperative day. This pain may be relieved by intra-arterial injection of a sympatholytic drug; and therefore, the return of pain should not be considered a complication.

Since arteriosclerosis obliterans is a progressive disease, any benefit derived from a sympathectomy may be lost when additional thrombosis occurs later.

Intermittent Claudication

Lumbar sympathectomy is not indicated for the treatment of uncomplicated intermittent claudication. However, controversy and confusion continue over the true value of the operation for this complaint. Some surgeons believe that it is definitely beneficial for intermittent claudication;[65,74,99-102] others hold that relief is so infrequent that it is unpredictable;[58] still others think that it is possibly harmful or will accomplish nothing.[57,59,103-108] Statistics on the results of lumbar sympathectomy range from a low figure of 5 per cent of patients improved to a high of 85 per cent.[1] The extreme discrepancy in statistics is probably due to the lack of standardized measures of improvement. A subjective evaluation would report a high figure of improvement, while an objective evaluation would indicate a much less favorable result. Much physiologic evidence supports the view that the sympathetic innervation of muscle blood vessels is negligible and that sympathetic denervation produces no more than a transitory increase in muscle blood flow.[57,106,109] Therefore, objective studies have not shown that a lumbar sympathectomy is warranted for intermittent claudication.[59,103,109-111] Why then should many surgeons continue to employ the procedure for intermittent claudication in occlusive vascular disease?

There are a number of reasons why some patients with claudication improve after sympathectomy. Intermittent claudication is prone in its natural history to wide spontaneous fluctuations in severity, and gradual improvement occurs if development of collateral circulation precedes the progression of the occlusive disease.[112] A control group will show equal improvement during the same period with subsidence of symptoms in the same percentage without operation.[108] The explanation for this is that patients can walk greater distances if they walk at a slower rate. Whether they do this naturally following surgery, discover this for themselves, or are instructed to stop for a short period prior to the anticipated claudication distance, their walking is quantitatively and qualitatively improved. Finally, analyzing the ambulatory pattern of these patients one often concludes that a patient who walks less rapidly shortens his distance between claudication symptoms. Many of these patients state that they disliked walking, not because of intermittent claudication but because of the foot discomfort which they had with each step. Studies have demonstrated that the blood flow increase to the lower extremity following lumbar sympathectomy is almost entirely due to increased blood flow to the skin and that muscle circulation is slightly affected.[61,71] In the patients who had improvement following sympathectomy, the improvement may be due indirectly to the relief of foot symptoms.[66,113] This relief encourages the patient to walk more, thereby stimulating increased muscle circulation by the best vasodilator known—the muscle metabolic waste products. The relief of pain may also reduce or eliminate vasospasm, for pain in an extremity usually induces vasoconstriction. Numerous clinical reports have revealed that improvement is gradual with the peak reached 6 or more months after surgery.[70,114,115] Similar results may be obtained in these patients when medical "sympathetic denervation" is used not for its vasodilatory effect but for relief of superficial foot pain.[66]

Judging from objective studies in the literature and personal clinical experience, lumbar sympathectomy is not indicated in the treatment of uncomplicated intermittent claudication.[61,112] We believe the wide range in the complication rate of failure can be explained by how the statistics were collected: by objective studies, by subjective evaluation, or a combination of both methods of measurement.

Regeneration

Until recently the return of sympathetic activity was loosely explained as the ability of the sectioned sympathetic nerves to regenerate. This concept has been challenged in recent years by several theories that will be discussed later in the chapter. "Regeneration" is extremely important relative to the limitations of sympathectomy when the surgery is performed in patients under 40. It is common for these patients to have at least some return of sympathetic activity within 2 years.[86,116,117] In patients with proper indications for sympathectomy who have an early return of preoperative findings after operation, it must be concluded that a more adequate or complete sympathectomy should have been performed.

Hope for Improvement

A surgeon may at some time overreact to the possible usefulness of a sympathectomy, for the procedure may be performed in the hope that some benefit will result or it may be a final attempt to save an extremity from amputation.[85,93,103,118] Patients who have

very borderline indications, such as those with rapidly progressive arteriosclerosis or severe concomitant disease, must be thoroughly studied preoperatively to avoid unnecessary surgery. It is more humane to remove a patient's hopelessly involved limb than to subject him to a sympathectomy followed by an amputation. The surgeon should avoid two extremes: a sympathectomy performed too early, when the patient has a segmental arterial occlusion with a patent distal segment when direct reconstructive surgery is indicated, or too late, when progressive gangrene is present and the limb is already doomed.

Methods of Selection

An objective method of assessing preoperatively what the operation will accomplish is needed to lessen the likelihood of results that are inconsistent, largely unpredictable, and easily misinterpreted.[70,71,119] In many patients the results may be predicted by history and clinical findings alone, depending upon the knowledge, experience, and capabilities of the surgeon.[120] Other patients may need more sophisticated methods of selection.

Upper Extremity Disorders

The primary indications for a sympathectomy apply to disorders that may occur in the upper extremity (Table 9-1).

Nasospastic Conditions. The most common vasospastic condition in the upper limb is Raynaud's phenomenon. In the selection of patients with this disorder for sympathectomy, the severity of the condition should be considered carefully. Sympathectomy is not advisable for the mild, nonprogressive form of the disorder nor for patients who respond well to medical therapies such as reserpine, sympatholytic drugs, and others. When Raynaud's phenomenon becomes more severe and in the late stages of the condition when painful superficial fingertip ulcers develop, sympathectomy may be expected to bring about healing of the lesions and subsidence of the pain.[87]

The results of sympathectomy for Raynaud's phenomenon affecting the upper limb are not very good, no matter which method of sectioning the sympathetic chain is used. The difference in results cannot always be blamed on the anatomic variations in the type of sympathectomy performed, for frequently the underlying cause of the disorder later becomes clear whether it be a collagen disease, such as scleroderma, or a mechanical entrapment, such as a thoracic outlet syndrome. Sympathectomy has no place in the treatment of scleroderma. It should not be the primary mode of therapy for patients who have thoracic outlet syndrome that does not respond to physiotherapy. However, it should be performed in addition to the first rib resection when any manifestation of causalgia-type pain accompanies the symptoms related to the thoracic outlet entrapment.[121]

Methods of studying Raynaud's phenomenon are directed towards an attempt to diagnose the primary lesion responsible for the phenomenon as well as assisting the clinician to have a better understanding of the circulatory and pain disturbance. Immersion of the affected hand in iced water of 15° C for 1 minute produces a cooling of the fingertips below the critical symptomatic level as well as a delay or absence in the hyperemic response. The rate at which rewarming occurs is an important index of the extent of the disorder.[94] A sympathectomy may improve these findings so that the fingertips do not cool to the critical level and the response to rewarming is more rapid. The emotional response that occurs during a stressful interview, (characterized by color changes and a drop in the skin temperature of the digits) is abolished by sympathectomy.[122]

Biopsy of a digital artery in patients suspected of having a diffuse collagen disease has been proposed by some clinicians.[98,123] This is never performed on the digit but may occasionally be undertaken in the temporal artery, in the deltoid muscle, or in the gastrocnemius muscle.

Arteriograms may be hazardous when done percutaneously in the upper limb. When one is performed, a vasodilator should be used with the contrast medium; otherwise vasoconstriction may be produced, and the studies will be difficult to interpret. Arteriograms are useful when there is more extensive digital arterial obstruction or arterial stenosis than expected or demonstrated by other studies. Arteriography is especially important when the patient is being considered for direct arterial surgery or relief of an entrapment syndrome rather than a sympathectomy. Digital plethysmography as well as the use of a Doppler flowmeter may reveal the status of peripheral and collateral circulation. (See Chap. 10 for a further discussion of disease evaluation in the upper extremities.)

Electroencephalography may be beneficial in separating patients who have a diencephalic discharge from those who have abnormalities due to vascular disease or who have normal patterns. Patients suitable for sympathectomy are those who have 6-second and 14-second positive spikes and rapid miniature discharges. Evidence of psychomotor seizures in patients with a diffuse collagen disease eliminates the indication for sympathectomy.[98]

Patients with Raynaud's phenomenon should routinely have a hypercoagulation screening study of their blood as well as investigation of cold agglutinins and cryoglobulins, and low-magnification study of the fingernail capillary beds.

Any suspicion of scleroderma or lupus erythematosus should be investigated before sympathectomy is undertaken, for these patients have the highest incidence of recurrence and failure.[87,92,98] This is especially important in patients with lupus erythematosus, who may experience a dramatic flareup of the disease after operation.

Hyperhidrosis. Hyperhidrosis, a pathologic condition of excessive sweating, is part of a symptom complex that apparently is caused by excessive stimulation of the sympathetic nervous system. Patients with essential idiopathic hyperhidrosis are distinguished from patients in whom excessive

TABLE 2

TABLE 2

LOWER EXTREMITY SYMPATHECTOMY

Methods of Selection

I. History and clinical findings

II. Evaluation of arterial circulation
   A. Palpation of pulses
   B. Oscillometer
   C. Doppler flowmeter distal to sphygmomanometer
   D. Foot elevation and dependency tests
   E. Arteriogram
   F. Specific tests
      1. Digital plethysmography
      2. Regional nerve block
      3. Radioactive studies
      4. Thermocouple in temperature-controlled room
      5. Combination of above tests
   G. Indications for sympathectomy
      1. Arteriogram shows inadequate run-off
      2. Slow progress and long history
      3. Vasodilatory response to tests
      4. Confirmation in more than one test

III. Evaluation of pain related to sympathetic nervous system
   A. Intra-arterial sympatholytic drug
   B. Oral sympatholytic drug
   C. Paravertebral block of lumbar sympathetic chain
   D. Determine per cent of relief for:
      1. Superficial pain–sympathetic origin
      2. Deep pain–somatic root origin
      3. Combination of deep and superficial
   E. Sympathectomy indicated if:
      1. Superficial pain relief more than 50 per cent
      2. No spontaneous progressive improvement of pain
      3. Medical therapy sporadic, hazardous, or burdensome
      4. Pain severe
      5. Additional indications present

sweating is the result of some underlying disorder (such as malaria, tuberculosis, and brucellosis) or is associated with alcohol intoxication, gout or disorders such as diabetes, hyperthyroidism, hyperpituitarism, obesity, and menopause; or is due to some deep-seated emotional disturbances; or a family history of hyperhidrosis. Asymmetrical hyperhidrosis may occur due to neurological lesions involving any part of the sympathetic pathway from the brain to the nerve ending. Sympathectomy is seldom indicated for any of these patients unless essential hyperhidrosis has been proved. Patients chosen for sympathectomy present evidence of excessive perspiration limited to the palmar surfaces of the hands, feet, and axillae. They may be selected on the basis of the clinical history and physical examination or when all attempts to treat the condition medically, including psychotherapy, have failed.

In essential hyperhidrosis serious psychologic and social problems invariably accompany the disorder. Psychotherapy, radiation, and topical preparations are not helpful. Only surgical removal of the sympathetic nerve pathways produces relief.[124-132]

Lower Extremity Disorders

The same primary indications for a sympathectomy listed for the upper extremity apply to disorders which may occur in the lower limb. However, the incidence of vasospastic conditions and possibly hyperhidrosis are less common while occlusive vascular disease and causalgia or causalgia-type pain are more common in the lower extremity.[130] Because the selection of patients with occlusive vascular disease is most difficult and controversial, the discussion in this section is weighted more to this disorder than to other conditions.

An established plan for screening must be available which meets the selection requirements of each patient and his disorder (Table 9-2).[66,116,137,138] The results of lumbar sympathectomy usually can be foretold by a competent clinician by history and clinical findings alone.[120] Only a small number of patients require additional methods of examination to determine selection for sympathectomy.

Arterial pulses are determined by palpation and oscillometry. The absence of a dorsalis pedis pulse is usually of little importance since from 8 to 12 per cent of normal patients do not have one. A third pulse may be informative when both the dorsalis pedis and posterior tibial pulses are not present; this is the perineal artery pulse occasionally located anterior to the lateral malleolus. Another means of establishing the presence and quality of the pulse is by the use of a Doppler flowmeter in combination with a sphygmomanometer applied proximally. Since the primary indication for sympathectomy in patients with arterial disease is an inadequate run-off distal to the occlusive site that precludes direct arterial surgery, all symptomatic patients with decrease or absence of distal pulse(s) should receive arteriography.[71]

Further studies for evaluation of the peripheral circulation may be indicated for patients who are not acceptable candidates for direct reconstructive arterial surgery. A sympathectomy is indicated when specific studies suggest there will be a vasodilatory response and/or some relief of pain if a lumbar sympathectomy is performed.[61]

The adequacy of collateral circulation and/or the status of the peripheral arterioles can be assessed by observing the degree of blanching on foot elevation, the presence or absence of rubor on dependency, and the rate of venous filling. The slower the return of adequate circulation during this maneuver, the poorer will be the outcome of a lumbar sympathectomy.[70,71,114]

After the collateral circulation and the degree of impaired arterial flow have been evaluated, it is important to determine whether an active vasoconstrictor mechanism is involved. The most reliable method of establishing the presence or absence of vasospasm in the limb is digital plethysmography. This apparatus measures the pulsatile blood flow to a digit by recording the character of the pulse deflection and pulse waves. Readings are made on the toes while the patient is exposed to a warm environment followed by a cold one.[110,135] If the plethysmographic recording in the cold environment is more than 50 per cent of the warm environment reading, the patients' collateral circulation can be interpreted as adequate enough to warrant sympathectomy.

Blocking of the posterior tibial nerve posterior to the internal malleolus may be informative.[2] Any increase in temperature and cutaneous circulation of the great toe indicates there is a good possibility that a sympathectomy will be successful. This procedure may be modified by combining the use of a plethysmograph and an ankle-occluding cuff.[58,61,62,136,139] Blood flow readings on the great toe of 10 to 18 cu. mm. per second may classify the patient as a good candidate; a reading of 1 to 3 cu. mm. per second establishes the patient as a poor candidate for sympathectomy.

General Comments

Procedures such as potential blood flow, inspiratory reflex, slow waves and pulse waves of the toe,[138] and radioactive material have been used by clinicians who desire additional means for screening patients. Lumbar sympathetic block and regional nerve anesthesia may also be used.[70,71,139] Because these procedures may be indicated for diagnostic reasons as well as for therapy, they are discussed later. It is essential that the examiner be cautious in his interpretation of each of the screening tests, especially when they are inconclusive. When borderline results are obtained more than one test should be used before the patient is scheduled for a sympathectomy.[65,70] No tests are infallible; in fact, several investigators have reported that they consider most tests unreliable for the purpose of predicting the outcome of any sympathectomy.[70,140] However, this pessimistic approach does little to aid us in evaluating the side effects and the risks of the operation and in pointing out the complications that are peculiar to the type of patient on whom it is performed. We therefore have concluded that the best method for selecting patients is simple to perform and economical in terms of time and money,[60] when utilized by a clinician who thoroughly understands the patient's disorder as well as the limitations of the procedure being advised for therapy.

Peripheral Arterial Disease. Peripheral arterial disease is the one disorder that may present any one or more of the indications for sympathectomy (i.e., vasospasm, inadequate small collateral vascular channels, causalgia or causalgia-type pain, and hyperhidrosis). This disease has therefore been the basis for more sympathectomies than any of the other disorders for which sympathectomy is designed. Conversely it is the cause of more unwarranted sympathectomies when the limitations of the procedure are not clearly understood, when proper methods for selection are not utilized, and when the course of the disease is not considered in the final outcome.

Thromboangiitis Obliterans. Thromboangiitis obliterans, or Buerger's disease, is the most controversial disorder of all occlusive diseases.[141,142] Confusion arises because of the possibility of thromboangiitis obliterans being caused by a local arteritis due to mechanical entrapment, or conditions of generalized vasculitis that result in peripheral gangrenous changes. Each of these conditions may be accentuated in a patient who has an acquired or congenital hypercoagulable state. Since the etiology of this condition continues to be an enigma, treatment is directed toward symptomatic relief, unless hypercoagulability indicates the continued use of an anticoagulant therapy. Vasospasm resulting from arterial occlusion is the primary indication for sympathectomy.[99,103] Since these patients go through remissions and exacerbations, complications from sympathectomy result when the procedure is performed during the acute stage of the disease. The association of this disease with the use of tobacco is well known, and elimination of this contributing factor should invariably precede consideration of sympathectomy.

Vasospasm. Vasospasm should not be considered as the sole cause for ischemia of tissue. Any vasospasm contributing to arterial insufficiency—whether it be due to trauma, embolus, thrombosis, or other vasospastic disorders—should be studied thoroughly.[71] There is no place for an emergency sympathectomy for any of these conditions unless it supplements definitive arterial surgery.

The most common vasospastic disorders are Raynaud's phenomenon, acrocyanosis, and livedo reticularis. Occasionally a lumbar sympathectomy is performed for Raynaud's phenomenon, never for acrocyanosis, and rarely for livedo reticularis.[143]

Causalgia. Causalgia or causalgia-type pain is a common entity with a highly predictable rate of success from sympathectomy. It may develop after any type of injury, accidental or surgical, infectious or noninfectious. Its presence may be localized to any surface area of the body, but it is most often noted in an extremity, especially the lower limb. It is frequently encountered by clinicians who treat peripheral vascular diseases, both in patients who have vascular disorders and those who do not.[83]

In general, diagnosis is based on (1) history of an overactive sympathetic nervous system; (2) superficial pain frequently described as burning and severe; (3) hyperesthesia localized to sensory nerve distribution; and (4) relief by medical or sympathetic denervation.[82,144]

Results of sympathectomy performed for relief of causalgia or causalgia-type pain are gratifying when patient selection is made on the basis of a diagnostic test of intra-arterial or intravenous sympatholytic drug, or a local anesthetic lumbar sympathetic block.[66] Two types of pain may be identified: one, of causalgic type, the other, of somatic root origin. Results of the removal of causalgia-type pain should be closely evaluated before treatment of somatic root pain is instituted by some other method. Pain in patients who have not been relieved by definitive and adequate sympathetic denervation should be studied further. The most common error in patient selection occurs when improper evaluation is made by sympathetic ganglion block or regional nerve anesthesia used to separate the two types of pain. When both types of nerves are anesthetized by the diagnostic procedure confusion results.[66]

Diagnostic and Therapeutic Regional Nerve Anesthesia

Sympathetic Blocks

Sympathetic nerve blocks to the cervical, thoracic, and lumbar ganglia were once popular diagnostic and therapeutic procedures,[70,71,139] but the objection to their use has been their unreliability, as judged by the patient's subjective response or the physician's interpretation of results. An acceptable test depends on the ability and knowledge of the clinician executing the block, the absence of anatomic variables in the sympathetic chain, and the availability of means to identify specific physiologic changes in the limb following the procedure.[133] Test facilities should include a skin resistor to verify obliteration of sudomotor activity, a plethysmograph to evaluate digital blood flow, and a temperature-controlled room where accurate thermocouple readings can be taken.[145]

Regional nerve anesthesia of the brachial plexus, spinal, or epidural areas may be employed, but relief of sympathetic-type pain may not be thereby distinguishable from somatic root pain, since these procedures usually result in complete sensory loss to the extremity.[146] Only a positive response is significant.[100] When an upper extremity is tested by injecting the stellate ganglion, a very common mistake is to conclude that the establishment of a Horner's syndrome identifies a successful sympathetic denervation of the upper limb. Even when a stellate ganglionectomy is performed, the presence of a Horner's syndrome does not assure that an adequate procedure was performed.

Certain technical dangers must be considered when doing sympathetic nerve blocks.[147] Paravertebral injection of alcohol or phenol for blocking sympathetic pathways is, in the author's opinion, not only hazardous but also frequently complicates pain problems. Complications such as Brown-Sequard paralysis, regional neuritis, and neuralgia have been reported when alcohol has been used for paravertebral sympathetic blocks. More serious complications have been reported following the injection of phenol: death from cardiac arrest, shock, renal or ureteric involvement, intrapleural injection, and neuritis.[148,149]

Hemometakinesia

Hemometakinesia, the borrowing-lending phenomenon described by DeBakey, Burch, Ray, and Ochsner, is one of the most interesting complications of sympathetic denervation that may occur from regional nerve anesthesia.[150] Following paravertebral, spinal, epidural, or caudal anesthesia or after a sympathectomy, there is a maximal degree of vasodilatation in the part.[152] Blood, therefore, shifts back and forth from one area of the body to another. The increase of blood volume in one part occurs at the expense of another, yet there is no variation in the total blood volume. Studies have demonstrated that the extremity with a sympathetic nerve block shows an increase in skin temperature while the opposite extremity has a drop in skin temperature. Other investigators have shown that vasodilatation produced by total body heating or by intravenous Tolazoline (Priscoline) is almost equal in normal subjects and in patients with vasospastic or ischemic disorders.[151] The greatest hemometakinesia effect is shown in patients who have had a sympathectomy and the sympathectomized extremities show a peripheral blood flow *decrease* when total body vasodilatation occurs. This is because the blood is diverted from the sympathectomized limb into the widespread new areas of reduced peripheral resistance.

Following lumbar sympathetic block, there is a marked vasodilatation in the lower extremity associated with increase in blood volume and rate of blood flow.[153] There may be as much as 75 per cent increase in extremity blood flow, and the venous pressure shows a decrease irrespective of a change in arterial pressure. There is "borrowed" blood flow to that extremity at the expense of the remainder of the body. The expense of this shift of blood is not borne entirely by the opposite limb, since its decrease is not as great as the other limb's increase.[150] Every organ that can afford to "lend" blood does so, and the amount depends on the quality and quantity of regional flow. When the shift is severe, such as in bilateral lumbar regional nerve anesthesia, death may occur from coronary insufficiency.

In addition, a patient with venous thrombosis in an extremity that has had a sympathetic block or spinal anesthesia demonstrates arterial dilatation, and more blood is forced into the extremity. Many of these cases have some manipulation of the limb, which increases muscle tone and compresses adjacent veins. This manipulation, when superimposed on an increased local circulation due to regional anesthesia, may precipitate embolism of the venous thrombus.[151,154]

Hazards of Regional Nerve Anesthesia

Two important factors may lead to a serious outcome during regional nerve anesthesia: (1) the borrowing of blood from the heart, and (2) the susceptibility of elderly patients to permanent vascular damage if hypotension develops during the regional anesthesia.[152]

Specific hazards associated with regional nerve anesthesia may be avoided by the following precautions: (1) Bilateral paravertebral sympathetic blocks or their equivalent should not be performed in elderly patients who are in congestive arteriosclerotic heart failure. (2) Patients with venous thrombosis in the lower extremities should have their blood volume restored before denervation of their sympathetics is undertaken. (3) Manipulation of the extremities should be minimal. (4) Any patient undergoing regional nerve anesthesia should be evaluated as to the risk of his having 500 to 1000 cc. of blood redistributed, mainly to the lower extremities and pelvis. (5) Any patient developing shock or having any evidence of pulmonary embolism during or immediately following sympathetic block

should not have the procedure repeated, and should be placed on anticoagulants. (6) Recognized preventive measures for thrombo-embolism should be instituted on all patients who are ultimately subjected to regional nerve anesthesia. Sympathetic denervation by regional nerve anesthesia is certainly not as popular as in the past, especially for thrombophlebitis. However, there are instances such as in causalgia-type pain and phlegmasia cerulea dolens where it may be indicated.

There are other complications from regional nerve anesthesia, such as pain at the site or distal to the injection, hemorrhage, infection, and injury to the specific nerve being infiltrated. A pneumothorax may easily be produced on the injected side while placing the needle for infiltration of the stellate ganglion and the second and third thoracic ganglion. Every patient should have a routine chest film following the block. During the same maneuver, the needle occasionally may be introduced into one of the large blood vessels resulting in a hematoma or in side effects that may occur from intravenous injection of a local anesthetic. A needle has been known to enter the esophagus or trachea when the clinician was not experienced or did not use due care. More hazardous complications have been a lateral spinal puncture with a fatal hemorrhage into the cord and a high spinal anesthesia with instant death in another patient.[147]

Anatomical Basis for Complications

A thorough knowledge of the normal anatomy and physiology of the sympathetic nervous system and its variables, and a clear understanding of the condition for which the procedure is being performed is essential to a critique of complications of sympathectomy.

The sympathetic nervous system is arranged segmentally, like its somatic counterpart. Sympathetic outflow extends from the first thoracic segment to the second lumbar segment with one paravertebral ganglion per segment which innervates the spinal nerve areas of that segment. The T_1 ganglion supplies the cervical nerves of the lateral aspect of the head and neck; T_2 innervates the T_2 dermatome to the upper limb. The first three lumbar ganglia supply the distribution of the femoral and sciatic nerves of the lower limb. The cell bodies of these efferent nerves are situated in the corresponding lateral horn of the grey matter of the spinal cord. Preganglionic nerves emerge from the spinal canal. The paravertebral sympathetic chain, lies on the lateral aspect of the vertebral column in the neck, on the neck of the ribs in the thorax, and on the lateral aspect of the vertebral bodies in the lumbar region. In the neck only three paravertebral ganglia are present, owing to fusion. The superior cervical ganglion is formed from the upper four cervical ganglia, the middle cervical ganglion by the fifth and sixth ganglia, and the inferior cervical ganglion by the fusion of the seventh and eighth ganglia. The "stellate ganglion" is the result of fusion of the inferior cervical ganglion with the first thoracic ganglion.

The cervical ganglia have two completely different sympathetic pathways to the upper extremities and the oculopupillary region. The preganglionic fibers supplying the oculopupillary apparatus arise in the lateral horn of the spinal cord, emerge with the anterior roots of T_1 and C_8, and traverse the stellate ganglion. They do not synapse with postganglionic fibers until they reach the superior cervical ganglion at which point postganglionic fibers pass on to the sheath of the internal carotid artery to the orbit. The skin of the neck and head as well as the salivary glands and the cervical plexus are supplied by preganglionic fibers that arise with the first and second thoracic nerves. They synapse in the superior cervical ganglion with postganglionic fibers that accompany the external carotid artery to the skin of the face, head, salivary glands and the cervical plexus. The anterior nerve roots in the cervical region have no accompanying sympathetic fibers, since the preganglionic

fibers begin at the T_1 level and preganglionic outflow to the upper limbs usually emerges from T_2 to T_9. These pathways and their variables are of interest to the surgeon, not only to accomplish the objective of sympathectomy but also to lessen the potential of unnecessary complications.[133]

In the thoracic area, the paravertebral ganglia are usually found adjacent to their somatic counterparts. In the lumbar region the ganglia are normally situated segmentally.

The upper extremity receives its sympathetic nerve supply via the brachial plexus. Its preganglionic fibers originate from the first or second thoracic segment to approximately the ninth thoracic segment of the spinal cord. They accompany the anterior spinal roots and ascend uninterrupted in the paravertebral chain until they synapse with postganglionic fibers in the stellate ganglion. In the upper extremity the median nerve carries the dominant sympathetic supply, occasionally the ulnar nerve, and, rarely, the radial nerve.

Anatomical Anomalies

Unexpected complications may occur when the surgeon is not completely familiar with the normal anatomy and its variables, especially in the cervicothoracic area. Ablation of the sympathetic outflow to the head alone may be accomplished by interrupting the cervical sympathetic chain. When sympathetic denervation of the head and upper extremity is desired, the sympathetic chain is interrupted by excision of the stellate ganglion. However, to avoid incomplete sympathectomy from possible anatomic variations, both the stellate ganglion and the second thoracic ganglion must be removed. A Horner's syndrome may be avoided in most patients by sectioning the sympathetic chain below the preganglionic fibers emerging from the first thoracic segment of the cord. Since there are many anatomic variables of sympathetic nerves to the brachial plexus, the upper limb has a high incidence of sympathectomy failure. An extreme anomaly is when the preganglionic fibers avoid the sympathetic chain completely and continue on to the brachial plexus via a somatic nerve. In this instance an upper thoracic sympathectomy would result in little, if any, change in the upper limb.

Law of Denervation

Ignorance on the part of the physician of Cannon's Law of Denervation is another reason for failure to achieve the desired benefit with a postganglionic sympathectomy.[155] This law maintains that in a series of efferent neurons, when a unit is interrupted, the isolated effector organ (sweat gland, smooth muscle) develops a hypersensitivity to humoral agents such as circulating epinephrine.[22] If the stellate ganglion and middle cervical ganglion are left intact (postganglionic fibers) and a preganglionic resection of T_2-T_5 is performed, the sympathetic fibers to the brachial plexus are preserved, and the hypersensitivity produced by epinephrine is avoided. A Horner's syndrome may also be avoided by leaving the preganglionic fibers to T_1 intact. Tilford and Smithwich advised that only a preganglionic ramisection for the upper extremity be performed.

The law of denervation is not universally accepted as the principal factor in a poor result. Some surgeons believe the failures are due to incomplete denervation when the stellate ganglion is not included in an upper thoracic sympathectomy; however, a better explanation may be the one patient in ten in whom the sympathetic outflow to the arm travels via T_1. In the author's experience there is some validity in the law when the indication for sympathectomy is causalgia-type pain with severe ischemia of the part or vasospasm alone. In addition, there is a higher incidence of failure to relieve causalgia when only a stellate ganglionectomy has been performed. We agree with Goetz who believes that some clinicians place too much emphasis on obtaining a Horner's syndrome and do not recognize the merits of producing

a permanent sympathetic paralysis to the upper extremity.[21]

The sympathetic outflow to the lower extremities is derived from the preganglionic fibers that arise in the lateral grey substance from T_{10} to approximately L_3. They accompany the anterior roots and join the paravertebral chain where they synapse with the postganglionic fibers in the ganglia adjacent to the roots of the femoral, obturator, and sciatic nerves. Fibers from the first four lumbar nerves supply the femoral and obturator nerves, while the sciatic nerve derives its fibers from the fourth and fifth lumbar roots, the first three sacral nerves, and occasionally, from the third lumbar root. Ablation of the sympathetic innervation to the lower extremities is generally not a problem. To completely denervate the sympathetic nervous system supplying the entire lower extremity, L_1, L_2, and L_3 ganglia must be sectioned. Since the sciatic nerve is the only nerve supplying the leg and foot, most emphasis is placed on removal of the second and third lumbar ganglia. Only occasionally is attention directed to sympathetic disorders of the femoral and obturator nerves.[133]

Operative Procedures and Related Complications

Complications arising from incomplete hemostasis at the time of operation and from infection are thoroughly appreciated by modern surgeons. Historically, hemorrhage was not uncommon during and after a periarterial sympathectomy. The fact that the procedure had to be performed on vessels containing plaques or severely sclerotic lumina contributed to the problem. The adventitia was so adherent to the vessel owing to the disease that a proper plane for dissection was difficult to establish. Where the vessel lumen was penetrated, permanent hemostasis usually was not obtained by suture closure. Severe hemorrhage, ligation of the iliac artery, amputation, and even deaths were reported.[156]

Upper Extremity Sympathectomy

The most controversial question involving sympathectomy for upper extremity disorders is whether to perform a preganglionic or a postganglionic section. The postganglionic operation, the procedure used thirty years ago, involved excision of the inferior cervical ganglion and the first, second, and third thoracic ganglia. Some surgeons extended the procedure up to the middle cervical ganglion to include some postganglionic fibers that originate in this area and pass to the brachial plexus, but this upward extension has since been abandoned. A significant objection to the postganglionic operation was the undesirable development of a Horner's syndrome, which occurs when the first thoracic white ramus communicans is divided.

The preganglionic operation was popular not only because it avoided a Horner's syndrome but also because there was both experimental and clinical evidence to suggest that it may be the better of the two procedures.[134] Physiologists have long known that a denervated organ becomes hypersensitive to the vasoconstrictor substance normally liberated at its nerve endings. This phenomenon has been used to explain why there is a return of function after a postganglionic sympathectomy for vascular disease. For example, in Raynaud's disease the results of a lumbar sympathectomy for the leg are much more favorable than those of a cervicothoracic ganglionectomy for the upper limb because a lumbar ganglionectomy is a preganglionic procedure. However, sensitization follows preganglionic section also. Ross believes that there is little to choose between the late results of the two operations, and therefore he prefers a preganglionic section, since it does not produce Horner's syndrome.[134] The leading proponents of the cervicothoracic ganglionectomy are Goetz[21] and de Takats.[67]

Operative Approaches

There are four approaches to denervating the cervical and/or upper thoracic sympathetic chain: (1) the posterior transthoracic route originally described by Adson[36] and later popularized by Smithwick;[157] (2) the supraclavicular approach developed by Gask and Ross[17] and Telford;[22] (3) the anterior transthoracic approach;[158] and (4) the axillary transthoracic route originally described by Goetz.[159]

The posterior transthoracic approach is seldom used because of limited visualization and the high incidence of performance of an inadequate procedure. Therefore, the procedure will not be described.

The supraclavicular approach to the cervicodorsal sympathetic chain is probably the most hazardous of all avenues used today to ablate the sympathetic nervous system. It is the author's opinion that this procedure should be abandoned because of the high potential for serious complications (especially in individuals with an overactive sympathetic nervous system). Injuries to the subclavian artery, carotid artery, jugular vein, thoracic duct, brachial plexus, phrenic nerve, and pleura have been observed by the author and reported by others.[160-162] Flye and Walkoff, reporting a mycotic aneurysm of the left subclavian and vertebral arteries, stated that even though the advantages of the supraclavicular approach were its simplicity, the surgeon's ability to remove more of the cephalic sympathetic chain, and less postoperative pain than from a thoracotomy, there were serious hazards.[160] These were limited caudad exposure, which permitted only a limited sympathectomy, and difficulties of exposure to control any hemorrhage that might cause ischemia of the limb after hemostasis was accomplished. Lord commented on a patient who developed gangrene of the hand following ligation of an inadvertently injured subclavian artery.[162] He also mentioned a brachial plexus injury. This writer has consulted on three patients with disabling ischemia of the hand following similar subclavian injuries by surgeons believed to be well qualified.

Positioning. The position of the patient may be supine or semi-sitting with the head hyperextended and turned away from the side of operation. The semi-sitting position is not recommended because of the potential for accidental air embolism.

Technique. The incision is made just above the clavicle and extends laterally from the medial border of the sternocleidomastoid for 2 to 3 inches. The skin, platysma, superficial fascia and descending supraclavicular nerves are divided. The external jugular vein may or may not be severed; the clavicular head of the sternocleidomastoid muscle is sectioned, leaving enough muscle inferiorly for repair. The omohyoid muscle is retracted and all vessels within the scalene fat pad are carefully ligated before they are divided. The scalenus anticus muscle appears and its fascia is left intact to avoid damage to the phrenic nerve lying on the medial border of the muscle and traversing it obliquely. Farther medially, the internal jugular vein is severed. Care is taken to avoid the thoracic duct on the left side. Laterally, the brachial plexus is recognized. The nerve to the subclavian muscle may be noted on the lateral border of the scalenus muscle.

The phrenic nerve is dissected free and carefully retracted medially without undue tension. At this point the scalenus anticus muscle is mobilized and transected just above its attachment to the first rib. At this area vessels such as the thyrocervical trunk may easily be cut, the subclavian artery and/ or the vetebral artery and vein damaged, and the phrenic nerve injured; on the left side the thoracic duct may easily be torn. The subclavian artery is separated from the internal jugular vein under which lies the vertebral artery as a branch of the subclavian just opposite to the internal mammary artery. The thyrocervical trunk coming off the subclavian distal to the vertebral artery should be carefully ligated to avoid injury and hazardous bleeding which often leads to damage of the subclavian artery. The vertebral artery usually leads to the stellate ganglion.

The subclavian artery is retracted and the

seventh cervical transverse process is exposed along with the dome of the lung, the pleural sac, and the suprapleural membrane (Sibson's fascia). The stellate ganglion lies on the neck of the first rib. The fascia is bluntly dissected from the rib to enter the retropleural space. The sympathetic chain emerges into view as a thick, cordlike structure transversing the neck of the first rib. The first intercostal artery and vein may be noted medially and should be avoided. The chain is then dissected inferiorly and sectioned below the third thoracic ganglion and removed along with the stellate ganglion; the connecting branches are clipped. Each of the structures in this area should be thoroughly visualized by drying the moist tissue with a dry sponge before cutting. If an isolated stellate block was performed preoperatively and a significant temporary relief of the upper extremity disorder was not obtained in spite of a Horner's syndrome, then the stellate ganglion may be spared.

If the subclavian artery or internal jugular vein is injured, the opening should be closed with fine nonabsorbable vascular sutures. The vein may be ligated. A thoracic duct injury requires careful ligature to prevent a lymphocoele or lymphorrhea in the wound postoperatively. Pneumothorax is treated by gentle suction using a catheter in the wound while the anesthetist keeps the lungs inflated. The catheter is slowly withdrawn as all structures except the scalenus anticus are closed in layers. Insertion of a chest tube may be necessary in some cases.

Anterolateral transthoracic approach through the fourth intercostal space gives the best exposure to the sympathetic chain. However, this approach necessitates a formal thoracotomy with the risk of the usual complications. The removal of the first rib from this approach in a thoracic outlet syndrome is not recommended, since it is overlapped by the second rib when the rib spreader is opened. One hazard of any transthoracic approach is postthoracotomy pain that may occur due to trauma to the intercostal nerve. This is especially likely in those patients who are "sympathetic reactors." Therefore the intercostal nerve is carefully protected during the procedure.

The axillary transthoracic approach has become increasingly popular since Goetz demonstrated it to Atkins, who described it in 1949.[21,163] This extrapleural or transpleural approach to the thoracic sympathetic chain has as its most serious hazard injury to the brachial plexus by overextension of the arm. This is prevented by placing the patient in the lateral position with the arm abducted 120° to 140° and drawn forward and placed on an armrest.[121] An assistant should prevent the shoulder from being displaced posteriorly, which could cause the clavicle to impinge on the thoracic outlet contents against the first rib. If the armrest does not accomplish this, the assistant should put tension on the arm while in the abducted position.

Technique. Two entries to the thorax may be made: one via the third intercostal space, the other via the bed of the first rib when its excision is indicated for a thoracic outlet syndrome. The incision is made at the base of the axilla below the hairline to avoid later problems with the scar and to avoid the lymph glands. It is directed towards the rib cage and extends from the pectoralis major anteriorly to the latissimus dorsi posteriorly. By finger dissection the chest wall is easily exposed. The intercostobrachial nerve lies in the center of the exposure exiting from the second intercostal space and it may be spared. If it is traumatized, there may be numbness and paresthesia in the axilla and medial aspect of the arm postoperatively. Posteriorly, the long thoracic and thoracodorsal nerves may be encountered and should be avoided.

During the procedure, the arm should be brought down to the patient's side for short periods to avoid prolonged tension and entrapment of the neurovascular bundle. Both the latissimus dorsi and pectoralis major muscles should be retracted. The pectoralis major may need to be incised for a short distance to give the operator better

exposure. The intercostal spaces are identified and counted. The third intercostal space is usually wide and allows easy exposure. The rib spreader is opened slowly to avoid fracturing any ribs; the lung is retracted over moist pads as it collapses. Unless dense adhesions are present, no damage to the lung should occur. The pleura is incised over the sympathetic chain lying on the neck of the ribs. The intercostal vessels, particularly the superior intercostal artery lying at the level of the stellate ganglion, should be avoided, or clipped and divided if necessary.

Beginning at the fourth ganglion, the trunk is transected and gently lifted from its bed, and as the dissection continues toward the first thoracic and the inferior cervical ganglia (stellate ganglion) all branches are divided. Each is clipped when there is any doubt that vascular structures may be incorporated nearby. The stellate ganglion is identified as a broad structure lying on the neck of the flat first rib. The first thoracic preganglionic fiber is identified. At this point the decision is made to remove the stellate ganglion and produce a Horner's syndrome or to section the chain just below the entrance of the first thoracic preganglionic fibers. The subclavian artery requires light retraction, and the vertebral artery must be carefully avoided during the dissection of the stellate ganglion. Inferiorly the thoracic duct may be visualized. If it is injured, no attempt should be made to repair it; nor should it be clipped, but securely ligated to prevent a chylothorax.

The lung is expanded, and the intercostal space and subcutaneous fat are closed over a catheter that is aspirated and withdrawn as the anesthetist maintains positive pressure. An intercostal catheter may be placed in the apex of the chest and brought out through the fifth intercostal space in the mid axillary line for underwater drainage when hemorrhage or pneumothorax is anticipated.

Similar exposure may be obtained retropleurally but with more difficulty, since the lung is not collapsed and occasionally a he-

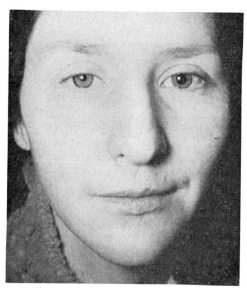

FIG. 9-1. Unilateral Horner's syndrome following cervicothoracic sympathectomy for Raynaud's phenomenon. Note ptosis of lid, enophthalmos, and constricted pupil on right.

matoma or serous loculation can occur postoperatively which may require aspiration. Visualization of the sympathetic chain may be a little difficult following a resection of the first rib for a thoracic outlet syndrome. Occasionally it may be necessary to resect the second rib for complete exposure if sympathectomy is essential.

Horner's Syndrome

Horner's syndrome is an inevitable complication of a complete stellate ganglionectomy. It is characterized by several ipsilateral signs including ptosis of the upper lid, enophthalmos, a constricted pupil, drying of the nasal mucosa of the face and loss of sweating on the face (Fig. 9-1).

The syndrome develops and becomes more marked 48 to 72 hours after ablation of the oculopupillary sympathetic tract anywhere, whether it be section of the first thoracic preganglionic tract, the sympathetic chain, or any of the ganglia traversed by the postganglionic fibers, especially the stellate or superior cervical ganglion. The pupil becomes small but retains its reflex movements. It cannot be dilated with atropine. The

ptosis, which disappears when the eyeball is raised, shows that it is due to the enophthalmos and not to an interference with the innervation of the levator palpebrae muscle. Neither the ptosis nor the enophthalmos ever completely disappears. If the ptosis is bilateral, it is hardly noticeable. In a myopic eye, however, Horner's syndrome seems to predispose to retinal detachment. Ross states that myopia therefore should be regarded as a contraindication to a postganglionic operation.[134]

A more disturbing effect of stellate ganglionectomy is the narrowed nasal passage on the corresponding side due to the vasodilatation of the nasal mucosa. When the narrowing is bilateral, it may result in mouth breathing which causes a great inconvenience to the patient for many years after operation. Treatment of the nasal mucosa with inhalation, nose drops, or cauterization is of little help.

There is no treatment for Horner's syndrome, only prevention. This can be accomplished by preganglionic section of the sympathetic chain just inferior to the stellate ganglion avoiding the first thoracic preganglionic fibers (Telford's operation).[22]

Gustatory Sweating and Pilomotor Changes

Following operations on the cervicodorsal sympathetic chain, gustatory sweating on half of the face is a fairly common occurrence.[116,164-166] It is a striking condition and occurs only after bilateral operations. The anomaly, an abnormal localized sweating associated with eating, has also been reported in syringomyelia, operations on the nose, infections, operations or injury to the parotid gland, or associated with congenital defects. Accompanying the gustatory sweating may be tingling and flushing, and vasoconstriction as well as pilomotor changes in the skin. The use of condiments, spicy or acid foods, or sweets may initiate the complaint.

The extent of the operation seems to have no influence on the incidence of the complication. It is more frequently noted whenever a cervicodorsal sympathectomy is performed for hyperhidrosis or Raynaud's phenomenon. It may be delayed, although most often it appears in the first 12 months postoperatively.

Sweating is produced by cholinergic sympathetic fibers while vasoconstriction and gooseflesh are adrenergic as well as gustatory responses. The tingling could be classified as a minor form of a postsympathectomy pain syndrome.

Flushing usually occurs on the upper chest and neck and is sharply demarcated and not associated with a rise in skin temperature. A similar condition is seen occasionally after a traumatic cord injury where the sweating, gooseflesh, and vasomotor disturbances occur in areas around the level where the injury of the cord occurred.[164,165] Causalgia-type pain has also been noted by the author in a patient who was making a successful recovery from quadraplegia.

It has been suggested that the findings may be due to regeneration of injured sympathetic fibers within the cord or as a result of sprouting.[165] One of the most interesting aspects of this phenomenon is why sudomotor, vasomotor, and pilomotor activity should return in an area of sypathectomized skin following a gustatory stimulus without the return of such activity as thermal response. Ashby questions how one reflex can regenerate without the other, unless they are served by different preganglionic fibers.[166]

Treatment for the complication includes the use of a ganglion-blocking drug, a stellate ganglion block with local anesthetic, and in some situations a sympathectomy, especially the excision of any residual stellate ganglion tissue.[116,166]

Thoracodorsal Sympathectomy and Splanchnicectomy

Around the middle of this century several thousand patients underwent various forms of sympathetic denervation for the relief of hypertensive vascular disease and splanchnicectomy for visceral disorders.[41,48,68,167-171] The majority of the procedures for hypertension involved resection of the sympathetic chain from the ninth thoracic through the second lumbar ganglion combined with bilateral resection of the splanchnic nerves. Splanchnicectomy consisted of removal of the splanchnic nerves that arise from the thoracic sympathetic chain. To obtain optimal results, surgeons began to extend their resections for hypertension as well as for visceral disorders. As with sympathectomies for other disorders, the more extensive the procedure the more numerous are certain problems associated with it.[111,167] The magnitude of these problems limited the use of the operative procedures about the time medical therapy began to produce more optimal results, and definitive surgery was being performed for the causes of hypertension and visceral disorders. Although sympathectomy for hypertension and visceral disorders was generally abandoned, some of its complications should be discussed for a more complete understanding of problems that can occur from sympathetic denervation in any area of the body. Those complications involving ablation of only the lumbar sympathetic trunk are listed in the section of lumbar sympathectomy.

Postural Hypotension

When sympathectomy was a popular treatment for hypertension most clinicians believed that postoperative postural hypotension was necessary to achieve a satisfactory reduction in blood pressure.[168-170] When any patient who had had extensive sympathetic denervation stood erect, the blood pressure usually fell to such a low level that syncope soon occurred, demonstrating the effective loss of vasoconstrictor tone. Patients with extensive atherosclerosis showed proportionately less significant postural hypotension. Postural hypotension seldom occurs from four-extremity sympathetic denervation, and it is not significant when a thoracolumbar splanchnic sympathectomy is performed on one side. Vasoconstriction in the enervated areas of the body usually compensates for extremity denervation while the abdominal splanchnic pool does not enlarge its vascular bed unless a bilateral denervation has been performed. Some patients may have temporary dizziness, faintness and lack of mental acuity after sympathetic denervation due to diminished cerebral flow and some degree of cerebral vasoconstriction.[168]

Postural hypotension can be prevented satisfactorily by compression stockings, a leotard, and a tight abdominal binder. A readjustment of sympathetic tone or compensatory processes occurs in a short time which makes compression measures unnecessary although many patients find that they must keep moving while on their feet in order to maintain an adequate blood pressure. Most patients with postural hypotension complain of a feeling of substernal fluttering or breathlessness early in their postoperative course, but not severe enough to suggest anginal pain. This is due to the increase in pulse rate to compensate for the decrease in venous return which in turn causes a fall in blood pressure. Postural hypotension seldom lasts for more than a few months, and patients in whom it persists longer do not find it uncomfortable.[168]

Hyperhidrosis

This uncomfortable condition may occur in enervated portions of the body and is most severe during the immediate postoperative period.[168] It is not persistent unless maximal sympathectomies are performed. Please see the discussion relative to sympathetic denervation of extremities elsewhere in this chapter.

Motor Dysfunction of the Intestinal Tract

Postoperative abdominal distension is not uncommon following extensive sympathectomies for hypertension. This occurs for a few days postoperatively owing to decreased intestinal mobility. A subsequent increase in gastric motility and secretion develops which may cause gastric or duodenal ulcers.

Some may go unnoticed until hemorrhage occurs due to elimination of visceral pain.[168]

Visceral Pain Loss. With a bilateral thoracolumbar sympathectomy or a bilateral splanchnicectomy, most visceral pain fibers from organs and tissues of the upper abdomen are destroyed. For diagnosic purposes the same effect may be obtained temporarily by blocking the sympathetic chain from the seventh thoracic through the second lumbar ganglion. Operations have been performed to remove this portion of the sympathetic nervous system to relieve intractable abdominal pain.[172,173] This loss of visceral pain may be a handicap if the patient develops an acute abdominal condition such as cholecystitis, perforated peptic ulcer, perforated bowel, or acute pancreatitis.[167,172] Such a patient may show evidence of being ill without the acute localizing signs, symptoms, and pain that usually signal an acute abdominal catastrophe. Therefore diagnosis may be delayed until the disorder has advanced sufficiently to cause irritation of the adjoining parietal peritoneum, where somatic root- rather than visceral nerve pathways are stimulated.

Paraplegia

Paraplegia is the most serious complication that can follow thoracolumbar sympathectomy.[174] Possible causes are: transverse myelitis, anterior spinal artery occlusion, venous thrombosis within the spinal canal, intraspinal hemorrhage, and arterial emboli to the cord. Recommendations for prevention are: avoidance of hypotension, ligation to control bleeding from intercostal vessels, and care in manipulating the aorta during surgery.

Other Complications

Additional complications which are largely technical include shock when bilateral procedures are undertaken, hemorrhage, neuralgia, and myalgia. The thoracic duct may be injured when this structure is mistaken for the major splanchnic nerve. Ligation with sutures instead of metal clips is advised if the thoracic duct is traumatized.[167]

Lumbar Sympathectomy

One of the major reasons a lumbar sympathectomy may fail to produce the expected results is the great anatomic variation in the sympathetic nervous system supplying the lower extremity. Fusion and splitting of ganglia and absence of ganglia are common.[75,175] Interconnections in the L_1 and L_5 region are frequent.[77] Widely scattered "intermediate ganglia" may be present in the plexus surrounding the aorta, posterior to the psoas muscle,[78] or contained in the spinal nerves that do not pass through the sympathetic chain or its ganglia.[111,116,131] The majority of lumbar sympathetic trunks show a textbook pattern, however. The outcome depends on the surgeon's knowledge of the anatomical variables and how the physiology of the sympathetic nervous system relates to the disorder for which the operation is being performed.

Since the sympathetic outflow from the spinal cord does not extend beyond L_2 or L_3, sectioning the trunk at this level should interrupt all of the fibers passing to the sciatic nerve and approximately half of those carried by the femoral and obturator nerves. Such a procedure would sympathetically denervate the limb below the knee, except for "islands" of sympathetic activity on the medial aspect of the leg and foot where the saphenous nerve is distributed.[116,156] This, therefore, would be considered an incomplete sympathectomy, and in some disorders a second procedure would be indicated at a higher level to interrupt the remaining fibers distributed by the femoral and obturator nerves.

It is, theoretically, better to remove a long segment of trunk than to excise a small portion and chance the possibility of persistent collateral pathways.[176] The usual procedure is a "low" lumbar sympathectomy in which the L_2 and L_3 ganglia are removed. A "high" sympathectomy is one in which the L_1 ganglion is also excised. A low thoracic–high lumbar sympathectomy, which includes additional excision of T_{12} and even T_{11} ganglia, has received controversial reports in the literature.[79,177,178] Proponents of a high sympathectomy believe that to increase the chances of interrupting an occasional aberrant pathway and lessen the possibility of missing an essential ganglion, a wide excision is necessary.[176,177] The argument against a high sympathectomy includes the possibility of loss of ejaculation and resultant sterility in the young male when L_1 is removed bilaterally.[178]

Operative Procedure

Lumbar ganglionectomy may be performed transperitoneally or extraperitoneally from the front or from the flank. Most surgeons use the transperitoneal approach only when a single bilateral operation is indicated or to complement definitive aortoiliac surgery for obliterative disease in the lower limbs. However, it should not be used (1) in patients over 60, especially in individuals with cardiac or pulmonary disease; (2) for obese patients owing to the difficulty of dissection, and (3) when dense adhesions are present from previous abdominal surgery.

A high sympathectomy requires general endotracheal anesthesia since the pleural cavity may be entered and a pneumothorax may be produced when ganglia are excised through the crus of the diaphragm.

Proper positioning of the patient on the operating table lessens the possibility of several complications. Optimal exposure and easy accessibility to the lumbar chain is obtained by a 30-degree tilt toward the supine with the area between the twelfth rib and pelvic crest centered over the kidney rest with a break in the operating table. The dependent limb is extended and the thigh of the uppermost limb flexed to relax the psoas muscle. Excessive elevation of the kidney rest or marked flexion of the table should be avoided in older patients since severe postoperative back pain may ensue due to injury of arthritic vertebrae. Any patient with an above-the-knee amputation who undergoes a lumbar sympathectomy (usually for causalgia in the phantom limb) must have the stump depressed by taping it to the table, since there is little weight to the remaining limb to tilt the pelvis inferiorly.

The incision is made transversely in the anterior superior lateral portion of the abdomen, avoiding the heavy flank musculature laterally and the rectus sheath medially. If reoperation or a high lumbar sympathectomy is planned, a more lateral approach and excision of the 12th rib may be necessary. The incision cuts across the external and internal oblique muscles. Only the transversus abdominis is separated in the direction of its fibers, because this lessens the demand for muscle relaxation. No hernia has been observed following this muscle cutting procedure. One or even two intercostal nerves may be cut unless care is exercised. This is not a serious matter unless three of these nerves are severed in sequence; however, later pain problems may appear in patients who are prone to causalgia. Between the internal oblique and the transversus abdominis muscle, the neurovascular plane meets the rectus sheath, and care must be taken at this area because the peritoneum may easily be entered. Any perforation is immediately closed, and tension is subsequently avoided in the area.

Attention is now directed laterally within the wound where the peritoneum is retracted medially, exposing the psoas muscle. This muscle is very prominent anteriorly because of hyperextension of the patient. Dissection must be carried out on the upper surface of the psoas muscle and not on the quadratus lumborum muscle, which lies posteriorly. The psoas muscle often lies closer to the midline and farther front than expected, and if the surgeon inadvertently dissects into the groove behind the psoas muscle, the operation is prolonged unnecessarily.

Each anatomical landmark is now identified: the kidney and ureter are displaced medially; the genitofemoral and ileoinguinal nerves lie on the psoas muscle posteriorly; and the vertebra is medial in the extreme depth of the operative wound. The sympathetic chain on the lateral border of the

vertebra may be palpated before it comes into view by rolling it against the vertebral body, where it feels cordlike, similar to a vas deferens. Any easily movable structure identified as a sympathetic chain should be avoided because these "fool's sympathetics" are not the true sympathetic chain.[147] These include the lymphatic chain on the vertebra, the ilioinguinal and genitofemoral nerves laterally, the obturator nerve inferiorly where the psoas muscle leaves the vertebra, fascial strips, and the ureter. On the right side the sympathetic chain lies just behind the lateral border of the inferior vena cava; on the left side, it is just beyond the lateral edge of the abdominal aorta. Dissection is continued superiorly and inferiorly along the lateral border of the vertebra. Harrington and Deaver retractors aid in isolating the chain, though care should be taken not to traumatize an atherosclerotic aorta or iliac artery.

In some patients lumbar veins may cross over the sympathetic trunk; in others, they are posterior to the sympathetic trunk. Ordinarily the L_4 ganglion is encountered first at the sacral promontory, just behind the iliac vessels. The L_3 ganglion is identified before the chain enters the crus of the diaphragm at the level of the second lumbar vertebra. The body of each vertebra is identified, and a long suture is passed beneath the chain with a right-angle clamp in an intervertebral space where lumbar vessels and preganglionic fibers traverse the foramen.

The sympathetic chain is held taut with the long suture or it is cut and a clamp is applied to the cut end being dissected. The chain is first traced inferiorly. The connecting fibers of the chain point caudad on the third and fourth ganglia and cephalad at the first and second ganglia.[147] The rami are sectioned inferiorly as they are identified until the trunk passes behind the iliac vessels, where it usually divides into two or three terminal branches from what appears to be a broad ganglion. Cross-over fibers communicating with the contralateral chain and intermediate ganglia on the aorta or iliac artery are identified and divided when present. The obturator nerve should be avoided as it emerges between the psoas muscle and vertebra. Retractors or other instruments should not be permitted to traumatize the genitofemoral or ilioinguinal nerves nor to press too firmly against an atherosclerotic aorta or iliac artery. After each terminal branch is identified, metal clips are applied and the chain divided inferiorly. Dissection is continued upward, and each intervetebral space is identified and the chain is gently dissected off of the lumbar vessels as they are encountered. If bleeding occurs, metal clips are applied for hemostasis. These vessels should not be clamped and tied, as they tear very easily and bleeding may become difficult to control. Veins crossing over the chain are clipped and divided but this may be avoided by passing the trunk beneath each of them.

As the trunk passes through the crus of the diaphragm the muscle and tendinous fibers are separated. Here the first or second lumbar ganglion is usually large and may be fixed to surrounding structures. The sympathetic trunk now begins to be displaced laterally. In this area the chain may be sectioned after a metal clip has been applied superiorly. Further dissection upward on the chain should be done carefully to avoid the pleural reflection.

Technical difficulties are uncommon when the procedure is performed properly, and postoperative complications are few, since hematoma and infection seldom occur. Mild abdominal distension from a dynamic ileus often accompanies retroperitoneal operations, but this usually subsides within 24 to 48 hours. If abdominal distension is persistent in aerophagic patients, it may be treated by nasogastric suction. Complications related specifically to ablation of the sympathetic nervous system are discussed below.

Derangement of Sexual Functions

Most surgeons fear that the bilateral removal of the L_1 and L_2 ganglia will produce loss of libido, failure of ejaculation, and even sterility. There is universal agreement, how-

ever, that preservation of the first lumbar ganglion on one side is a good safeguard against this complication.[145,179] Bilateral lumbar sympathectomy which includes L_1, L_2, and L_3 ganglia has been reported to cause permanent loss of seminal emission in 54 per cent of patients and temporary reduction or permanent loss of erection in 63 per cent of cases.[179] Fowler and de Takats believed that the high incidence of impotence reported could be the result of factors other than sympathectomy. They believed it was unwise to question the patient directly about this occasional undesirable complication of sympathectomy during the postoperative followup, and therefore they obtained their findings only by casual questioning or information volunteered by patients. Their conclusions are supported by Alnor, who found no close correlation between the extent of denervation and sexual ability or libido.[167,180]

Whitelaw and Smithwick[179] carefully questioned a group of male sympathectomy patients. In a very interesting, detailed clinical report they reviewed the normal anatomic pathway and the physiologic mechanisms involved in erection and ejaculation and how often these functions were deranged after various types of sympathectomy. They concluded that when a transthoracic procedure was performed for hypertension there was no permanent loss of ejaculation, but 57 per cent of cases did have a disturbance of erection. This was not complete enough to interfere seriously with sexual intercourse. All phases of sexual function could be preserved in a lumbodorsal operation by not removing any ganglion below L_1 on one side and T_{12} on the other. In a bilateral lumbar procedure, it was their impression that sexual function was not deranged if the operation was not extended to include L_1 on either side. However, when L_1, L_2, and L_3 ganglia were removed on both sides there was significant change in sexual function in at least 63 per cent of the patients.

These findings have been misunderstood and misrepresented to patients, and it is essential to know exactly what effect a bilateral excision of the first lumbar ganglion may have on the sexual activity of a potent male. A considerable number of patients are unable to ejaculate externally following a first lumbar ganglionectomy. The internal vesical sphincter is unable to close at the moment of ejaculation, and therefore the discharge is directed into the bladder instead of through the urethera. Sterility always follows failure to ejaculate, but sensations and potency remain unchanged.[156]

Apparently sympathectomy has no adverse effect on the female genital tract when L_1 is included in the procedure bilaterally. Reports of its effect on menses and on sexual desire and sensory response of intercourse vary.[145,156,167]

An interesting observation in the Whitelaw and Smithwick study was that 7 per cent of their male patients reported that sexual function had increased.[179] Several years ago this author was quite surprised when two patients who had undergone bilateral high lumbar sympathectomy volunteered information that their sexual desire and ability had become more frequent since operation. Kuntz comments that patients with functional impotence who undergo bilateral lumbar sympathectomy may have marked improvement in erections, but the ability to discharge semen through the urethra is lost.[156]

The Aortoiliac Steal Syndrome

Some surgeons routinely perform bilateral lumbar sympathectomies;[181] others believe a bilateral procedure may increase the likelihood of blood being shunted from the affected extremity causing a steal phenomenon. In bilateral vascular disease, a unilateral sympathectomy may cause a steal from the contralateral limb.[100,150] Kountz et al. reported a case of necrosis of the small bowel following sequential lumbar sympathectomy and iliofemoral bypass grafts. They theorized that a reflex redistribution of blood had occurred in which blood was "stolen" from the mesenteric vasculature by

the iliofemoral system; they named the phenomenon the aortoiliac steal syndrome.[182]

Vascular surgeons have accepted De Bakey's idea that the carotid system should be evaluated and revascularized prior to extensive aorto-iliac reconstruction if obliterative disease is present. This procedure is not only a precautionary measure against cerebrovascular insufficiency during aortic surgery; it also protects against any shunting or "stealing" of blood from the cerebral arterial system to the lower extremities following aortoiliac surgery.[182]

Another type of steal phenomenon has been reported when asymmetric lumbar sympathectomies were performed.[183] This resulted in a shunting of blood away from the incompletely sympathectomized extremity.[184,185] It has been advised that if a bilateral lumbar sympathectomy was indicated, the same amount of sympathetic chain should be excised bilaterally.[186] This is disputed by advocates of a high lumbar sympathectomy who advise that the L_1 ganglion be spared on one side in a bilateral procedure performed on a sexually potent patient.[176,177]

Further clinical studies of steal syndromes are needed for a better understanding of how they occur. As with sexual derangement and "paradoxical gangrene," it is believed that factors other than sympathectomy either influence or cause this complication.

Paradoxical Gangrene—A Myth

The concept of paradoxical gangrene was first described by Atlas in 1942.[187] He reported three cases of this catastrophic complication that immediately followed lumbar sympathectomy and necessitated amputation. It received little attention until 1947 when Freeman resurrected and popularized the concept that the worsening of ischemic manifestations after lumbar sympathectomy was directly related to the procedure.[188] Freeman explained its occurrence as due to the opening of arteriovenous shunts that permitted blood to be shunted from the arterioles to the venules thus critically reducing cutaneous capillary flow. Blood flow to the limb was increased at the expense of irreversible distal tissue ischemia, and gangrene ensued. Others published similar cases of the so-called "paradoxical gangrene," and some reported an incidence as great as 2 to 4 per cent of lumbar sympathectomies for vascular disease.[1,3,73,189] Several authorities denied its existence and large series of lumbar sympathectomies were reported with no mention of such a severe complication.[65,69,103-105]

The belief that paradoxical gangrene is a myth is supported by several explanations.[73] Patients may have acute onset of severe ischemic manifestations immediately after sympathectomy because a major arterial occlusion develops during or immediately after operation. The occlusion may develop from manipulation of a brittle abdominal aorta and iliac artery by heavy retractors, dislodgement of an atheromatous plaque with embolization to a distal arterial segment, or thrombosis of critical collateral lumbar arteries. Hypotension from hypovolemia is a contributory factor to any one of these occlusive lesions. The occurrence of gangrene could be identified as faulty technique by the surgeon. Some patients have an insidious increase in ischemia postoperatively. These patients have widespread arterial occlusive disease and demonstrate progression of their disease. Sympathectomy neither benefits nor harms the extremity. Often there has been short duration of ischemic symptoms prior to sympathectomy which would progress to amputation unless revascularization is performed. De Takats thought it possible that gangrene occurred because the distal bed of the artery was incapable of dilation or a transient reflex vasoconstriction developed during section of the sympathetic chain.[69]

Other explanations have suggested that sympathectomy in these cases was generally done with "hope for improvement." These patients demonstrated all or some of the following: clinical evidence of atherosclerotic involvement of other organs, marked atrophic changes in the foot and leg, evidence of a progressing process with widespread arterial involvement, and severe pain in the distal portion of the limb.[114] Gangrene can occur after sympathectomy, after other operations, and without any operation when diseased arteries are present.

For the prevention of postsympathectomy paradoxical reaction and gangrene, we and others suggest the following:[3] (1) Select patients to conform to the indications for sympathectomy. (2) Do not compress the limb on the operating table. (3) Place retractors carefully and hold them gently during sympathectomy to avoid contusion of the aorta and iliac arteries. (4) Avoid hypotension or correct it during and after the operation. (5) Observe the limb closely in the immediate postoperative period and institute aggressive measures if severe ischemia develops. This usually requires a definitive vascular procedure to improve distal blood flow.

Ureteral Injuries

The actual incidence of injuries to the ureter during lumbar sympathectomy is difficult to determine from a review of the literature, and Higgins reported only one instance in his review.[190] Even though the complication is highly unlikely when a retroperitoneal approach is used, prophylaxis is of paramount importance. The easiest means to prevent injury is to have the ureter always contiguous with the peritoneum as it is bluntly dissected from the psoas muscle. The ureter should be protected with moist sponges when the peritoneum is retracted. Higgins comments that "the venial sin is injury to the ureter, but the mortal sin is failure of recognition."

Vesicoureteral reflux may follow unilateral lumbar sympathectomy, as paralysis of the ipsilateral trigonal muscle may occur, since it is supplied by the sympathetic nerves. This reflux condition may appear in animals from 5 to 22 days after a lumbar sympathectomy and is manifested by lateral displacement of the ureteral orifice on the operated side, shortening of the intravesical ureter, and reflux.[191] The literature infers that it can occur in man, but sympathectomy alone is not the cause. Since the only study of vesicoureteral reflux involved just 12 patients and was not found to be present, it is listed only to identify its possibility as a complication.[192]

Regeneration

The concept of the regeneration of sympathetic nerve fibers is controversial. Surgeons have attributed their failures to its occurrence. This notion so plagued the profession several years ago that surgeons routinely covered the severed portion of the sympathetic trunk with silk, cellophane or tantulum, redirected the cut chain into nearby muscle tissue, or applied a metal clip to the end of the trunk.[193]

Numerous theories have been proposed to explain return of sympathetic activity following surgical ablation of the sympathetic nerve trunk: (1) Inadequate sympathectomy performed (early).[88,93] (2) An anatomically complete sympathectomy impossible to perform because of variations in anatomy of the sympathetic trunks, the pattern of distribution of branches and communications,[79,95,194,195] and the presence of so-called intermediate ganglia that do not lie in normal pathways of the sympathetic nervous system early, 8 to 10 weeks.[78,111,131] (3) Sympathetic pathways may readjust from "crossover fibers" from the contralateral side, (early–within 1 year).[77] (4) Remaining intake nerve fibers may "sprout" in response to a stimulus from neighboring degenerating fibers (late–1 year or more).[76] (5) The disease process may continue and further reduce circulation, which can be mistakenly attributed to regeneration of a sectioned sympathetic trunk (early or late). (6) Abnormal sensitivity of the vessels to circulating catecholamines may accompany a decrease in the amino-oxidase content of the arterial wall and elimination of normal synthesis of acetylcholine in the wall of the artery (early or late).[80,196]

Sympathetic innervation of the upper limb via the brachial plexus is complex and does not arise only from the stellate and vertebral ganglia. Simeone believes that sympathetic denervation should include the T_1 or C_8 ganglion; otherwise, there may be recurrence of vasomotor activity in a year or more.[197] The recurrence, due to "sprouting" of preganglionic cells, is not always complete. These sprouts may reach ganglion cells in the stellate ganglion and establish a successful functional union.

Goetz maintains there is no difference between the somatic and the sympathetic nervous systems regarding degeneration and regeneration of severed nerve fibers.[21] There is no documented proof that sympathetic ganglion cells regenerate. When an axis cylinder is cut and separated from the ganglion cell, Wallerian degeneration occurs and new fibers begin to regenerate from the ganglion cell. Therefore, preganglionic fibers can regenerate from ganglion cells of the lateral horn when only the rami communicans is sectioned and the chain is not removed. However, this is not possible if there is a large separation between these divided fibers. Goetz has reported that if preganglionic fibers regenerate and the severed ends join, they cannot relay function through postganglionic pathways, because postganglionic fibers are adrenergic in function and preganglionic fibers are cholinergic.[21] Therefore, regeneration has little place when the proper paravertebral ganglia are removed.

But sympathetic activity does return, and the most acceptable explanation is that functional reorganization, called sprouting, occurs in the sympathetic chain where intact nerve fibers give off "sprouts" in response to a humoral stimulus from nearby degenerating fibers. These side branches unite with denervated ganglion cells. An example of this phenomenon may occur when T_2 and T_3 preganglionic fibers to the upper limb are severed but the preganglionic fibers of T_1 and C_8 which traverse the stellate ganglion to supply the oculopupillary apparatus are left undisturbed. These latter fibers may form "sprouts" and reinervate the ganglion cells in the stellate ganglion. When this occurs, sympathetic activity returns.

Goetz believes this "regeneration" is reason enough not to perform a preganglionic sympathectomy for upper extremity disorders.[21] He advocates a cervicodorsal sympathectomy including T_2, T_3 and the entire stellate ganglion, thereby lessening failures in sympathetic denervation due to: (1) leaving unsectioned fibers of T_1 passing through the stellate ganglion; (2) not interrupting Kuntz's nerve, which bypasses the stellate ganglion; (3) regeneration of preganglionic fibers; and (4) permitting the "sprouts" of T_1 and C_8 preganglionic fibers to join with denervated ganglion cells as they pass through the stellate ganglion. Goetz maintains that the extremity is permanently denervated in organic vascular disease but some vascular tone recurs when sympathectomy is performed for Raynaud's phenomenon.[21] The Raynaud's phenomenon failure is probably due to hypersensitivity to circulating catecholamines. Failures in patients with causalgia of the upper limb may be attributed to the need for more than an upper thoracic sympathectomy. An objection to cervicodorsal sympathectomy is Horner's syndrome.

Unlike the lumbar sympathetic pathways, the presence of intermediate ganglia in the upper thoracic and cervical area is questionable, since sudomotor escape areas have not been noted in the face, neck, and upper extremity following ganglionectomy.[21]

The Crossover Fiber Syndrome

A simultaneous bilateral lumbar sympathectomy is advocated by many surgeons for patients with unilateral symptoms.[181,198] They maintain that patients often fail to achieve expected beneficial results following a unilateral procedure, owing to the high incidence of crossover sympathetic fibers,[77,95] and that bilateral sympathectomy affords some protection to the contralateral extremity.[199] In addition, they have noted

greater symptomatic improvement after a bilateral procedure.[100]

Performing a bilateral lumbar sympathectomy routinely for unilateral symptoms does not appear justified. A more logical approach is to perform a bilateral lumbar sympathectomy only when an adequate unilateral procedure fails to produce the expected beneficial outcome or if relief of symptoms is only temporary. If, after a paravertebral block on the opposite side, there is relief of symptoms, the possibility of crossover fibers is considered, and sympathectomy on the contralateral side may be performed. The patient may also be considered for a higher sympathectomy on the previously operated side.

Sudomotor Changes

Dry limbs due to loss of sweating is a necessary consequence of any extremity sympathectomy. When the hands or feet become dry after sympathetic denervation the patient experiences a considerable inconvenience. Some complain of cracked skin as well as an inability to grasp smooth objects. Frequent applications of lubricating lotions are helpful to minimize these complaints. Occasionally when upper thoracic sympathectomies are performed for hyperhidrosis both feet also become dry or show decreased sweat activity.[125,127] Sweating activity may recur after two years due to "regeneration."[125,128]

Compensatory body sweating may be a complication of sympathetic denervation of large surface areas of the body and may alter its heat control.[125,130] These physiologic disturbances of heat control and normal sweat patterns are not usually a problem when bilateral sympathectomy is performed. However, when a four-extremity sympathectomy or an extensive thoracolumbar sympathectomy has been performed, the heat regulatory and sudomotor mechanisms of other body parts must assume those functions for areas no longer capable of sweating. Patients exhibit excessive sweating in nondenervated areas usually only immediately after surgery. In hyperhidrosis, compensatory sweating may follow an operation on two limbs or may especially affect the axilla unless the thoracic sympathectomy includes T_2 through T_5 ganglia. Excision of the axillary skin may be required when the procedure involves fewer ganglia.[128,132]

Four extremity sympathectomies for hyperhidrosis or rare pain problems may be staged at 6-month intervals, or three extremities may be denervated separately during a short period, such as 3 months or less.[128] The patient is usually not disabled by increased sweating in the nondenervated areas, since the return of sudomotor activity to the thigh and arm usually appears in 3 months by readjustment of the sympathetic nervous system.[77,171]

Postsympathectomy Pain Syndromes

The most common complication following sympathectomy is unexpected pain that is poorly defined, difficult to understand, and may be difficult to treat. The most common type of pain and the only type usually mentioned in the literature is postsympathetic neuralgia;[145, 200-205] however five postsympathetic pain syndromes may be identified.[66,86]

"Rebound" Rest Pain. Type 1, "rebound"

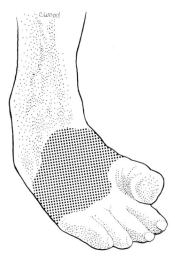

Fɪɢ. 9-2. Type 1: "Rebound" rest pain—appearance 4 to 6 days.

rest pain (Fig. 9-2) is the recurrence of preoperative foot pain within 4 to 6 days after what was considered an adequate sympathectomy. Its appearance apparently is limited to patients who have severe rest pain and dependent rubor. Several theories have been proposed to explain "rebound" rest pain. Maximal vasodilatation occurs immediately after sympathectomy but subsides on the fifth or sixth day when vessels become hypersensitive to circulating ephedrine, catecholamines, or to an unknown hormone or when there is an intrinsic change in the smooth muscle of the vessels.[80,98] Another theory is that there are changes in the enzyme content of the arterial wall. After an initial increase in blood flow, arteries regain tone and blood flow decreases.[196] These changes may cause the temperature of the foot to drop and may also cause reappearance of pain, particularly in an extremity with marked ischemia.

Rest pain may be confused with ischemic neuritis of somatic root origin where sympathectomy is contraindicated, and amputation is usually inevitable if definitive vascular surgery cannot be performed. Injection of the femoral artery or an arm vein with a sympatholytic drug such as 25 mg. tolazoline hydrochloride (Priscoline) is effective for "rebound" rest pain. Therefore therapy should be directed chiefly toward relieving the patient's pain rather than toward acting on the erroneous belief that further sympathetic denervation of the limb may increase circulation.

Case History. An example of "rebound" rest pain is the intermittent claudication in the left calf and burning discomfort of the foot that developed in a 41-year-old man. A left lumbar sympathectomy produced relief of the foot discomfort and progressive improvement of the calf claudication. Ten years later the foot pain reappeared in a pulseless left leg that had dependent rubor, trophic skin changes, and sweating of the foot as well as hyperesthesia of the sole and toes. Intra-arterial di-hydro ergot alkaloids (Hydergine), 0.3 mg., relieved the superficial burning pain for 12 hours. A higher sympathectomy was undertaken at T_{11}, T_{12}, and L_1. A few fibers of the chain, which apparently regenerated below L_1, were also excised. Postoperatively there was increased warmth and relief of foot pain. The patient was ambulatory on the first postoperative day. On the sixth postoperative day, the previous pain returned to the foot and it became quite cool; another injection of Hydergine into the left femoral artery alleviated the pain. On the tenth postoperative day, postsympathectomy neuralgia appeared on the thigh and was successfully treated with oral sympatholytic drugs. Eight months later, the deep foot pain became intense, and a large ischemic ulcer appeared on the dorsum of the foot. Only heavy sedation relieved the pain. A below-the-knee amputation was required. This patient demonstrated three postsympathectomy pain syndromes, "rebound" rest pain, "regeneration" pain, and postsympathectomy neuralgia.

Inadequate Sympathectomy. The recurrence of the preoperative pain within three months of a supposedly adequate procedure may result from inadequate sympathectomy (Fig. 9-3). Six possible reasons for this recurrence are proposed: (1) The original sympathectomy was technically adequate, but owing to anatomic variables, the procedure should have included denervation of an adjacent area.[75,195] (2) A less than adequate sympathectomy was performed. (3) "Crossover" fibers were present and bilateral sympathectomy may be indicated.[77,95] (4) The process of readjustment of sympathetic pathways occurred.[77] (5) Probably none of the present methods of sympathectomy could produce a complete interruption of sympathetic pathways.[197] (6) The vessels became hypersensitive to circulating catecholamines, "intrinsic tone" developed in the smooth muscles of the arterial vessels, or another hormone was the offending mechanism.[80,98]

Following are a few explanations for an inadequate upper extremity sympathectomy.

Pain may recur after excision of T_2, T_3, and T_4 ganglia. To insure denervation of the upper limb, it is essential to divide the sympathetic chain below the third ganglion and to remove any rami associated with the second. Poor visibility afforded by the dorsal approach may permit the third thoracic ganglion to be mistaken for the second thoracic ganglion and T_3, T_4, and T_5 being excised. This may leave a branch passing from the second thoracic ganglion to the lowest trunk of the brachial plexus (Kuntz's nerve).[15] Accessory (ectopic) sympathetic trunks to the upper limb may lie in the spinal canal and emerge with higher brachial plexus nerve roots.[25]

In the lower extremity there are numerous possible causes for pain to reappear 3 months later. Even when L_2, L_3, and L_4 ganglia have been removed, the postoperative pain-free interval may have been the period before readjustment of sympathetic pathways,[77] or an incomplete denervation may have mimicked complete denervation for a period of 3 months.[78] Ray and Console maintain that complete denervation of the lower extremity is not determined by preservation or removal of the L_1 ganglion

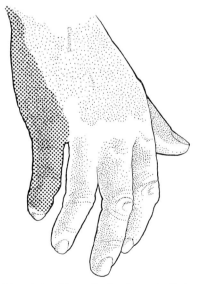

FIG. 9-3. Type 2: Inadequate "adequate" sympathectomy – appearance within 3 months.

or any part of the paravertebral ganglionated chain above it,[77] while others emphasize the importance of extending a lumbar sympathectomy to the first lumbar or even to the tenth dorsal segment.[177] These and other possibilities have been discussed previously. Relief of this type of recurrent pain is obtained with a more extensive sympathectomy, unilateral or bilateral. Another approach is oral, intravenous, or intra-arterial reserpine or sympatholytic drugs.[86]

Case History. Inadequate "adequate" sympathectomy occurred in the case of a 38-year-old milkman who received a spider bite on the right ring finger, which became extremely painful and swollen. Two weeks later the finger was incised over the dorsal aspect of the third phalanx with negative findings. The swelling remained for a month, but the pain, which was initially described as deep, changed to an intolerable superficial burning pain with hyperesthesia localized to the injured finger. The patient was unable to work and received industrial compensation. Seven months after the injury he underwent an upper thoracic sympathectomy through a posterior approach. A Horner's syndrome was not noted postoperatively. The pain was not relieved after operation although the hand was warm and dry. On the tenth postoperative day the

patient developed a postsympathectomy neuralgia with hyperesthesia and burning pain over the shoulder and anterior chest; he was unable to abduct his arm over 70 degrees from his body. One month after the sympathectomy amputation of the finger produced no change in the character of the pain. Twelve months after the initial injury the patient was found to have painful hyperesthesia of the hand localized to C_6, C_7 ulnar nerve distribution. He held the hand constantly with his left hand and refused to shake hands for fear of producing intolerable pain in the affected site. Intravenous Priscoline relieved both shoulder and hand pain almost completely for 12 hours. A right stellate ganglion block also relieved the pain for a similar period. Oral Ilidar, 100 mg. four times a day, produced significant relief. The patient later reduced the dosage of the medication and was able to attend school to learn a new trade. His only complaint was occasional discomfort in the right shoulder joint. This patient is an obvious example of an incomplete sympathectomy where the stellate ganglion should have been included in the resection.

Type 3—"Regeneration." Regeneration syndrome appears more than 1 year after an adequate sympathectomy (Fig. 9-4). If patients are relieved of their preoperative symptoms for several years, it must be assumed that an adequate sympathectomy was performed, but "regeneration" by some method has occurred. (For a detailed discussion, refer to the section on "regeneration" and the references listed.) An interesting observation is that if "regeneration" occurs it is likely to produce an irregular pattern with islands of low skin resistance appearing in any of the denervated dermatomes particularly about the foot and toes and hands and fingers, where the density of innervation is greatest.

Relief of this pain syndrome may be obtained with intra-arterial Priscoline or oral sympatholytic drugs (such as Ilidar, Hydergine, or Dibenzyline), a higher sympathetic block, or a more extensive sympathectomy.

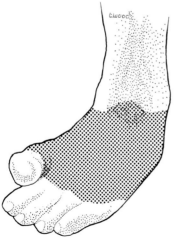

FIG. 9-4. Type 3: "Regeneration"–appearance 1 year or more.

Case History. A case of "regeneration" pain occurred in a 60-year-old woman who suffered a comminuted fracture of the left calcaneus. Three months after the fracture she began to show evidence of Sudeck's atrophy with coldness, burning pain, hyperesthesia of the foot, and demineralization of bones of the foot. Repeated paravertebral lumbar blocks gave temporary relief of pain until a left lumbar sympathectomy was performed 2 months later at L_1 through L_4. Postoperatively, she experienced loss of superficial pain and increased warmth of the involved foot. Skin resistance studies at this time confirmed sympathetic denervation of the extremity. Somatic pain due to traumatic arthritis at the talocalcaneal joint was present on motion. Almost 4 years later, burning pain and subjective coolness returned to the foot, particularly at night. Skin resistance studies showed some return of sweating to the foot and mild hyperesthesia. Sympathetic "regeneration" was confirmed when paravertebral blocks at T_{11}, T_{12}, and L_1 relieved pain for 2 to 3 months. Physiotherapy was continued, and fusion of the ankle and a higher sympathectomy were refused. Occasional paravertebral blocks were done for 3 years when pain was reported as being only very mild for short periods.

Postsympathetic Neuralgia. Type 4, postsympathectomy neuralgia (Fig. 9-5) is the most common complication; it occurs in the vast majority of patients who have undergone what is generally accepted as an adequate sympathectomy. It is characterized by a gradual or sudden onset of mild to severe aching, burning, or stabbing pain which is more intense at night, with varying manifestations of hyperesthesia. In lumbar

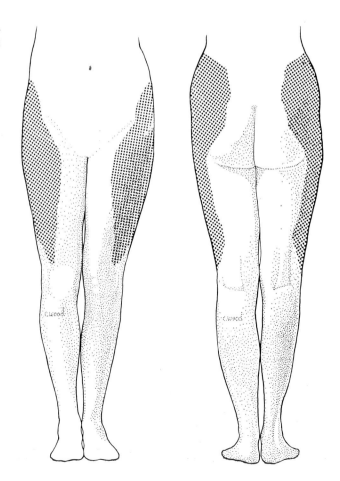

Fig. 9-5. Type 4: Postsympathectomy neuralgia, front and back views—appearance 5 to 20 days.

sympathectomy, the pain is localized to the lateral, anterior, or medial aspect of the thigh and often includes the sacroiliac area and buttocks of the involved side. After a cervicodorsal or upper thoracic sympathectomy, pain is present on the lateral aspect of the neck, shoulder, arm, anterior chest, or a combination of these areas. The patient may describe the pain as both superficial and deep.

Although various theories have been advanced for this type of pain problem, the etiology of the complication is not clear. Litwin reported the incidence of postsympathetic neuralgia varying from 2 per cent to 100 per cent.[200] This author has observed an incidence of at least a 90 per cent. This is undoubtedly related to the inclusion of the L_2 ganglion in every lumbar sympathectomy procedure and L_1 in many. In recent years, higher and more extensive sympathectomies have been performed. The high incidence of postsympathectomy neuralgia after lumbar sympathectomy has led some vascular surgeons to remove no ganglia above L_3,[206] or to do no sympathectomy at all when considering it as a supplement to definitive vascular surgery. This approach should avoid the postsympathectomy neuralgia since the L_1 and L_2 ganglia supply the iliac and femoral vessels as well as the skin and soft tissues of the thigh. However, to be considered adequate, a sympathectomy should include L_2 and L_3 ganglia. Some authors report that preganglionic fibers may not be present below L_2.[116,156] Therefore patients who receive a low lumbar sympathectomy would have a postganglionic rather than a preganglionic resection of the sympathetic chain. In these patients one might expect the results of the procedure to be inadequate and temporary as in the case history of the Type 2 pain syndrome.

Performing a postganglionic resection or a limited sympathectomy does not obviate postsympathectomy neuralgia in sympathetic denervation of the upper limb, since the complication occurs frequently after an upper thoracic sympathectomy or cervico-

dorsal sympathectomy and less often after stellate ganglionectomy. Cooley and Herman predicted that pain could be prevented by ligation of the sympathetic chain with silk.[204] Others state that pain patterns would remain despite ligation.[86,207]

Onset almost invariably occurs around the tenth day. However, some have reported the onset from 5 to 20 days after operation.[200,203]

Sedation is usually not required when oral, intravenous, or intra-arterial sympatholytic drugs are administered. Relief may be achieved, at least temporarily, by a paravertebral block central to the denervated area. Even without treatment, the pain usually subsides in 3 months. It is important to reassure the patient and the referring physician that the onset of the pain does not signify aggravation of the disease.

Maculoerythematous rash and cyanotic mottling have been reported in the site of postsympathectomy neuralgia. Ray and Console believed the cyanotic mottling of the skin represented compensatory vasoconstriction of nondenervated areas in postural hypotension.[77] Litwin and First, who reported maculoerythematous rash accompanying postsympathectomy neuralgia, had no explanation for it.[208] Both conditions have been noted to disappear simultaneously with remission of postsympathectomy neuralgia.

Case History. A 56-year-old man who had a 12-year history of intermittent claudication in both calves which progressed to both legs, suffered post sympathectomy neuralgia. The patient complained of a burning sensation in the soles of both feet. Examinaton confirmed obstruction of both common iliac arteries at the aortic bifurcation (Leriche syndrome). There were moderately advanced trophic changes on both feet with hyperesthesia. An aortogram revealed extensive arteriosclerosis obliterans of the abdominal aorta and iliac and femoral arteries with poor distal vessel runoff. Definitive surgery was considered inadvisable at the time; therefore a bilateral lumbar sympathectomy was performed via a transperitoneal approach excising L_2, L_3, and L_4 ganglia on each side. Ten days postoperatively there was a sudden onset of severe burning and aching pain, beginning at both sacroiliac joints and radiating bilaterally to the lateral and anterior aspect of both thighs. The pain was worse just before bedtime. Complaints were confirmed by tenderness over both sacroiliac joints and marked hyperesthesia over the lateral and anterior aspects of both thighs. Priscoline, 25 mg., was administered intravenously with 90 per cent relief of pain in all areas for 3 hours. Oral Ilidar, 50 to 100 mg. four times a day, resulted in prompt relief of the pain. Six weeks later there was minimal tenderness and aching over the sacroiliac joints and no hyperesthesia on the thighs. Oral medication was used only at bedtime. Within a month all pain had resolved and medication was discontinued.

Postsympathectomy Causalgia. Type 5, Postsympathectomy causalgia (Fig. 9-6) is localized to the operative site and occurs months after operation. This pain is probably the easiest to explain. Certain patients develop causalgia with injury to any somatic nerve group that is accompanied by sympathetic nerve fibers. Intercostal nerves may certainly be damaged during sympathectomy, and they are a common cause of post-thoracotomy pain.[144] Besides causalgia-type pain, other causes for pain can be ruled out when the complaint is temporarily relieved by 25 mg. of Priscoline. Medical sympathetic denervation utilizing oral medication then affords relief. Blocking the nerve with phenol or alcohol or by section of the neuroma gives only temporary relief and complicates the problem with additional pain of traumatic neuritis which makes specific treatment more difficult.

Case History. Postsympathectomy causalgia occurred in a 51-year-old man who complained of discomfort in the area of his left thoracolumbar sympathectomy 10 months after his operation (Fig. 9-6). Hyperesthesia was present over the course of

the 10th, 11th, and 12th intercostal nerve distributions. Intravenous Priscoline, 25 mg., produced significant relief of pain for a few hours. Left paravertebral block at T_8, T_9, and T_{10} also gave similar relief but only for a few days. Oral sympatholytic drugs were required, especially at night, for about 2 years. Six years after sympathectomy, the pain was minor.

Medicolegal Problems and "Sympathetic Reactors"

"Sympathetic reactors" are certain individuals who present moist palms and feet and unstable personalities. When sympathectomy is performed, the surgical trauma results in a high incidence of postsympathectomy pain patterns. Industrial compensation and medicolegal problems are heavily weighted. Such individuals complaining of intolerable pain, are frequently involved in litigation over medical treatment and disability compensation. As others have noted, the postoperative complaint is frequently described in terms reminiscent of causalgia-type pain.[145,203] Patients with causalgia-type pain are often unjustly classified as malingerers, assigned to a psychiatrist for therapy,

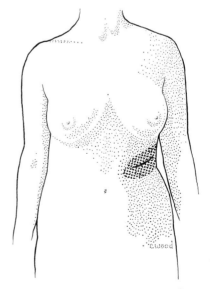

FIG. 9-6. Type 5: Postsympathectomy causalgia—appearance months postoperatively.

or awarded a financial settlement with or without court action. Causalgia-type pain should be properly identified and treated before any such decisions are made. Patients with this disorder are often noted to have seen a large number of physicians before the correct diagnosis and treatment was instituted.

Postthrombotic Postsympathectomy Syndrome

This complication was first described by Linton in 1938 after he noted that some patients with a postphlebitic syndrome become more disabled after lumbar sympathectomy.[209] He and others have pointed out that there is increased edema and while arterial inflow is increased, venous pressure is higher and ambulation causes further swelling.[145] Linton also reported chronic painful ulcerations on the dorsum of the foot and on the toes in contradistinction to the original lesion in the area of the medial malleolus.

Sympathectomy may be warranted when an ulcer fails to heal following accepted treatment, when the pain localized to the ulcer is of causalgia-type and medical sympathetic denervation is not sufficient to permit the patient to wear an elastic support with comfort, and when excessive sweating of the foot is present. It should be understood that sympathectomy is not done solely for chronic venous ulcers that fail to heal. Since lumbar sympathectomy is not considered a part of the standard care of a postphlebitic syndrome and is contraindicated for any patient having acute venous thrombosis, this complication is rarely seen.

Mortality Rate

The incidence of undesirable side effects and mortality following sympathectomy procedures varies with the type of procedure performed, the condition of the patient, the disorder for which sympathectomy is undertaken, and the anatomical variables of the system and the knowledge and judgment of the surgeon. Fulton and Blakeley wrote a strong condemnation of lumbar sympathectomy; they questioned its value in the treatment of arteriosclerosis obliterans of the lower extremities. It was their opinion that sympathectomy did not alleviate intermittent claudication, or salvage gangrenous limbs, did not have any effect on amputation rate or level of amputation, and did have a significant mortality.[210] A review of the mortality rate for lumbar sympathectomy in a large series for many diseases was 0.13 per cent in all cases and 0.78 per cent in patients over 50 years of age.[211] Others have reported death rates of 2.9 per cent[212] and 3.5 per cent.[181] Baffes et al. had a mortality rate of 4.4 per cent, though 20.2 per cent had ancillary vascular procedures in conjunction with lumbar sympathectomy.[213] Fulton and Blakeley reported the highest death rate which was 11.1 per cent, none of which were operative deaths.[210]

Complications that contributed to the deaths in most reports were delay in amputation myocardial infarction, cerebrovascular ischemia, pulmonary emboli, cardiac decompensation, and wound sepsis. One report mentioned that all infected wounds had incisional Penrose drains at the time of initial operation.[213]

Mortality rates for upper limb sympathectomy have been negligible, though complications have been as high as 23.9 per cent in transpleural and 13.5 per cent in extrapleural procedures.[87] Complications most commonly noted were pleural effusion, atelectasis, hemothorax, pneumothorax, hemopneumothorax, atrial fibrillation, and pulmonary embolism.

Although there are numerous possible complications following a sympathectomy, many of which are bizarre and complex, very few are common, and even fewer appear frequently enough to be considered a serious hazard to the patient. Therefore, the sympathectomy procedures that are accepted today have much to offer patients when their limitations are clearly understood and the operation chosen is properly indicated.

References

1. DeBakey, M. D., Creech, O., and Wood-hall, J. P.: Evaluation of sympathectomy in arteriosclerotic peripheral vascular disease. JAMA, *144*:1227, 1950.
2. de Takats, G.: Place of sympathectomy in the treatment of occlusive arterial disease. Arch. Surg., *77*:655, 1958.
3. Balas, P., Plessas, S., Segditsas, T., and Antonopoulous, J.: Post lumbar sympathectomy gangrene. Angiology, *21*:552, 1970.
4. Jennesco, T.: Rescetia totala di bilaterala a simpaticului cervical in cazuri: de epilepsi si gusa exoftalmica. Romania Med., *4*:479, 1896.
5. Jaboulay, M.: Le traitement de quelques troubles trophiques du pied et de la jambe par la denudation de l'artere femorale et la distension des nerfs vasculaires. Lyon Med., *91*:467, 1899.
6. Leriche, R.: De l'elongation et de la section des nerfs perivasculaires dans cetains syndromes douloureaux d'origine arterielle et dans quelques troubles trophiques. Lyon Chir., *10*:378, 1913.
7. Leriche, R., and Heitz, J.: Des effets physiologiques de la sympathectomic peripherique. Compt. Rend. Soc. de Biol., *80*:66, 1917.
8. Leriche, R., and Fontaine, R.: Experimental researches on vasomotoricity. Amer. J. Surg., *85*:641, 1927.
9. Leriche, R., Jung, A., and DeBakey, M.: The surgical treatment of scleroderma. Surgery, *1*:6, 1937.
10. Kramer, J. G., and Todd, T. W.: The distribution of nerves to the arteries of the arm with a discussion of the clinical value of results. Anat. Rec., *8*:243, 1914.
11. Woollard, H. H., and Norrish, R. E.: The anatomy of the peripheral sympathetic nervous system. Br. J. Surg., *21*: 83, 1934.
12. Jennesco, T.: Traitement chirurgical de l'angine de poitrine par la resection du sympathetique cervico-thoracique. Presse Med., *1*:193, 1921.
13. Brüning, F.: Weitere Erfahrungen uber den Sympathicus. Klin. Wochnschr., *2*: 1872, 1923.
14. White, J. C. :Progress in the surgery of the sympathetic nervous system. New Eng. J. Med., *203*:226, 1930.
15. Kuntz, A.: Distribution of the sympathetic rami to the brachial plexus. Arch. Surg., *15*:871, 1927.
16. Brown, G. E., and Adson, A. W.: Physiologic effects of thoracic and of lumbar sympathetic ganglionectomy or section of the trunk. Arch. Neurol., *21*:322, 1929.
17. Gask, G. E., and Ross, J. P.: The Surgery of the Sympathetic Nervous System. London, Balliere, Tindall and Cox, 1934.
18. Simmons, H. T., and Sheehan, D.: An inquiry into "relapse" following sympathectomy. Lancet, *2*:788, 1937.
19. ———: The causes of relapse following sympathectomy on the arm. Br. J. Surg., *27*:234, 1939.
20. Fulton, J. F.: Vasomotor and reflex sequelae of unilateral cervical and lumbar ramisectomy in a case of Raynaud's disease with observations on tonus. Ann. Surg., *88*:827, 1928.
21. Goetz, R. H.: Sympathectomy for the upper extremities. *In* Dale, ?. (ed.): Management of Arterial Occlusive Disease. Chicago, Year Book, 1971.
22. Telford, E. D.: The technique of sympathectomy. Br. J. Surg., *23*:448, 1935.
23. Smithwick, R. H.: The problem of producing complete and lasting sympathetic denervation of the upper extremity by preganglionic section. Ann. Surg., *112*: 1085, 1940.
24. Harman, N. B.: The anterior limit of the cervico-thoracic visceral efferent nerves in man. J. Anat. Physiol., *34*: 359, 1900.
25. Ray, B. S.; Hinsey, J. C.: and Geohegan, W. A.: Observations on the distribution of the sympathetic nerves to the pupil and upper extremity as determined by stimulation of the anterior roots in man. Ann. Surg., *118*:647, 1943.
26. Goetz, R. H.: The surgical physiology of the sympathetic nervous system with special reference to cardiovasulcar disorders. Surg. Gynecol., Obstet., *87*:17, 1948.
27. Royle, N. D.: A new operative procedure in the treatment of spastic paralysis and its experimental basis. Med. J. Aust., *1*:77, 1924.
28. Hunter, J. I.: The influence of the sympathetic nervous system in the genesis of the rigidity of striated muscle in spastic paralysis. Surg., Gynecol., Obstet., *39*: 721, 1924.
29. ———: Relationships of sympathetic innervation to tone of skeletal muscle. Amer. J. Med. Sci., *170*:469, 1925.

30. ——: Sympathetic innervation of striated muscle. Br. Med. J., *1*:197, 1925.

31. Hunter, J. I., and Latham, O.: A contribution to the discussion of the histological problems involved in the conception of a somatic and sympathetic innervation of voluntary muscle. Med. J. Aust., *1*:27, 1925.

32. Royle, N. D.: The treatment of spastic paralysis by sympathetic ramisection. Surg., Gynecol., Obstet., *39*:701, 1924.

33. ——: Operations of sympathetic ramisection. Med. J. Aust., *1*:587, 1924.

34. Ewing, M.: The history of lumbar sympathectomy. Surgery, *70*:790, 1971.

35. Greenwood, B.: The origins of sympathectomy. Med. Hist., *11*:165, 1967.

36. Adson, A. W., and Brown, G. E.: The treatment of Raynaud's disease by resection of the upper thoracic and lumbar sympathetic ganglia and trunks. Surg., Gynecol., Obstet., *48*:577, 1929.

37. ——: Treatment of Raynaud's disease by lumbar ramisection and ganglionectomy and perivascular sympathecteurectomy of the common iliacs. JAMA, *84*: 1908, 1925.

38. White, J. C., Smithwick, R. M., and Simeone, F. A.: The Autonomic Nervous System: Anatomy, Physiology and Surgical Application. ed. 3. New York, Macmillan, 1941.

39. de Takats, G., Fowler, E. F., Jordan, P., and Resley, T. C.: Sympathectomy in the treatment of peripheral vascular sclerosis. JAMA, *131*:495, 1946.

40. Grimson, K. S., et al.: Results of treatment of patients with hypertension by total thoracic and partial or total lumbar sympathectomy, splanchnicectomy and celiac ganglionectomy. Ann. Surg., *129*: 850, 1949.

41. de Takats, G., Graupner, G. W., Fowler, E. F., and Jensik, R. J.: Surgical approach to hypertension. Second Report. Arch. Surg., *53*:111, 1946.

42. White, J. C., and Bland, E. A.: Surgical relief of severe angina pectoris; methods employed and results in 83 patients. Medicine, *27*:1, 1948.

43. Lindgren, I., and Olivecrona, H.: Surgical treatment of angina pectoris. J. Neurosurg., *4*:19, 1947.

44. Shumacker, H. B., Jr.: Sympathectomy in treatment of peripheral vascular disease. Surgery, *13*:1, 1943.

45. Southworth, J. C.: Role of sympathectomy in treatment of immersion foot and frostbite. New Eng. J. Med., *233*:673, 1945.

46. Taylor, J.: Discussion on Hirschsprung's disease. Proc. Roy. Soc. Med., *42*:221, 1949.

47. Mallet-Guy, P.: La splanchnicic tonic gauche dans le chronic pancreatitis chroniques. Presse Med., *51*:91, 1943.

48. Ray, B. S., and Console, A. D.: The relief of pain in chronic (calcareous) pancreatitis by sympathectomy. Surg., Gynecol., Obstet., *89*:1, 1949.

49. Palmer, A. J.: Hyperhydrosis. Study of a Case. Arch. Neurol. Psychol., *55*:582, 1947.

50. Wan, F. E.: Sympathetic causalgia. Report of twenty cases treated by sympathectomy. Chinese Med. J., *61*:1, 1946.

51. Mayfield, F. H.: Causalgia. W. Va. Med. J., *43*:201, 1947.

52. Lempert, J.: Tympanosympathectomy: a surgical technic for the relief of tinnitus aurium. Arch. Otolaryngol., *43*:199, 1946.

53. Passe, E. R. G., and Seymour, J. S.: Meniere's syndrome: successful treatment by surgery on sympathetic. Br. Med. J., *2*:812, 1948.

54. Leriche, R.: Des causes d'echec de la surrenolectomie et de la gangliectomic dans la thrombo-angeite d'apres 898 operations. Presse Med., *57*:539, 1949.

55. ——: De la surrenalectomic secondaire a une ganglionectomie et une splanchnicectomie inefficaces chez les thrombo-angeitiques. Lyon Chir., *44*: 513, 1949.

56. ——: Physiologic pathologique et traitement chirurgicale des maladies arteriolles de la vasomotricite. Paris, Masson et Cie, 1945.

57. Fulton, R. L., and Blakeley, W. R.: Lumbar sympathectomy: A procedure of questionable value in the treatment of arteriosclerosis obliterans of the legs. Amer. J. Surg., *116*:735, 1968.

58. Strandness, D. E., and Bell, J. W.: Critical evaluation of the results of lumbar sympathectomy. Ann. Surg., *160*:1021, 1964.

59. Verstraete, M.: A critical appraisal of lumbar sympathectomy in the treatment of organic arteriopathy. Angiologica, *5*: 333, 1968.

60. Hardy, J. D., and Conn, J. H.: Surgical procedures for leg ischemia in 549 con-

secutive cases. Surg., Gynecol., Obstet., *117*:686, 1963.

61. Strandness, D. E., Jr.: Long-term value of lumbar sympathectomy. Geriatrics, *21*:144, 1966.

62. Gillespie, J. A.: Late effects of lumbar sympathectomy on blood flow in the foot in obliterative vascular disease. Lancet, *1*:891, 1960.

63. White, A. E., Flasher, J., and Drury, D. R.: The effect of lumbar sympathectomy on the collateral arterial circulation. Surgery, *37*:567, 1955.

64. Rutherford, R. B., and Valenta, J.: Extremity blood flow and distribution. The effects of arterial occlusion, sympathectomy and exercise. Surgery, *69*:332, 1971.

65. Robertson, H. F.: Lumbar sympathectomy: A long-term followup on 124 operations done for arteriosclerosis and Buerger's disease of the lower limbs. Can. J. Surg., *1*:253, 1958.

66. Owens, J. C.: Indications for lumbar sympathectomy. *In* Dale, ?. (ed.): Management of Arterial Occlusive Disease. Chicago, Year Book, 1971.

67. de Takats, G.: Sympathectomy revisited: Retrospect and prospect. Rush-Presbyterian-St. Luke's Med. Bull., *12*:188, 1973.

68. ———: Surgical physiology of hypertension. Surg. Clin. No. Amer., *42*:91, 1962.

69. ———: The place of sympathectomy in the treatment of arterial occlusive disease. Arch. Surg., *77*:655, 1958.

70. Hoerner, M. T.: Lumbar sympathectomy for peripheral obliterative arteriosclerosis. Geriatrics, *17*:765, 1962.

71. McGarity, W. C.: The role of sympathectomy in peripheral vascular diseases. J. Med. Assoc. Ga., *51*:364, 1962.

72. Boucher, J. R., et al.: Le reflexe sympatho-galvanique (RSG) et la sympathectomic. Can. Anaesth. Soc. J., *17*:504, 1970.

73. Bergan, J. J., and Trippell, O. H.: Arteriograms in ischemic limbs worsened after lumbar sympathectomy. Arch. Surg., *85*:135, 1962.

74. McAllister, F. F.: The place of lumbar sympathectomy in the light of recent advances in vascular surgery. Bull. N.Y. Acad. Med., *37*:433, 1961.

75. Pick, J.: The identification of sympathetic segments. Ann. Surg., *144*:355, 1957.

76. Murray, J. C., and Thompson, J. W.: Collateral sprouting in response to injury of the autonomic nervous system and its consequence. Br. Med. Bull., *13*:213, 1957.

77. Ray, B. S., and Console, A. D.: Residual sympathetic pathways after paravertebral sympathectomy. J. Neurosurg., *5*:23, 1948.

78. Boyd, J. D.: Intermediate sympathetic ganglia. Br. Med. Bull., *13*:207, 1957.

79. Gillespie, J. A.: Extent and permanence of degeneration produced by lumbar sympathectomy. Br. Med. J., *1*:79, 1961.

80. Parks, V. H., Sandford, L. S., and Whelan, R. F.: Mechanisms in the return of vascular tone following sympathectomy in man. Circ. Res., *9*:1026, 1961.

81. Barcoft, H., and Swan, H. J. C.: Sympathetic Control of Human Blood Vessels. London. Edward Arnold and Co., 1953.

82. Owens, J. C.: Causalgia. Amer. Surg., *23*:636, 1957.

83. de Takats, G., Walter, L. E., Lasner, J.: Splanchnic nerve section for pancreatic pain. Ann. Surg., *131*:44, 1950.

84. Raney, R. B.: Hitherto undescribed surgical procedure relieving attacks of angina pectoris. Anatomic and physiologic basis. JAMA, *113*:1619, 1939.

85. Julian, O. C.: Surgery of the sympathetic nervous system. Surg. Clin. N. Amer., *34*:1173, 1954.

86. Owens, J. C.: Postsympathectomy pain syndromes. Bull. Soc. Inter. Chir., *23*:500, 1964.

87. Baddeley, R. M.: The place of upper dorsal sympathectomy in the treatment of primary Raynaud's disease. Br. J. Surg., *52*:426, 1965.

88. Barcroft, H., and Walker, A. J.: Return of tone in blood vessels of upper limb after sympathectomy. Lancet, *1*:1035, 1949.

89. Hall, K. V., and Hillestad, L. K.: Raynaud's phenomenon treated with sympathectomy. Angiology, *10*:186, 1960.

90. Montorsi, W., Chiringhelli, C., Mascetti, M., and Gallo, G.: A contribution to the study of clinical relapses after thoracic ganglionectomy for Rayanud's disease affecting the upper limbs. Parnminerva Med., *2*:538, 1960.

91. Owens, J. C.: Peripheral arterial disease. *In* Conn, ?. (ed.): 1972 Current Therapy. Philadelphia, W. B. Saunders, 1972.

92. Johnston, E. N. M., Summerly, R., and Bernsting, M.: Prognosis in Raynaud's phenomenon after sympathectomy. Br. Med. J., *1*:962, 1965.

93. Popkin, R. H.: Sympathectomies in peripheral vascular diseases: followup studies in twenty years. Angiology, *85*: 156, 1957.

94. de Takats, G., and Fowler, E. F.: Raynaud's phenomenon. Bull. Int. Soc. Chir., *21*:73, 1962.

95. Webber, R. H.: An analysis of the sympathetic trunk, communicating rami, sympathetic roots and visceral rami in the lumbar region in man. Ann. Surg., *141*:399, 1955.

96. Romeo, S. G., Whalen, R. E., and Tindall, J. P.: Intra-arterial administration of reserpine. Arch. Intern. Med., *125*: 825, 1970.

97. Abboud, F. M., Eckstein, J. W., Lawrence, M. S., and Hook, J. C.: Preliminary observations on the use of intra-arterial reserpine in Raynaud's phenomenon Circulation. *36*:[Supplement II]: 49, 1967.

98. de Takats, G., and Fowler, E. F.: The neurogenic factor in Raynaud's phenomenon. Surgery, *51*:9, 1962.

99. Palaschi, G., and Lynn, R. B.: The role of sympathectomy in the treatment of obliterative peripheral vascular disease. Can. Med. Assoc. J., *90*:1147, 1964.

100. Flotte, C. T.: Evaluation of lumbar sympathectomy. Amer. J. Cardiol., *4*:644, 1959.

101. Laufman, H.: Surgical management of chronic ileofemoral arterial occlusion. Surg. Clin. N. Amer., *40*:153, 1960.

102. Enjalbert, A., Gedeon, A., and Castany, R.: Indications and results of lumbar sympathectomy. J. Cardiovasc. Surg., *9*: 146, 1968.

103. Abramson, D. I., Edinburg, J. J., and Lu, S. W.: Clinical evaluation of lumbar sympathectomy in chronic occlusive arterial disorders. Geriatrics, *20*:563, 1965.

104. Stanford, W., and Lawrence, M. S.: Results of sympathectomy for arterial occlusive disease at University Hospitals, Iowa City, 1954-1964. J. Amer. Geriatr. Soc., *14*:1122, 1966.

105. Szilagyi, D. E., Smith, R. F., Scerpella, J. R., and Hoffman, K.: Lumbar sympathectomy: current role in the treatment of arteriosclerotic occlusive disease. Arch. Surg., *95*:753, 1967.

106. Hill, A. V. L., Lyall, I. G., and Barnett, A. J.: Sympathectomy for occlusive arterial disease of the lower limb. Med. J. Aust., *49*:901, 1962.

107. Taylor, G. W., and Calo, A. R.: Atherosclerosis of arteries of lower limbs. Br. Med. J., *1*:507, 1962.

108. Shaw, R. S., Austen, W. G., and Stega, S.: A ten-year study of the effect of lumbar sympathectomy in the peripheral circulation of patients with arteriosclerotic occlusive disease. Surg., Gynecol., Obstet., *119*:486, 1964.

109. Hoffman, D. C., and Jepson, R. P.: Muscle flow and sympathectomy. Surg., Gynecol., Obstet., *12*:12, 1968.

110. Strandness, D. E., Jr.: Peripheral Arterial Disease: A Physiologic Approach. Boston, Little, Brown, 1969.

111. Kuntz, A., and Alexander, W. F.: Surgical implications of lower thoracic and lumbar independent sympathetic pathways. Arch. Surg., *61*:1007, 1950.

112. Gillespie, J. A.: Further place of lumbar sympathectomy in obliterative vascular disease of lower limbs. Br. Med. J., *2*: 1640, 1960.

113. Ozeran, R. S., Wagner, G. R., Reimer, T. R., and Hill, R. A.: Neuropathy of the sympathetic nervous system associated with diabetis mellitus. Surgery, *68*:953, 1970.

114. Berry, R. E. L., Flotte, C. T., and Coller, F. A.: A critical evaluation of lumbar sympathectomy for peripheral arteriosclerotic vascular disease. Surgery, *37*: 115, 1955.

115. Smithwick, R. H.: Lumbar sympathectomy in the treatment of obliterative vascular disease of the lower extremities. Surgery, *42*:415, 1957.

116. Monroe, P. A. G.: Sympathectomy: An Anatomical and Physiological Study with Clinical Applications. London, Oxford University Press, 1959.

117. Adel, A. El-Etrr.: Relief of arterial spasm by epidural block in a sympathectomized patient. Anesthesia, *28*:1107, 1967.

118. Baffes, R. E. L., Carney, A. L., Baffes, E. C., Kottke, F. J.: Blood flow in postsympathectomy patients. Angiology, *10*: 139, 1960.

119. Theis, F. V.: Role of lumbar sympathectomy in treatment of vascular disease. JAMA, *164*:1302, 1957.

120. Blain, A., Zadek, A. T., Teres, M. L., and Bing, R. J.: Lumbar sympathectomy for arteriosclerosis obliterans. Surgery, *53*:165, 1963.

121. Roos, D. B., and Owens, J. C.: Thoracic outlet syndrome. Arch. Surg., *93*:71, 1966.

122. Mittleman, B., and Wolff, H. G.: Affective states and skin temperatures; experimental study of subjects with cold hands and Raynaud's syndrome. Psychosom. Med., *1*:271, 1939.

123. Goetz, R. H.: Raynaud's Disease and Raynaud's Phenomenon. *In* Samuels, S. S. (ed.): Diagnosis and Treatment of Vascular Disorders. Baltimore, Williams & Wilkins, 1956.

124. Veal, J. R., Shadid, J. N.: Hyperhidrosis: Observations on the study of sixty-one cases. Surgery, *26*:89, 1949.

125. Cloward, R. B.: Hyperhydrosis. J. Neurosurg., *30*:545, 1969.

126. Ellis, H., and Morgan, M. N.: Surgical treatment of severe hyperhidrosis. Proc. Roy. Soc. Med., *64*:768, 1971.

127. Dohn, D. F., and Zraik, O.: Essential hyperhidrosis—pathogenesis and treatment. Cleveland Clinic Quart., *36*:79, 1969.

128. Harris, J. D., and Jepson, R. P.: Essential hyperhidrosis. Med. J. Aust., *2*:135, 1971.

129. Renwick, S., and Loewenthal, J.: Cervicodorsal sympathectomy in the management of essential hyperhidrosis in the upper limb. Aust. N.Z. J. Surg., *38*:221, 1969.

130. Shelley, W. B., and Florence, R.: Compensatory hyperhidrosis after sympathectomy. New Eng. J. Med., *263*:1056, 1960.

131. Leivy, D. M., Tovi, D., and Krueger, E. G.: Failure of lumbar sympathectomy in the relief of hyperhidrosis. J. Neurosurg., *29*:65, 1968.

132. Greenhalgh, R. M., Rosengarten, D. S., and Martin, P.: Role of sympathectomy for hyperhidrosis. Br. Med. J., *1*:332, 1971.

133. Fairbairn, J. F., Juergens, J. L., and Spittell, J. A., Jr.: *In* Allen, E., Barker, N. W., and Hines, E. A. (eds.): Peripheral Vascular Diseases. ed. 4. Philadelphia, W. B. Saunders, 1972.

134. Ross, J. P.: Surgery of the Sympathetic Nervous System. London, Balliere, Tindall and Cox, 1958.

135. Gilbertsen, V. A., Emerson, E. C., and Kottke, F. J.: Blood flow in postsympathectomy patients. Angiology, *10*:139, 1960.

136. Knox, W. G.: The value of digital plethysmography in evaluating patients with peripheral arteriosclerosis for lumbar sympathectomy. Ann. Surg., *149*:539, 1959.

137. Myers, K. A., and Irvine, W. T.: An objective study of lumbar sympathectomy. II. Skin Ischemia. Br. Med. J., *54*:943, 1966.

138. Winsor, T.: Peripheral Vascular Diseases. Springfield, Ill., Charles C Thomas, 1959.

139. Harridge, W. H.: Diagnostic and therapeutic uses of sympathetic block. Surg. Clin. N. Amer., *39*:203, 1959.

140. DeMedeiras, A., Pinto-Rebeiro, A., Porente, E., and DeMedina, A. L.: The role of lumbar sympathectomy in the era of direct arterial surgery. Vasc. Dis., *4*:353, 1967.

141. Wessler, S., Ming, S., Gurewich, V., and Freeman, D. G.: A critical evaluation of thromboangiitis obliterans. The case against Buerger's disease. N. Eng. J. Med., *262*:1149, 1960.

142. Haimovici, H.: Thromboangiitis obliterans. A nostalgic reappraisal. J. Cardiovasc. Surg., *4*:83, 1963.

143. Gifford, R. W.: Arteriospastic disorders of the extremities. Circulation, *27*:970, 1963.

144. Richards, R. L.: Causalgia: A centennial review. Arch. Neurol., *16*:339, 1967.

145. de Takats, G.: Vascular Surgery. Philadelphia, W. B. Saunders, 1959.

146. Julian, O. C., and Dye, W. S.: Treatment of vascular disease. Surg. Clin. N. Amer., *32*:263, 1952.

147. Pratt, G. H.: Cardiovascular Surgery. Philadelphia, Lea & Febiger, 1954.

148. Reid, W., Watt, J. K., and Gray, T. G.: Phenol injection of the sympathetic chain. Brit. J. Surg., *57*:45, 1970.

149. Roedling, H. A., Roth, G. M., Osborn, J. E., Shick, R. M., and McCarty, C. S.: Paravertebral alcohol block of lumbar sympathetic nerves. JAMA, *165*:799, 1957.

150. DeBakey, M. E., Burch, G., Ray, T., and Ochsner, A.: The "borrowing-lending" hemodynamic phenomenon (Hemometakinesia) and its therapeutic application in peripheral vascular disturbances. Ann. Surg., *126*:850, 1947.

151. Owens, J. C., and Smith, A. J.: Fatal pulmonary embolism during regional nerve anesthesia. Angiology, *4*:23, 1953.

152. Murphy, T. O., and Piper, C. A.: Hematometakinesia effects upon the sympathectomized extremity. Am. Surg., *31*:437, 1965.

153. Prinzmetal, M., and Wilson, C.: The nature of the peripheral resistance in arterial hypertension with specific reference to the vasomotor system. J. Clin. Invest., 15:63, 1936.
154. Weamer, A. A.: Role of anesthesiologist in prevention and treatment of thrombophlebitis. Rocky Mtn. Med. J., 43:376, 1946.
155. Cannon, W. R.: A law of denervation. Am. J. Med. Sci., 198:737, 1939.
156. Kuntz, A.: The Autonomic Nervous System. ed. 4. Lea & Febiger, 1953.
157. Smithwick, R. H.: The rationale and technic of sympathectomy for the relief of vasospasm of the extremities. New Eng. J. Med., 222:699, 1940.
158. Palumbo, L. T.: Upper dorsal sympathectomy without Horner's syndrome. Arch. Surg., 71:743, 1955.
159. Goetz, R. H., and Marr, J. A. S.: The importance of the second thoracic ganglion for the sympathetic supply of the upper extremities with a description of two new approaches for its removal. Clin. Practice (Cape Town), 3:102, 1944.
160. Flye, M. W., and Wolkoff, J. S.: Mycotic aneurysm of the left subclavian and vertebral arteries. Am. J. Surg., 122:427, 1971.
161. Gifford, R. W., Jr., Hines, E. A., and Craig, W. M.: Sympathectomy for Raynaud's phenomenon. Followup study of 70 women with Raynaud's disease and 54 women with secondary Raynaud's phenomenon. Circulation, 17:5, 1958.
162. Lord, J. W.: Post-traumatic vascular disorders and upper extremity sympathectomy. Orthop. Clin. N. Amer., 1:393, 1970.
163. Atkins, H. J. B.: Peraxillary approach to the stellate and upper thoracic sympathetic ganglionectomy. Ann. Surg., 72:659, 1956.
164. Haxton, H. A.: Gustatory sweating. Brain, 71:16, 1948.
165. Bloor, K.: Gustatory sweating and other responses after cervico-thoracic sympathectomy. Brain, 92:137, 1969.
166. Ashby, W. B.: Gustatory sweating and pilomotor changes. Br. J. Surg., 47:406, 1960.
167. Fowler, E. F., and de Takats, G.: Side effects and complications of sympathectomy for hypertension. Arch. Surg., 59:1213, 1949.
168. Poppen, J. L., and Lemmon, C.: Surgical treatment in hypertension. JAMA, 134:1, 1947.
169. Smithwick, A. H., and Thompson, J. E.: Splanchnicectomy for essential hypertension. JAMA, 152:1501, 1953.
170. Peet, M. M.: Results of supra-diaphragmatic splanchnicectomy for arterial hypertension. New Eng. J. Med., 236:270, 1947.
171. McGregor, A. L.: Surgery of the Sympathetics. Bristol, John Wright and Sons, 1955.
172. Bronson, R. S., and Neil, C. L.: Abdominal visceral sensation in man. Ann. Surg., 126:709, 1947.
173. Grimson, K. S., Hesser, F. H., and Kitchen, W. W.: Early results of transabdominal celiac and superior mesenteric ganglionectomy, vagotomy, or transthoracic splanchnicectomy in patients with chronic abdominal pain. Surgery, 22:230, 147.
174. Shallat, R. F., and Klump, T. E.: Paraplegia following thoracolumbar sympathectomy. J. Neurosurg., 34:569, 1971.
175. Yeager, G. H., and Cowley, R. A.: Anatomical observations on the lumbar sympathetics with evaluation of sympathectomies in organic peripheral vascular disease. Ann. Surg., 127:953, 1948.
176. Barker, W. F.: Surgical Treatment of Peripheral Vascular Disease. New York, McGraw-Hill, 1962.
177. Hohf, R. P., Dye, W. S., Olwin, J. H., and Julian, O. C.: Low thoracic–high lumbar sympathectomy for vascular diseases of the legs. JAMA, 156:1236, 1954.
178. Listerud, M. B., and Harkins, H. N.: A clinical analysis of experiences with lumbar sympathectomy at the King County Hospital, 1948-1955. Western J. Surg., Obstet., Gynecol., 64:189, 1956.
179. Whitelaw, G. P., and Smithwick, R. H.: Some secondary effects of sympathectomy, with particular reference to disturbance of sexual function. New Eng. J. Med., 245:221, 1951.
180. Alnor, P.: The influence of lumbar sympathetic chain resection upon sexual function. Z. Chirurgie, 269:506, 1951.
181. Palumbo, L. T., and Lulu, D. L.: Lumbar sympathectomy in peripheral vascular diseases. Arch. Surg., 86:512, 1963.
182. Kountz, S. L., Laub, D. R., and Connolly, J. E.: "Aortoiliac steal" syndrome. Arch. Surg., 92:490, 1966.
183. Carey, J. P., Stemmer, E., Heber, R., and Connolly, J. E.: Evaluation of lumbar

sympathectomy for obliterative arterial disease. Rev. Surg., *26*:148, 1969.

184. Goetz, R.: Discussion of Edwards, E. A., and Crane, C.: Lumbar sympathectomy for arteriosclerosis. Arch. Surg., *72*:32, 1956.

185. May, A. G., DeWeese, J. A., and Rob, C. G.: Effect of sympathectomy on blood flow in arterial stenosis. Ann. Surg., *158*: 182, 1963.

186. Carey, J. P., Stemmer, E. A., Heber, R. E., and Connolly, J. E.: The effectiveness of bilateral sympathectomy for unilateral occlusive arterial disease. Amer. Surg., *33*:772, 1967.

187. Atlas, L. N.: Lumbar sympathectomy in the treatment of peripheral arteriosclerotic disease. II Gangrene following operation in improperly selected cases. Amer. Heart J., *23*:493, 1942.

188. Freeman, N. E., Leeds, F. H., and Gardner, R. E.: Sympathectomy for obliterative arterial disease. Indications and contraindications. Ann. Surg., *126*:873, 1947.

189. Passler, H. W.: New experiences with the treatment of acute ischemia (paradoxical reaction) following sympathectomy. Med. Welt, *15*:808, 1966.

190. Higgins, C. C.: Ureteral injuries during surgery. A review of 87 cases. JAMA, *199*:118, 1967.

191. Tanagho, E. A., Hutch, J. A., Meyers, F. H., and Rambo, O. N., Jr.: Primary vesicoureteral reflux: experimental studies of its etiology. J. Urol., *93*:165, 1965.

192. Fryjordet, A., Jr.: Sympathectomy and ureteral reflux. Scand. J. Urol. Nephrol., *2*:196, 1968.

193. White, J. C., and Hamlin, H.: New uses of tantalum in nerve suture, control of neuroma formation, and prevention of regeneration after thoracic sympathectomy. Illustration of technical procedures. Neurosurg., *2*:402, 1945.

194. Randall, W. C., Pickett, W. J., Folk, F. A., and McNally, H. J.: The effective level of lumbar sympathectomy. As determined by direct electrical stimulation at operation. Ann. Surg., *148*:51, 1958.

195. Kirgis, H. D., and Kuntz, A.: Inconstant sympathetic neural pathways. Arch Surg., *44*:95, 1942.

196. Marinescu, V., Pausescu, E., Parvlescu, I., and Fagarasanu, D.: Functional and structural changes of the arterial wall after sympathectomy. J. Cardiovasc. Surg., *9*:54, 1968.

197. Simeone, F. A.: Intravascular pressure, vascular tone, and sympathectomy. Surgery, *53*:1, 1963.

198. Busch, W.: Beitrag zur Anatomie und Topographie des lumbalen sympatheschen Grenzstranges. Helvet. Chir. Acta., *17*: 143, 1950.

199. Fisher, M. M., and Ross, M. E.: Simultaneous contralateral prophylactic sympathectomy with amputation to protect the remaining limb. Angiology, *15*:471, 1964.

200. Litwin, M. S.: Postsympathectomy neuralgia. Arch. Surg., *84*:121, 1962.

201. Pirogov, A. I.: On the recurrence of pain after lumbar ganglionectomy in obliterating endarteritis. Khirurgiia (Moskova) *36*:106, 1960.

202. Hallen, L. G.: Postoperative pain syndrome after lumbar sympathectomy. Nord. Med., *56*:1440, 1956.

203. Policoff, L. D.: Postsympathectomy neuralgia. New York J. Med., *58*:2388, 1958.

204. Cooley, D. A., and Herman, B. E.: Simple means for prevention of postsympathectomy neuralgia. Surgery, *53*: 587, 1963.

205. Tracy, C. D., and Crockett, F. B.: Pain in the lower limb after sympathectomy. Lancet, *1*:12, 1957.

206. Sanders, R.: Personal communication.

207. Barker, W. F.: Peripheral Arterial Disease. Philadelphia, W. B. Saunders, 1966.

208. Litwin, M. S., and First, R. A.: Maculoerythematous rash after lumbar sympathectomy. New Eng. J. Med., *265*:484, 1961.

209. Linton, R. R.: The communicating valves of the lower leg and the operative technique for their ligation. Ann. Surg., *107*:582, 1938.

210. Fulton, R. L., and Blakeley, W. R.: Lumbar sympathectomy: a procedure of questionable value in the treatment of arteriosclerosis obliterans of the legs. Am. J. Surg., *116*:735, 1968.

211. Shumacher, H. B.: Sympathetic denervation of extremities. Operative technique, morbidity, and mortality. Surgery, *24*: 304, 1948.

212. Haimovici, H., Steenman, C., and Karson, I. H.: Evaluation of lumbar sympathectomy. Arch. Surg., *89*:1089, 1964.

213. Baffes, T. G., Carney, A. L., Baffes, C. G., and Guy, C. C.: Lumbar sympathectomy. A five-year survey of 185 patients. Ind. Med. Surg., *36*:593, 1967.

Chapter 10 | Complications of Treatment for

J. W. Lord, Jr., M.D. | # Thoracic Outlet Syndrome

The pitfalls and avoidable errors which confront surgeons caring for patients troubled by symptoms involving the upper extremity seem endless and frustrating. Proper selection of patients for operative intervention is the foundation of a favorable outcome. Yet this initial process is the most difficult. Careful observation, appropriate testing and critical, deliberate evaluation are the rule; however, in occasional instances a major decision must be made to act promptly if, in a few patients, a favorable outcome is to be achieved. Ultraconservatism and wishful thinking may be disastrous in cases of acute arterial thrombotic or embolic episodes. The same error may also be perpetrated in patients with venous thrombosis.

Diagnostic Errors

Organic Lesions

Numbness, tingling, pain and aching discomfort are the predominant complaints of most patients with pressure from any cause on the neurovascular structures in the thoracic outlet. Coldness, fatigue, pallor or cyanosis of the arm and hand are frequently noted. Unfortunately many of these complaints have their origin in the cervical root area wherein a protruded intervertebral disc, an arthritic spur, or other boney abnormality is the causative mechanism. Sectioning of the scalenus anticus muscle or resection of the first rib in patients with cervical root

compression can only lead to a poor postoperative result and in some instances worsen the situation. With patients in whom neurologic symptoms predominate and arterial and venous involvement is either absent or minimal, the clinician should be cautious.

If on examination, maneuvers to determine arterial and venous obstruction by boney and fascial structures of the thoracic outlet show little or no interference with flow, and neurologic examination shows interference with normal function of one or more of the cervical roots or brachial plexus, even the seasoned clinician should be on guard. Under these circumstances the aid of an experienced neurologist who is particularly interested in problems of the thoracic outlet should be obtained. Electrodiagnostic testing is often helpful under such circumstances. In recent years the more frequent use of electrodiagnostic testing has been of great help in locating organic pressure on one or more of the nervous elements of the upper extremity and also in the elimination of those patients who might have been subjected to an unnecessary and possibly unfortunate surgical procedure on the thoracic outlet.

If the issue remains in doubt as to the site of neural compression then a trial of cervical traction, use of a collar and physiotherapeutic measures are indicated. The assessment over a period of time of response

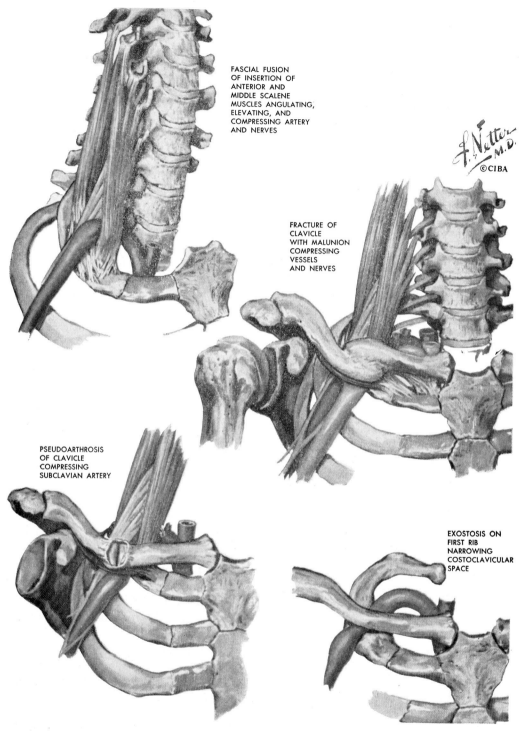

FASCIAL FUSION
OF INSERTION OF
ANTERIOR AND
MIDDLE SCALENE
MUSCLES ANGULATING,
ELEVATING, AND
COMPRESSING ARTERY
AND NERVES

FRACTURE OF
CLAVICLE
WITH MALUNION
COMPRESSING
VESSELS
AND NERVES

PSEUDOARTHROSIS
OF CLAVICLE
COMPRESSING
SUBCLAVIAN ARTERY

EXOSTOSIS ON
FIRST RIB
NARROWING
COSTOCLAVICULAR
SPACE

PLATE VI   STRUCTURAL ABNORMALITIES CAUSING COMPRESSION

FIG. 10-1. Some of the structural abnormalities that may result in compression of the contents of the thoracic outlet. (Lord, J. W., and Rosati, L. M.: Thoracic-outlet syndromes. Clin. Sympos., *23*:3, 1971. © Copyright 1971 CIBA Pharmaceutical Company, Division of CIBA-GEIGY Corporation. Reproduced with permission, from the CLINICAL SYMPOSIA, illustrated by Frank H. Netter, M.D. All rights reserved.)

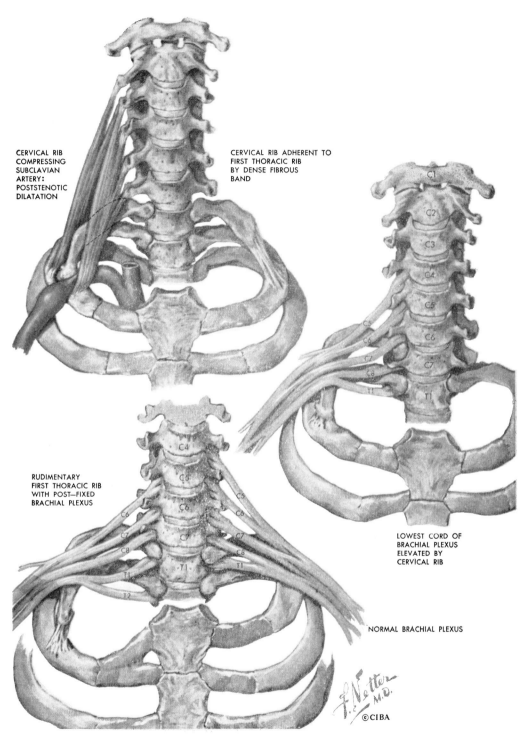

CERVICAL RIB
COMPRESSING
SUBCLAVIAN
ARTERY:
POSTSTENOTIC
DILATATION

CERVICAL RIB ADHERENT TO
FIRST THORACIC RIB
BY DENSE FIBROUS
BAND

RUDIMENTARY
FIRST THORACIC RIB
WITH POST—FIXED
BRACHIAL PLEXUS

LOWEST CORD OF
BRACHIAL PLEXUS
ELEVATED BY
CERVICAL RIB

NORMAL BRACHIAL PLEXUS

©CIBA

PLATE VII   COMPRESSION CAUSED BY CONGENITAL RIB ABNORMALITIES

FIG. 10-2. Compression of the contents of the thoracic outlet by congenital rib abnormalities. (Lord and Rosati, *op. cit.* © Copyright 1971 CIBA Pharmaceutical Company, Division of CIBA-GEIGY Corporation. Reproduced with permission, from the CLINICAL SYMPOSIA, illustrated by Frank H. Netter, M.D. All rights reserved.)

TABLE 10-1. PARTIAL DIFFERENTIAL
DIAGNOSIS OF THORACIC OUTLET SYNDROME

Herniated Intervertebral Disc
Degenerative Cervical Spine Disease
Osteoarthritis
Spinal Cord Tumor
Superior Pulmonary Sulcus Neoplasm
Post-traumatic Cervical Injury
Entrapment Neuropathy
Tardy Ulnar Palsy
Carpal Tunnel Syndrome
Alcoholism
Diabetes Mellitus
Psychoneurosis
Arteriosclerosis
Causalgia
Vasculitis
Collagen Disease
Arterial Embolism
Raynaud's Disease

to these measures, particularly cervical traction, may reveal sufficient improvement to clearly suggest cervical root origin of symptoms. Lastly, myelographic studies may be required to rule in or rule out cervical root compression.

In one unfortunate instance a patient whose upper extremity pain and numbness were thought initially by a neurosurgeon to be due to compression of the brachial plexus by the scalenus anticus muscle was studied further because he also developed similar complaints of lower extremity difficulty. Further neurological consultation and a myelogram led to the diagnosis of cervical cord pressure by a boney spur. Laminectomy by an experienced neurosurgeon was followed by a near complete paraplegia. Ultimately the diagnosis proved to be multiple sclerosis. Operative intervention probably hastened the inexorable course of this patient. This case serves to illustrate the major diagnostic difficulty which some patients will cause the clinician interested in upper extremity problems.

Another patient was a woman with left upper extremity pain and paresthesia located in the ulnar distribution of the hand and forearm. The Adson maneuver was positive and a neurologic consultant agreed that no

other offending mechanism was involved. Complete symptomatic relief followed section of the scalenus anticus muscle and lasted for two years when the old complaints recurred. Repeated examination by neurologists over a period of two more years led to cervical cord exploration and the discovery of a slowly growing cord tumor. Undoubtedly this patient had two distinct lesions causing her symptoms.

To summarize the above comments, one cannot be too careful in the study and observation of patients whose predominant complaints are neurologic and not clearly related to arterial and/or venous involvement (Table 10-1).

Functional States

Few areas in the body are target sites of psychosomatic complaints as commonly as the upper extremities. Symptoms such as numbness, tingling, weakness and aches and pains frequently have as their underlying basis personality disorders and emotional derangement. Relief of such patients' symptoms may occasionally be spontaneous or may require considerable management by an internist or psychiatrist. If operative intervention is delayed until objective evidence, clinical and laboratory, shows mechanical compression of the neurovascular structures, mistakes will be few. Occasionally the association of organic compression and emotional disturbance is present and such patients, although diagnostically challenging, should not be denied surgical help.

The following case of a 27-year-old woman, is a sad but informative one. When seen for the first time in October, 1950 she had had a symptomatically unsuccessful left scalenotomy by one surgeon in 1948. Later the pain had been relieved by a left upper thoracic sympathectomy by the transthoracic approach. In 1949 section of the right scalenus anticus muscle for pain in the right arm was without help and an upper thoracic sympathectomy by the White-Smithwick approach was also without help. A fifth operative procedure earlier in 1950 consisting of division of some scar tissue, brought temporary relief of pain in the right hand and arm. Examination in October, 1950 was essentially negative for thoracic outlet maneuvers and it seemed clear that she was an emotionally unstable patient and needed psychiatric care. It was possible that this should have been considered in the first place. Further operations were advised against, but in spite of this a vascular surgeon in another hospital explored the right supraclavicular area. Massive hemorrhage developed and ligation of the subclavian artery with partial claviculectomy was required. Without explanation the patient's symptoms abated for a few months. When they recurred, her physician advised total claviculectomy which was carried out with temporary relief of pain. Finally when the pain recurred, she was referred to a psychiatrist in December, 1951. Unfortunately by this time her life pattern had become so disturbed that in July, 1953 she committed suicide.

A 27-year-old nun, an accomplished pianist and teacher, was seen by an experienced vascular surgeon in January, 1958 because of coldness and painful swelling of the left hand and distal forearm of a few days' duration. Coolness and cyanosis of all four extremities had been noted intermittently for several years. Physical examination showed marked swelling of the fingers, hand and distal forearm stopping abruptly above the wrist. The left radial pulse was weaker than the right one. Several stellate ganglion blocks were temporarily helpful, but the edematous changes and pain recurred shortly thereafter. Operative intervention included sectioning of the scalenus anticus, resection of a 1.5 inch segment of the first rib anteriorly and an upper thoracic sympathectomy by a supraclavicular approach. Symptomatic relief was noted for three months when once again the swelling and pain in the left hand recurred. In May, 1958 the patient underwent a partial claviculectomy and lysis of scar tissue from around the subclavian artery. Short-lived help was followed by a recurrence of edema and then a transthoracic sympathectomy in

July 1958 achieved relief of pain for six weeks. The same symptoms recurred and she was referred to a medical center in New York for study. It seemed possible that the remaining outer segment of clavicle may have compressed the neurovascular bundle so the remaining clavicle was completely removed. Relief of edema and pain was noted for two months. She was again admitted to the hospital on two occasions during the next twelve months. Eventually the conclusion was reached for the first time that the patient's symptoms and signs were self induced. One sister who accompanied her gave assurance that she was "happy, contented, talented and successful at her work." No one had observed any suspicious action. It was recommended that she be admitted to a semi-private room and observed closely. Later it was learned that she had been using constriction of her forearm and arm to induce the changes from the very first. Psychiatric study was undertaken without avail, and the patient committed suicide early in 1960.

These two patients cited in some detail emphasize the great need to withhold operative intervention in patients with unusual complaints and physical findings. Careful testing and observation will lessen the chance for error and occasionally tragic outcomes. The concept of exploration without clear indications has only an occasional place in patients suspected of having problems with their thoracic outlets (Figs. 10-1 and 10-2).

Patients who have been in automobile accidents and sustained "whiplash" injuries to their necks may experience symptoms similar to those caused by thoracic outlet syndrome. The situation is frequently confused by the influence of associated litigation, the awards and rewards of which are sometimes proportionate to "suffering" and objective changes. This type of case will tax the ingenuity and thoroughness of the clinician, and such comments hold equally well for workmen's compensation cases. "Make haste slowly" is perhaps the best axiom, and objective testing should be thoroughly employed.

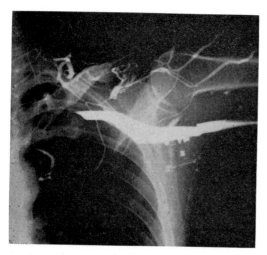

FIG. 10-3. Left-arm phlebogram obtained with the arm in abduction and external rotation in a 34-year-old man who complained of aching forearm pain and dysesthesia in the ulnar distribution of his left hand. The arm and shoulder were normal in appearance with the arm *adducted*, but with arm in *abduction* a prominent venous plexus appeared about the shoulder. There was no edema of the arm or hand. (Courtesy H. G. Beebe, M.D.)

Selection of Diagnostic Tests

The selection of appropriate radiographic examinations should routinely include cervical spine films with oblique projections and chest films. These will serve to identify the patient whose symptoms arise from a Pancoast tumor or a cervical rib and to alert the surgeon to the presence of bony abnormality in the cervical spine. Beyond these routine roentgenograms, contrast studies of arteries or veins may be considered depending on the patient's symptoms and physical findings. In patients with typical thoracic outlet syndromes arteriography is not a necessary examination. Although compression of the subclavian artery as it crosses the first rib to become the axillary artery can frequently be demonstrated by arteriograms taken with the arm in abduction, it is also true that such findings may not be present even when thoracic outlet compression is the true cause of the disorder. Thus, arteriography should be selected only when the presenting clinical signs suggest arterial occlusion as the predominant feature. Arteriographic delineation of the subclavian artery and its branches including the small vessels of the hand is of inestimable value in patients with thrombotic or embolic complications. Eastcott has emphasized the nature of thromboembolic episodes associated with cervical rib, formerly considered by many to be vasospastic in origin.[1] Only by the frequent use of arteriographic studies has this observation been made.

Venous compression is very common in patients with thoracic outlet syndromes and may be demonstrated by phlebography with injection in the basilic vein of the arm.[2] This is a simpler procedure than arteriography and will often demonstrate local abnormality at the thoracic outlet. So-called "effort thrombosis" or Paget-Schroetter syndrome may often result from pre-existing venous compression by a narrowed thoracic outlet which can readily be shown by upper extremity phlebography. Observation for the appearance of prominent veins about the shoulder during arm abduction and external rotation or for forearm venous distention during Adson's maneuver will help indicate which patients may be usefully subjected to phlebography. Phlebographic study combined with pressure data obtained by the passage of a catheter to the superior vena cava and withdrawal into the axillary vein complement each other in the location of pressure points causing intermittent compression of the venous system of the arm. (Fig. 10-3).

Possible complications related to phlebographic and arteriographic studies are discussed in Chapter 1. Such studies should be employed only when the information to be derived is required for accurate diagnosis which in turn aids in the selection of appropriate operative and nonoperative procedures. Further, these tests, whenever possible, should be carried out by experienced "angiographers" or by trainees under their careful supervision. Even under these circumstances complications will occasionally occur and represent the risks which must be accepted if the patient's condition is to be treated properly.

Electrodiagnostic testing should be considered whenever the patient complains of symptoms which are primarily neurologic and unaccompanied by coincident signs of vascular compromise. The value of nerve conduction studies is variable depending upon the experience and skill of the physician conducting the examination. This is especially true when evaluating deficits of nerve impulse transmission across the region of the thoracic outlet. The stimulus must be applied in the supraclavicular fossa where the brachial plexus is variously distributed. The recording electrode is placed below the shoulder joint over a more discreetly located upper arm nerve. Therefore the limitation of the method at the shoulder level is an anatomic one, and requires experienced interpretation. Urschel[3] has reported that such studies showing nerve conduction rates under 60 meters per second have been of great value in selecting patients with neurologic symptoms due to compression in the thoracic outlet. For identification of patients with tardy ulnar palsy occurring at the elbow level or with carpal tunnel syndrome occurring at the wrist level, such diagnostic techniques are uniformly valuable and accurate in distinguishing these conditions from thoracic outlet syndrome. Complications from the use of electrodiagnostic testing are virtually nonexistent.

Errors in Selection of Patients for Operative Intervention

All of the considerations previously discussed apply here. There are also other points to note, however. Mild symptoms related to the thoracic outlet may, after careful examination, be observed without treatment in many instances, or if symptoms persist, be helped by physical therapy. In fact, spontaneous remission often occurs. Although reliable objective data to support this hypothesis are lacking, it is the author's impression that less than 10 percent of patients with complaints in their upper extremities require operative intervention.

For all patients with predominantly neurologic symptoms where pain and paresthesia are the dominant clinical presentation, neurologic consultation is a must. Ischemic pain of arterial origin is diffuse without neural distribution. Venous obstruction is usually readily identifiable on physical examination. In selected patients, psychiatric consultation should be considered.

At the other end of the spectrum, undue delay in operative intervention may result in permanent changes including tissue loss due to arterial obstruction. Thromboembolic episodes are best surgically corrected within hours rather than in days. However, as long as the hand is viable, delayed thrombectomy or embolectomy will not infrequently be successful. Arteriographic study is required only in those cases wherein exact localization of the embolus is not possible by physical examination. If the source of the embolus is from an abnormal heart with arrhythmia such as auricular fibrillation or with myocardial infarction, angiographic study may be withheld. However, in some patients the site of thrombus formation is in a poststenotic aneurysm in the region of the thoracic outlet not detectable by palpatation and only delineated by angiographic study.

When thrombosis of the axillosubclavian vein is acute, delay in operative intervention may lessen the opportunity for complete restoration of venous flow from the arm to the superior vena cava.[4,5] Fortunately the development of collateral circulation will relieve many patients sufficiently and tide them over, allowing for consideration of definitive procedures to eliminate pressure on the subclavian vein by a narrowed costoclavicular space. As an emergency procedure, transbrachial removal of the thrombus by a Fogarty catheter with maintenance of continuity of the vein by careful suture followed by transaxillary resection of the first rib or resection of the costocoracoid liga-

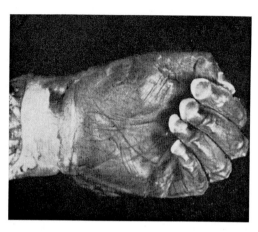

FIG. 10-4. Gangrenous hand from reflex anteriospasm following an upper thoracic sympathectomy carried out by the supraclavicular approach. This approach should not be used in a patient with vascular impairment. (Lord and Rosati, *op. cit.* © Copyright 1971 CIBA Pharmaceutical Company, Division of CIBA-GEIGY Corporation. Reproduced with permission, from the CLINICAL SYMPOSIA, illustrated by Frank H. Netter, M.D. All rights reserved.)

ment and section of the scalenus anticus represents ideal management of the problem. Whether the two procedures should be carried out at one time or be staged, must be left to the judgment of the surgeon in each case.

Long-term anticoagulant therapy along with elevation and compression of the hand and arm for control of edema should be reserved for patients in whom operative intervention is contraindicated or in those where operation has failed. Patients whose symptoms indicate the presence of venous thrombosis for longer than one week should probably be treated by nonoperative means, as the likelihood of complete and lasting thrombus removal is slight.

Patients with predominantly neurologic symptoms who can be demonstrated to have these due to thoracic outlet syndrome may be managed deliberately without great concern for the development of permanent nerve deficit. The major problem in delayed management of thoracic outlet syndrome is usually the development of subsequent arterial or venous vascular complications.

Selection of the Appropriate Operative Procedure

Selection of the best operation for a given thoracic outlet problem rests on an accurate diagnosis of where the trouble lies. Complicating this matter is the occasional patient with two offending mechanisms. Another factor in selecting the "best" operation for a specific patient is the relative risk of a procedure from a technical viewpoint. In the hands of some skilled surgeons all operations are relatively safe and complications are few, but for most of us, an analysis of the good to be derived from an operative procedure must be balanced against possible complications which may develop as a result of it.

An example illustrating these comments is selection of approach for sympathetic denervation of the upper extremity for vasospastic or arterially insufficient hands. Based on current concepts, the posterior paravertebral exposure of White and Smithwick results in a partial denervation in most patients. Complications are few and usually not serious, but the morbidity of the operative approach is excessive. The supraclavicular (Telford) approach is favored by many British and some American surgeons in affording removal of the stellate and second thoracic ganglion along with correction of associated abnormality of the scalenus anticus and medius muscles or cervical rib when present.[6] However, there are several reports in the literature of injury to the subclavian artery associated with this approach requiring ligation for control of hemorrhage. The writer has observed one instance of gangrene of the hand requiring amputation from such a complication (Fig. 10-4). For exposure of the ganglia, retraction of the subclavian artery is necessary and in vasospastic individuals this is potentially hazardous.

The inframammary, transthoracic, transpleural approach of Palumbo[7] allows for excellent exposure and complete sympathectomy with removal of the lower one-half of the stellate ganglion (or all of the ganglion if one so desires), and the second, third and fourth upper thoracic ganglia. This approach would seem to be the safest of all but of course requires a separate procedure, at the same time or sequentially, for correction of any boney or fascial points of pressure in the thoracic outlet.

The transaxillary approach described by Goetz[8] is a safe and adequate one, and may be combined with transaxillary resection of the first rib and section of the scalenus anticus and medius muscles.

From the viewpoint of completeness or adequacy of an operative procedure, simplicity and safety should serve as guidelines only when the selected operation will assure a satisfactory outcome. In some patients an operative procedure with greater chance of risk will be necessary for the relief of symptoms. For instance, section of the scalenus anticus or of the pectoralis minor tendon is easier and safer than transaxillary resection of the first rib. But, unless a precise diagnosis of this site of neurovascular pressure has been made preoperatively, the minimal operation will fail and cast an unfavorable light on operative intervention for the relief of true thoracic outlet syndromes.

Under some circumstances thorough exploration of the supra- and retroclavicular structures is necessary for the detection of fascial anomalies of the scalenus medius muscle and of rudimentary cervical rib with a ligamentouslike extension of the first rib. If at this time marked narrowing of the costoclavicular space is detected, then total claviculectomy along with complete removal of the periosteum can be carried out with clinically satisfactory results. If periosteum is left behind, bone regeneration and subsequent recurrent compressive symptoms may be encountered. Although several authors have stated that claviculectomy is unsatisfactory from functional and cosmetic viewpoints, the evidence for those comments is not well documented. In 32 patients who had 40 total claviculectomies (bilateral in eight), with complete removal of the periosteum to prevent regeneration, there has not

been a major complaint either functionally or cosmetically.[9]

Patients who have classical symptoms of thoracic outlet syndrome with clear physical findings with the Adson maneuver and negative physical findings with arm elevation and abduction may be considered for scalenus anticus muscle section alone. However, transaxillary removal of the first rib is usually a better choice of procedure for the patient suffering from thoracic outlet syndrome because it relieves compression from multiple causes, the precise preoperative anatomic understanding of which may be impossible.[10] It is a fortunate circumstance that the first rib comprises the "floor" of the thoracic outlet and the fact that the insertions of the scalenus anticus and medius muscles are freed during its removal. Patients who have a cervical rib anomaly may be treated by resection of this structure along with the accompanying fascial extension to the first rib.

Technical Considerations

In supraclavicular operations, the author's preference is to position the patient in a semi-upright position with the back elevated 30 degrees from the horizontal and a thinly folded sheet placed behind the scapulae. The neck is thereby extended a little and the chin is turned away from the operative site. The anterior chest is prepared along with the entire neck and shoulder. A suction apparatus should be available prior to making the incision. The structure with the greatest potential for catastrophe is the subclavian vein which may be accidentally torn behind the clavicle in the region of the scalenus anticus muscle. In addition to extensive blood loss, air embolism is an added hazard. Careful, painstaking dissection is the keynote when working in this region. If hemorrhage from the subclavian vein occurs in the position described above, venous pressure is low and gentle packing will often control it. If the surgeon will now allow ten minutes to pass, often venous bleeding will remain controlled following removal of the

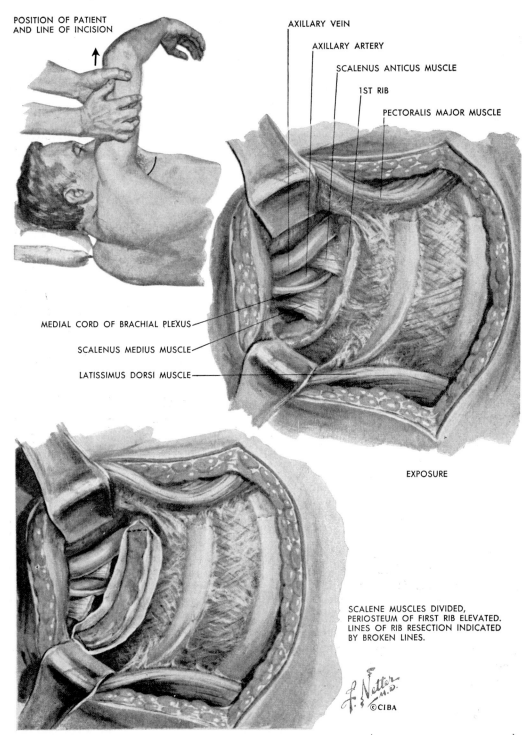

POSITION OF PATIENT
AND LINE OF INCISION

AXILLARY VEIN

AXILLARY ARTERY

SCALENUS ANTICUS MUSCLE

1ST RIB

PECTORALIS MAJOR MUSCLE

MEDIAL CORD OF BRACHIAL PLEXUS

SCALENUS MEDIUS MUSCLE

LATISSIMUS DORSI MUSCLE

EXPOSURE

SCALENE MUSCLES DIVIDED,
PERIOSTEUM OF FIRST RIB ELEVATED.
LINES OF RIB RESECTION INDICATED
BY BROKEN LINES.

PLATE IV   RESECTION OF FIRST RIB (TRANSAXILLARY APPROACH)

FIG. 10-5. Transaxillary approach to first-rib resection for relief of thoracic outlet syndrome. (Lord and Rosati, *op. cit.* © Copyright 1971 CIBA Pharmaceutical Company, Division of CIBA-GEIGY Corporation. Reproduced with permission, from the CLINICAL SYMPOSIA, illustrated by Frank H. Netter, M.D. All rights reserved.)

packing since a thrombus will have sealed the opening. During this time instruments for the removal of the clavicle including a Gigli saw and bone holding clamps can be obtained for prompt use if necessary. If vigorous bleeding persists after removal of the packing, the area should be repacked and the clavicle quickly resected. The subclavian vein can then be readily visualized and repaired.

Injury to the subclavian artery is a possibility especially when unduly forceful maneuvers during dissection may avulse one of its branches. This is more likely to occur when exposure of the stellate and second thoracic ganglia is attempted than during section of the scalenus muscles or resection of a cervical rib. When arterial hemorrhage occurs, temporary packing may be effective, but gently applied suction and irrigation will usually permit successful suture of the opening. If these techniques fail then resection of the clavicle and other steps described under control of hemorrhage from the subclavian vein may be necessary. If a segment of the artery has been severely traumatized, a vein graft, preferably from the saphenous vein, should be inserted between healthy ends of the subclavian-axillary artery.

In transaxillary first rib resection, injury to the brachial plexus may occur in two ways. The common hazard is the use of long metal retractors placed too deep within the wound, particularly on the superior and lateral or "arm" side of the incision impinging on the medial cord of the brachial plexus in particular. The other notable hazard occurs during rongeuring of the posterior aspect of the first rib where limited exposure and visualization dictate great care in performance of this maneuver. Late symptoms of nerve irritation may be caused by leaving a sharp spicule of bone from the posterior point of first rib division which impinges upon the brachial plexus. Numbness of the inner aspect of the arm may follow transaxillary operation even though the intercostobrachial nerve has been preserved,

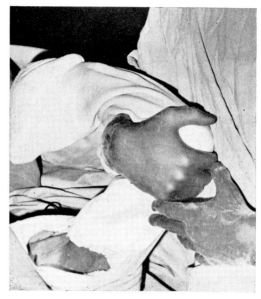

FIG. 10-6. The patient's left arm is prepared and draped free for left transaxillary first-rib resection. The arm should be held so as to avoid prolonged traction with pressure applied at the elbow which may result in continuing postoperative symptoms and ulnar nerve palsy.

which is usually possible in most cases (Fig. 10-5).

The pleura may be inadvertently entered during transaxillary first rib resection, and routine irrigation of the wound prior to closure along with forceful respiration by the anesthesiologist will demonstrate this. This is managed simply by aspiration of air with a catheter that is removed at skin closure.

During transaxillary operations the arm, with appropriate sterile draping, should be held freely mobile by an assistant. During operation, manipulation of the arm to distract the shoulder will materially aid exposure of the first rib. This should be done with due care so as to place no undue pressure on the ulnar nerve at the elbow or to apply no excessive stretch to the brachial plexus in the anesthetized patient (Fig. 10-6).

Rough retraction of the brachial plexus must be avoided during removal of a cervical rib by the supraclavicular approach.

However, in some instances postoperative neuritis will follow even when great pains are taken to handle brachial plexus structures as gently as possible. Gentle retraction by an encircling thin Penrose drain is preferable to a metal retractor. Attention should also be paid to irrigation with lukewarm, isotonic saline during the procedure to prevent dehydration of neural tissues. Although the pain experienced by patients with postoperative neuritis may be severe, it usually clears in a few weeks. During this time narcotics should be withheld if at all possible as addiction may occur too easily. Tranquilizing medication in adequate dosage may prove helpful in avoiding narcotics.

Injury to the thoracic duct may follow extensive dissection proximally along the subclavian artery and vein. Lymph drainage on such occasions may be controlled by careful suture, including thoracic duct ligation, without sequelae. Persistent lymph drainage, an annoying complication, may subside promptly and permanently following immobilization and elevation of the extremity by pulley and weight and compression of the forearm and arm with an Ace bandage.

The phrenic nerve should be identified and retracted before sectioning of the scalenus anticus muscle. In spite of such care, a paralyzed diaphragm occasionally may be found in an asymptomatic patient on a routine chest film as late as one year postoperatively.

Postoperative Care

Operative complications have been discussed in "Selection of the Appropriate Operative Procedure" and some of the postoperative problems noted. In spite of detailed efforts directed at complete hemostasis, postoperative accumulation of blood will frequently fill the "dead space" following section of the scalenus anticus muscle with or without removal of a cervical rib. The empirical use of dexamethasone (Decadron) and promethazine (Phenergan) for a few days may lessen the tendency for scar formation that may entrap the very structures released by the operative procedure. Postoperative oozing following transaxillary resection of the first rib is of less importance as gravity will allow the blood to dissect inferiorly and posteriorly without accumulation in the region of the brachial plexus and subclavian vessels.

If the pleura has been entered, a postoperative chest film will serve as a guide for the need for aspiration of a significant amount of air, if present.

Although active gradual use of the extremity is encouraged postoperatively, vigorous activities are banned for a period of two to three months. A few patients have been observed who were doing well until they engaged in strenuous work or sport followed by a recrudescence of their preoperative symptoms. A further period of guarded activity has usually sufficed to enable a complete recovery.

In many patients, symptoms are substantially relieved but in some, especially those whose primary problem has been that of nerve pressure, only partial improvement is noted. In these patients reassurance is vital with the graceful acceptance by the patient of some residual discomfort. The task is made much easier for the surgeon and internist if preoperative psychological preparation has been adequate. "Promising too much" may lead postoperatively to a less than satisfactory result.

Late Failures and Long Term Problems

Late failures and poor postoperative results will be few if the physician and surgeon have followed the suggestions outlined above. Nevertheless certain problems do occur in spite of careful selection of patients for operation and proper performance of an appropriate and thorough procedure.

Occasionally partial regeneration of the clavicle, in spite of diligent efforts to remove all periosteum, is followed by recurrence of costoclavicular symptoms. A second claviculectomy with removal of all suspicious surrounding soft tissue is followed by an improved result.

Numbness of the anterior chest wall following a supraclavicular approach is annoying, but reassurance usually suffices and reinnervation will take place in a few months.

Of great importance is the patient who has had a good result for one to three or more years when symptoms recur. It is vital not to overlook the development of a new cause of symptoms and not to fault the adequacy of the first procedure. Five patients have been seen with six involved extremities who had either a primary thoracic outlet syndrome followed later by a genuine carpal tunnel syndrome or vice versa. All of these patients were helped by secondary operative intervention in the new region. Re-exploration of the primary site would have been ineffectual and possibly harmful.

The cornerstone for the avoidance of complications in the treatment of the thoracic outlet syndrome is an accurate differential diagnosis. A detailed history with particular consideration of the emotional and psychosomatic problems is vital. A thorough physical examination of the arterial and venous circulations should be supplemented by a careful neurologic examination.

Useful diagnostic tests include arteriography, phlebography and electrodiagnostic studies. These studies should be selectively applied with the patient's full understanding of possible complications. Consultation with an experienced neurologist interested in all aspects of the thoracic outlet syndrome is most helpful. With the exception of acute arterial and venous problems, an unhurried and thoughtful approach to the selection of patients for operative intervention is recommended. Haste is seldom necessary.

The surgical procedure and its extent should be individualized, employing that particular operation best suited to the patient and his condition. Finally careful and painstaking dissection will lessen the chances of an operative mishap.

References

1. Eastcott, H. H. G.: *In* Arterial Surgery p. 220, Philadelphia, Lippincott, 1969.
2. Adams, J. T., DeWeese, J. A., Mahoney, E. B., and Rob, C. G.: Intermittent subclavian vein obstruction without thrombosis. Surgery, *63*:147, 1968.
3. Urschel, H. C., Jr., Paulson, D. L., and McNamara, J. J.: Thoracic outlet syndrome. Ann. Thor. Surg., *6*:1, 1968.
4. Adams, J. T., McEvoy, R. K., and DeWeese, J. A.: Primary deep venous thrombosis of the upper extremity. Arch. Surg., *91*:29, 1965.
5. DeWeese, J. A., Adams, J. T., and Gaiser, D. L.: Subclavian venous thrombectomy. Circulation 41, Suppl. *2*:158, 1969.
6. Telford, E. D., and Mottershead, S.: Pressure at the cervicobrachial junction. J. Bone Joint Surg., *30B*:249, 1948.
7. Palumbo, L. T.: Anterior transthoracic approach for upper thoracic sympathectomy. Arch. Surg., *72*:659, 1956.
8. Goetz, R. H., and Marr, J. A. S.: Importance of second thoracic ganglion for sympathetic supply of the upper extremities, with description of two new approaches for its removal in cases of vascular disease; preliminary report. Clin. Proc., *3*:102, 1944.
9. Rosati, L. M., and Lord, J. W.: *In* Neurovascular Compression Syndromes of the Shoulder Girdle, p. 123, New York, Grune and Stratton, 1961.
10. Roos, D. B.: Transaxillary approach for first rib resection to relieve thoracic outlet syndrome. Ann. Surg., *163*:354, 1966.

Chapter 11

Hugh G. Beebe, M.D.

Deep Venous Thrombosis and Complications of Peripheral Venous Procedures

Diagnosis of Deep Venous Thrombosis

It is difficult to estimate the frequency with which the diagnosis of deep venous thrombosis is in error. Depending on the severity of clinical criteria utilized, the clinical impression of deep venous thrombosis is falsely positive somewhere between 20 and 66 percent of the time. The false negative incidence is harder, of course, to estimate. Considering the large numbers of patients having autopsy findings of pulmonary emboli who were not thought to have deep venous thrombosis before death, this must be an uncomfortably high number.

Clinical Symptoms

Symptoms are generally less striking than their accompanying signs. Depending on the level of involvement, patients with even extensive thrombosis may have surprisingly minimal symptoms. The commonest symptom is pain with active motion of the affected part, which is usually in proportion to the amount of edema present. For the same reason, a sense of heaviness is also present particularly with more proximal occlusion, associated with aching discomfort of the involved leg.

Clinical Signs

The commonly helpful and usually reliable signs of deep venous thrombosis are swelling and tenderness. Other signs may also accompany the process, but are not necessarily

to be relied upon. In 100 patients proved by DeWeese and Rogoff to have unequivocal phlebographic demonstration of thrombosis within the deep venous system, a significant percentage of them had absence of the usual clinical findings.[1]

As pointed out by DeWeese, swelling bears a direct relationship to the degree to which collateral venous return is impeded resulting in elevation of the venous pressure. In patients with calf vein thrombosis, he found only 3 of 43 patients had significant calf swelling and that the venous pressure in the foot of such patients was minimally elevated. Patients with femoral vein thrombosis demonstrated calf swelling of significance 86 percent of the time and venous pressure was approximately three times normal. Almost all patients with iliofemoral venous thrombosis can be expected to have leg swelling and their venous pressures may be as high as ten times normal. McLachlin, *et al.* have emphasized the importance of swelling in a careful study of clinical signs compared with postmortem findings.[2]

However, the patient who develops deep venous thrombosis during the course of complete bedrest or with the affected extremity elevated throughout the development of the process may have extensive thrombosis with virtually inapparent swelling. An example is illustrated in Figure 11-1. This was a young, previously healthy woman with no history of venous disease or leg swelling.

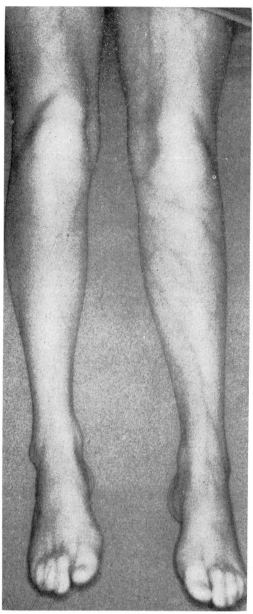

A

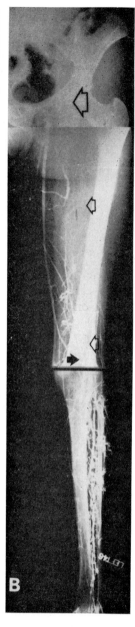

B

FIG. 11-1. (A) Infrared photograph taken at the same time as the phlebogram shown in (B), illustrates the similarity of gross appearance of the legs despite extensive deep venous thrombosis on the left. The prominence of superficial venous flow, which was not striking clinically, is well shown by the technique of infrared photography. (B) Left-leg phlebogram showing iliofemoral venous thrombosis extending proximally from the knee as marked by the solid arrow. The open arrows indicate the course of the thrombosed deep system which did not visualize.

Two weeks after an uncomplicated lumbar laminectomy and spinal fusion, during which time she had been at complete bedrest, an unexplained low grade fever developed and minimal calf tenderness and Homans' sign were found to be present. Bilateral phlebography demonstrated a normal right leg and extensive occlusion in the deep veins of the left leg. There was no noticeable difference in the appearance of the legs, and calf measurements showed only 1.5 cm. difference at the calf level and 2 cm. difference in the thigh.

The location of tenderness may be diffuse throughout the leg, but generally parallels the location of the thrombus itself. A useful technique in assessing calf muscle tenderness is to position the patient with the knees half drawn up permitting easy palpation of the relaxed calf muscles. Often gentle ballottement of the posterior compartment will also give a sense of induration on the involved side. Tenderness in the anterior compartment is easily elicited when thrombosis of the anterior tibial veins is present. This is fortunate since these veins may commonly fail to be visualized on phlebography due to compression of the small entrance to the anterior compartment by a low-lying tourniquet.

The cause of pain and tenderness in the limb with deep venous thrombosis is not fully understood. Tenderness is observed in areas of superficial venous thrombosis without marked edema and, therefore, it may be presumed that the inflammatory change associated with a blood clot is responsible in like manner for some of the tenderness seen in deep vein thrombosis. There is no ready explanation for the cause of inflammation by stagnant, clotted blood, however. Or, the tenderness and pain of deep venous thrombosis may also be due to stretched "C" fiber nerve endings in edematous muscle compartments. In pelvic thrombophlebitis, lower abdominal tenderness may be the only physical finding suggesting further pursuit of the diagnosis.

Skin changes are not reliable guides to the diagnosis, but may help to increase the index of suspicion. At times a faint generalized blush of erythema may be seen accompanied by an impression of increased cutaneous warmth. Superficial venous distension may be present, presumably due to an increased blood flow through subcutaneous collateral veins. Evidence of arteriovenous shunting in deep venous thrombosis has been demonstrated by femoral vein blood gas determinations.[3] Mild cyanosis may also be seen due to very slow flow of deoxygenated blood in the subcapillary venous plexus of the skin. Patients who are suffering from phlegmasia alba dolens demonstrate pallid appearance because of their edema, which gives rise to the colloquialism "milk leg." Skin changes in phlegmasia cerulea dolens or venous gangrene may be dramatic, with almost complete envolvement of the extremity by obvi-

ous, advanced, gangrenous change. Usually, however, the progression of iliofemoral thrombosis to phlegmasia cerulea dolens is heralded by small, isolated, irregular patches of faint, milder, pre-gangrenous changes.

Homans' sign is so frequently in error, that it cannot be relied upon, and yet it is known to practically every medical student and house officer.[2] There are two variations on this theme: The patient's foot may be dorsiflexed passively, and when this is accompanied by pain in the calf muscle, the sign is considered to be present. Specifically, Homans' sign does not refer to accompanying pain or discomfort along the course of the hamstring tendons behind the knee. Another way of eliciting Homans' sign is to ask the patient to actively dorsiflex his great toe and foot. When the involved foot is dorsiflexed less than the uninvolved foot because this causes the patient accompanying calf pain, the sign is present. At least half of the time, patients proved to have deep venous thrombosis by phlebography, do not have Homans' sign. This sign may also be seen in patients who have sustained a ruptured plantaris longus tendon, tear of the medial head of the gastrocnemius muscle, after blunt trauma to the leg, in viral illnesses, in patients who have recently changed to unaccustomed footwear, in trichinosis, and in apparently normal individuals.

The sphygmomanometer cuff pain test described by Lowenburg has been used as a method of eliciting calf tenderness with a uniform stimulus. Pain caused by inflation of a blood pressure cuff about the calf at a pressure below 180 mm. Hg is considered a pathologic finding. However, this test was found unreliable by Barner and DeWeese, who encountered an incidence of 26 percent false positive and 22 percent false negative incidence.[4]

Typical factors which predispose to the development of deep venous thrombosis include age, obesity, a previous history of thromboembolic disease, congestive heart failure, prolonged limb immobilization or bed rest, malignancy, trauma, recent pelvic surgery and certain predisposing drugs, such as the oral contraceptive agents. The enormity of the failure to appreciate the occurrence of deep venous thrombosis in hospitalized patients is indicated by the frequency with which pulmonary embolism can be found at autopsy, when carefully searched for.

The greatest aid to diagnosis of deep venous thrombosis is a suspicious physician armed with the knowledge of predisposing conditions, who frequently seeks to find clinical signs of the disorder. The importance of having good ancillary methods for supporting the clinical impression of deep venous thrombosis should be apparent from the foregoing discussion of the rather protean clinical presentation. A rational approach to the diagnosis of deep venous thrombosis in the lower extremity would be to evaluate the patient with the idea of answering the question; "Does this patient have sufficient signs or symptoms to warrant a phlebogram?" rather than asking whether the clinical presentation warrants the *diagnosis* of deep venous thrombosis. Considering how involved and expensive the current ideal treatment for deep venous thrombosis is, it hardly seems rational to base treatment on frequently erroneous clinical signs when phlebography is such an easily performed and well-tolerated examination. A number of additional laboratory methods of proving the diagnosis of deep venous thrombosis are currently under development, including isotopic detection of thrombi, impedance phlebography, and the use of Doppler ultrasonic techniques. None of these techniques has wide usage at the present time, and furthermore all of them are associated with a significantly lower incidence of diagnostic accuracy than phlebography, which must remain the standard against which all other methods are judged.

Aids to Diagnosis

Phlebography

By far the most informative examination is functional ascending phlebography, as described by DeWeese and Rogoff.[5,6] This simple technique has become a routine radiographic procedure in most hospitals, and offers the distinct advantage over the other methods mentioned, by permitting visual inspection of the lumen of the veins in question.

When properly performed, the leg phlebogram will almost always accurately reflect the status of the deep venous system. False negative results will be few, if the technique employed results in adequate amounts of contrast medium injected under conditions which favor flow into the deep system and delay the rate of venous emptying of the leg. False positive results usually are due to inexperienced interpretation, compounded by poor technique, causing "flow artefacts" or streaming of the dye. Multiple views should routinely be obtained, and a typical filling defect should be demonstrated on more than one film.

The notion that phlebography may result in pulmonary embolism, aggravation of existing phlebitis, or initiation of phlebitis, is unfounded if proper technique is used. Phlebography is never performed using high pressure injection, and the use of a continuous infusion technique as described in Chapter 1 will obviate irritation of the vein wall. Phlebography may be readily performed on an outpatient basis, and in the author's clinic, is routinely done prior to admitting a patient for the primary diagnosis of deep venous thrombosis.

Radioisotopic Techniques

Two approaches to the use of radioisotopes for detection of deep venous thrombosis have been used. Spar, Goodland and Schwartz[7] demonstrated that radioactive fibrinogen antibody could be used to detect experimental thrombi in dogs, and proceeded to a clinical trial in 1965, of a small series of patients. Deep venous thrombi in the legs were demonstrated using ^{131}I labelled rabbit antihuman fibrinogen, and confirmed by phlebography. Both false positives and false negatives may occur with this technique. The antibody will localize in areas of inflammation, wound healing, fracture or hematoma, and is thus nonspecific for acute venous thrombosis. If very small areas of calf vein thrombus exist, these may be undetected by this method.

Another test reagent has been employed by Kakkar after Hobbs and Davies showed that a developing thrombus will incorporate ^{131}I labelled fibrinogen.[8] This method may be the earliest presently available technique for clot detection, since it depends upon the active process of thrombus formation. It has the limitation of being less useful if the process is not suspected clinically at an early enough time to be evaluated during thrombus formation. In 25 patients controlled by phlebography, Kakkar showed positive correlation in 17.[9] More recently, Kakkar has used ^{125}I labelled fibrinogen in 88 patients also evaluated phlebographically with 92 percent accuracy.[10]

Browse feels that ^{125}I scanning of the leg is perhaps a more sensitive method of detecting small calf vein thrombi than phlebography, since not all such veins are well shown by phlebography. This is, of course, dependent upon the quality of phlebography. But, also, since he does not treat such patients, the practical value of such sensitivity is questionable.[11]

The disadvantages mentioned for this technique include the failure to detect iliac or pelvic thrombi, owing to the high amount of isotope contained in adjacent patent vessels, the risk of serum hepatitis from the injected fibrinogen, and the practical difficulty of a test requiring specially trained personnel and involved equipment. Beyond this, the isotope used is not generally available in this country.

Ultrasound

The use of Doppler ultrasound instrumentation to assess venous blood flow has received recent attention from a number of groups. This technique takes advantage of the frequency shift that occurs when an ultra high frequency sound wave is reflected from a moving surface. Differences in velocity of

wave forms can be demonstrated in patients with patent or occluded veins. The advantage of the Doppler technique lies in its ease of application and innocuous, noninvasive nature. Comparing results of Doppler and phlebographic assessment of deep venous thrombosis, Sigel, *et al.*[12] found only a 60.7 percent sensitivity of the ultrasonic technique in calf vein occlusion and 83.6 percent in femoral level disease.

This method does not distinguish between new and old occlusions, and requires a high degree of experienced interpretation. The large number of false negatives with a limited extent of thrombosis is disturbing, but the ease of performance stimulates interest in this as a screening device.

Plethysmography

Wheeler and his colleagues have developed an ingenious approach to detection of venous occlusion by employing a device to detect changes in the electrical impedance of the leg in relation to venous blood flow.[13] Since the electrical conductivity of the leg is variable, depending on its fluid content, the rate of emptying of venous blood from the leg can be related to the rate of change of electrical resistance. Patients are tested by inducing a mild Valsalva maneuver, during breath holding, which causes pooling of blood in the leg veins. Upon release of breath holding, the rate of change of electrical impedance is related to patency of the leg veins.

Although not extensively compared with phlebography in all types of patients, Wheeler's studies indicate a high degree of sensitivity in showing abnormality when "clinically significant" deep venous thrombosis was present.[14]

Limitations of this method include false normal results in patients with limited calf vein involvement, and false positive results if the test is not very precisely controlled in terms of leg position, amount of knee flexion or extension and electrode placement. It is a noninvasive, simple technique which is readily acceptable to patients and apparently free of complications.

The fact remains that to date, no technique equals the diagnostic accuracy of contrast phlebography, though other methods may prove to be more suitable for screening large groups of patients.

Differential Diagnosis of Deep Venous Thrombosis

In the patient who has not recently had a vascular reconstructive operation, the development of acute clinical signs and symptoms of deep venous thrombosis should prompt additional diagnostic maneuvers such as those discussed above. Such tests may fail to confirm the presence of deep venous thrombosis, and the list of conditions which may simulate deep venous thrombosis includes all of those mentioned in Table 11-1, and others. Even retroperitoneal fibrosis has been described as presenting with a typical appearance of deep venous thrombosis.[15] Not infrequently patients with rest pain from advanced arterial disease will present with edematous legs due to the long-standing passive dependency they have maintained in an effort to relieve their symptoms.

Considering the associated conditions occurring in a patient with lower extremity arterial insufficiency, it is surprising that the natural course of arterial disease is not more frequently complicated by deep venous thrombosis. All of the factors predisposing

TABLE 11-1. CONDITIONS THAT MAY SIMULATE DEEP VENOUS THROMBOSIS

Postphlebitic Syndrome
Congestive Heart Failure
Nephrotic Syndrome
Other Renal Disease
Severe Hypoproteinemia
Pelvic Tumor
Lymphedema
Pregnancy
Gastrocnemius Muscle Tear
Plantaris Longus Tendon Rupture
Allergic Reaction
Arteriovenous Fistula

the thrombosis identified by Virchow some 120 years ago, to which very little new information about etiology has been added, are present in the patient with arterial disease in the legs. There is low inflow, moderately severe hypoxia of venous blood and an immobile, dependent limb. Hypoxia has been implicated as a precipitant of endothelial injury and platelet aggregation. This is a setting where the development of deep venous thrombosis would hardly be surprising, and yet it is uncommon to see clinical stigmata of deep venous thrombosis in the patient with arterial insufficiency.

Treatment

Management of the patient with uncomplicated deep venous thrombosis is discussed below followed by special consideration of the patient who has an accompanying arterial lesion.

Uncomplicated Deep Venous Thrombosis

A treatment regimen which is commonly employed is outlined below. As soon as the diagnosis has been established, the patient is placed at bedrest for seven to ten days. The choice of ten days is a somewhat arbitrary one, but has a rational basis in the experimental observation that thrombi become adherent to the venous wall within that period of time. The lower half of the bed is elevated to raise the feet approximately 15 or 20° above horizontal. It is important to also use the knee gatch with which most hospital beds are equipped so as to support the knee which would otherwise lie in hyperextension. Permitting the knee to rest in a position of hyperextension without posterior support will result after about 24 hours in symptoms of greater discomfort from stretching of the hamstring tendons than the original deep venous thrombosis. Furthermore, the positioning of the leg in complete extension has been shown to interfere with venous flow from the lower leg.[14] If there is concern over flexing the bed at the hip level to achieve leg elevation, 20 to 35 cm. blocks are available in most hospitals to place under the foot of the bed. Pillows under the legs should be avoided.

The mainstay of treatment is anticoagulation with heparin. There is a great deal of controversy over the choice of route of administration and control monitoring of this drug. Intravenous heparin may be given at six-hour intervals in sufficient dosage to prolong the Lee-White clotting time to approximately 2½ times the control value; however, more recent clinical trends seem to be in favor of less emphasis on laboratory control by this means. This is partly because of the great variability and inaccuracy of this clotting test when done at the bedside and also because of the difficulty of systematic accomplishment of it in most hospitals. The partial thromboplastin time may be used to monitor heparin anticoagulation as a substitute for the questionable Lee-White clotting time. When this method of control is used, two times the control value represents a therapeutic range.

An alternative form of heparin anticoagulation commonly employed is administration of 15,000 to 20,000 units of heparin given subcutaneously every 12 hours. So long as the patient is not hypotensive this results in a prolonged absorption of the drug. It has also proved a useful route of administration in avoiding irregular anticoagulation so often seen in hospitals where heparin must be administered by a physician if given intravenously, which usually results in erratic dose schedules. A Lee-White clotting time may be usefully employed in the 12-hour subcutaneous method immediately preceding a dose, at least to establish that an excessive residual from the preceding dose is not present.

Continuous intravenous heparin administration has at least four criticisms which limit its usefulness. It requires a significant added volume of fluids to be given which would not otherwise be necessary and may be poorly tolerated, particularly in patients who have sustained a pulmonary embolus. The rate of administration may be irregular, resulting in wide variations in anticoagulation because of the vagaries of intravenous flow rates. Most patients with straight forward deep venous thrombosis would not otherwise require intravenous fluid administration and finally, the unusual development of heparin antibody formation is said to be somewhat more common in patients given heparin by this method.

Additional symptomatic treatment may also be considered, but the anti-inflammatory properties of heparin make prompt improvement in leg discomfort the rule, without additional measures such as local application of moist heat. Aspirin and Butazolidin have both been employed to relieve symptoms of deep venous thrombosis, but their tendency to cause gastrointestinal hemorrhage makes them a doubtful adjunct in patients receiving anticoagulants. The common clinical observation that pulmonary embolism is frequently associated with the act of defecation suggests the importance of venous pressure changes during a Valsalva maneuver in dislodging a loosely attached thrombus from the leg. For this reason, the routine employment of some sort of regimen to facilitate bowel function is theoretically useful.

The legs are not wrapped with any sort of elastic support during the time the patient is at bed rest. Specifically Ace bandages are scrupulously avoided because of their tendency to be rolled up into tourniquets by leg motion during sleep. When the patient is free of significant edema, the legs can be measured for below knee elastic stockings which can be ordered in time to be available when ambulation is to be permitted.

After ten days of heparin, this drug is tapered over 48 hours and discontinued during which time warfarin is given in sufficient dosage to reduce the prothrombin time to below 30 percent of normal. How long warfarin anticoagulation should be continued after an episode of uncomplicated deep venous thrombosis remains unsettled. Indeed, it is not clear that such continued anticoagulation has any distinct value at all. It seems rational to employ warfarin routinely whenever a patient has developed

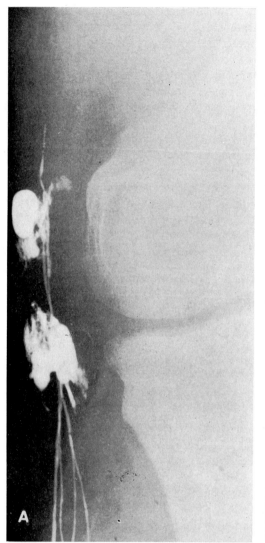
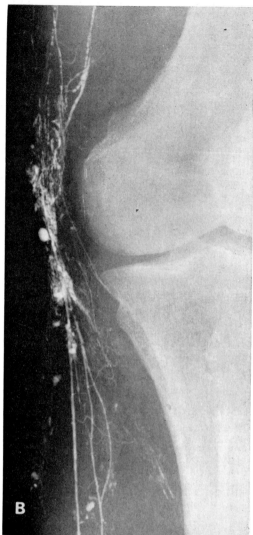

FIG. 11-2. (A) Lymphangiogram taken one week after femoropopliteal bypass in a 62-year-old man. All superficial lymphatic trunks on the medial side of the knee were divided, and extravasation of iodized oil was evident. (B) The same patient six weeks later. Although an extensive anastomosis is visible, the iodized oil ascended slowly and dermal backflow, indicating lymphedema, is displayed in the calf. (Vaughan, B. F., *et al.*: Edema of the lower limb after vascular operations. Surg. Gynec. Obstet., *131*:282, 1970)

deep venous thrombosis and will have a prolonged period of limited mobility such as that required in treatment of an associated fracture. However, it remains a moot point whether such continued anticoagulation is of value in the patient who can resume full, normal ambulation promptly. Many sur-

geons feel that three to six months of anticoagulation with the warfarin drugs is useful in preventing early recurrence of acute thrombophlebitis. Controlled data to support this view are lacking. Further discussion of this unsettled area is reviewed in Chapter 12.

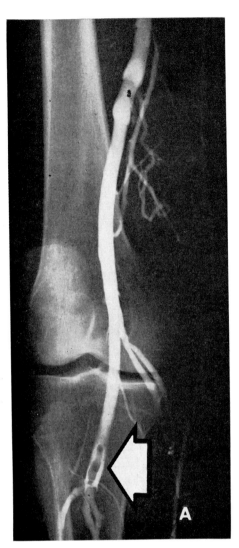

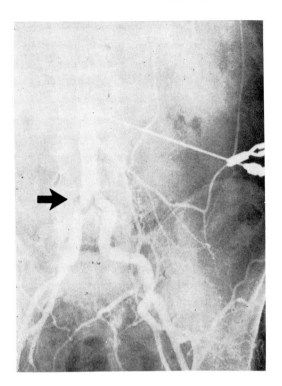

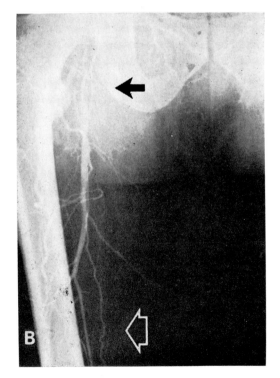

FIG. 11-3. (A) Right-leg phlebogram showing acute deep venous thrombosis of the popliteal vein. A semi-attached thrombus, noted to change position slightly on serial films, is indicated by the arrow. (B) Translumbar aortogram of patient whose phlebogram is shown in (A).

Edema After Arterial Reconstruction

Patients who have had a recent lower extremity arterial reconstruction will often show moderate degrees of leg swelling beginning within a few days of operation and lasting weeks, or occasionally many months. This can be seen after either aortofemoral bypass grafting or after femoropopliteal operations. Some surgeons have the impression that this problem is more commonly associated with transverse groin incisions than with longitudinal incisions.

The commonly held belief that such leg edema so frequently accompanies a successful arterial operation as to herald a good result has been investigated by Simeone and Husni.[16] They found that hyperemia and edema were present in 32 extremities usually when extensive and long-standing ischemia had been present, and only when the arterial operation had been successful. Therefore, they postulated that the "set" of smooth muscle tone and arterial resistance required time to adjust to the influences of suddenly increased flow and pressure. Phlebograms were not included in that study.

Others have felt that lymphedema secondary to the operative trauma was a likely explanation, particularly when phlebograms obtained after arterial reconstruction failed to show evidence of deep venous occlusion. Vaughan and his colleagues performed lymphangiograms in a series of 22 patients after arterial reconstructive surgery, many of whom also had phlebograms.[17] As illustrated in Figure 11-2 there was clear evidence of lymphatic obstruction and disruption as a result of the operative trauma. Further discussion of leg edema after arterial reconstruction can be found in Chapter 3.

Deep Venous Thrombosis and Arterial Reconstruction

Management of the patient with deep venous thrombosis also known to have arterial occlusive disease for which operation is planned can be undertaken as outlined above. Additional consideration should be given to venous interruption at the time of arterial reconstruc-

tion. The necessity for withholding anticoagulants immediately after arterial operation suggest the wisdom of prophylactic measures against pulmonary embolism.

The following case illustrates this point. A 57-year-old man with severe claudication and foot rest pain developed right leg swelling one week prior to his scheduled admission. A phlebogram, shown in Figure 11-3A, showed popliteal vein thrombosis. He was kept at bed rest and given heparin for eight days, after which time a translumbar aortogram, shown in Figure 11-3B, was obtained during a 12-hour interruption of heparin. Two days later his heparin was tapered and he underwent uneventful aortofemoral bypass grafting. A partially interrupting clip was prophylactically applied to the inferior vena cava just below the renal veins at that time. He made an uneventful recovery until the eighth postoperative day, when he developed 3+ edema of both legs over a period of eight hours. It was presumed that his clip had trapped an embolus. His edema was controlled by elevation and elastic stockings, and he was discharged on the 14th postoperative day. At one year follow up, he was edema free without stockings.

Leg edema following arterial reconstruction is so common and so seldom evaluated by phlebography in most clinics that the possibility exists that some cases of deep venous thrombosis are missed. Perhaps these patients should routinely be screened by impedance plethysmography or Doppler ultrasonic means. If there is accompanying tenderness, thigh swelling or Homans' sign, a phlebogram may be indicated.

If deep venous thrombosis is proved in the early postoperative period, heparin should be withheld because of the risk of hemorrhage. Dextran, as mentioned below, is a reasonable alternative treatment. If thrombophlebitis arises late after arterial surgery, anticoagulants may be safely used in the routine manner.

Occasionally the development of extensive deep venous thrombosis following successful arterial reconstruction has resulted in sufficient compromise of venous flow that failure of the arterial graft has ensued. This uncommon complication should prompt consideration of early venous thrombectomy, and arterial thrombectomy followed by cautious anticoagulation and/or the use of dextran.

Complications of anticoagulation have been well summarized by Macon, Morton and Adams, who extensively reviewed the literature in 1970.[18] Hodin and Dass have focused attention specifically on retroperitoneal hemorrhage associated with the use of Coumadin.[19] Other mention of the complications associated with the early postoperative use of anticoagulants is made in Chapter 12 and Chapter 17.

Alternative Treatment

Dextran

Over the past ten years, a large number of publications have reported the use of dextrans of various molecular weights for a variety of conditions. Some of the properties of dextran in the 42,000 and 75,000 molecular weights which suggest its use as treatment for deep venous thrombosis are its viscosity-reducing effects on blood, its bioelectric property in coating the intima with negatively charged molecular moieties, its enhancement of the rate of venous flow and its reduction of blood sludging. All of these effects may be transiently achieved without giving sufficient dextran to cause direct anticoagulation effects. Dextran has been employed as an alternative to heparin as the primary treatment in deep venous thrombophlebitis, with apparent success.[20]

Since the objective of anticoagulation and dextran therapy in phlebitis is the same—to prevent extension of an existing thrombus—both may be effective but by different means. A theoretical objection to dextran is that its primary effect may reside in increasing the rate of venous flow[21] which could be impossible in a severely occluded venous system.

Thrombolysins

Thrombolytic drugs are currently being investigated for the treatment of venous blood clots. Streptokinase, urokinase and Arvin are all being evaluated. Kakkar has compared the use of streptokinase, a plasminogen activator, and Arvin, an extract of snake venom which converts fibrinogen to an altered form, and found the former encouraging in seven of nine patients.[22] Arvin was not effective in that study. Others have reported varying results in the use of streptokinase.[23] Mavor has indicated preference for streptokinase over urokinase and suggested that this drug may ultimately replace venous thrombectomy.[24]

At present such drugs are available only on an investigational basis in this country, and hence are not a currently practical alternative. Among the limitations currently mentioned in connection with their use are allergic reactions, frequent associated bleeding complications, rethrombosis after cessation of treatment, the probable necessity for very early treatment if it is to be effective, and the poor results in very extensive occlusions, with low flow to involved veins.

Prophylaxis

Measures used to reduce the development of post operative deep venous thrombosis have included: early ambulation, avoidance of sitting, use of elastic stockings, elevation of the legs, adequate hydration, anticoagulation with warfarin drugs or heparin, and the use of dextran.

All of these measures have in common either reduction in venous stasis or interference with blood coagulation. Most of the clinical studies evaluating the prophylactic use of anticoagulants have relied upon clinical signs to determine the presence of thrombophlebitis, which makes their interpretation difficult.

Physical measures such as avoidance of passive limb dependency, exercises in bed, early ambulation, manual leg massage, and elastic compression, are of variable usefulness, depending on the method of employment. All too often the result of physician instructions to "ambulate" the patient, is a few steps from bed to chair followed by a prolonged interval of sitting. The use of physical measures prophylactically were evaluated by Flanc, Kakkar and Clarke, using ^{125}I fibrinogen leg scanning, and found to be of very limited value.[25] Other British workers have employed electrical muscle stimulation with more encouraging results, especially when used intraoperatively.

An excellent study of the usefulness of physical measures in prophylaxis was conducted by Eckert and his group who controlled their clinical observations with the use of phlebography and ^{125}I labelled fibrinogen scans.[26] They found that only 2 of 51 treated patients had evidence of deep thrombophlebitis, as contrasted with 6 of 44 control patients.

Many of the more recent studies which have approached the problem through the use of anticoagulants or dextran have been collected by Haller and his associates at the time of reporting a prospective, double-blind inquiry into the use of dextran prophylaxis.[27] They found no value in prevention of pulmonary embolism, but suggestive evidence of a reduced incidence of thrombophlebitis.

More recently, the use of antiplatelet-aggregation drugs such as dipyridamole or aspirin have attracted attention. To date, insufficient trials are available on which to judge their value.

Upper Extremity Deep Venous Thrombosis

The occurrence of thrombophlebitis in the arm is relatively uncommon as compared with the leg. As pointed out by Coon and Willis, no single physician is likely to see many cases and therefore the ideal treatment of this condition is still unsettled.[69]

Some generalizations can be made about this disorder and its natural history, however. First, it usually occurs in younger, otherwise healthy adults in association with abnormal amounts of exercise requiring hyperabduction. It may be that most of these patients have thoracic outlet syndrome underlying their acute condition. Second, prompt resolution of edema is usually seen with ordinary conservative treatment. Third, the

incidence of pulmonary embolism is probably 5 to 17 percent, but some patients who have embolized have also had leg thrombophlebitis. Fourth, venous gangrene of the arm is very rare and usually associated with a generalized coagulopathy. Fifth, the incidence of this condition may be expected to increase with the current greater use of central venous catheters and prolonged intravenous alimentation.

Late persistent symptoms have been reported in 68 percent of 25 patients studied by Adams, McEvoy and DeWeese.[70] If they are significant symptoms and interfere with work activity, operation should be considered. The most frequent complication of the several procedures used for late sequelae of axillary-subclavian venous thrombosis is failure to relieve the compression when anterior scalenotomy is employed. This is also true in patients with intermittent subclavian vein obstruction without thrombosis as discussed by Adams, DeWeese, Mahoney and Rob.[71] If operation is recommended for such patients, either claviculectomy or first rib resection would seem a better choice than scalenotomy from the reports mentioned above.

Superficial Thrombophlebitis

The common opinion that superficial thrombophlebitis is only of symptomatic importance may often be an incorrect one. Aside from the diagnostic implications suggested by this process in patients with occult visceral malignancy or Buerger's disease, superficial venous clots may have important complications in their own right.

The increasing use of prolonged intravenous cannulation, particularly in intensive care units where the resident bacterial flora is antibiotic resistant, has resulted in a higher incidence of septic complications. These cases are usually associated with contaminated equipment and adherent small thrombi. Furthermore, although superficial venous clots very rarely are thought to become pulmonary emboli, the extension of a superficial clot into the deep venous system is not rare. Galloway, Karmody and Mavor have documented several such instances as have others, and this suggests that superficial thrombophlebitis deserves serious attention.[28]

Although anticoagulants are not necessary in the management of superficial thrombophlebitis, if the process is ascending in the limb, especially in the greater saphenous vein of the leg, or if the process arises in the thigh, interruption of the offending vein flush with the common femoral vein has been considered of help in limiting the potential for extension into the deep system.

Venous Thrombectomy

Rationale and Indications

One of the more controversial procedures employed in managing deep venous thrombosis is thrombectomy. Currently the procedure is criticized both in terms of the results obtained and in terms of largely theoretical concern over potential inducement of pulmonary embolism. Much of the debate surrounding this operation arises from a lack of clear understanding of the objectives desired by such treatment, compounded by wide variations in patient selection. The greatest misunderstanding lies in postoperative evaluation, however.

The two major objectives of venous thrombectomy are prevention of late sequelae of the postphlebitic syndrome and reduction in morbidity of the acute episode. Although prevention of pulmonary embolism has been mentioned as an objective by some, this is not a generally accepted indication for thrombectomy since there is no evidence available that this procedure reduces the incidence of this complication below that achieved by nonoperative means alone.

Following the early report by Mahorner[29] in 1957, DeWeese, Jones, Lyon and Dale, in 1959, refined the indications in an excellent study of 23 patients of whom 11 were submitted to thrombectomy.[30] Their initial suggestion that thrombectomy be reserved for patients whose thrombosis was localized to the iliac and femoral veins has been sup-

ported by a subsequently reported larger experience.

A later report by Haller in 1963 indicated the great difficulty of effecting a satisfactory outcome if thrombectomy is not performed early in the course of the disease.[31] Presently most surgeons feel that good results are seldom if ever obtained beyond five days after the onset of thrombosis.

In considering whether this procedure is of value, it is important to realize that the objective of the operation is not merely venous patency. Since the large majority of thrombosed veins subsequently recanalize, patency is usually restored in the natural course of the disorder anyway. The rationale for thrombectomy is the preservation of competent valves within the veins, thus reducing or preventing postphlebitic morbidity. The natural course of recanalization after phlebitis usually destroys these valves by fibrosis and scarring of the vein wall.

Late follow-up studies of patients treated by thrombectomy have given conflicting information on whether or not the venous valves have been preserved. DeWeese showed phlebographic documentation of preserved valves to some degree in patients studied one to five years postoperatively.[30] Lansing consistently failed to demonstrate functional valves in 15 patients studied five years or longer after thrombectomy.[32] Edwards, *et al.* commented on 58 patients with a one to nine year follow-up and, although recommending greater use of phlebography in evaluating postoperative status, mentioned only one phlebogram showing competent valves following thrombectomy.[33]

Clinical assessment of symptoms and appearance of the leg are insufficient guides as to the efficacy of this procedure, for at least two reasons. A good clinical result is not infrequently accompanied by phlebographic evidence of re-occlusion or absent valves, thus indicating that the operation may fail in its primary objective without apparent signs. Secondly, the development of the postphlebitic syndrome takes a variable and often prolonged period of years to become clinically apparent. Thus, destroyed valves may ultimately result in significant morbidity which is not appreciated in its full extent for five or ten or more years.[34]

The secondary objective of reducing morbidity of the acute process is usually attainable if patients are seen early, and particularly if selection is made of patients with more proximal limited extent of thrombosis. Since this goal depends on patency alone, and not valve preservation, the early results are reliable estimates of this value of thrombectomy. The prompt improvement in most patients with phlegmasia alba dolens with

elevation and heparin alone is indicated in Figure 11-4A compared with a typical course after thrombectomy shown in Figure 11-4B.

Although some patients will have unusually prolonged and severe symptoms of acute iliofemoral thrombosis, the rapid improvement in the majority even without operation suggests that limitation of acute morbidity should be viewed as a secondary benefit derived from thrombectomy and not as a primary indication for surgery.

The uncommon development of phlegmasia cerulea dolens or frank venous gangrene is considered a firm indication for

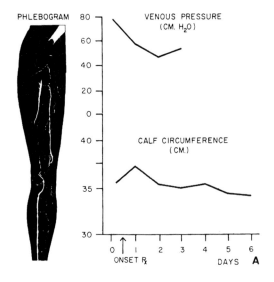

FIG. 11-4. (A) This illustrates the usual prompt resolution of edema in the leg following elevation and anticoagulation alone. (B) Usual prompt resolution of edema in the leg following thrombectomy for iliofemoral thrombosis. (DeWeese, J. A., *et al.* Surgery, *47*:140, 1960)

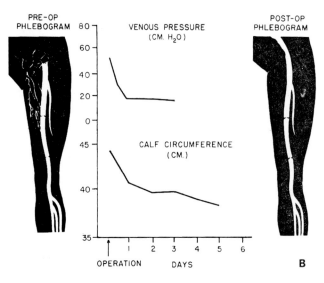

venous thrombectomy in most clinics, although Haimovici has recommended a trial of conservative measures first.[35]

In patients who have uncomplicated ilio-femoral venous thrombosis, the generally accepted indications for considering thrombectomy at the present time are:

1. Phlebographic evaluation showing extent of thrombosis limited to iliac and proximal femoral systems, not involving calf veins.

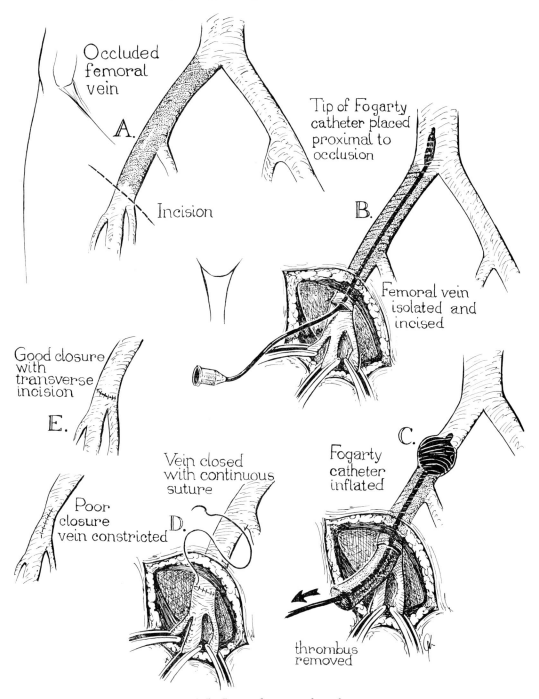

FIG. 11-5. Steps of venous thrombectomy.

2. Duration of thrombosis of less than five to seven days, ideally less than three days.

3. Expectation of patient survival for long enough period of time to warrant prevention of postphlebitic sequelae.

4. An otherwise stable patient who can tolerate the operative procedure and its usual accompanying requirement for 500 to 1000 ml. blood loss and replacement transfusion.

Technique

Preoperative preparation should include availability of adequate cross-matched blood, since the usual transfusion requirement for this procedure is 500 to 1000 ml. and occasionally more. The patient should be adequately sedated to facilitate the use of local anesthesia. Anesthesia standby should be mandatory for monitoring of the patient and administration of blood replacement.

Local plain lidocaine anesthesia is employed. A small groin incision is used to expose the common femoral vein and all of its tributaries which are dissected free and preserved. When occluding vascular clamps are applied to all except the common femoral vein, this vessel is opened through a transverse venotomy extending across the entire anterior surface.

The distal thrombus in the leg may best be removed by manual or elastic compression. Passage of the Fogarty catheter distally in the leg is irrational if it destroys the valves that thrombectomy serves to preserve. Use of curved common duct stone forceps is helpful in removing iliac vein clot. A Valsalva maneuver performed during iliac clot extraction may aid removal and theoretically add protection against embolism of a fragment.

Vigorous back bleeding indicates improvement, but is no guarantee of complete thrombus removal. Occasionally, back bleeding cannot be obtained from a patent iliac vein unless the valve in it is rendered incompetent briefly by holding it open with the common duct stone forceps.[36] Often thrombus material will exude from the vein immediately. A Fogarty balloon catheter can then be passed upward into the vena cava and withdrawn, removing iliac vein thrombus. The previously recommended technique of occluding the vena cava by advancing a Fogarty catheter from the contralateral, uninvolved side[37] has been abandoned by most surgeons, including Fogarty.[38] Alternatively a suction catheter may be employed. DeWeese prefers applying suction by use of a large-bore syringe, to the use of a tubing connected to wall suction, in order to limit blood loss.

Operative phlebography is the best method of establishing when complete thrombectomy has been accomplished.[39] Congenital and acquired anomalies, particularly of the left common iliac vein, which may be encountered have been summarized by Bales.[40]

The vein is closed with 50 silk with great care, and meticulous hemostasis is secured because of the anticipated use of postoperative anticoagulants.

Complications

Hume, Levitt and Thomas[41] have collected four probable instances of pulmonary embolism "provoked by thrombectomy", but this must be exceedingly rare, as most surgeons with a large experience with this procedure have not encountered it. The use of a Valsalva maneuver to increase vena caval pressure during clot removal from the iliac vein is of theoretical benefit. Some surgeons have routinely applied a partially interrupting vena cava clip prior to iliofemoral venous thrombectomy, as indicated in Chapter 12. If preoperative phlebography shows clot extending into the vena cava, or if bilateral disease exists, such a measure would seem prudent.

The commonest complication is postoperative hemorrhage and hematoma formation in the wound. This is related to the early use of anticoagulants. The use of dextran for 24 to 48 hours before instituting heparin may help reduce this frequent cause of delayed healing. Some series have encountered this complication in nearly 50 percent of patients and have felt that strict control of heparin by using small doses was of preventive value.

Rethrombosis of the operated vessel is uncommon if early thrombectomy is accomplished before intimal roughening by adherent clot has occurred, and if complete thrombus removal has been accomplished. Conversely, failure to remove all thrombus has frequently been associated with rethrombosis to the original extent or greater.[42] Occasional successful re-operation in a favorable situation has been reported.[33]

Shock occurring during operation from excessive blood loss is an entirely preventable complication resulting from inexperience with venous surgery as contrasted with arterial surgery. The use of suction equipment to extract clot will quickly remove a much larger volume of blood than is immediately apparent. Moreover, the low pressure bleeding from veins does not always compel attention as does arterial bleeding. Ordinarily, blood transfusion will routinely be required during this operation, and should be anticipated before hypotension ensues, which may predispose to other venous thrombosis.

Varicose Veins

Patient Selection

The indications for surgical treatment of varicose veins include improvement in cosmetic appearance of the leg, decrease in the risk of developing both superficial or deep venous thrombosis, relief of symptoms of aching discomfort in the leg and treatment of the uncommon leg ulcer which may be accurately ascribed to the underlying varicosity.

The surgeon should assure himself that the leg symptoms, when present, which he seeks to relieve may be attributed to varicose veins. When prominent varicosities are obviously cosmetically deforming, a good result may also be anticipated. But, the neurotic patient with an unrealistic body image who seeks surgical care for small or insignificant varices should be dealt with cautiously. Such patients, frequently middle-aged women whose complaints of pain are out of proportion to the physical findings, are apt to remain dissatisfied after an operation and present a challenging management problem.

When extensive varicosities are seen, operation should be advised before they continue to enlarge and multiply making excision inordinately difficult. The patient shown in Figure 11-6 was seen 15 years previously and no operation was advised for his moderate-sized varicose veins. He continued to pursue an occupation requiring prolonged standing and was seen again when aching pain in his legs became moderately severe. His varicosities required multiple staged procedures and excessive hospitalization compared to what would have been possible 15 years previously.

Concern is sometimes expressed over the wisdom of operating for varicose veins in a female patient in childbearing years because of the presumed risk that subsequent pregnancy may result in recurrence. Lofgren and Lofgren reported that about half the women they had seen who had recurrent varicose veins had had one or more intervening pregnancies since their original operation.[43] Others have indicated a liberal operative approach when young women have had significant varices. Fanfera and Palmer reported 87 women operated on for varicose veins three days postpartum without complications except recurrent varices in two patients.[44] Haeger has even suggested operating on women with prominent varices during pregnancy and had 90 percent or better satisfactory results in 21 patients treated during the first trimester and 33 patients treated during the second trimester.[45]

These and other reports tend to indicate that female patients with symptomatic varicosities should not be denied surgery simply because they are in the child-bearing age range and may have a subsequent pregnancy. Rather, it would appear that recurrent varicosities associated with pregnancy occurring after a vein stripping are more likely due to inadequate removal of diseased veins at the original operation.

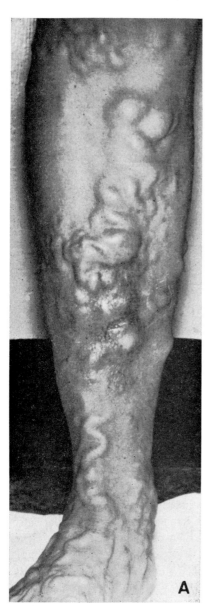

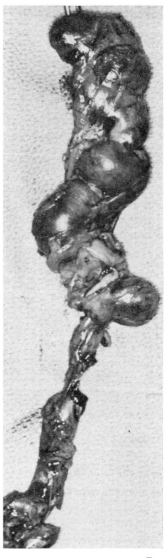

Fig. 11-6. (A) Varix that need not have been permitted to enlarge to this degree if earlier operation had been advised. (B) Operative specimen removed from patient shown in (A). (Courtesy of Harry C. Hull, M.D.)

A

B

Technique of Operation

Stripping and excision are the accepted standard treatment of varicose veins in this country. Other therapeutic alternatives are discussed in the following section.

The patient's varicosities are marked with a suitable semi-indelible solution preoperatively during a period of dependency. Carbolfuchsin or brilliant green in alcohol are excellent solutions for this. The currently available felt-tipped marking pens are usually not suitable since their ink is too often water soluble. Care should be taken to identify incompetent perforating veins if present and to mark major tributaries of the saphenous system to facilitate direct, separate removal at operation.

A transverse incision above and anterior to the medial malleolus is used to expose the greater saphenous vein and to dissect it free from the adjacent saphenous nerve. Some authors have recommended approaching the

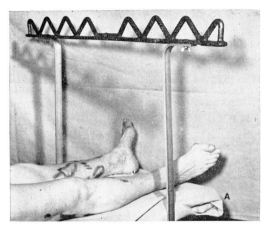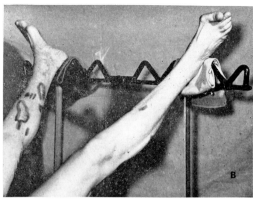

FIG. 11-7. (A) Slotted rack device for leg elevation in varicose vein surgery. The veins have been marked previously. (B) The legs are elevated before skin preparation and draping, and the entire operative procedure is carried out in this position. The lesser saphenous vein can be approached without turning the patient. (Dale, W. A.: Ligation, stripping and excision of varicose veins. Surgery, *67*:389, 1970)

saphenous vein from the dorsum of the foot, but this has not gained wide acceptance.

A flexible stripper of a wide variety of types, almost all of them satisfactory, is inserted and passed to the groin or to a point of obstruction usually due to extreme tortuosity. Care should be taken to palpate the stripper throughout its passage to insure that it does not enter the deep system through an abnormal communication. Failure to observe this step may result in trauma to the deep system or mistaken confusion between femoral and saphenous veins which has occasionally been reported by inexperienced operators.

If the stripper can be passed to the fossa ovalis a transverse groin incision is made to expose the saphenofemoral junction. Intervening incisions are made as required. The groin exposure is important since the commonest cause of "recurrent" varicosities is failure to adequately divide the superficial branches at the groin.[43] A reliable landmark to locate the fossa ovalis, and avoid placing the incision too low as is commonly done, is to center a 5 cm. incision two finger-breadths lateral and two finger-breadths below the pubic tubercle.

Considerable variation in the number of branches at the saphenofemoral junction exists as documented by Haeger in a study of 181 legs.[46] His investigation of 54 patients with recurrent varices showed evidence that recurrence could be attributed to poor anatomic dissection at the fossa ovalis.

All superficial venous tributaries joining the saphenous vein at the groin should be individually divided. The saphenous vein is divided so as to leave a flush surface at the femoral vein without a stump for thrombus formation in communication with the deep system.

Dale has recommended conducting the entire operative procedure with the legs elevated on a rack device which he has described in his discussion of technique.[47] If the patient is operated on supine, the legs should be elevated after the internal stripper is positioned prior to removal. Dale also suggests the use of tightly applied Ace bandages temporarily placed before removing the stripper and left on for a full ten minutes. These measures will largely eliminate significant subcutaneous hematoma formation.

In patients with a normal blood clotting mechanism, no significant bleeding should occur after stripping. Occasional major blood loss has been described when a mis-

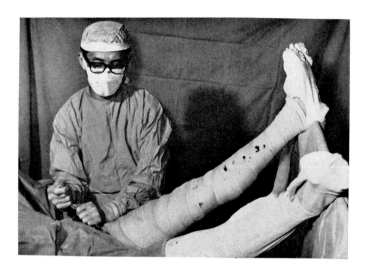

FIG. 11-8. The legs have been tightly wrapped prior to removal of the previously placed stripper to prevent hematoma. (Dale, W. A.: *op. cit.*)

diagnosis of varicose veins was applied to a leg with an arteriovenous fistula, but this complication should be avoidable. Schriabman has reported an investigation of the contribution of arteriovenous fistula to varicose vein formation in 62 patients studied by blood gas analysis and 12 patients studied by dye dilution methods. He concluded, as had John Gay in 1867, that there was no evidence to support the notion that such arteriovenous communication was involved in varicose veins at all.[48]

Liberal use of intervening incisions to effect direct excision of significant tributaries should be the rule. Incompetent perforating veins, which usually communicate with tributaries rather than the major saphenous veins directly, should be ligated subfascially to prevent recurrent varices.

The lesser saphenous vein may be approached laterally with the patient supine and the leg elevated while the surgeon sits. Alternatively, the patient may be turned prone. However, this carries the risks of accidental limb or nervous injury when turning the anesthetized patient along with other possibilities for complication such as airway compromise.

Exposure of the lesser saphenous vein is made behind the lateral malleolus taking care to avoid the sural nerve. The stripper passed from below in this vein must also be guided by careful palpation since the entrance of the lesser saphenous vein into the popliteal vein is quite variable.

Some authors have described a large and satisfactory experience with varicose vein stripping performed as an ambulatory procedure on out-patients.[49] In this day and age of increasing concern over rising costs of health care, it is interesting to note that Haeger estimates a saving of nearly three quarters of a million dollars in hospital costs in treating 4,462 patients on an ambulatory basis in Scandinavia.[50]

Complications of Vein Stripping

Recurrent varicose veins, wound infection and hemorrhage or hematoma formation are the most frequent complications. Less commonly seen are deep venous thrombosis, pulmonary embolism, nerve damage and bizarre injuries to adjacent vascular structures.

Recurrent varicose veins have been studied by Lofgren and Lofgren who have had occasion to investigate a large number of patients referred to their institution after previous treatment elsewhere.[43] In 43 of 121 patients they found that an inadequate dissection at the groin level had resulted in residual persistence of significant tributaries. Figure 11-9 summarized their findings in 488 operations for recurrent varicosities. It seems clear that recurrent varicosities are largely a preventable complication if sufficient exposure of the saphenofemoral junc-

FIG. 11-9. Findings in 488 operations for recurrent varicosities showing how inadequate groin dissection contributes to recurrent varicosities. (Lofgren, E. P., and Lofgren, K. A.: Recurrence of varicose veins after the stripping operation. Arch. Surg., *102*:111, 1971)

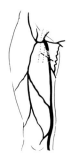 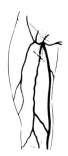 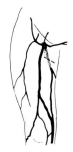 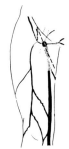

Ligation Too Low 48%   Persistent Greater Saphenous Vein 8%   Persistent Accessory Saphenous Vein 4%   Adequate Ligation Above 40%

tion is obtained, and care is taken to divide individually the groin branches near the fossa ovalis.

Extensive varicosities of the type shown in Figure 11-5 must be approached directly. They are often adherent to the dermis requiring undermining of flaps for removal. Failure to adequately excise prominent tributaries beyond the main channel will leave residual varicosities at any level of the leg.

Although simple ligation of varicose veins was practiced in the past, this treatment can only be considered inadequate today. Lofgren, Ribisi and Myers have evaluated the results of stripping versus ligation in 400 patients and found a 55 percent poor result immediately postoperatively in 200 patients treated by ligation.[51] Moreover, there was a 36 percent reoperative rate subsequently required in patients ligated, but no reoperation at all required in patients whose veins were removed by stripping.

Wound infection, bleeding and hematoma formation are related since groin wound infection is usually associated with the presence of a hematoma. Precautions recommended by Dale using elevation and temporary tight wrapping of the leg, as shown in Figure 11-7, will prevent significant bleeding in the calf and thigh. Direct hemostasis by ligatures in the groin wound should be complete. Since venous pressures in the saphenous vein stump may exceed systemic arterial pressures during vigorous straining such as coughing in the standing position, suture ligature of this vessel may be well advised.

The following case illustrates the significant morbidity which may follow infection developing after a saphenous vein stripping. A 56-year-old diabetic man entered the hospital for stripping of prominent varicose veins of the left leg. A more extensive procedure than usual was required to remove the varicosities, and lasted three and one half hours. On the second postoperative day he became febrile and soon thereafter demonstrated typical findings of extensive inflammation over the entire course of the excised greater saphenous system. Despite prompt antibiotic treatment, he required multiple drainage procedures of abscesses and two skin grafting procedures to accomplish eventual wound healing. His five-week hospitalization resulted in a hospital bill of $4,304.

Among the miscellaneous complications of vein stripping, deep venous thrombosis and pulmonary embolism are very uncommon. This may be due to the beneficial effects of leg elevation and elastic support usually practiced after stripping operations. Damage to the saphenous nerve or to the sural nerve can be aovided by careful dissection when inserting the stripper. Even so, transient hypesthesia in the distribution of the saphenous nerve, along the medial calf and over the medial malleolus may be observed. The anatomic distribution of the sural nerve is highly variable, usually lying alongside and medial to the lesser saphenous vein. Despite adequate precautions, transient numbness along the posterolateral leg may result from edema around the area of vein stripping.

In many communities accounts of inadvertent stripping or injury to the superficial femoral artery or vein can be heard. It is difficult to imagine how such misadventure can occur, and thorough knowledge of anatomy should be completely sufficient to prevent this tragedy. Reports of such injury are understandably rare, but Tera[52] has described one case of femoral vein injury with successful repair and summarized a world experience with 12 similar injuries.

Injection-Compression Treatment

Although there has been little enthusiasm for it in this country, injection-compression treatment of varicose veins has been popularized in England and Ireland where this practice was reintroduced a decade ago by Fegan.[53] The stimulus for use of this procedure in the British Isles may result from the prolonged waiting periods for elective hospitalization rather than from inherent benefits of the technique itself.

Hobbs compared conventional surgical stripping with injection-compression treatment in a random trial with comparably good results in both groups who had ordinary saphenous varicosities.[54] However, pa-

tient and doctor tolerance for the continuing and involved outpatient care may be limited in the United States. The patient usually must wear elastic stockings without removing them at all for four to five weeks, 10 injections are required on the average, but may be as high as 38, and an average of six office visits per patient were required. The complications of injection include skin necrosis from extravasated sclerosing solution, allergic and toxic reactions to the solution, and the risk of deep venous thrombosis.

Postphlebitic Syndrome
Diagnosis and Pathophysiology

The term "postphlebitic syndrome" implies the conditions commonly recognized as sequelae of previous thrombosis involving the deep venous system of the leg. Varying degrees of severity range from mild edema to chronic, circumferential leg ulcers which may even undergo malignant degeneration. Many patients with postphlebitic legs will describe an episode of acute leg swelling occurring years previously in association with pregnancy or an illness which forced recumbency. However, it is not uncommon for such a history to be lacking despite the fact

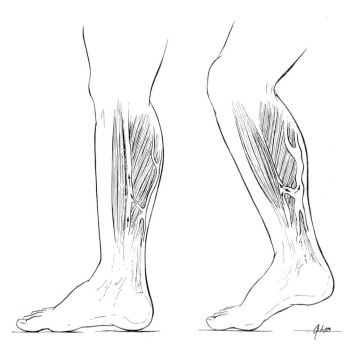

FIG. 11-10. As contraction of the calf muscles occurs with walking, high venous pressures are transmitted to superficial veins through incompetent perforating veins.

that deep venous thrombophlebitis occurred in the past. The consequences of abnormally high pressures resulting from deranged venous hemodynamics may take 5 to 15 years to develop. Thus the true causative events may be lost to recollection.

The most important feature of the postphlebitic syndrome is the destruction of venous valves by the process of recanalization. This results in excessively high venous pressure in the leg of the ambulatory patient. The valves of perforating veins which communicate with the superficial veins are rendered incompetent by dilatation due to this high pressure. Sometimes the valves of perforating veins are destroyed by the original thrombotic process. Thus the stage is set for persistently high venous pressure throughout the leg and even more important, for focal points of even higher pressure in the region of incompetent perforating veins. As illustrated in Figure 11-10, whenever the patient takes a step, contraction of the calf muscles adds to the high pressure transmitted by reversed flow through the incompetent perforating veins. This causes the so-called "stasis" changes most commonly seen along the medial lower leg where incompetent perforating veins transmit the highest pressures to the thinnest skin of the leg. Such pressures have been measured at levels in excess of 100 mm. Hg.[55]

Understanding of this process is essential before attempting treatment of patients suffering from postphlebitic syndrome. Unfortunately, the commonness of inadequate treatment for this condition indicates that many surgeons have failed to grasp the underlying physiologic changes and have undertaken measures which are not wholly logical or at best only incomplete. It is insufficient treatment, for example, to apply skin grafts alone to heal a postphlebitic ulcer without taking measures to control the underlying cause of the ulcer. Recurrence will almost always ensue unless the problem is attacked from its etiologic aspect.

While it is true that some venous ulcers of the leg are due to varicose veins and may properly be termed "varicose ulcers" it is also true that these are a distinct minority and should be distinguished from the far more common postphlebitic ulcer. Varicose ulcers always occur in association with advanced superficial varicose veins and overlie them, usually in the pretibial region. Postphlebitic ulcers occur along the medial or lateral aspects of the lower leg in the region of underlying incompetent perforators. They are often seen in patients without varicose superficial veins at all.

Conservative Treatment

In mild and moderately severe cases of postphlebitic syndrome, even including patients with small ulcers, nonoperative measures may suffice to permanently control the morbidity of the disease. These measures include:

1. Strict avoidance of passive dependency, even changing occupations if necessary to accomplish this.

2. Elevation of the legs whenever possible including the use of 30 cm. blocks under the foot of the bed.

3. Faithful use of properly fitted, adequately strong elastic stockings whenever ambulatory. (Jobst Stockings made by the Jobst Institute, Inc., Toledo, Ohio, are preferred by the author.)

4. Use of sponge rubber pressure pads beneath elastic stockings over areas of marked trophic change or ulceration.

5. Careful skin care and prompt treatment of fungal infection to which such patients are prone.

The commonest complication of conservative management is failure to control postphlebitic changes due to lack of effort on the part of the patient or the physician, usually both. This is a difficult condition to treat and requires a great deal of time and effort spent in educating the patient to understand his disease. Many doctors fail to pursue this beyond recommending "elastic stockings" without specifying adequate ones. The persistent morbidity due to half measures is avoidable. Perhaps the growing appearance of nurse practitioners and such allied health personnel will help reduce this incidence.

Another common probem in management of these patients is untoward reaction to various topical medications. A large variety of agents are applied to the skin of post-phlebitic legs and the fact is that practically none of them is helpful. The skin in the leg of these patients seems to be very sensitive and atopic reactions to local medication are common.

Operative Treatment

When varicose veins are present and complicating the postphlebitic syndrome, it may be helpful to remove them. However, care should be taken to insure that a patent deep venous system exists prior to stripping what may be the major venous channel. The majority of patients who develop deep ve-nous thrombosis will ultimately "recanalize" their occluded veins. This process may take a considerably longer time than is generally appreciated as suggested by Bergvall and Hjelmstedt.[56] They obtained serial phlebo-grams on 24 patients with deep venous thrombosis and indicated that the recanaliza-tion process takes many months or even years. Some occluded veins do not recover patency at all.

Some patients who have thrombosed their deep venous system and not recanalized will have a cramping sensation when they walk, so-called "venous claudication." They can be identified by placing several tourniquets on the thigh to occlude the superficial veins and asking the patient to walk. If three minutes of ambulation can be tolerated with-out significant pain, the deep venous system can be confidently assumed to be patent.

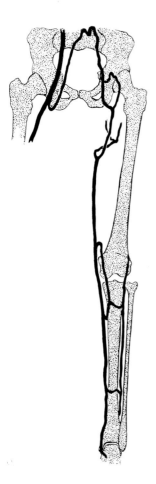

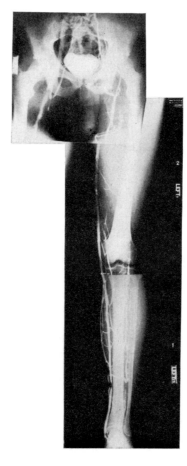

Fig. 11-11. Phlebogram obtained by injecting dye only into the left leg. The deep calf veins are filled, but empty into a dilated saphenous vein which drains into the right femoral vein by epigastric collaterals crossing at the umbilicus. The left femoral vein is chronically occluded.

The following case illustrates the importance of superficial veins in unrecanalized old deep venous occlusion. This 31-year-old dentist was referred for varicose vein stripping because he had some mild aching discomfort in his leg and prominent superficial veins. On examination, the greater saphenous vein was varicose and there were several large collaterals particularly along the posterior thigh. He gave a history of having had a swollen leg two years before after a skiing injury. Ambulation with a thigh tourniquet caused discomfort throughout the leg in 30 seconds. A phlebogram was obtained which is shown in Figure 11-11. Because of these findings indicating the importance of his superficial system, vein stripping was not advised. He improved with below-knee elastic stockings alone.

Simple removal of varicose veins will not improve the patient whose complaints are due to postphlebitic syndrome unless additional measures are taken. In addition to the conservative measures already mentioned, operative treatment includes:

1. Local subfascial excision of an ulcer-bearing area, including ligation of the perforating vein, and skin grafting.

2. Extensive subfascial ligation of the perforating veins throughout the lower leg using one of several techniques along with appropriate ulcer excision and grafting.

3. Radical excision of the skin, subcutaneous tissue and crural fascia over an extensive area of the leg with immediate skin grafting.

The choice of procedure depends on the necessity for radical versus more limited measures. The most radical operation, total excision of all diseased skin, subcutaneous tissue and fascia, following by immediate grafting was recommended over 50 years ago by Homans. Despite the excellent symptomatic results obtained by these somewhat heroic measures, the procedure has not been widely popular. It is an extensive undertaking and the cosmetic appearance of the leg when healed may cause concern. In terms of controlling the disease, the results are good. Andersen and McDonald reported good results in 85 percent of ulcers treated by this approach in a series of 33 patients.[57]

Complications of this procedure mentioned in their report were largely related to inadequate excision, particularly of the underlying fascia. In four patients with recurrent ulceration, reoperation with complete removal of the fascia was successful. In another patient with recurrent ulceration, more aggressive resection of disease skin and subcutaneous tissue at reoperation yielded a good result.

A less radical operation which directly approaches the cause of venous hypertension acting on the skin has been advocated by Linton.[58] In this operation, the perforating veins are ligated through a large subfascial flap incision without excising the overlying tissues. A medial approach is favored by many using an incision extending from the upper calf to below the medial malleolus. Others have preferred a posterior approach as reported by Lim, Blaisdell, et al.[59] and illustrated in Figure 11-12.

Some authors have recommended delaying this operation in the presence of open ulceration until the ulcers are healed because of concern over potential infection. Others have felt that operation may be safely conducted in the presence of a clearly granulating ulcer as soon as leg edema has been controlled.[60]

The most frequent complication of this procedure, whether carried out through a medial or posterior approach has been delayed wound healing from necrosis of skin edges. This appears to be far more frequent when the medial approach is used since 72 percent of the 51 patients reported by Field and Van Boxel had delayed wound healing from two weeks to over three months.[61] In contrast, only 10 percent of the 29 limbs treated through a posterior approach had delayed healing. This difference may reflect variations in patient selection or preoperative state, but theoretically a higher rate of wound complications might be expected in the medial approach which is made through

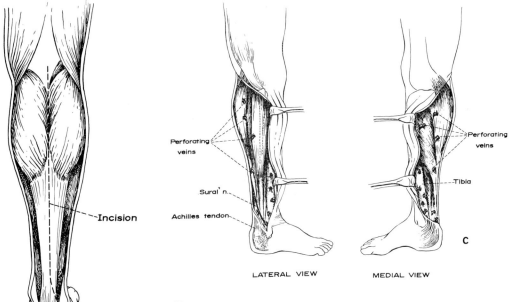

LATERAL VIEW MEDIAL VIEW

Fig. 11-12. Technique of radical subfascial division of communicating veins. (A) Location of posterior incision which curves away from achilles tendon distally. (B) The perforating veins are ligated and divided in the subfascial plane. The sural nerve is preserved. (C) Extent of medial and lateral subfascial plane. (D) Closure of fascia and skin by meticulous technique. (Lim, R. C., Jr., *et al.*: Subfascial ligation of perforating veins in recurrent stasis ulceration. Amer. J. Surg., *119*:246, 1970)

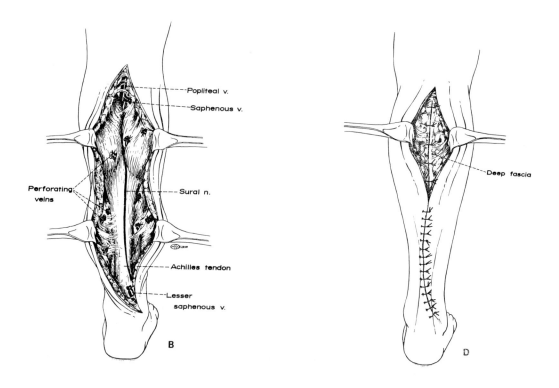

more abnormal skin and subcutaneous tissue than is the posterior approach.

All measures which will help reduce wound complications in these patients should be taken. The leg should be rendered as edema free as possible by use of bed rest, elevation, and diuretics when appropriate. Preoperative skin care should be enthusiastic. The most important measure is careful operative technique emphasizing three points: no dissection in the subcutaneous plane *above* the fascia, meticulous hemostasis, and gentle technique including use of skin hooks and no application of forceps to the skin. Postoperatively, continued bedrest with elevation for seven to ten days and posterior splint, plaster immobilization has been beneficial. These points have been emphasized in a comparative study of variations in technique and postoperative care in such patients by Haeger.[62]

If more limited, local excisions of an ulcer and subfascial ligation of its accompanying perforating vein are elected, precise localization of the incompetent perforating vein should be made. If there is extensive induration of the subcutaneous tissue or ectopic bone formation, this may be difficult. The combined use of clinical testing using the Trendelburg principle, infra-red photography and phlebography will correctly localize incompetent perforators in most cases.[63]

Autogenous Venous Grafts in the Venous System

Autogenous venous grafts have been sporadically employed for a variety of occlusive conditions of the venous system. Superior and inferior vena caval grafts have been reported with greater success in the superior vena cava. The postphlebitic syndrome has been similarly treated by several techniques including insertion of competent saphenous autografts into an incompetent deep system[64] and the use of crossover grafts to relieve persistent iliofemoral occlusion as reported by Dale.[65]

The complications of venous autografts are chiefly related to the high rate of post-operative thrombosis. Haimovici and his colleagues have reviewed the recent literature concerning both experimental and clinical grafts in the venous system and summarized the factors which influence patency.[66] Among those factors identified are: site of implantation and the associated external pressures, internal venous pressure and rate of blood flow, rigidity or motion of the graft and a critical period of time up to approximately two weeks after which thrombosis appears less likely.

Femoral Vein Ligation

Femoral vein ligation has been employed for prevention of pulmonary embolism in acute deep venous thrombosis and for treatment of late sequelae of postphlebitic syndrome. Recent reports have tended to cast doubt on the benefits of this procedure for either condition.

In prevention of pulmonary embolism, superficial femoral vein ligation has been the preferred site of ligation because common femoral vein ligation has led to distressing changes secondary to venous hypertension. This level of interruption leaves unprotected the 10 percent of patients whose superficial and deep veins are interconnected and an additional unknown number of patients whose pulmonary emboli arise primarily in the deep system. A recent report by Nabatoff, Blum and Touroff describes a 90 percent incidence of postphlebitic sequelae in 73 patients whose course after common femoral vein ligation was assessed from 6 months to 15 years later.[67] Forty-six percent had moderate to severe changes. If femoral level venous interruption is preferred for treatment of a patient whose poor general condition precludes vena cava interruption, it would seem prudent to use a partial interruption technique by suture plication of the common femoral vein.

Femoral vein or popliteal vein ligation was employed by Buxton and Coller and by others in an attempt to reduce venous hypertension in patients with chronic postphlebitic legs. Although some authors indicated improvement, the critical review of Straffon and Buxton which reported a series of 72 patients followed for an average of eight years postoperatively indicated that improvement was slight and more likely due to general measures than to the operative procedure.[68] At present this operation has been abandoned.

References

1. DeWeese, J. A., and Rogoff, S. M.: Phlebographic patterns of acute deep venous thrombosis of the leg. Surgery, *53*:99, 1963.
2. McLachlin, J., Richards, T., and Paterson, J. C.: An evaluation of clinical signs in the diagnosis of venous thrombosis. Arch. Surg., *85*:58, 1962.
3. Flotte, C. T., and Cox, E. F.: Dextran in treatment of thrombophlebitis. Trans. Southern Surg. Assoc., *74*:114, 1963.
4. Barner, H. B., and DeWeese, J. A.: An evaluation of the sphygmomanometer cuff pain test in venous thrombosis. Surgery, *48*:915, 1960.
5. DeWeese, J. A., and Rogoff, S. M.: Clinical uses of functional ascending phlebography of the lower extremity. Angiology, *9*:268, 1958.
6. ———: Functional ascending phlebography of the lower extremity of serial long film technique; evaluation of anatomic and functional detail in 62 extremities. Amer. J. Roentgen., *81*:841, 1959.
7. Spar, I. L., Varon, M. I., Goodland, R. L., and Schwartz, S. I.: Isotopic detection of thrombi. Arch. Surg., *92*:752, 1966.
8. Hobb, J. T., and Davies, J. W. L.: Detection of venous thrombosis with ^{131}I-labelled fibrinogen in the rabbit. Lancet, *2*:134, 1960.
9. Kakkar, V. V.: The problems of thrombosis in the deep veins of the leg. Ann. Roy. Coll. Surg. Eng., *45*:257, 1969.
10. ———: The diagnosis of deep vein thrombosis using the ^{125}I fibrinogen test. Arch. Surg., *104*:152, 1972.
11. Browse, N. L.: The ^{125}I fibrinogen uptake test. Arch Surg., *104*:160, 1972.
12. Sigel, B., Felix, R., Jr., Popky, G. L., and Ipsen, J.: Diagnosis of lower limb venous thrombosis by Doppler ultrasound technique. Arch. Surg., *104*:174, 1972.
13. Wheeler, H. B., Millick, S. C., Anderson, J. N., and Pearson, D.: Diagnosis of occult deep vein thrombosis by a noninvasive bedside technique. Surgery, *70*:20, 1971.
14. Wheeler, H. B., Pearson, D., O'Connell, D., and Millick, S. C.: Impedance phlebography. Arch. Surg., *104*:164, 1972.
15. Larson, R. E., and Doan, R. E.: Retroperitoneal fibrosis—Presenting as acute iliofemoral thrombophlebitis. Minn. Med., *53*: 251, 1970.
16. Simeone, F. A., and Husni, E. A.: The hyperemia of reconstructive arterial surgery. Ann. Surg., *150*:575, 1959.
17. Vaughan, B. F., Slavotinek, A. H., and Jepson, R. P.: Edema of the lower limb after vascular operations. Surg. Gynec. Obst., *131*:282, 1970.
18. Macon, W. L., Morton, J. H., and Adams, J. I.: Significant complications of anticoagulant therapy. Surgery, *68*:571, 1970.
19. Hodin, E., and Dass, T.: Spontaneous retroperitoneal hemorrhage complicating anticoagulant therapy. Ann. Surg., *170*: 848, 1969.
20. Cox, E. F., Flotte, C. T., and Buxton, R. W.: Dextran in the treatment of thrombophlebitis. Surgery, *57*:225, 1965.
21. Schwartz, S. I., Shay, H. P., Beebe, H. G., and Rob, C.: Effect of low molecular weight dextran on venous flow. Surgery, *55*:106, 1964.
22. Kakkar, V., Flanc, C., Howe, C. T., O'Shea, M., and Flute, P. T.: Treatment of deep vein thrombosis: A trial of heparin, streptokinase and Arvin. Brit. Med. J., *1*:806, 1969.
23. Robertson, B. R., Nilsson, I. J., and Nylander, G.: Value of streptokinase and heparin in treatment of acute deep venous thrombosis—A coded investigation. Acta Chir. Scand., *134*:203, 1968.
24. Mavor, G. E.: Surgical management. Brit. Med. J., *4*:680, 1969.
25. Flanc, C., Kakkar, V., and Clarke, M. B.: Postoperative deep vein thrombosis: Effect of intensive prophylaxis. Lancet, *1*:477, 1969.
26. Tsapogas, M. J., Goussous, H., Peabody, R. A., Karmody, A. M., and Eckert, C.: Postoperative venous thrombosis and the effectiveness of prophylactic measures. Arch. Surg., *103*:561, 1971.
27. Brisman, R., Parks, L. C., and Haller, J. A.: Dextran prophylaxis in surgery. Ann. Surg., *174*:137, 1971.
28. Galloway, J. M. D., Karmody, A. M., and Mavor, G. E.: Thrombophlebitis of the long saphenous vein complicated by pulmonary embolism. Brit. J. Surg., *56*:360, 1969.
29. Mahorner, H., Castleberry, J. W., and Coleman, W. O.: Attempts to restore func-

tion in major veins which are the site of massive thrombosis. Ann. Surg., *146*:510, 1957.

30. DeWeese, J. A., Jones, T. I., Lyon, J., and Dale, W. A.: Evaluation of thrombectomy in the management of iliofemoral venous thrombosis. Surgery, *47*:140, 1960.

31. Haller, J. A., Jr., and Abrams, B. L.: Use of thrombectomy in the treatment of acute iliofemoral venous thrombosis in forty-five patients. Ann. Surg., *158*:249, 1963.

32. Lansing, A. M., and Davis, W. M.: Five-year follow-up study of iliofemoral venous thrombectomy. Ann. Surg., *168*:620, 1968.

33. Edwards, W. H., Sawyers, J. L., and Foster, J. H.: Iliofemoral venous thrombosis: Reappraisal of thrombectomy. Ann. Surg., *171*:961, 1970.

34. Baner, G.: Roentgenological and clinical study of the sequels of thrombosis. Acta Chir. Scand., *86*: Suppl. 74, 1942.

35. Haimovici, H.: Ischemic Forms of Venous Thrombosis. Springfield, Thomas, 1971.

36. Wilson, H., and Britt, L. G.: Surgical treatment of iliofemoral thrombosis. Ann. Surg., *165*:855, 1967.

37. Fogarty, T. J., Dennis, D., and Krippaehne, W. W.: Surgical management of iliofemoral venous thrombosis. Amer. J. Surg., *112*: 211, 1966.

38. Fogarty, T. J.: Personal communication, 1972.

39. Reeves, C. D., Madison, J., and Longerbeam, J. K.: Use of operative venography during iliofemoral venous thrombectomy. Amer. Surg., *34*:114, 1968.

40. Bales, C., and DeWeese, J. A.: Iliac vein stenosis: A case report and review of literature. Vasc. Diseases, *3*:373, 1966.

41. Hume, M., Levitt, S., and Thomas, D. P.: *In* Venous Thrombosis and Pulmonary Embolism, p. 416, Cambridge, Harvard Univ. Press, 1970.

42. Smith, G. W.: Iliofemoral venous thrombectomy. Circulation, *37*:847, 1968.

43. Lofgren, E. P., and Lofgren, K. A.: Recurrence of varicose veins after the stripping operation. Arch. Surg., *102*:111, 1971.

44. Fanfera, F. J., and Palmer, L. H.: Pregnancy and varicose veins. Arch. Surg., *96*: 33, 1968.

45. Haeger, K.: The treatment of varicose veins in pregnancy by radical operation or conservatively. Acta Obst. et Gynec. Scandinav., *47*:233, 1968.

46. ————: The surgical anatomy of the saphenofemoral and the saphenopopliteal junctions. J. Cardiov. Surg., *3*:420, 1962.

47. Dale, W. A.: Ligation, stripping and excision of varicose veins. Surgery, *67*:389, 1970.

48. Schraibman, I. G.: Blood oxygen saturation and dye dilution studies in the investigation of the aetiology of varicose veins. Aust. New Zeal. J. Surg., *36*:136, 1966.

49. Carleson, R., and Gotham, B.: Results of stripping in about 2500 ambulatory patients. Acta Chir. Scand., *125*:423, 1963.

50. Haeger, K.: Complications after outpatient surgery for varicose veins and perforator incompetence. Vasc. Surg., *4*:238, 1970.

51. Lofgren, K. A., Ribisi, A. P., and Myers, T. T.: An evaluation of stripping versus ligation for varicose veins. Arch. Surg., *76*: 310, 1958.

52. Tera, H.: Emergency repair of femoral vein accidentally divided at operation for varicose veins. Acta Chir. Scand., *133*:283, 1967.

53. Fegan, W. G.: Continuous compression technique of injecting varicose veins. Lancet, *2*:109, 1963.

54. Hobbs, J. T.: The treatment of varicose veins: A random trial of injection-compression therapy versus surgery. Brit. J. Surg., *55*:777, 1968.

55. Arnoldi, C. C.: Venous pressure in patients with valvular incompetence of the veins of the lower limb. Acta Chir. Scand., *132*: 628, 1966.

56. Bergvall, U., and Hjelmstedt, A.: Recanalisation of deep venous thrombosis of the lower leg and thigh. Acta Chir. Scand., *134*:219, 1968.

57. Andersen, M. N., and McDonald, K. E.: Results of surgical therapy of severe stasis ulceration of the legs. Ann. Surg., *157*:281, 1963.

58. Linton, R. R.: The communicating veins of the lower leg and the operative technique for their ligation. Ann. Surg., *107*:582, 1938.

59. Lim, R. C., Blaisdell, F. W., Zubrin, J., Stallone, R. J., and Hall, A. D.: Subfascial ligation of perforating veins in recurrent stasis ulceration. Amer. J. Surg., *119*:246, 1970.

60. Harjola, P., Tala, P., Ketonen, P., and Tolvanen, E.: Surgical treatment of incompetent perforating veins of the lower limb. Ann. Chir. et Gyn. Fenn., *57*:213, 1968.

61. Field, P., and Van Boxel, P.: The role of the Linton flap procedure in the management of stasis dermatitis and ulceration in the lower limb. Surgery, *70*:920, 1971.

62. Haeger, K.: Variations in operative technique, wound dressing and postoperative care in subfascial ligation of incompetent ankle perforator veins. Acta Chir. Scand., *133*:277, 1967.

63. Beesley, W. H., and Fegan, W. G.: An investigation into the localization of incompetent perforating veins. Brit. J. Surg., *57*: 31, 1970.

64. Husni, E. A.: In situ saphenopopliteal by-pass graft for incompetence of the femoral and popliteal veins. Surg. Gynec. Obstet., *130*:279, 1970.

65. Dale, W. A., and Harris, J.: Crossover vein grafts for iliac and femoral venous occlusion. Ann. Surg., *168*:139, 1968.

66. Haimovici, H., Hoffert, P. W., Zinicola, N., and Steinman, C.: An experimental and clinical evaluation of grafts in the venous system. Surg. Gynec. Obst., *131*:1173, 1970.

67. Nabatoff, R. A., Blum, L., and Touroff, A. S. W.: Long-term sequelae of common femoral vein ligation in the treatment of thromboembolic disease. Surgery, *67*:272, 1970.

68. Straffon, R. A., and Buxton, R. W.: Deep vein ligation in the postphlebitic extremity. Surgery, *41*:471, 1957.

69. Coon, W. W., and Willis, P. W.: Thrombosis of the deep veins of the arm. Surgery, *64*:990, 1968.

70. Adams, J. T., and McEvoy, R. K.: Primary deep venous thrombosis of upper extremity. Arch. Surg., *91*:29, 1965.

71. Adams, J. T., DeWeese, J. A., Mahoney, E. B., and Rob, C. G.: Intermittent subclavian vein obstruction without thrombosis. Surgery, *63*:147, 1968.

Chapter **12** | *Management of*

William H. Moretz, M.D.
Charles H. Wray, M.D.

Pulmonary Embolism and Complications of Vena Cava Interruption Procedures

Pulmonary embolism is a common, very serious complication of vascular surgery and occupies a unique position. Not only is it a complication which may follow vascular procedures, but the surgical procedure most often used in treating this condition, interruption of the inferior vena cava, not infrequently exposes the patient to additional complications. This chapter is in two parts; the first deals with pulmonary embolism, the second specifically with complications of inferior vena cava interruption.

Management of Pulmonary Embolism

Pathogenesis

Present day understanding of pulmonary embolism is attributed to Virchow[1] who, in 1846, clarified the relationship between thrombus in pulmonary arteries and thrombosis of peripheral veins. He recognized that pulmonary artery thrombi originated elsewhere, became dislodged and were carried as emboli through intervening veins and the right ventricle to come to rest in appropriate-sized pulmonary arteries. Virchow's triad of venous stasis, vein wall injury and hypercoagulability of the blood are still generally accepted as the factors responsible for the formation of thrombus within veins, and efforts to prevent thrombosis are based upon these concepts.

Hypercoagulability is known to be associated with trauma, including surgery and childbirth, certain blood dyscrasias such as polycythemia, severe dehydration and advanced malignancy. Increased platelet adhesiveness has been demonstrated by many observers in patients with thrombophlebitis, but the causative significance of this finding remains obscure.[2]

Venous stasis, or a condition of low blood flow, occurs in many situations. Slowing of arterial flow through extremities, as with occlusive arterial disease, reduces the rate of flow through veins. Conditions which increase venous pressures decrease the velocity of flow by making the normally flattened venous channels more cylindrical. Also, veins which are abnormally dilated by previous disease, such as varicosities, result in local venous stasis. Thrombosis is encouraged by strict bed rest, dependent position of the legs, relative immobility due to casts or postoperative pain, general debilitation, dehydration, shock, abdominal distention and congestive heart failure.

Abnormal vein walls result from previous thrombosis and phlebitis, varicosities, local trauma such as adjacent surgery or intravenous injections and adjacent inflammatory processes such as an abscess in the pelvis or an infected wound.

It is probable that thrombi begin at selective foci such as an area of relative stasis behind a valve cusp, a spot of roughened intima, or a dilated area associated with stasis, turbulent flow or eddy currents. Platelets may aggregate to form a nidus for thrombosis which is then built up by successive layers of platelets and fibrin incorporating red cells and leukocytes.

Most thrombi originate in the lower extremities, probably in the veins of the soleus muscle of the calf. The specific veins involved in a series of injured and burned patients coming to autopsy were: intramuscular calf (48 percent), post-tibial (39 percent), common femoral (27 percent), popliteal (20 percent), superficial femoral (20 percent), external iliac (17 percent) and common iliac (8 percent).[3] The larger veins were affected more often in patients with longer periods of bed rest prior to death, suggesting that many thrombi begin in small veins and progress into larger ones. Thrombi probably originate in multiple areas simultaneously. They propagate proximally and may be attached primarily only distally, thus subject to breaking off and becoming emboli.

Incidence

Pulmonary embolism has been described as the most frequent acute pulmonary illness seen in general hospitals, as one of the most common lethal processes seen at necropsy, and the third most common nonlethal lung affliction, pneumonia and emphysema being more frequent. The true incidence of pulmonary embolism, and of its predecessor, deep venous thrombosis, is most difficult to ascertain. The routine type of autopsy sheds no significant light on the frequency of venous thrombosis in the extremities but does reflect the incidence of major pulmonary embolism.

The overall incidence of thrombophlebitis reported following operative procedures varies between 0.5 percent and 0.9 percent. The incidence increases to 5 or 6 percent when only major surgery is considered. From the Phlebitis Registry at Boston City Hospital, Byrne[4] reported an incidence of phlebitis of 0.79 percent, or 167 cases in

20,938 operations. Predisposing conditions, in order of decreasing importance were: cardiac disease, postoperative state, trauma, idiopathic, infection, pregnancy and hemiplegia.

Further discussion of the diagnosis and management of deep venous thrombophlebitis is contained in Chapter 11.

Operations involving laparotomy, the kidneys, bladder and prostate or the femoral neck are more likely to be followed by phlebitis and embolism than are lesser and more superficial procedures. In a report by Lassen, with no specific program of prophylaxis in effect, death due to embolism occurred in 0.8 percent following laparotomy, 0.56 percent following operations on the kidney, bladder and prostate, and 3.1 percent following operations on the femoral neck.[5]

Estimates of the incidence of pulmonary embolism based upon clinical criteria are undoubtedly low, as illustrated by the frequency with which unsuspected emboli are found at necropsy. A recent, carefully studied series of 61 consecutive adult autopsies, revealed old or recent thromboemboli in 64 percent of cases.[6] The reported incidence of fatal embolism varies widely, usually ranging from one fatal embolus for each 150 medical, surgical and obstetric cases to one in 3,000 such cases. DeBakey, in reviewing reports totaling over three million surgical patients found a mean incidence of 0.14 percent postoperative fatal emboli (range 0.01 to 0.87 percent).[7] At autopsy, however, he found the range of fatal embolism to vary from 0.21 percent to 23.1 percent with a mean of 2.8 percent. Most prospective studies show an overall incidence of 13 to 25 percent. The frequency of pulmonary embolism found at autopsy varies tremendously with type of hospital, type of patient in the hospital and how long the patient had been immobile prior to death.

There probably has been a real increase both in deep venous thrombosis and in pulmonary embolism in recent years. Among the related factors accounting for this are: increase in major surgery in older and poorer risk patients; increase in survival of severely ill patients following surgery; prolongation of life in the severely ill with respirators, drugs and blood; and institution of therapy for formerly fatal conditions allowing longer survival and development of venous thrombosis.

Diagnosis and Misdiagnosis

A clear and concise account of the typical clinical picture seen with a pulmonary embolus would be helpful to the clinician. However, the symptoms and signs of a pulmonary embolus are widely variable depending on the number and size of emboli, the location of the pulmonary artery blocked, the physiologic status of the lungs and heart and the general status of the patient. There are four main groups of major pulmonary embolism: massive emboli, major emboli in lobar vessels, multiple small emboli and multiple microemboli. Small and microemboli are usually insidious in onset and may be manifest primarily as pulmonary hypertension with symptoms of fatigue and dyspnea, while large and massive emboli give rise to the more commonly recognized signs and symptoms of pulmonary embolism. A major embolus has been defined by Crane and his associates[8] as one with two or more of the following four features: hypotension, hypoxemia by blood gas assay or clinical cyanosis, main stem or first subdivision filling defects on pulmonary angiogram, and a mean pulmonary artery pressure of 25 mm. of mercury or more.

The clinical, radiologic and electrocardiographic features of pulmonary embolism may imitate and are most commonly confused with those of pleurisy, pneumonia and coronary occlusion. Postoperative atelectasis, pulmonary neoplasm, angina pectoris, asthma, uremia, and hyperventilation syndrome also simulate, and may be simulated by pulmonary embolism. Most emboli produce pulmonary hypertension which may be transient with small emboli, but more persistent with large ones. As the embolus blocks a segment of the pulmonary artery, vasospasm and bronchospasm may be reflexly or chemically induced. Recent evidence has tended to implicate vasoactive amines re-

leased from the embolus, or perhaps from a platelet coat residing on it, as being causative in producing local constrictive changes of pulmonary embolism by use of serotonin[9,10,11] and experimental studies showing marked survival improvement in platelet-deficient animals with pulmonary emboli.[12] This results in ventilation-perfusion imbalance in the affected lungs which accounts for many of the clinical symptoms of pulmonary embolism. Inadequate perfusion of lung situated peripheral to the block may lead to atelectasis and to impaired gas exchange. The dual blood supply of the lung protects against infarction.

The clinical feature most commonly associated with pulmonary embolism is dyspnea when unassociated with other signs or symptoms should suggest embolism. Hypotension is common, and with a large embolus blocking more than 50 percent of the pulmonary arterial tree, shock is usual. Chest pain is frequently characterized by a vague substernal discomfort which may closely mimic that of a coronary occlusion. A feeling of marked apprehension or of impending doom is common and a dry nonproductive cough is a frequent early symptom. Pleuritic pain is delayed over 24 hours and coincides with the onset of pulmonary infarction or reactive pleuritis. Hemoptysis, also a later sign, is present in less than half of cases, but cyanosis is frequent.[13] There may be splinting of the chest, fine rales and wheezing. Tachycardia is common, as is accentuation of the second pulmonic sound which may also develop a bell-like quality. Increased cervical venous pressure may be noted reflecting increased right ventricular end diastolic pressures.

Less than half of patients with pulmonary emboli show evidence of phlebitis of the lower extremities. The occurrence of Homans' sign, calf tenderness, mild swelling of an extremity or the less frequently observed evidences of massive venous thrombosis lends support to an otherwise questionable diagnosis of pulmonary embolism.

The diagnosis of pulmonary embolism is often difficult in patients who have recently

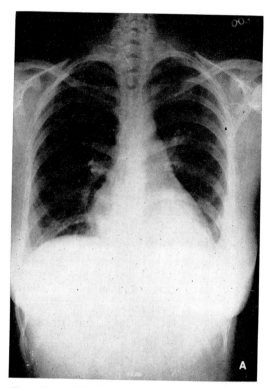
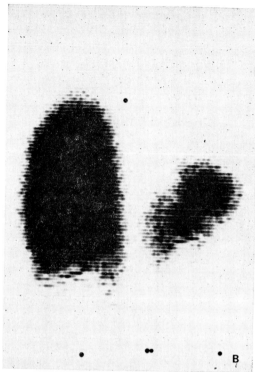

FIG. 12-1. (A) Relatively clear upper lung field on the right side in a 30-year-old woman with right chest pain of two weeks' duration. (B) Postero-anterior lung scan taken the same day showing absence of uptake in the right upper lung field and right base. (Moretz, W. H.: Pulmonary embolism. Hosp. Med., 7:128, 1971)

undergone vascular surgery, because of the effects of operation or coincident disease. The diagnosis must be entertained in any patient developing any of the above signs or symptoms for which there is no other ready explanation. The condition is more often under-diagnosed than over-diagnosed, but errors are common in both directions. When pulmonary embolism is suspected, careful examination, arterial blood gases, chest x-ray and electrocardiogram are indicated.

In normal, young patients the arterial Po_2 should be 100 mm. Hg. An arterial Po_2 below 80 mm. Hg should suggest the diagnosis of pulmonary embolism. The normal arterial Po_2 decreases gradually with age and may be 70 mm. Hg in the elderly. Patients with chronic obstructive pulmonary disease may have chronically low arterial Po_2 values. A drop from previous values with appropriate clinical signs should suggest pulmonary embolism.

A normal chest x-ray, in the face of arterial oxygen unsaturation is very suggestive of pulmonary embolism. Demonstrated enlargement of the pulmonary artery is almost diagnostic. The classical "wedge-shaped" peripheral density appears coincident with infarction in 24-48 hours. If the initial chest film shows atelectasis, pneumonic infiltration or pneumothorax, pulmonary embolism may be tentatively excluded.

Tachycardia, right ventricular overload patterns and atrial arrhythmias characterize the electrocardiographic changes of pulmonary embolism. A normal electrocardiogram does not exclude the diagnosis. Positive changes of myocardial infarction are helpful in differentiation from embolism. Probably less than 2 percent of patients with pulmonary embolism will have typical electrocardiographic changes.

Sequential recording of physical examination, blood gases, chest x-rays and ECG's are more helpful than single studies to establish an accurate diagnosis.

Special Studies

Various special studies are often required to establish the diagnosis. Most helpful is the lung scan. Injected macroaggregated human serum albumin tagged with ^{131}I is blocked by the embolus and cannot reach the area of hypoperfused lung. However, similar areas of poor perfusion may be seen with pneumonic consolidation, atelectasis, neoplasm, or pleural fluid or bullous cysts. A normal chest film with a positive scan is characteristic of pulmonary embolism. The lung scan is a sensitive detector of small peripheral lesions. This is particularly true of the gamma

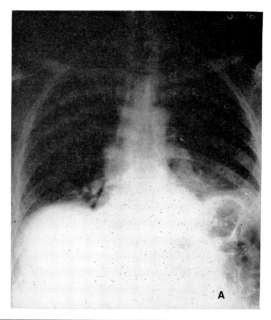

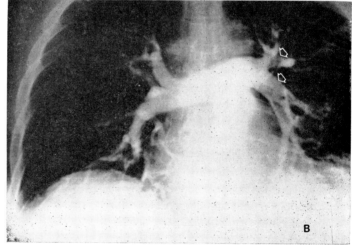

Fig. 12-2. (A) Chest film shows evidence of atelectasis in right base and density in left lower lobe. (B) Arteriogram established diagnosis of pulmonary embolism, showing filling defects in pulmonary arteries feeding left lower and upper lobes. (Moretz, W. H., *op. cit.*)

camera scan. Repeated scans help further both in diagnosis and in following the resolution of known emboli.

The relatively recent development of the gamma camera technique for pulmonary scanning has been helpful in another important way. The time required for obtaining the test is very much reduced by the newer techniques. Thus patients who have sustained a pulmonary embolus are away from the nursing area a briefer period of time.

The pulmonary arteriogram is the most reliable means of diagnosing emboli in major channels of the pulmonary arteries and to establish the diagnosis prior to pulmonary embolectomy. Prior to injection of radiopaque material, the pulmonary artery pressure should be determined. Since these patients may be critically ill, hypotensive and hypoxic, injection should not be made if the pressure is extremely high. Experienced personnel are required to perform this procedure. The procedure is less time consuming than rectilinear scanning, but more time consuming and more dangerous than gamma camera studies.

Not all patients thought to have pulmonary embolism need pulmonary arteriography. In general, patients who are considered for pulmonary embolectomy should always have a pulmonary arteriogram. In addition, for patients in whom the risk of other forms of treatment for embolism, such as anticoagulation or vena cava interruption, would be very high, and the diagnosis is unclear after simpler measures, pulmonary arteriography may be indicated.

The lung scan and pulmonary arteriogram are complementary studies. The scan is safe and capable of diagnosing major or smaller peripheral emboli. The arteriogram is more definitive and is necessary in selecting patients for embolectomy procedures.

Pulmonary arteriography may eventually be replaced by the development of dynamic imaging with radioisotopes and the gamma camera. With this technique radioisotopes are followed during intravenous injection through the vena cava, the right side of the heart, the arterial and venous circulation of the lung, the left side of the heart and out the aorta. The definition of pulmonary arterial flow may be satisfactory enough to clearly identify major obstructions.

Diagnostic measures which establish the existence of deep venous thrombosis in patients being evaluated for pulmonary embolism are strongly supportive of the diagnosis. These tests include phlebography, radioactive leg scanning, Doppler flow measurement and impedance phlebography. These and other diagnostic features of deep venous thrombosis are discussed in Chapter 11.

Wacker, *et al.*[14] reported that there was an increased LDH (serum lactic acid dehydrogenase) with normal SGOT (serum glutamic oxaloacetic transaminase) in patients with pulmonary infarctions. Others, who subsequently studied the relationship of LDH, SGOT, and serum bilirubin in patients with pulmonary infarction found much less specific differences. Coodly[15] found that CPK (creatine phosphokinase) was rarely, if ever, elevated in patients with pulmonary infarction. An elevated LDH, without elevations of its HBD component (hydroxybityrate dehydrogenase—a measure of the cardiac

isoenzymes of LDH) is strong evidence against myocardial necrosis. LDH is also elevated in pneumonia, carcinoma, renal and liver disease, anemia and leukemia, and is not of great value in diagnosis of pulmonary infarction. Enzyme determinations in the differential diagnosis of pulmonary embolism are of relatively little value at present.

The recent development of the ventilatory lung scan appears very promising. The conventional lung scan using radioactive macro-aggregated particles assesses the regional pulmonary blood flow or perfusion. The ventilation lung scan, using radioactive xenon, gives information regarding ventilation of that portion of lung. After deep inspiration of ^{133}Xe (5 milli-curies per liter) in air and a 5 to 15 second period of breath holding, images with 100,000 counts are obtained. Obstructive airway disease causes abnormalities in pattern.[16] The combined use of radioactive xenon together with conventional lung scanning aids in the differential diagnosis of pulmonary embolism. The conventional scan delineates the size, shape and positions of perfusion abnormalities while the xenon scan shows whether those areas are associated with abnormal ventilation. Normally ventilated lung associated with a perfusion defect suggests pulmonary embolism.

Studies have also been done obtaining scintiphotographs after the intravenous injection of ^{133}Xe with promising results. Scintiphotographs made during breath holding after injection of ^{133}Xe depict perfusion while those made during clearance of the radioactive xenon by breathing represent regional ventilation.[17]

Treatment of Pulmonary Embolism
Anticoagulants

The preferred treatment of pulmonary embolism, as for venous thrombosis, is prompt anticoagulation with heparin. While oral anticoagulants, dextran and other agents have some preventive effect on thrombosis, heparin is specifically favored for treating the patient who has just had a pulmonary embolus. When given intravenously, it is effective immediately in preventing thrombosis and may have important antihumoral effects as well.

Heparin, by preventing the activation of Factor IX (Christmas factor), of Factor XI (plasma thromboplastic antecedent) and by being a potent antithrombin, stops coagulation of blood. It also has an anti-inflammatory action which may be helpful in relieving symptoms in the extremities and possibly also in the lungs. Heparin may be partially inactivated in the liver or bound by tissue proteins and only 30 to 40 percent is excreted by the kidney.

Observation of bronchoconstriction accompanying pulmonary embolism has been made in both experimental studies and in man. The improvement in this bronchoconstriction which accompanies heparin administration is thought to be due primarily to the interference with serotonin release from platelets in and coating the surface of acute pulmonary emboli.[18]

Heparin is relatively contraindicated in patients with thrombocytopenia, except when resulting from disseminated intravascular coagulation. It must also be used with caution when glomerular filtration is impaired. The primary contraindication to heparin, however, is the presence of an open lesion which is likely to bleed, such as recently bleeding peptic ulcer or a recent surgical procedure, particularly procedures involving the central nervous system, prostate gland or extensive retroperitoneal dissection. The danger of excessive bleeding is great when emergency surgery is required in the early postembolism period, as for example, when caval interruption is required because of recurrent embolism. In such instances full heparin dosage is contraindicated for at least 24 and preferably 48 hours following operation, and may be contraindicated altogether.

Heparin has been administered intramuscularly, subcutaneously and intravenously. There is some danger of local bleeding at the injection site when given intramus-

cularly or subcutaneously, and hematoma formation associated with intramuscular administration represents a contraindication to the use of that route. More importantly absorption of heparin from these sites is relatively unpredictable making strict control more difficult. Neutralization is also less precise because heparin is sequestered from circulating protamine. If the patient requires intravenous fluids because of his general condition, the desired amount of heparin can be injected every four to six hours, using the existing infusion. However, when only heparin is needed intravenously, repeated venipunctures may be avoided by inserting a pediatric scalp-vein infusion set with a winged, 21 gauge needle, and plastic tubing sealed by a rubber cap. This is left in the vein without a continuous infusion, and heparin is injected through it at intervals. A continuous infusion of heparin may be given with a suitable infusion pump if low volumes of fluid and very accurate administration is required.

A Lee-White clotting time should be performed prior to institution of therapy. When the initial dose is given, a clotting time should be done after one or two hours to determine that the patient is anticoagulated by that dose. If heparin resistance is discovered by this method, then the dose should be increased until satisfactory anticoagulation has occurred. The clotting time should remain prolonged to approximately twice normal at the time of the next dosage in four to six hours. After the dose has been stabilized, daily clotting times are adequate to provide guidance.

The dosage of heparin is higher in the initial treatment of pulmonary embolism than in the treatment of peripheral vein thrombosis. There is a growing body of evidence suggested by such studies as those of Crane and his colleagues[8] that the dosage of heparin needed to treat pulmonary embolism adequately is far greater than that usually employed in management of uncomplicated deep venous thrombosis. Intravenous injections of 15,000 units to 20,000 units every four to six hours to achieve a 24 hour total dosage of 80,000 to 100,000 units, resulted in sufficient improvement in their patients with major pulmonary emboli that the indication for embolectomy became restricted to continuing refractory systemic hypotension.

The employment of vigorous, aggressive heparin anticoagulation in pulmonary embolism may result in greater patient improvement because the higher dose levels exert a greater antihumoral effect.[19,20] The effectiveness of antihumoral measures in pulmonary embolism is a currently active field at present, and may be expected to add to future therapy.

Occasionally, heparin resistance is seen and larger dosages are required, up to 20,000 or even 30,000 units every four hours to prolong the clotting time to more than two and one-half times normal. Initially higher dosages are indicated to make certain that secondary thrombosis in lung vessels does not occur.

It is preferable to continue heparin at least seven to ten days to allow thrombi remaining peripherally to become adherent to the vein wall and to encourage thrombolysis. If the patient is immobile, if sepsis continues or if intercurrent episodes of thrombophlebitis occur, longer periods of treatment are indicated. Prolonged therapy is indicated not only to prevent further embolization, but also to minimize future residual postphlebitic difficulties.

The warfarin anticoagulants are very useful for long-term therapy: of which the most commonly used is Coumadin (warfarin sodium). Unlike heparin, which has a direct and immediate effect on blood, the mode of action of warfarin is to affect the liver and is thus delayed. The warfarin drugs inhibit liver production of four clotting Factors, VII, IX, X and II (including prothrombin itself), which are involved in changing prothrombin to thrombin. They may also interfere in some manner with platelet function. The effect of these anticoagulants is antagonized by administering vitamin K, especially the water-soluble vitamin K_1.

The amount of vitamin K synthesized in the bowel by bacterial action, which in turn is influenced by oral antibiotics, may affect the dose of warfarin anticoagulants required. Warfarin drugs may be a part of the initial anticoagulant therapy, but most physicians prefer to start them just three to five days before discontinuing heparin to assure a continuous anticoagulant effect. A base line prothrombin time should be obtained. Initial doses for loading vary with the patient's age, weight, sex and general condition and require intelligent estimation by the physician, aided by previous experience. In the case of Coumadin (warfarin sodium) the usual oral loading dose for the first day is 15 to 30 mg. and for the second day 10 to 20 mg., the maintenance dose of 5 to 10 mg. being started on the third day. In the case of Phenindione, the oral loading dose is 100 to 250 mg. the first day and 50 to 150 mg. the second day, the maintenance dose being 50 to 100 mg. Both of these drugs are intermediate acting, requiring one and one-half to two days to become effective. Prothrombin times should be obtained daily initially and then at appropriate intervals for guidance on dosage.

Coumadin (warfarin sodium) is available in parenteral form for intravenous or intramuscular use and doses are similar. The principal excretion of warfarin appears to be in the urine in an altered form and patients known to have altered liver function should be given this drug with caution.

Continued weekly and later bi-weekly prothrombin times are desirable to direct the dosage required to maintain the preferred therapeutic range of between two to three times normal control values or 20 to 30 percent of normal prothrombin activity. Regular hemoglobin or hematocrit determinations are helpful in detecting possible occult hemorrhage.

Warfarin anticoagulants probably may be stopped abruptly without real danger of "rebound thrombosis" but many prefer to gradually reduce them over a period of a week or so, which certainly can do no harm. This point remains controversial however, and some reports have emphasized the clinical implications of a rebound hypercoagulable state following abrupt cessation of anticoagulation.[21]

Contraindications to warfarin anticoagulants include, in addition to those which contraindicate heparin (special risk of bleeding, ulcers, recent operation on brain, spinal cord, prostate or hemorrhagic diathesis) liver disease, jaundice and pregnancy. For long-term therapy, contraindications include severe anemia, chronic alcoholism, inadequate laboratory facilities and a patient who is incapable or unwilling to follow directions.

Complications resulting from the use of anticoagulants are discussed in Chapter 11.

General Supportive Measures

Since the clinical features of pulmonary embolism vary so much from patient to patient, any plan of treatment including general supportive measures must be flexible and adaptable to individual management. In addition to beginning therapy aimed at prevention of further emboli, consideration must be given to measures to maintain or improve cardiopulmonary function and to relieve pain or discomfort and apprehension. These general supportive measures include adequate oxygenation and circulatory support to correct hypotension and minimal sedation.

Oxygen should be administered in most instances since hypoxemia is commonly present in all but the most minor episodes. Administration may be by nasal catheter or face mask with precautions that the oxygen not exceed 50 percent of the inspired air except for short periods. Monitoring the Po_2 content of arterial blood is very helpful in maintaining an optimal Po_2 level of between 70 and 90 mm.

Circulatory support is indicated if the patient is in shock or hypotensive. Hypotension is usually present with major pulmonary emboli and is an indication of the seriousness of the episode. Papaverine, in addition to its pain relieving qualities, may be useful in producing vasodilatation of the pulmonary vessels. It is contraindicated in the presence of cardiac arrhythmias. Atropine is also used for this purpose, but its effectiveness is doubtful. Isoproterenol is helpful both for its inotropic effect on the heart and its dilating effect on the pulmonary vessels and bronchi. With right ventricular failure, digitalis is useful. Should hypotension persist in spite of other measures, vasoconstrictors, such as levarterenol or metaraminol, may be tried, but they should be used very cautiously and for only short periods of time. If hypotension is severe or progressive and prolonged use of vasoconstrictors is required, pulmonary embolectomy should be considered.

Morphine in low dosage is very helpful both to relieve pleuritic pain, if present, and to relieve anxiety. Demerol may be used instead.

Supportive measures should be continued until all acute symptoms subside. Ambulation should be permitted and encouraged, if the patient feels strong enough, any time after the first week when danger of re-embolization from nonadherent venous thrombi should be minimal.

Pulmonary Embolectomy

Pulmonary embolectomy for massive emboli, suggested by Trendelenburg[22] in 1908, was first successfully performed by Kirschner[23] in 1924. After a long relatively dormant period, this procedure was brought into prominence by the advent and common usage of cardiopulmonary bypass techniques. Although the procedure is now technically feasible there is still considerable disagreement as to when an attempt at embolectomy is indicated.

Trendelenburg stated in 1908, "Two conditions are necessary for embolectomy: first, the diagnosis must be right; second, there must be enough time to remove the obstruction." No one would disagree with the requirement that the diagnosis must be correct. The advent of the lung scan and the pulmonary arteriogram has made accurate diagnosis possible. Partial cardiopulmonary bypass initiated at the bedside under local anesthesia can increase available time for diagnosis and preparation for surgery. Yet despite these advances there remains considerable disagreement over the need for pulmonary embolectomy. Most agree that if the patient will survive without embolectomy the operation is not indicated, because eventual spontaneous thrombolysis and restoration of pulmonary artery patency will occur in a high percentage of cases. The difficulty arises in selecting accurately from those who survive long enough to allow embolectomy, those patients who will not survive without it.

The degree of pulmonary artery blockage relates to the severity of the embolism and the chance of survival. It has been stated that emboli involving 50 percent or less of the pulmonary arterial tree will not be fatal if the patient survives the immediate vasomotor and respiratory insult, and that those with more than 50 percent occlusion and hypotension are unlikely to survive without pulmonary embolectomy. The usual experiences of those performing pulmonary embolectomy with assistance of the cardiopulmonary bypass has been that about 50 percent of patients are salvagable. If this truly represents salvage in that all such patients selected for embolectomy would otherwise die, then operation certainly is warranted. However, this is questionable since some, and probably most, of those surviving long enough to permit embolectomy would survive if treated strenuously by nonoperative means.

Del Guercio et al.[24] reported on their observations in 19 patients in shock from pulmonary embolism. Eleven of these 19 patients died of the embolic episode while eight survived. Hemodynamic variables were studied in each group, and they felt that patients who would die of pulmonary embolism could be identified by markedly elevated mean right ventricular pressures

and low cardiac output. This was true even when systemic blood pressure and arterial oxygen tension were maintained near normal levels with vasopressors and oxygen therapy.

Crane studied 13 patients who qualified as possible candidates for embolectomy.[8] Eleven were treated initially with high dose intravenous heparin and two were treated by embolectomy. All 11 patients treated by heparin and subsequent caval interruption did well, while the two treated by embolectomy did not survive. They indicated that three indications for pulmonary embolectomy previously advocated were no longer valid. The first was a high degree of pulmonary arterial obstruction seen on angiography; the second indication felt not to be valid was assigning a critical level to pulmonary arterial, right ventricular end diastolic or right auricular pressure above which recovery is unlikely. They felt that while critical levels might exist for each individual patient, it was not feasible to establish critical levels that would apply to all patients. The third indication questioned was "hypotension not responding *promptly* to vasopressor infusion." Several of their patients who survived had initial hypotension for several hours despite vasopressor infusion. For the great majority of patients with major pulmonary embolism, they favored immediate high dose intravenous heparin with prompt interruption of the inferior vena cava after stabilization of circulation.

Sauter, Emanuel and Winzel reported on their experience with 14 patients undergoing pulmonary embolectomy, six of whom had been placed on partial cardiopulmonary bypass using peripheral cannulation prior to thoracotomy.[25] Seven of the eleven patients operated upon with cardiopulmonary bypass died. Their experience using urokinase to treat ten patients with pulmonary embolism was promising. In three patients, thought to fulfill the criteria previously established for performing pulmonary embolectomy, urokinase was used instead to induce a fibrinolytic state. A loading dose of 1,650

CTA units per pound in a ten minute period and a similar amount per hour by continuous infusion for eight hours was given. All three patients survived with clinical results comparable to those who survived pulmonary embolectomy.

It is estimated that about 75 percent of those who have fatal massive embolism die within one hour, which is the minimum time required in most institutions for assembling the surgical team, obtaining necessary pulmonary arteriograms and moving the patient to the operating room. The remaining 25 percent who might be potential candidates for embolectomy, would be further reduced by excluding those whose primary disease, such as metastatic cancer, was lethal, those whose clinical state had deteriorated so far that they would not survive operation, and those with irreversible anoxic brain damage. After all these exclusions it is obvious that very few patients in whom embolectomy is justified will live long enough to allow it. It is probable that more patients will be saved by routinely giving massive doses of heparin and supportive treatment in the period immediately following embolism, reserving embolectomy for those who survive beyond the first hour, but do not maintain a favorable response to full supportive measures. With the best medical care including vasopressors and massive doses of heparin, if systemic hypotension persists or becomes more marked, embolectomy is indicated.

Pulmonary embolectomy is occasionally indicated for chronic pulmonary embolism with pulmonary hypertension as reported by Moor and Sabiston in a 31-year-old patient suffering from chronic cor pulmonale from repeated pulmonary emboli.[26] Removal of an organized thrombus from the left pulmonary artery and the branches distal to this, resulted in improvement.

Technique of Pulmonary Embolectomy. Partial cardiopulmonary bypass is very helpful as a means of improving the patient's condition prior to the time of instituting total cardiopulmonary bypass. Partial

bypass is accomplished by cannulating the femoral artery and vein under local anesthesia at the bedside. The patient is then taken to the operating room and total cardiopulmonary bypass instituted after opening the chest through a median sternotomy incision. The main pulmonary artery is opened with an incision extending almost to its bifurcation. All accessible embolic material is removed by sponge forceps and suction. Removal of more distal emboli is aided by manually massaging the lung toward the hilus and by forceful overdistention of the lungs by the anesthesiologist. After removal of all embolic material the air is evacuated from the arterial tree and right ventricle and the pulmonary artery is repaired. Subsequent to embolectomy, and at the same procedure, the inferior vena cava should be interrupted.

Septic Pulmonary Emboli

There are few similarities between pulmonary embolism of bland thrombi and septic pulmonary emboli. Septic pulmonary emboli are usually quite small and multiple and tend to occur in showers. The emboli contain thrombus and bacteria and usually arise in infected systemic veins such as pelvic veins in young females who have had septic abortions or inflammatory involvement of their pelvic structures. Another increasingly common source is infected injection sites of drug abusers. Endocarditis of the right side of the heart as may occur with certain congenital anomalies is an additional source. In contrast to bland thromboembolism, septic pulmonary embolism is quite rare and usually occurs in adults less than fifty years of age who are usually septic with shaking chills and high fever. The sputum is sometimes purulent but may be bloody. Chest films usually show numerous small nodular or patchy infiltrates often with cavitation. The roentgenographic appearance is similar to that of miliary lung abscesses secondary to staphylococcal bacteremia or the nodular infiltrates of some patients with pneumonia due to Pseudomonas or Proteus. New scattered infiltrates seen on serial films and the presence of a distant septic focus favor the diagnosis of septic pulmonary emboli.

Pulmonary scans are of relatively little value since tiny septic emboli are not shown. If the scan is abnormal, it does not differentiate between the various other diseases commonly considered in the differential diagnosis. Pulmonary arteriograms are also disappointing because the arteries blocked are often too small to be detected. In doubtful cases, however, lung scan and pulmonary arteriograms may be helpful.

Treatment is frequently unsatisfactory. Anticoagulants alone are disappointing. Specific antibiotics, in large dosages, are indicated and may be successful, if blood cultures are positive or organisms are grown from a septic focus. In drug addicts, right-sided endocarditis is a common source and antibiotic therapy is the primary treatment. In women who are not drug addicts, suppurative thrombophlebitis of the pelvic veins is a more likely source even if pelvic examination is not revealing. When a septic focus is found in the lower extremities or thought to be the pelvic veins, the venous pathway should be interrupted. The inferior vena cava is the preferred level with additional ligation of the ovarian veins for pelvic thrombophlebitis. For the occasional superficial arm or leg vein grossly involved with septic thrombosis, excision of the affected vein is most likely to succeed.

Complications of Vena Cava Interruption Procedures

These may be considered from several viewpoints. General complications which may occur after any major operation such as pneumonia, paralytic ileus, wound infection or urinary tract infection are not peculiar to the operative procedure of caval interruption, the method of caval interruption or the presence or absence of continued caval blood flow, and are therefore not discussed.

Complications which will be discussed are those related to the act or method of interrupting the inferior vena cava. Some are

related to whether caval blood flow is totally or only partially occluded, some to the state of coagulability of the blood, the adequacy of collateral pathways, the pre-existence or later development of thrombophlebitis, the site of caval interruption and to whether or not thrombosis occurs at the site of interruption.

Indications for Interruption of the Vena Cava

Indications for interrupting the vena cava vary with different surgeons. Although a few feel that the mere presence of deep venous thrombosis is sufficient justification for interrupting the cava, most surgeons feel that immediate heparinization is the treatment of choice and reserve surgical interruption for specific indications. Specific indications include:

1. Failure of anticoagulants to prevent embolism
2. Contraindication to anticoagulation
3. Embolism occurring while the patient is normally ambulatory
4. Ancillary to pulmonary embolectomy
5. Ancillary to iliofemoral thrombectomy
6. Incidental at the time of laparotomy for other disease in the embolus-prone patient.

Failure of Anticoagulation. The vast majority of patients with pulmonary embolism respond favorably to heparinization. Theoretically, perhaps all should respond well to adequate heparin therapy, and some physicians state that they have seen no patients who required surgical interruption. Nevertheless, the best heparin therapy attainable in most situations is less than perfect, and, despite the best efforts of physicians and surgeons, occasional failures are encountered. If further embolism occurs in the face of the best available efforts at anticoagulation with heparin, then for practical purposes this is assumed to be a failure of anticoagulants and vena cava interruption is justified.

Failure of anticoagulants is by far the most common indication for surgical interruption of the vena cava. There are two groups of anticoagulation failures. The first and more common is the group with further embolization occurring while on active heparin therapy for an embolus. The second and smaller group includes those who had early successful heparin therapy, but on subsequent Coumadin therapy, have recurrent embolism, often after having become ambulatory. If embolism recurs with heparin therapy which is obviously poorly controlled and inadequate, better controlled and more adequate heparinization prior to considering surgery should be recommended. But, when heparin therapy is well managed with a clotting time of two and one-half to three times normal, recurrent embolism justifies surgical interruption. In most reported series failure of anticoagulation is the indication for surgery in from one-third to one-half the patients, and was the indication for surgery in 30 of the 72 patients in our series at the Medical College of Georgia.

Contraindication to Anticoagulation. The contraindication of heparin is usually a relative matter, and is infrequently the indication for surgery. This was the indication in only six of our 72 patients. Heparin is strongly contraindicated in patients with severe blood dyscrasias, with intracranial injuries or recent surgery, and with severe renal disease. It is relatively contraindicated in patients with active peptic ulcer disease, especially those who have had recent bleeding, and those who have active ulcerative colitis or other gastrointestinal lesions which are prone to bleed. Occasionally, the patient who is already on heparin for embolism will develop an acute condition which requires surgery, such as a perforated ulcer or acute appendicitis. In these instances, heparin must be discontinued and surgical interruption of the vena cava gives the greatest assurance of protection against embolism. Occasionally, the patient who has had pulmonary emboli in the past and who is facing a series of operative procedures, as in those with severe third degree burns or those who need a series of operative procedures, is best protected by surgical caval interruption.

Embolism While Ambulatory. This is an uncommon indication. The patient whose occupation requires much sitting such as a secretary or highway patrolman may be such a candidate. Six of our 72 patients were in this category. The patient who is seemingly perfectly healthy and normally ambulatory when he has a pulmonary embolus represents a problem. He has no warning signs and no evidence of phlebitis. Should he be placed on anticoagulants permanently? It has been our feeling in these rare instances that the best protection would be offered by interrupting the vena cava, and treating with anticoagulants for a period of several months.

Ancillary to Pulmonary Embolectomy. It is generally agreed that when pulmonary embolectomy is indicated the vena cava should be interrupted at the same procedure. These patients are critically ill, and maximum protection against the further possible insult of repeated embolism is mandatory. Failure to interrupt the cava in this situation has led to fatalities.

Ancillary to Iliofemoral Thrombectomy. Occasionally, during or following thrombectomy for iliofemoral thrombosis, notably with acute phlegmasia cerulea dolens, a pulmonary embolus occurs. Although there is some disagreement, many surgeons feel that the inferior vena cava should be interrupted either immediately before or just after the thrombectomy.

Incidental in the Embolus-Prone Patient. This indication for caval interruption is becoming more common as experience and confidence is gained in the use of partial interruption techniques. Because of the possible deleterious effects on the lower extremities, one would hesitate to ligate the vena cava unless it were known to be required. The same reticence is not felt about partial interruptions which give similar protection without the possible late sequelae effects of caval ligation. In 30 of our 72 patients the inferior vena cava was partially occluded as an incidental procedure in patients undergoing laparotomy for other disease. The presence of a history of previous pulmonary embolism, the presence of severe varicose veins, or evidence of previous deep phlebitis justifies this procedure. It also is justified in the embolus-prone group of elderly or debilitated patients undergoing major abdominal surgery with anticipated prolonged recovery periods. Present evidence indicates fairly conclusively that the externally applied plastic clip does not produce thrombosis at the application site and that any elevation of venous pressure distally is minimal. We feel confident that an externally applied smooth teflon clip with a 3.0 mm. or 3.5 mm. gap is most unlikely to do any harm unless it catches an embolus in which case any harmful effects of caval occlusion are more than offset by its having prevented a possibly fatal pulmonary embolus.

Site and Methods of Vena Cava Interruption

Because of the high incidence of recurrent emboli after ligations at more distal sites (superficial femoral, common femoral and iliac veins), the preferred site for interrupting the venous pathway is the inferior vena cava. Rarely, in patients too ill to withstand caval interruption, one may elect to interrupt the common femoral veins bilaterally under local anesthesia. With this possible exception, the inferior vena cava is the site chosen for interrupting the venous pathway to prevent pulmonary embolism.

Opinions differ as to whether the interruption should be at the lower, middle or infrarenal level of the inferior vena cava. In one of the few studies of this question, Dale[27] showed in dogs a somewhat higher femoral vein pressure following low ligation than following ligation at the infrarenal level. In monkeys, Beltz and Condors[28] found no significant differences in distal venous pressures or in the development and competence of venous collaterals in ligations at the infrarenal and the low caval levels. Due to high flow from the renal veins, less stasis would be expected above the point of ligation in the high infrarenal level interruption than in the cul-de-sac above a low caval ligation. This

is especially true if the vena cava is divided to allow the cul-de-sac to retract upward. However, the midportion of the cava is more easily approached by the usual retroperitoneal route and, if care is taken to place the interruption just caudad to a sizeable vein, stasis is minimized. For routine use, most surgeons favor the low or mid inferior vena cava level.

The time-honored and proved method of caval interruption was complete ligation, often with heavy umbilical tape, doubly applied with the cava transected between the two ties. Dissatisfaction with postligation sequelae of edema and stasis changes in the lower extremities led to modifications in the methods of interrupting the vena cava. Early trials with temporary occlusions using absorbable catgut and removable clips were superseded by various methods of producing permanent but incompletely occluding caval interruptions. Among the methods other than ligation which have been evaluated clinically are: *smooth teflon clip,* Moretz, Rhode and Shepherd[29] 1959; *plication,* Spencer, Quattlebaum, J. K., Quattlebaum, J. K., Jr., Sharp, Jude[30] 1962; *harp-string filter,* DeWeese and Hunter[31] 1963; *serrated teflon clip,* Miles, Fenwick and Renwer[32] 1964; and *intravascular umbrella,* Mobin-Uddin, Kazi and Jude[33] 1969.

Mortality

There is an appreciable mortality, both early and late, in most sizeable series of vena caval interruptions. Mortality from pulmonary embolism has been shown to vary with the predisposing condition: with cardiac disease 29.1 percent, postoperative state 15.7 percent, trauma 9.7 percent, idiopathic 2.2 percent, infection 6.7 percent, pregnancy 6.7 percent, and with hemiplegia 53.8 percent.[4] Operative mortality is not only related to associated diseases, but also to the precarious condition of the patient at the time of operation. This precarious state is due to the underlying disease usually present, and also to altered cardiopulmonary physiology pro-

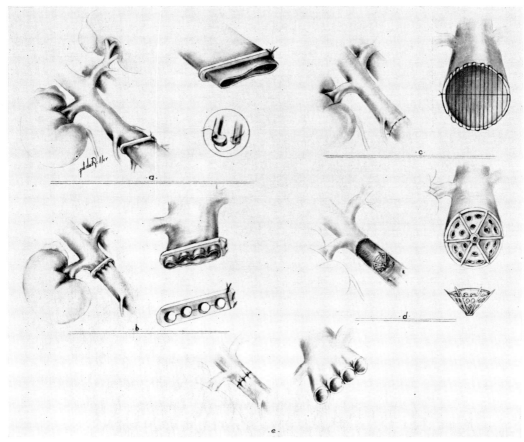

F<small>IG</small>. 12-3. Methods of partial occlusion. Five procedures representative of the many being used to occlude partially the inferior vena cava. (A) Smooth Teflon clip (Moretz), (B) Serrated Teflon clip (Miles), (C) Harp-string filter (DeWeese), (D) Umbrella (Mobin-Uddin), (E) Plication (Spencer).

duced by recent pulmonary embolism particularly in patients with pre-existing, serious cardiovascular disease. Comparisons of overall mortality of total versus partial caval occlusion are not very meaningful. Reported deaths within 30 days of caval interruption vary between 4 percent and 23 percent, usually 10 to 18 percent. Late mortality, with the exception of the very rare fatal pulmonary embolus, is due exclusively to the underlying patient disease, and is unrelated to the fact or method of caval interruption.

Intolerance to Vena Cava Occlusion

Occasionally death occurs shortly after sudden occlusion of the inferior vena cava, usu-

ally in those with reduced cardiac reserve. Observations upon the acute effects of sudden occlusion of the inferior vena cava, both in dogs and humans, demonstrate a significant reduction in cardiac output primarily due to decreased return of venous blood to the heart. In dogs, Maraan and Tabor[34] demonstrated a 47 percent decrease in cardiac output after inferior vena cava occlusion. Williams, Roding and Schenk showed a 21.6 percent reduction in cardiac output, a 17.6 percent reduction in aortic pressure and a 13-fold increase in inferior vena cava pressure.[35] Similar changes have been demonstrated by others.[36,37] In patients, an increase in venous pressure distally is common[38-41] and occasional massive sequestration of blood in the lower extremities has been described.[42]

Benavides and Noon [43] compared the relative hemodynamic effects of interrupting the inferior vena cava by ligation, plication, silk suture screen and smooth teflon clip. Neither the silk suture screen nor the clip interferred significantly with venous return, while plication interferred moderately and ligation significantly with venous return. In the dog, this interference with venous return after ligation leads to appreciable mortality of between 20 percent in our own studies and 22 and 37.5 percent in those of others.[34,43]

Many reports[34,37,42,44-46] include an occasional instance of death within a few hours of caval ligation which seem attributable to sudden caval occlusion. Such occurrences are unlikely following partial caval occlusion even in patients with poor cardiac function. We have observed one such instance 24 hours after application of a smooth clip when it was suddenly occluded by a large embolus.

Several authors[47,48] have noted the increased risk to life of sudden caval occlusions in those with cardiac disease, particularly those with low output myocardial failure. While the poor general condition of many of these patients makes any operative procedure relatively dangerous, the combination of poor cardiac reserve from myocardial disease plus the embarrassed cardiopulmonary function from pulmonary embolism, makes any further acute reduction in cardiac output particularly hazardous. Occlusions occurring later in the postoperative period have been observed, but these are better tolerated than when associated with the precarious state so often present at the time of operative caval interruption.

Re-embolization

Making a diagnosis of pulmonary embolism following caval interruption is fraught with the same difficulties as making the diagnosis originally. No doubt some recurrent pulmonary emboli go unrecognized while many episodes are wrongly diagnosed pulmonary emboli. Lacking conclusive objective evidence, the individual physician's beliefs, prejudices and hopes assume greater importance in the diagnosis. Compounding these biases with the know difficulty of accurate diagnosis makes meaningful statistics on the incidence of recurrent embolism, especially smaller, nonfatal ones, difficult or impossible to obtain.

Pulmonary embolism occurring after caval interruption may be either a complication of the vena cava interruption itself, or it may be instead simply a failure of the procedure to stop further embolization. Numerous instances have been reported of embolizations recurring after caval interruption with the source of emboli found at autopsy to be mural thrombi in the right side of the heart or, less commonly, a vein in the upper part of the body. Other recurrent emboli have been identified as having arisen from, or below the area of caval interruption. Rare occurrences from thrombosis just above the site of interruption have been reported following both ligation and partial interruption.[49-51] In four of 37 autopsies reported by Amador, Khi and Crane[52] in a series of 119 patients treated by inferior vena cava ligation, thrombosis was noted cephalad to the inferior vena cava tie and in two of these four had led to recurrent pulmonary emboli.

Recurrent fatal pulmonay embolism was documented in one instance[38] as having arisen from thrombus cephalad to an inferior vena cava ligature placed 18 days previously. In five of ten autopsies reported by DeMeester[40] there was thrombus at the site of plication extending cephalad for distances of a few centimeters and in one instance up to the renal vein.

A fatal complication recently occurred in a 65-year-old man who had undergone a successful carotid artery endarterectomy.[53] He suffered a massive pulmonary embolus and while being treated with heparin had another large embolus. An umbrella was placed without difficulty in the inferior vena cava and heparin was continued for seven days while he was still hospitalized. Heparin was then discontinued and he was allowed to go home without anticoagulation. Fourteen days later he had a sudden fatal pulmonary embolus. Autopsy revealed complete occlusion of the inferior vena cava below the umbrella with the thrombus extending through the apertures of the umbrella into the cava proximally (Fig. 12-4), presumably the site of origin of the large fresh thrombus found in the pulmonary artery.

Some degree of stasis, which encourages thrombosis, occurs in the blind cul-de-sac above the point of ligation or an occluded partial interruption. To avoid or reduce this stasis the site of caval interruption, regardless of method, should be just caudad to a sizeable tributary, either a lumbar or renal vein. Ideally there should be a sizeable tributary just below the point of interruption as well, to avoid stasis there. The possibility of propagation through a partial occlusion

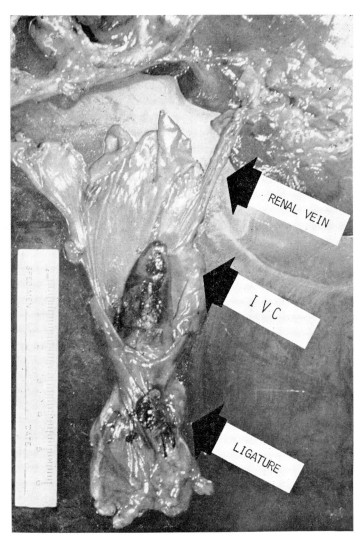

FIG. 12-4. Autopsy specimen from a patient who underwent successful pulmonary embolectomy and vena caval ligation. Then three weeks later he died with recurrent pulmonary embolism. Clot arising above the ligature is clearly evident. (Courtesy of H. G. Beebe, M.D.)

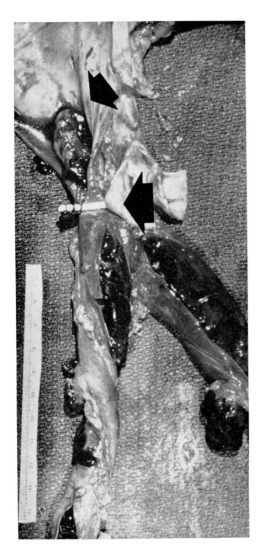

FIG. 12-5. Clot arising above a serrated clip which was placed just immediately above the bifurcation of the vena cava. (Courtesy of H. G. Beebe, M.D.)

from an embolus trapped below should also be lessened by reduced stasis resulting from a properly selected site.

The narrow apertures remaining with partial occlusion techniques may allow passage of tiny emboli but, at least with externally applied clips, these channels do not enlarge with time. With ligation, collaterals invariably develop after a few weeks which are larger than the 3 mm. channels and may

allow passage of larger emboli. Parrish[54] and his associates have shown the prompt development of such collaterals in the dog and have demonstrated that they are capable of transmitting emboli from the lower extremities. This seemed to be the mechanism in the recurrent embolus reported by McIntyre, *et al.*[55] in a ligated patient who noted pain in the leg and groin and could feel the "clot moving up" just prior to the event. Therefore, the early theoretical advantage of completely occluding the cava is lost within a few weeks.[45,46]

Coupland has documented experimentally in the sheep that suture plication may ultimately fail to compartmentalize the vena cava if the sutures pull through the vessel wall permitting full re-expansion of the lumen.[56]

Recurrence from ovarian or spermatic veins is possible after caval interruption by any method. To prevent this possibility the specific vein harboring the thrombus must be interrupted, or in the case of the right ovarian or spermatic vein, the caval interruption must be cephalad to where this vein enters the vena cava.

Reported recurrence rates following partially occluding methods are shown in Table 12-1. Reported recurrences after complete caval ligations are shown in Table 12-2.

The true incidence of recurrent pulmonary embolism is difficult or impossible to ascertain. Objective studies should be used in all cases to document carefully the occurrence as clinical suspicion is not adequate. Recurrent pulmonary embolism probably occurs with about equal frequency after either complete or partial caval occlusion. Fatal embolism following either is extremely rare. In a large collected series, recurrent emboli were more common (4.6% vs. 2.3%) after partial interruptions.[68] Small emboli may be more frequent in the first few weeks after partial occlusions, but this possible early advantage of ligation is soon reversed as the collaterals about a total occlusion enlarge.

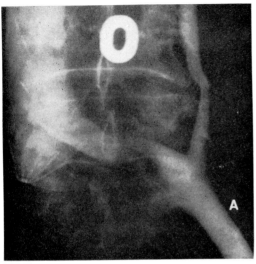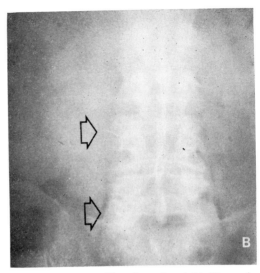

FIG. 12-6. (A) Phlebogram showing placement of the vena cava filter into the right iliac vein which resulted in right iliofemoral venous thrombosis and necessitated placement of a second "umbrella." (B) Flat plate of the abdomen showing position of the first and second "umbrellas." (Gaston, E. A., III: Incorrect placement of prosthesis for pulmonary embolism, JAMA, *214*:2338, 1970)

Lower Extremity Sequelae

The chief complications of vena cava interruption occurring in the lower extremities relate to venous thrombosis, recurrent phlebitis and chronic postphlebitic syndrome. Patients with venous thrombosis and phlebitis prior to caval interruption may be expected to have these after caval interruption. The primary question is whether the lower extremity sequelae are worse after complete than after partial caval interruptions.

Review of the literature is confusing because individual interpretations vary considerably. What is "significant" to one may be "insignificant" to another. One individual may continue working with moderate incapacity while another may stop work with almost no postphlebitic changes. One patient may develop ulcers because of poor care, while another with worse disease and better care will not ulcerate. Some patients continue to wear elastic stockings who could easily do without them; others will not wear them who should. Marked differences also

TABLE 12-1. REPORTED RECURRENCE RATES FOLLOWING PARTIAL OCCLUSION

Author	Type of Interruption	Recurrence Rate %
Leather[57]	Smooth clip	6.5
Mandel[58]	Smooth clip	17
Moretz[59]	Smooth clip	4.8
Miles[60]	Serrated clip	4.1
Moran[61]	Serrated clip	14
DeWeese[31]	Harp string filter	4
Little[62]	Plication	3
DeMeester[40]	Plication	9

TABLE 12-2. REPORTED RECURRENCE RATES FOLLOWING COMPLETE OCCLUSION

Author	Type of Interruption	Recurrence Rate %
Ochsner[46]	Ligation	0
Shauble[63]	Ligation	5
Crane[64]	Ligation	1
Stevens[65]	Ligation	10
Nabseth[42]	Ligation	2.7
Amador[52]	Ligation	8.1
Moran[61]	Ligation	12
Piccone[66]	Ligation	50
Gurewich[67]	Ligation	20

exist in the groups of patients treated, some having a much higher proportion with old deep venous thrombosis, and some having far more essentially "normal" extremities. Reports of postoperative sequelae, therefore, vary markedly, from almost a complete absence of sequelae to some stasis problems in nearly all patients.

In most reports of ligations since 1960, new ulcerations occur in five to ten percent of patients, while only an occasional new ulceration is reported following partial occlusions. Significant late lower extremity morbidity is reported in 20 to 50 percent of vena cava ligations, considerably higher than with partial occlusions. Furthermore, much of the morbidity occurring after partial occlusion techniques is in those found to be occluded, a relationship supported by several reports DeMeester,[40] Bergan,[44] and Moretz,[59] but not by others. One of the few reports comparing results in sizeable groups of ligations with partial occlusions in the same institution is that of Adams, Feingold and DeWeese.[47] They showed significant late extremity morbidity in 43 percent following ligation, as compared with 16 percent after partial interruption. In the group with partial interruptions morbidity was higher in those that became completely occluded, than in those that remained patent.

Pre-existing deep vein pathology is a very important factor in late morbidity after vena cava interruption. Extremities with previous phlebitis are prone to have recurrent difficulties, with or without caval interruption, and the possible role played by a superimposed proximal, complete or partial, caval interruption is very difficult to evaluate. The role

of the proximal occlusion is often overshadowed by a more obvious relationship with pre-existing thrombophlebitis. A recent study illustrating such a dual relationship showed that not only the previous state of the extremity, but also proximal venous interruption influenced the fate of the extremity.[59] After application of a partially occluding clip to the inferior vena cava, 130 extremities, 60 of which were involved with thrombophlebitis before operation, were followed. The status of the proximal veins, both the inferior vena cava and the iliac veins, was studied in 79 extremities, with occlusion demonstrated proximally in 24 extremities. The results are shown in Table 12-3.

These findings clearly implicate the importance of proximal veins as well as pre-existent thrombophlebitis in the fate of the extremity after caval interruption.

A few patients have extremely severe postphlebitic sequelae with gross involvement of the entire lower half of the body and legs and obvious large collateral veins of the abdominal wall. They have extensive, old, postphlebitic involvement of the entire inferior vena cava below the renal veins, as well as extensive involvement of the iliac veins and veins of the lower extremities. Attempted cavagrams show no patency of the original iliac veins and vena cava, and exploration reveals only small fibrotic cords in place of the vena cava and iliac veins. This situation is found occasionally in patients who have had no caval surgery. We have seen it in two patients who had had caval ligations years before, but have not yet seen it following partial occlusion of the

TABLE 12-3.
FATE OF EXTREMITY CORRELATED WITH PROXIMAL VENOUS OCCLUSION
AND PRE-EXISTING PHLEBITIS

| | Proximal Veins | | Pre-existing Phlebitis | |
	Occluded (24)	Patent (55)	Present (60)	Absent (70)
Significant Edema	17% (4)	4% (2)	8% (5)	3% (2)
Recurrent Phlebitis	21% (5)	11% (6)	17% (10)	1% (1)
Massive Venous Thrombosis	38% (9)	0% (0)	10% (6)	6% (4)

inferior vena cava. Currently available elastic support, although of the the made-to-measure "leotard" type are inadequate. Moderate limitation of activities is of little or no help. Anticoagulants continuously or intermittently for control of recurrent thrombophlebitis may be required. Such patients remain incapacitated regardless of the best therapeutic efforts. Proximal venous occlusion is certainly not beneficial to the extremity, and in theory should be detrimental. By increasing the distal venous pressure, even though only slightly, the cross sectional area of leg veins, normally partially collapsed, is increased which slows the rate of blood flow and increases any tendency toward venous thrombosis. One would expect therefore, other factors being equal, a greater incidence of venous thrombosis and stasis difficulties in extremities distal to an occluded vena cava than to an open one.

A few generalities may be stated. With good care, most patients, particularly with anticoagulants given postoperatively, do not have serious postphlebitic difficulties following either ligation or partial occlusion of their inferior vena cava. Extremities which are already postphlebitic at the time of caval interruption are likely to have further trouble whether the cava is completely or only partially occluded. Both an already involved extremity or a clinically normal extremity is more likely to develop sequelae if there is obstruction of the venous drainage proximal to the extremity. Fewer and less severe sequelae are reported following partial than following complete caval occlusions.

Massive Venous Thrombosis

Extensive thrombosis in the veins below the site of caval interruption is not rare. In one series[59] ten of 140 extremities developed massive venous thrombosis, analogous to phlegmasia cerulea dolens, in the early postoperative period. This complication is apparently more common with complete occlusion of the cava than with partial occlusion, since in the series cited, a report on smooth clip partial occlusion, the nine instances studied by venography each showed complete occlusion proximally in either the iliac vein or the inferior vena cava. In one instance of massive thrombosis occurring on the third day, after application of a partially occluding clip, thrombectomy was performed with marked improvement. Others were treated with elevation, anticoagulants and elastic supports with gradual improvement in most. One patient with bilateral involvement expired on the 28th postoperative day and was shown at autopsy to have massive thrombosis involving not only all the major veins below the clip, but also the external jugular vein and the superior vena cava. This example of what has been called "malignant coagulopathy" has also been observed on rare occasions following caval ligation and without preceding surgery. Moses, *et al.*,[69] noted this in two of 74 caval ligations with one being accompanied by severe shock and death.

Miles in 1971 observed 19 instances (15%) of acute thrombophlebitis after 121 clip applications.[60] Seven of these had thrombectomy. DeMeester, *et al.* noted of 49 patients surviving plication, 15 who developed extensive iliofemoral thrombosis with five requiring thrombectomy.[40] Ten of these 15 demonstrated occlusion at the plication site. There is practically no information at hand on the very late effects of these acute episodes of extensive thrombosis.

The frequency of postinterruption venous thrombosis and its significant morbidity emphasize the need of postoperative efforts to prevent its development. Since heparin is dangerous in the early postoperative period, a common practice is to use Dextran for the first three days, followed by heparin and later Coumadin (warfarin sodium). In addition, early ambulation, elevation of legs while at rest and good elastic leg supports are useful. If thrombosis occurs, bed rest with maximal leg elevation and elastic wrappings are indicated as well as carefully controlled heparin, unless contraindicated.

Most complications occurring at the site of interruption relate to operative errors, to

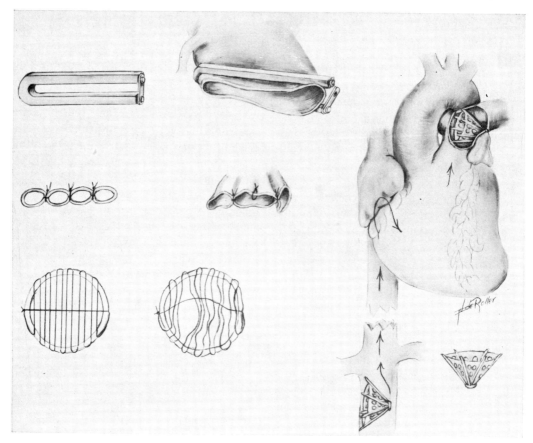

FIG. 12-7. Complications at site of interruption. (*Left Upper*) The end piece of a smooth Teflon clip is unfastened. (*Left Middle*) Plication suture has pulled through one wall of cava and channels have enlarged. (*Left Lower*) Disalignment of strands in harp-string filter. (*Right*) Dislodgement and migration of "umbrella" filter from inferior vena cava to pulmonary artery.

thrombosis in that area or to postoperative bleeding.

Operative Errors

Occasional accidents occur during operation which can be troublesome. A lumbar vein can be torn as the vena cava is being dissected. If the vein is injured at its junction with the cava, the caval junction can be identified and sutured with a fine vascular suture. This can be very troublesome and it may be necessary to occlude the cava above and below the site in order to find the tear. Once found, a partially occluding clamp may be used to isolate the tear. Injury to a tributary away from the cava is usually more easily found and ligated. Moderate care during the

caval dissection usually prevents this injury. Occasionally the cava seems adherent to its surroundings, making dissection tedious. Since the lumbar veins are not evenly spaced and paired, one cannot assume that a lumbar vein laterally has its mate at the same level medially. It may be caudad or cephalad and subject to injury when dissecting behind the cava for passage of a suture, tape or clip. It is during this dissection that injury is most likely. After a tie or tape has been drawn around the cava upward traction allows better visualization of the tributaries and lessens the danger of injury if further dissection is needed for proper placement of the occluding device. In the retroperitoneal approach, inadvertent peritoneal tears may occur, but these require only recognition and simple closure.

Errors in Placement of the Occlusion

Congenital anomalies may account for some incorrectly placed occlusions. A left-sided inferior vena cava has been described, either as the sole inferior cava or as part of a duplication with both a right- and a left-sided cava. Much less rare is an unusually high confluence of the two common iliac veins to form the vena cava. Venacavagrams should demonstrate these anomalies. A "pelvic" kidney with its renal vein emptying into the iliac vein would probably be damaged by ligation of the inferior vena cava. Although this has not yet occurred in our experience, a routine intravenous pyelogram has been advised prior to ligation to exclude this possibility.

One recurrent embolus was noted following the erroneous placement of a serrated clip on the common iliac vein.[60] This was successfully managed by placing a second clip on the inferior vena cava. In one instance, reported by Gaston, an "umbrella" was inadvertently pushed to the right common iliac vein and could not be withdrawn.[71] A phlebogram showed the prosthesis to be in the right common iliac vein. A second "umbrella" was placed in the inferior vena cava above the first, both prostheses being visible in Figure 12.7.

Of the more than 880 implantations of the Mobin-Uddin "umbrella," nine were erroneously placed in the iliac vein.[33,70,71] An additional three had misplacement of the "umbrella" filter in the renal vein (in two the filter was removed by operation). The "umbrella" filter became dislodged and migrated from the site of placement in eight patients, one lodging in the right atrium and four lodging in a pulmonary artery. Two of these were surgically removed from the pulmonary artery, two patients died within 36 hours primarily from nonprevented pulmonary emboli, and another, an 83-year-old man, died three months later of heart disease, the filter remaining in the left pulmo-

nary artery. One instance was reported of recurrent embolization presumably through a clip found at autopsy to be open and not effectively narrowing the vena cava.[58] This was an old model, smooth, teflon clip with a snap-on end piece.

There have been rare instances of the ligature slipping off the end of the divided vena cava. Although some continue to doubly ligate the vena cava, only a few surgeons still divide the cava between ligatures except as a means of flattening out the small cul-de-sac otherwise present when ligating just below the renal vein.

In one patient the "umbrella" filter is known to have perforated the third portion of the duodenum. There have been no instances reported of a clip causing any harm to the adjacent aorta, a fear expressed by some.

Thrombosis of Vena Cava

Thrombosis occurring at the site of either ligation or partial occlusion is considered a complication since it may lead to recurrent embolism or to increased obstruction and greater postphlebitic difficulties. Following ligation, thrombosis may occur above and below the ligature in an appreciable number of patients. In 37 autopsies following ligation reported by Amador, *et al.,* four had thrombosis cephalad to the tie, two of which led to recurrent embolism, and ten had thrombosis caudad to the tie.[52] Ferris, *et al.* showed by cavagrams that in ten of 20 cavas ligated, the cava was thrombosed below the tie.[41] In their series there was none with thrombus above the tie. In 16 autopsies after ligation two had thrombus above the ligation, and one had thrombus below.[66] In ten patients coming to autopsy after plications, five had thrombus extending cephalad to the plication site, of which four might well have been the result of local thrombosis.[40]

Partial occlusions may become completely occluded either by catching an embolus or by thrombosis occurring at the site. The frequency with which spontaneous thrombosis at the site of partial occlusion occurs varies considerably with the method of interruption. It should be least with externally applied, nonreactive teflon clips, and probably less with smooth than with serrated clips.[20] Methods which necessitate injury to the vein wall such as plication with sutures or staples, sieve construction, or an intraluminal element probably have a higher incidence of thrombosis.[33] Using teflon clips, late patency, either maintained or regained after earlier occlusions and recanalization, has been reported in 67 to 94 percent of cases.[32,48,57,59] With plication, patency was demonstrated in 60 percent of 35 patients and in 82 percent of 17 patients.[72] It is noteworthy that by serial cavagrams, some which had earlier shown complete occlusion later regained some degree of patency.[48,59,73] With the Mobin-Uddin "umbrella" filter, all apparently become occluded within a few weeks, some by stopping emboli, the remainder by gradually becoming thrombosed.

Postoperative Bleeding

Bleeding in the postoperative period is usually related to the use of anticoagulants, especially when heparin is begun within a few hours of operation, and can be a serious complication. In one instance, we began heparin within two hours of closing the wound after the usual muscle splitting, retroperitoneal approach. Even though hemostasis was thought to be adequate prior to wound closure, a very large hematoma developed requiring blood transfusions and cessation of heparin.

Miles reported postoperative hemorrhage in 12 patients of 121, 11 of whom were receiving anticoagulants at the time.[60] One retroperitoneal hematoma required evacuation. In seven patients bleeding was not from the operative site. Five bled from the gastrointestinal tract and one from the genitourinary tract, and represent complications of anticoagulants rather than of caval interruption.

Stevens, *et al.* reported five instances of hematomas following caval ligation in 41 patients.[65] Each of the five had received anticoagulants postoperatively, one beginning immediately after operation, two after an interval of 12 hours and two after intervals of 24 hours.

Because of this experience with heparin, we rely upon dextran in the early postoperative period and begin heparin only after 48 to 72 hours. While some begin heparin immediately following a midline, transperitoneal approach to the vena cava this seems dangerous and unnecessary for the routine case. Exceptions might be justified in the occasional instance where the inferior vena cava is interrupted in conjunction with ileofemoral thrombectomy for acute phlegmasia cerulea dolens. Even here, it would seem preferable first to partially occlude the vena cava, give dextran and delay thrombectomy at least 12, and preferably 24 hours, until heparin could be more safely utilized.

References

1. Virchow, R.: Die Verstopfung der Lungenarterie unde Ihre Folgen. Beitr. Exp. Path. Physiol., *2*:1, 1946.
2. Hume, M.: Platelet adhesiveness and other factors in thrombophlebitis. Surgery, *59*: 110, 1966.
3. Sevitt, S., and Gallagher, N. G.: Venous thrombosis and pulmonary embolism: A clinico-pathological study in injured and burned patients. Brit. J. Surg., *48*:475, 1961.
4. Byrne, J. J., and O'Neill, E. E.: Fatal pulmonary emboli, a study of 130 autopsy proven fatal cases. Amer. J. Surg., *83*:47, 1952.
5. Lassen, M.: Heat, denaturation of plasminogen in fibrin plate method. Acta Physiol. Scandinav., *27*:371-376, 1952.
6. Freiman, D. C., Suyento, J., and Wessler, S.: Frequency of pulmonary thromboembolism in man. New Eng. J. Med., *272*:1278, 1965.
7. DeBakey, M. D.: Collective review: Critical evaluation of problem of thromboembolism. Int. Abstr. Surg., *98*:1, 1954.
8. Crane, C., Hartsuck, J., Birtch, A., Couch, N. P., Zollinger, R., Matloff, J., Dalen, J., and Dexter, L.: The management of major pulmonary embolism. Surg. Gynec. Obst., *128*:27, 1969.

9. Comroe, J. H., VanLingen, B., Stroud, R. C., and Roncoroni, A.: Reflex and direct cardiopulmonary effects of 5-OH-tryptamine (serotonin): Their possible role in pulmonary embolism and coronary thrombosis. Amer. J. Physiol., *173*:379, 1953.

10. Stone, N. H., and Nemir, P.: Study of the role of 5-OH-tryptamine (serotonin) and histamine in the pathogenesis of pulmonary embolism in man. Ann. Surg., *152*:890, 1960.

11. Webster, J. R., Jr., Saadeh, G. B., Eggum, P. R., and Suker, J. R.: Wheezing due to pulmonary embolism: Treatment with heparin. New Eng. J. Med., *274*:931, 1966.

12. Hume, M., Sevitt, S., and Thomas, D. P.: *In* Venous Thrombosis and Pulmonary Embolism, pp. 260-268, Cambridge, Harvard University Press, 1970.

13. Just-Viera, J. O., Norwood, T., and Yeager, G. H.: Importance of shock and cyanosis in pulmonary embolism. Amer. Surg., *165*: 528, 1967.

14. Wacker, W. E. C., Rosenthal, M., Snodgrass, P. J., and Amador, E.: Triad for diagnosis of pulmonary embolism and infarction. JAMA, *178*:8, 1961.

15. Coodley, E. L.: Enzyme profiles in the evaluation of pulmonary infarction. JAMA, *207*:1307, 1969.

16. Wagner, H. N., Jr.: Current status of lung scanning. Radiology, *91*:1235-7, 1968.

17. Medina, J. R., L'Heureux, P., Lillehei, J. P., and Lkaer, M. K.: Regional ventilation in the differential diagnosis of pulmonary embolism. Circulation, *39*:831, 1969.

18. Thomas, D. P., Tanabe, G., Kahn, M., and Stein, M.: Humoral factors mediated by platelets. *In* Sasahara, A. A., and Stein, M.: Experimental Pulmonary Embolism in Pulmonary Embolic Disease. A Symposium. New York, Grune & Stratton, 1965.

19. Gurewich, V., Thomas, D. P., and Stuart, R. K.: Some guidelines for heparin therapy of venous thromboembolic disease. JAMA, *199*:116, 1967.

20. Price, T. B., Wray, C. H., Callahan, A. B., and Moretz, W. H.: Effect of ellagic acid on thrombosis of vena cava after partial interruption. Rev. Surg., *27*:60, 1970.

21. Sise, H. S., Moschos, C. B., Gauthier, J., and Becker, R.: The risk of interrupting long term anticoagulant treatment. Circulation, *24*:1137, 1961.

22. Trendelenburg, F.: Ueber Bie Operative Behaudlung der Emboli der Lungenarterie. Arch. Klin. Chir., *86*:686, 1908.

23. Kirschner, M.: Ein Durch die Trendelenburgische Operation Geheilter Fall von Emboli der Art. Pulmonalis. Arch. Klin. Chir., *133*:312, 1924.

24. Del Guercio, L. R. M., Cohn, J. D., Feins, N. R., Coomaraswamy, R. P., and Mantle, L.: Pulmonary embolism shock. JAMA, *196*:71, 1966.

25. Sautter, R. D., Emanuel, D. A., and Wenzel, F. J.: Treatment of acute pulmonary embolism. Ann. Thorac. Surg., *4*:95, 1967.

26. Moor, G. F., and Sabiston, D. C., Jr.: Embolectomy for chronic pulmonary embolism and hypertension. Case report and review of the problem. Circulation, *41*:701, 1970.

27. Dale, W. A., Pualwan, F., and Bauer, F. M.: Ligation of the inferior vena cava with absorbable gut. Surg. Gyn. Obst., *102*:517, 1956.

28. Beltz, W. R., and Condon, R. E.: Influence of level of ligation on the results of vena caval interruption. Surg. Gyn. Obst., *133*: 257, 1971.

29. Moretz, W. H., Rhode, C. M., and Shepherd, M. H.: Prevention of pulmonary emboli by partial occlusion of the inferior vena cava. Amer. Surg., *25*:617, 1959.

30. Spencer, F. C., Quattlebaum, J. K., Quattlebaum, J. K., Jr., Sharp, E. H., and Jude, J. R.: Plication of inferior vena cava for pulmonary embolism: Report of 20 cases. Ann. Surg., *155*:827, 1962.

31. DeWeese, M. S., and Hunter, D. C.: A vena cava filter for prevention of pulmonary embolism. Arch. Surg., *86*:852, 1963.

32. Miles, R. M., Fenwick, C., and Renwer, O.: A partially occluding clip for prevention of pulmonary embolism. Amer. Surg., *20*:40, 1964.

33. Mobin-Uddin, Kazi, McLean, R., and Jude, J. R.: A new catheter technique of interruption of the inferior vena cava for prevention of pulmonary embolism. Amer. Surg., *35*:889, 1969.

34. Maraan, B. M., and Taber, R. E.: The effects of inferior vena caval ligation on cardiac output: An experimental study. Surgery, *63*:966, 1968.

35. Williams, B. T., Roding, B., and Schenk, W. G., Jr.: Experimental evaluation of haemodynamic effects of inferior vena cava ligation. J. Cardiov. Surg., *11*:454, 1970.

36. Adams, J. T., and DeWeese, J. A.: Experimental and clinical evaluation of partial vein interruption in the prevention of pulmonary emboli. Surgery, *57*:82, 1965.

37. Gazzaniaz, A. B., and MacArthur, J. D.: Blood volume, cardiac output, and renal

function changes after plication of the inferior vena cava. Ann. Surg., *169*:483, 1969.

38. Carrol, S. E., Coles, J. C., Gergely, N., and Ross, C. C.: Ligation of the inferior vena cava. Canad. J. Surg., *6*:18, 1963.

39. Dale, W. A.: Ligation of the inferior vena cava for thromboembolism. Surgery, *43*:24, 1958.

40. DeMeester, R. T., Rutherford, R. B., Blazek, J. V., and Zuidema, G. D.: Plication of the inferior vena cava for thromboembolism. Surgery, *62*:56, 1967.

41. Ferris, E. J., Vittemberga, F. J., Byrne, J. J., Nabseth, D. C., and Shapiro, J. H.: The inferior vena cava after ligation and plication. Radiology, *89*:1, 1967.

42. Nabseth, D. C., and Moran, J. M.: Reassessment of the role of inferior vena cava ligation in venous thromboembolism. New Eng. J. Med., *273*:1250, 1965.

43. Benavides, J., and Noon, R.: Experimental evaluation of inferior vena cava procedures to prevent pulmonary embolism. Ann. Surg., *166*:195, 1967.

44. Bergan, J. J., Kaupp, M. A., and Trippel, O. H.: Critical evaluation of vena cava plication—Prevention of pulmonary embolism. Arch. Surg., *88*:1016, 1964.

45. Moretz, W. H., Naisbitt, P. F., and Stevenson, G. P.: Experimental studies on temporary occlusion of the inferior vena cava. Surgery, *36*:384, 1954.

46. Ochsner, A., Ochsner, J. L., and Sanders, H. S.: Prevention of pulmonary embolism by caval ligation. Ann. Surg., *171*:923, 1970.

47. Adams, J. T., Feingold, B. E., and DeWeese, J. A.: Comparative evaluation of ligation and partial interruption of the inferior vena cava. Arch. Surg., *103*:272, 1971.

48. Moran, C., and Callow, A. D.: Vena cava interruption for thromboembolism: partial or complete. Influence of cardiac disease upon results. Supplement to Circulation XXIX & XL: 263, May, 1969.

49. Mullick, S. C., and Wheeler, H. B.: Recurrent pulmonary emboli after inferior vena caval clipping. Amer. J. Surg., *119*:746, 1970.

50. Case Records of the Massachusetts General Hospital. New Eng. J. Med., *277*:360, 1967.

51. Amador, E., Khi, T. K., and Crane, C.: Ligation of inferior vena cava. Arch. Surg., *103*:272, 1971.

52. ———: Inferior vena cava ligation for thromboembolism clinical and autopsy correlations in 119 cases. JAMA, *206*:1758, 1968.

53. Cornett, V. E.: Personal communication, 1972.

54. Parrish, E. H., Pories, W. J., Adams, J. T., Burget, D. E., and DeWeese, J. A.: Pulmonary emboli following vena cava ligation. Arch. Surg., *97*:899, 1968.

55. McIntyre, K. M., Belko, J. S., and Sasahara, A. A.: Pulmonary embolism. Premonitory signs and recurrence after vena cava ligation. Arch. Surg., *98*:671, 1969.

56. Coupland, G. A. E., and Reeve, T. S.: Recurrent pulmonary emboli following inferior vena caval plication. Surgery, *67*:639, 1970.

57. Leather, R. P., Clark, W. R., Powers, S. R., Parker, F. B., Bernard, H. R., and Eckert, C.: Five year experience with the Moretz vena cava clip in 62 patients. Arch. Surg., *97*:357, 1968.

58. Mandel, S. R., Johnson, G., Jr., and Capps, J. H.: Angiographic, hemodynamic and clinical evaluation of partial occlusion of the inferior vena cava. Southern Med. J., *64*:647, 1971.

59. Moretz, W. H., Still, J. M., Jr., Griffin, L. H., Jennings, W. D., and Wray, C. H.: Partial occlusion of the inferior vena cava with a smooth teflon clip: Analysis of long term results. Surgery, (In Press) 1972.

60. Miles, R. M., and Elsea, P. W.: Clinical evaluation of the serrated vena caval clip. Surg. Gyn. Obst., *132*:581, 1971.

61. Moran, J. M., Kahn, P. C., and Callow, A. D.: Partial versus complete caval interruption for venous thromboembolism. Amer. J. Surg., *117*:471, 1969.

62. Little, J. M.: Inferior vena caval interruption for pulmonary embolism. Ann. Surg., *171*:250, 1970.

63. Shauble, J. F., Stickel, D. L., and Anlyan, W. G.: Vena caval ligation for thromboembolic disease. Arch. Surg., *84*:35, 1962.

64. Crane, C.: Femoral vs. caval interruption for venous thromboembolism. New Eng. J. Med., *270*:819, 1964.

65. Stevens, L. E., Fitzpatrick, W. K., Stewart, G. K., and Burdette, W. J.: Ligation of the inferior vena cava. Arch. Surg., *90*:578, 1965.

66. Piccone, V. A., Jr., Vidal, E., Yarnoz, M., Glass, P., and LeVenn, H. H.: The late results of caval ligation. Surgery, *68*:980, 1970.

67. Gurewich, V., Thomas, D. P., and Robinov, K. P.: Pulmonary embolism after ligation

of the inferior vena cava. New Eng. J. Med., *274*:1350, 1966.

68. Schowengerdt, C. G., and Schreiber, J. T.: Interruption of the vena cava in the treatment of pulmonary embolism. Surg. Gyn. Obst., *132*:645, 1971.

69. Moses, M., Adar, R., Bogokowsky, H., and Agmon, M.: Vein ligation in the treatment of pulmonary embolism. Surgery, *55*:621, 1964.

70. Mobin-Uddin, K.: Personal communication, 1972.

71. Gaston, E. A., III: Incorrect placement of prosthesis for pulmonary embolism. JAMA, *214*:2338, 1970.

72. Burget, D. E., Jr., Henzel, J. H., Smith, J. L., and Pories, W. J.: Inferior vena cava plication for prevention of pulmonary embolism: results in 24 cases. Ann. Surg., *165*:437, 1967.

73. Siegel, B., Popky, G. L., Mapp, E. M., Feigl, P., Felix, W. R., Jr., and Ipsen, J.: Evaluation of Doppler ultrasound examination. Arch. Surg., *100*:535, 1970.

Chapter 13 | Complications of

Seymour I. Schwartz, M.D. | ## Portal-Systemic Shunting Procedures

Decompression of the portal venous system to reduce hypertension was initially performed on an experimental basis by Nicolai Eck in 1877. The modern era of clinical application dates from 1945 when Whipple[1] and Blakemore and Lord[2] demonstrated the clinical feasibility of a shunting procedure. The ensuing quarter century saw an initial increase of enthusiasm as indications were extended from therapy for bleeding esophagogastric varices to treatment of ascites and prophylactic shunts for varices which had not bled. Subsequently, it became apparent that the prophylactic portacaval shunt was inappropriate, and enthusiasm for portal decompressive procedures as treatment for ascites waned when it was shown that most cases could be managed medically. This has left bleeding esophagogastric varices as essentially the sole indication for decompressive procedures. In addition, during the past 25 years concern for the immediate postoperative consequences and the long-term effects has increased. This discussion presents a general assessment of the efficacy of the various decompressive procedures and considers specific intraoperative problems, as well as complications which become apparent in the early postoperative period and those which persist.

Major Portal-Systemic Shunts

A wide variety of portal-systemic shunts, employing major and smaller vessels within the portal venous system, have been performed to reduce portal hypertension and decompress esophagogastric varices. The use of either small vessels or "makeshift shunts" which employ larger collaterals is inappropriate since the reduction of portal pressure is relatively insignificant and rarely permanent. Figure 13-1 offers a diagrammatic representation of the shunting procedures which have been shown to significantly and persistently reduce portal pressure. These include: (1) the end-to-side portacaval shunt; (2) the side-to-side portacaval shunt performed either directly, as a double-barreled shunt, or employing an H-graft between the portal vein and the inferior vena cava; (3) the splenorenal shunt, using the central end of the splenic vein; (4) the central side-to-side splenorenal shunt; (5) the reverse splenorenal shunt using the splenic end of the splenic vein, usually combined with ligation of the coronary vein and devascularization of the stomach; and (6) anastomoses between the inferior vena cava and superior mesenteric vein either as a direct end-to-side anastomosis or with the interposition of an H-graft.

Functionally, portal-systemic shunts have been categorized as either totally or partially diverting portal venous flow away from the liver and also as decompressing or failing to decompress intrahepatic venous hypertension.

The end-to-side portacaval shunt prevents blood from reaching the liver by providing

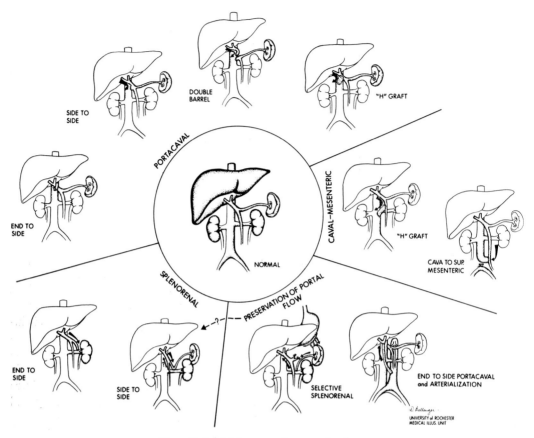

Fig. 13-1. Major portal systemic shunts.

complete drainage of the splanchnic venous circulation into the vena cava. The argument that this shunt deprives the liver of an important source of blood has been refuted by Madden.[3] The alteration of hepatic blood flow associated with this shunt is extremely variable, ranging from an increase of 34 percent to a decrease of 53 percent.[4] The end-to-side portacaval shunt also prevents the portal vein from serving as an efferent conduit from the liver. Regarding decompression of hepatic sinusoidal hypertension, Gliedman, *et al.*[4] have shown that following an end-to-side shunt, the wedged hepatic vein pressure and the prehepatic vein pressure declined in all of a series of 5 patients. Interestingly, ascites cleared in all of these patients. Ekman's series[5] has provided confirmation of these findings. Proponents of the end-to-side portacaval

shunt have indicated this as best preventing recurrent bleeding since it most completely decompresses the portal venous system's splanchnic circulation, including esophagogastric varices. However, Ferguson,[6] comparing the end-to-side and side-to-side portacaval shunts, demonstrated equal portal flow increases and equivalent reductions of portal pressure.

The concept that the side-to-side portacaval shunt provides the liver with portal venous flow is erroneous in most circumstances. It is true that when large boluses of radiopaque material are injected into the portal vein small amounts may be demonstrated in the intrahepatic tree. Longmire and associates[7] demonstrated by portal venography, employing 15 ml. radiopaque performed at surgery in patients with side-to-side portacaval shunts, that there was no material in the proximal vein while, using about 30 ml., some material could be identified in the cephalad portion of the portal vein. Radioisotope injected into the distal portal vein resulted in minimal recovery in the portal vein cephalad to a side-to-side anastomosis.

Evidence has accumulated that the side-to-side portacaval shunt converts the cephalad portion of the portal vein to an outflow tract from the liver. Britton, *et al.*,[8] Kraft and Fry,[9] and Viamonte and associates[10] have all provided angiographic demonstration of reverse flow from the liver through the side-to-side shunt. Whether decompression of the sinusoidal hypertension is greater with the side-to-side shunt than with the end-to-side shunt has not been defined. There is also concern whether the portal vein is beneficial or harmful as an efferent conduit. Longmire, *et al.*,[7] following injection of radioisotope into the hepatic artery, have shown rapid demonstration of the isotope in the cephalad limb of the portal vein and evidence of reflux of arterial blood, suggesting that the proximal portal vein may provide a siphon effect and reduce the blood available to the hepatic cell. On the other hand, Warren and Muller's[11] analysis of 3 patients exhibiting reversal of flow following a side-to-side shunt presented oxygen saturation data indicating that the blood leaving the portal vein was not arterial in nature and concluded that it had been used for hepatic function.

The classic end-to-side splenorenal shunt using the central end of the splenic vein also prevents flow of portal venous blood to the liver if it adequately performs its prescribed function of decompressing esophagogastric varices. The side-to-side anastomosis between the central splenic vein and the renal vein, proposed by Britton,[12] presumes that the shunt will selectively drain the lesser portal circulation, including varices, and that the kinetics of laminar flow in the superior mesenteric vein will favor flow into the liver rather than retrograde flow through the shunt. Salam and associates[13] have shown

that the side-to-side splenorenal shunt is similar to the side-to-side portacaval shunt in that it decompresses the portal circulation and does convert the portal vein into an outflow tract, completely abolishing portal venous flow. In addition, the side-to-side splenorenal shunt less completely decompresses portal venous hypertension.

The other functional side-to-side shunts, including the end-to-side inferior vena cava —superior mesenteric shunt and the interposition of an H-graft, have been thought by Read, *et al.*[14] and Drapanas,[15] based on angiographic evidence, to permit significant portal venous flow to enter the liver. This is contrary to hemodynamic expectations since the flow within the cephalad portion of the portal vein also should be away from high pressure hepatic venous sinusoids into the low pressure inferior vena cava if the functioning shunt is adequately decompressing esophagogastric varices within the portal venous system.

The distal splenorenal shunt proposed by Warren and associates[16] is the one precedure which can be classified as truly selective because it decompresses the esophagogastric varices while maintaining portal hypertension within the portal veins and hepatic sinusoids. Portal venous perfusion has been demonstrated in over 90 percent of patients with selective distal splenorenal shunts, and the total hepatic blood flow has been shown to be unchanged while splenic venous circulation and esophagogastric veins have been reasonably decompressed.[18]

Selection of Procedure

In most instances, preference for a surgical procedure is based on emotional and visceral reactions rather than on statistically valid data. With a readily accessible and "shunt-able" portal vein, the end-to-side portacaval shunt is most commonly performed. As it is the easiest shunt to perform, it is generally associated with the lowest incidence of thrombosis, which occurred in only four of 200 patients recorded by Child and Turcotte.[17] The presence of a large caudate lobe is less compromising to this procedure than to the side-to-side shunt. Mikkelsen, *et al.*[18] arbitrarily compared equal numbers of patients subjected to end-to-side or side-to-side shunts and concluded that the end-to-side shunt was associated with the lowest operative mortality. Malt reported in the discussion following the presentation of Jackson, *et al.*[19] that a three-year study revealed a significant difference in survival between patients with bleeding varices treated with end-to-side anastomosis and those medically treated. Patients with side-to-side shunts were no different from the control group.

The selection of a specific shunting procedure has been related to technical or pathologic factors, in addition to the specific manifestations of portal hypertension. In some cases with extensive adhesions from previous operative procedures in the right upper quadrant, the splenorenal or mesocaval shunts are the preferred procedures. Thrombosis with or without recanalization of the portal vein (cavanomentous transformation) generally precludes the portacaval anastomosis, although the author has performed a portal vein thrombectomy and an end-to-side portacaval anastomosis in two patients with fresh thrombi defined at surgery. The Budd-Chiari syndrome, whether related to a web in the inferior vena cava or to endophlebitis of the hepatic veins, dictates a side-to-side shunt to decompress the liver. To define whether the portal vein has been acting as a significant outflow tract requiring a side-to-side shunt to decompress hepatic sinusoids in the patient with cirrhosis, one can determine the portal pressure, apply a vascular clamp, and then remeasure the pressure on the cephalad limb. In the event that the portal vein is serving as a natural decompressive channel for the liver, portal pressure in the cephalad limb will be significantly increased, but in the author's experience, this is extremely rare. Reynolds[20] collated observations on the frequency of spontaneous reversal of portal vein flow

in portal hypertension. Only 20 of 286 patients had evidence of reversed flow.

In addition to bleeding esophagogastric varices, the other significant manifestations of portal hypertension include hypersplenism, ascites, and encephalopathy. Hypersplenism rarely dictates a splenorenal shunt, for several reasons. The splenorenal shunt is generally associated with a higher incidence of recurrent bleeding,[21] and in the majority of patients, hypersplenism is reversed following an adequate portacaval shunt. If the platelet count approaches zero, it is reasonable to perform a splenectomy and a splenorenal shunt in an attempt to reduce portal hypertension and obviate significant postoperative bleeding complications, holding the portacaval shunt in reserve for those patients with splenorenal shunt thrombosis.

It has been suggested that the side-to-side shunt, which decompresses the liver, is indicated for the patient with bleeding varices and ascites. This is largely based on the experimental model for ascites which employs partial obstruction of the suprahepatic inferior vena cava or direct obstruction of the hepatic veins. Sherlock in the Discussion following Orloff's report[22] has pointed out that one cannot extrapolate from this experimental model because it employs pure outflow block while the mechanism of cirrhosis is far more complex. Warren and Muller[11] could find no correlation between the level of intrahepatic pressure and the development of ascites. Of three patients with reversed flow in the portal vein, none had ascites, but one of four patients with normal directional flow had massive ascites. As mentioned previously, Gliedman and associates[4] reported that the end-to-side shunt significantly reduced hepatic sinusoidal pressure. Barker and Reemstma,[23] in an early report from Presbyterian Hospital, noted that the end-to-side shunt relieved the ascites of the majority of patients with bleeding esophagogastric varices and significant ascites, and in very few patients was ascites accentuated. A later report by Voorhees and associates[24] from the same hospital indicated that 39 percent of patients with end-to-side shunts who had preoperative ascites experienced postoperative relief, and in 12 percent of patients, ascites appeared after the shunt. All patients with side-to-side shunts and ascites had relief of ascites, and no ascites appeared later in this group. Interestingly, the splenorenal shunt, which is a functional side-to-side shunt, failed to relieve ascites in 12 percent of cases, and ascites appeared after the shunt in 16 percent of cases. Dispassionate evaluation of these figures indicates that ascites is not a significant factor in determining the type of shunt to be performed, except that it should preclude performance of the selective splenorenal shunt.[25]

Similarly, whether previous encephalopathy or the presence of asterixis is an important determinant of the type of shunt has not been resolved. While Hallenbeck, *et al.*[26] reported ammonia intoxication followed the end-to-side portacaval shunt in 25 percent of patients compared to a 5 percent incidence following splenorenal decompression, Mikkelsen and associates reported only 9 percent incidence of encephalopathy following the end-to-side shunt compared to 27 percent incidence after side-to-side shunting.[18] Zuidema, *et al.*[27] noted a significantly greater incidence of postoperative encephalopathy with the side-to-side than with the end-to-side portacaval shunt. Compilation of these figures does not provide conclusive data, but there is abundant evidence that the reduction in total effective hepatic blood flow is the important factor in the development of encephalopathy. This, combined with the now-accepted fact that the side-to-side shunt does not provide the liver with effective portal venous flow, suggests that there is no logical explanation for the advantage of either the end-to-side or the side-to-side portacaval shunt. The only procedures which specifically attack the problem of encephalopathy are the selective splenorenal shunt or the portacaval shunt with arterialization of the distal portal vein.[28]

Selection of Patients

Linton[29] was one of the first to emphasize the importance of the status of liver function on the patient's ability to tolerate portal systemic decompressive procedures. Ascites which failed to respond to medical therapy, a prothrombin time which remained prolonged after parenteral vitamin K, a serum albumin less than 3, a bilirubin greater than 1, and a bromsulphalein retention greater than 10 percent were all associated with poor operative prognosis. Zuidema and Child[30] divided patients into three groups, including those with good hepatic function (A), those with moderate hepatic function (B), and those with advanced disease and poor reserve (C). In group A are patients with serum bilirubin below 2, albumin above 3.5, no ascites, no neurologic disorders, and excellent nutrition. Patients in the B group have bilirubin between 2 and 3, albumin between 3 and 3.5, easily controlled ascites, minimal neurologic disorder, and good nutrition. In the C group, the bilirubin is above 3, the albumin is below 3, and the ascites are poorly controlled with advanced coma and wasting. The operative mortality following portacaval shunts in the A group was 0, in the B group 9 percent, and in the C group 53 percent.[30] Although Orloff[31] has reported early survival of 38 percent and long-term survival of 45 percent for patients subjected to emergency portacaval shunt for bleeding varices regardless of the presence of significant ascites, jaundice, or encephalopathy, it has been this author's general assessment that increasing jaundice, tense ascites, asterixis, or encephalopathy are all associated with a prohibitive mortality. At present, we do not shunt such patients.

In addition to evaluation of hepatic function, efforts have been made to assess the dynamics of hepatic flow when selecting both surgical patients and the appropriate shunt. Warren and associates[32] combined estimation of hepatic flow with radioactive gold, hepatic vein catheterization, splenoportography, visceral angiography, and occasional umbilical vein catheterization. Warren and other associates[33] divided patients into three groups according to hepatic vein wedge pressure. In stage 1, the hepatic vein wedge pressure is less than 15, and this group generally tolerates shunting poorly. Patients with established hypertension reflected in elevated wedge pressures greater than 15 tolerate the shunts more easily. Unfortunately the techniques of estimating hepatic blood flow are less reliable in patients with cirrhosis, and angiographic evaluation is qualitative and imprecise. In addition, there are crossovers between categories. Thus, it is still difficult to determine either which patients will tolerate shunting or the appropriate shunt.

Intraoperative Problems

Bleeding. Diffuse bleeding during the operative procedure may be related to technical factors, coagulation defects which frequently accompany cirrhosis, or a combination of the two. Preoperative assessment of the patient requires a platelet estimate or preferably a direct platelet count and evaluation of the coagulation factors. The most common hematologic cause of intraoperative bleeding is thrombocytopenia, and it is generally felt that the count must be below 70,000 to be significant. This may be corrected by administering frozen platelet packs, repeating the platelet count following 10 or 20 packs to determine the effect. If there is little change in the platelet count, removal of the spleen, which acts as a platelet sequestering or destructive organ, may be required. After this, additional platelet packs should be used. Deficiencies in specific coagulation factors can be corrected by administering the lacking factors. Fresh frozen plasma or fresh whole blood can be given if necessary. Fresh whole blood is certainly preferable to banked blood since it contains platelets and all coagulation factors and does not have the significant increase in ammonia level noted in banked blood, i.e., in which ammonia increases from a base of 50 micrograms to 580 micrograms within 21 days. Although

Grossi and associates[34] reported that a large proportion of surgical patients with cirrhosis had increased fibrinolytic activity which could be reversed by ϵ-aminocaproic acid, there is hesitancy to use this drug because of its potential for causing diffuse clotting and embolization. Mechanical control of the bleeding site is most important, since failure of control is the cause of diffuse bleeding in most instances.

Nonshunting Situation. An unusual complication, determined intraoperatively, is caval hypertension caused by hypertrophy or nodularity of the caudate lobe. This may be determined after shunting when what appears to be an excellent shunt does not reduce portal pressure to the level expected for normal caval pressure. However, it may be anticipated when an extremely large caudate lobe is encountered. In this case, it is imperative to determine pressure in the infrahepatic inferior vena cava before progressing with the shunt. The author has encountered one patient in whom elevated pressure in the infrahepatic cava prevented a shunting procedure; a recent case report by Welling and McDermott[35] recorded two such cases. This pathophysiologic situation precludes any conventional portal decompressive procedure. The only remaining approaches to bleeding varices in this circumstance are either transesophageal ligation, gastric devascularization, or esophagogastrectomy. Fonkalsrud, *et al.*[36] have successfully decompressed the portal venous system by anastomosing the splenic vein to the isolated pulmonary artery of the left lower lobe of the lung by means of an interposed teflon graft, a procedure applicable to this situation.

The Shunt

The usual principles which apply to vascular surgical procedures are particularly applicable to the establishment of a portal-systemic anastomosis. Kinking and extreme angulation of the portal vein are to be avoided, and occasionally splitting the pancreas is required to permit a gentle curve in the proximal por-

Fig. 13-2. End-to-side porta-caval shunt. (Schwartz, S. I.: Surgical Diseases of the Liver, New York, McGraw-Hill, 1964)

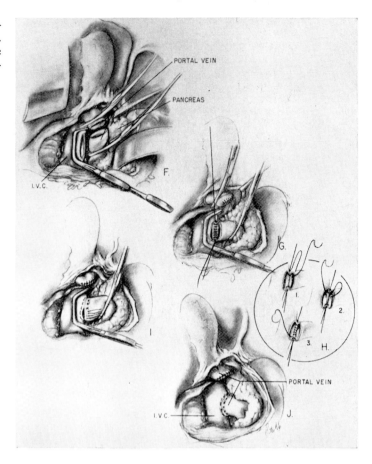

tal vein. An appropriate venotomy in the cava is one which is one and one-half times the diameter of the portal vein. Studies in our laboratory employing pressure determinations and latex casts have indicated that there is no need to remove an ellipse from the cava since an equivalent stoma results when a simple longitudinal venotomy one and one-half times the width of the portal vein is performed. The shunt is generally accomplished with a continuous silk suture interrupted at the craniad and caudad ends (Fig. 13-2). Following removal of the clamp, shunt patency should be assessed. Turbulence of caval flow is noted. Even if this is readily apparent, it is imperative to measure pressures with a spinal manometer in the infrahepatic cava and in the portal vein to demonstrate the absence of a significant gradient.

Postoperative Complications
Early Postoperative Complications

Rebleeding. Upper gastrointestinal bleeding after a shunt for acutely bleeding varices generally represents a continuation of the preoperative bleeding. This occurs more frequently in patients with advanced hepatocellular dysfunction and is related largely to a coagulation defect. The management of these patients is essentially the same as that prescribed for the nonoperative management of acutely bleeding varices.[37] We use iced saline gastric lavage, combined with continuous infusion of pitressin, 0.2 units/ml./min.,[38] directly into the superior mesenteric artery. If these measures fail, the Sengstaken-Blakemore triple lumen balloon is used to establish tamponade. The prognosis for this group of patients is extremely poor.

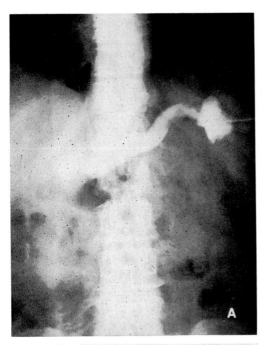

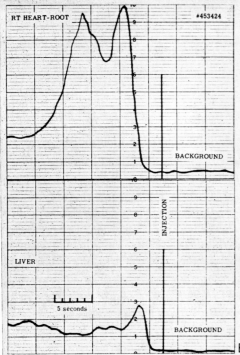

FIG. 13-3. Definition of shunt patency. (A) Splenoportagram showing patent end-to-side shunt and absence of collaterals. (B) Simultaneous tracings (50μ curies ^{131}I hipputope). Patent portacaval shunt. Transient peak recorded by hepatic probe reflects flow through retrohepatic inferior vena cava.

For the electively shunted patient, i.e., one whose varices have ceased bleeding prior to the operation, who rebleeds in the early postoperative phase, a differential diagnosis must be established between thrombosis of the shunt and peptic ulceration. In the great majority of cases, rebleeding is due to thrombosis of the shunt.[19,39] Duodenal ulcer infrequently causes early postoperative bleeding, and when peptic ulceration is indicted, it is usually of the stress ulcer variety.[40] The site of bleeding may be established by esophagoscopic evaluation of the esophagus and stomach or by angiographic studies, injecting the celiac artery to define gastric bleeding and injecting the superior mesenteric artery and noting the venous phase to define esophageal bleeding and persistence of collaterals. The yield from these angiographic procedures has been extremely low in our experience. The shunt patency may be assessed by determining the urinary excretion of a test dose of orally administered fructose.[41] For a more definitive assessment, splenic pulp manometry and a splenoportogram can determine patency of a portacaval shunt, or isotopic evaluation of the circulation can be performed by injecting a bolus of 0.5 ml. radioactive material directly into the spleen and counting simultaneously over the liver and the esophagus (Fig. 13-3).[42] These techniques pertain only to the portacaval and mesocaval shunts and, of course, cannot be applied to the splenorenal shunt. In the latter instance, it is possible to cannulate the left renal vein via the inferior vena cava and attempt to catheterize the shunt area, but this is usually very difficult.

If the shunt is assessed to be patent, therapy is directed at stress ulceration. This generally includes iced saline lavage and continuous pitressin infusions into the celiac artery, with which we have had significant success. If surgery is required, it should include a high subtotal gastrectomy combined with vagotomy. If shunt thrombosis is defined in a good risk patient, re-operation should be considered. One can directly take down a recently performed shunt, perform a thrombectomy, and anastomose the vessels or perform another decompressive procedure such as a mesocaval or splenorenal shunt.

Ascites. The appearance or persistence of ascites following a portal-systemic shunt suggests either insufficient reduction of hepatic sinusoidal pressure or impairment of hepatocellular function, both of which contribute to the formation of ascitic fluid. As mentioned previously, the theoretic advantage of the side-to-side shunt is decompression of sinusoidal venous hypertension. However, in the experience of Sherlock, et al.,[43] Mikkelsen and associates,[18] and Resnicoff and Schwartz,[39] the subsequent accentuation of ascites is unusual if an end-to-side shunt remains patent. Orloff, in a review of the literature,[44] has reported that 81 percent of survivors in whom end-to-side portacaval shunts were established for relief of ascites were subsequently free of ascites, and 90 percent of patients with side-to-side shunts for ascites were persistently clear of ascites. The difference between the two figures is not statistically significant. Wolfman and associates[45] studied the effects of side-to-side portacaval anastomoses on urinary sodium, water, and aldosterone excretion in a group of patients with cirrhosis of the liver and portal hypertension. Of four patients who retained 38 to 98 percent of sodium given preoperatively, sodium excretion was enhanced postoperatively; in two of these patients, this was not associated with decreased urinary excretion of aldosterone. These patients also showed definite improvement in excretion of sodium loads following side-to-side portacaval shunt. The sodium concentration in the urine increased while the urine volume showed no appreciable change from preoperative levels.

The management of patients with ascites is based on measures to improve hepatic function and treat the factors implicated in the formation of intraperitoneal fluid. A dietary regimen of low sodium intake (10 to 20 mEq daily) and a high protein, high caloric intake is essential. Although impaired water diuresis after water loading is well documented in the cirrhotic,[46] fluid restriction is not usually required. If there are symptoms of water intoxication associated with severe hyponatremia, water must be restricted and an osmotic diuretic administered.[47] Potassium supplements are provided to treat potassium depletion which frequently accompanies the formation of ascites. Salt-poor albumin is administered to raise the colloidal osmotic pressure. Albumin has also been administered by the intravenous infusion of autogenous ascitic fluid which has been concentrated or merely collected in vacuum tubes and reinfused.[48] However, this technique has limited practical value.[49] Wilkinson and Sherlock[50] have demonstrated in a controlled study that human albumin infusion over many months did not control fluid retention of patients receiving aldosterone antagonists, chlorothiazide and low salt diet. The diuretics generally employed include chlorothazide, spirinolactone, Furosemide, and ethacrynic acid. Although repeated adbdominal paracenteses in the ascitic patient with depleted albumin are to be condemned because of accentuated hyponatremia and danger of peritonitis, there is a distinct place for paracentesis in the patient who develops tense ascites in the immediate postoperative period. Since portal pressure directly parallels intraperitoneal pressure, removal of ascitic fluid results in reduction of the existing portal hypertension.[51]

Eisenmenger and Nickel[52] considered the complexity of salt, water, and steroid metabolism in the cirrhotic patient and reported several patients in whom peripheral edema developed following the shunting procedure although ascites did not recur. Read, et al.[53] reported edema of the ankle to be an extremely frequent complication of effective portal-systemic shunting, occurring in 10 of 20 patients in their series. These authors relate the process to a reduction in portal venous pressure so that fluid is no longer retained in the peritoneal cavity, accompanied by a reduction in colloid osmotic pressure related to the deterioration of hepatocellular function after surgery and impairment of albumin synthesis. Since inferior vena cava pressure does not increase following a successful portacaval or splenorenal shunt, venous hypertension does not contribute to the edema. The classic mesocaval shunt in the cirrhotic is associated with a high incidence of leg edema in the early postoperative course since caval flow is interrupted, compounding the problem.

Hepatic Failure. Hepatic function may deteriorate after a shunting procedure, and the incidence of postoperative hepatic failure is significantly higher in patients with advanced impairment of hepatic function prior to surgery.[30] Child's group A and B patients[30] normally tolerated decompressive procedures well. Although the serum bilirubin may become slightly elevated and serum albumin level depressed for a brief period of time, both generally return to normal without specific treatment. By contrast, group C patients may show startling elevations of the serum bilirubin and reductions of the serum albumin, requiring as much as 200 Gm. of albumin daily for two weeks following surgery in order to maintain a normal level. Coagulation factors may also be markedly reduced.

The relationship between anesthesia and hepatic damage is difficult to assess. Hypoxia, hypercapnea, and hypotension all contribute to hepatocellular damage. Whether the development of hepatic necrosis following halogenated anesthetic agents is statistically significant has not been totally resolved. Most studies suggest that the surgical procedure *per se* is a more significant factor than the anesthetic agent in the genesis of postoperative abnormalities of liver function.[54] Muscle relaxants do not contribute to hepatic damage.

The clinical manifestations of hepatic failure may include increasing jaundice and ascites, fetor hepaticus, oliguria, hypotension, asterixis, and encephalopathy. When coma occurs in the postoperative period, a mortality rate of 67 percent can be anticipated; if the coma is associated with continual postoperative variceal bleeding, the mortality rate is over 90 percent.[19]

The major discussion of postshunt encephalopathy will be presented in the section on Late Complications. General management of this complication in the early postoperative period includes maintenance of good nutrition with protein restriction. Studies by Crews and Faloon[55] have demonstrated that fat is not injurious to the liver and can provide significant calories. Nitrogenous materials should be eliminated from the gastrointestinal tract and neomycin administered to control the bacterial flora. Narcotics should be used sparingly, if at all. Improvement of a patient in postshunt hepatic coma has been reported with the use of L-dopa.[56] Use of this drug is based on the theory that hepatic coma is due to central neuronal derangement by replacement with false neurochemical transmitters. Since L-dopa represents a normal precursor material, administration in large doses may restore normal central nervous system stores of norepinephrine and dopamine. The author's experience with this drug is limited, but in the few patients to whom it was applied, no improvement in the coma was noted.

The various proposed treatments for Stage IV hepatic coma, including exchange transfusion,[57] pig liver perfusion,[58] baboon and human liver perfusion,[59] and recently popularized asanguineous hypothermic total body perfusion,[60] are logistically difficult and not applicable to the cirrhotic patient in the postshunt period since regeneration of normal liver tissue is not anticipated.

Hepatorenal Syndrome. This term has been applied to the occurrence of azotemia and oliguria in patients with severely decompensated liver disease unassociated with primary renal disease or obstructive uropathy. Renal failure following a portal-systemic decompressive procedure is not predictable from either clinical or laboratory data, but it is extremely uncommon in patients without ascites. Garrett, *et al.*[61] reported a 3 percent incidence in a series of 113 patients; all four patients developed ascites and gastrointestinal hemorrhage, and the complication represented 27 percent of the total operative mortality.

Suspected etiologic factors are renal sympathetic vasoconstriction, alteration in intrarenal blood flow, diminished effective plasma volume, and increased renal venous pressure, but none of these have been proved. Lack of consistent changes in renal histology suggests a functional defect, which has been substantiated by the fact that kidneys from patients dying with the hepatorenal syndrome are capable of normal function after transplantation.[62]

The syndrome is characterized by normal blood volume, high cardiac output with cardiac indices ranging between 4 and 6 L./min./M.[2], low peripheral resistance, and low urinary sodium excretion which is characteristically less than 10 mEq. There is dilutional hyponatremia and an elevation in the BUN which is out of proportion to the elevation of creatinine.

Renal failure associated with hepatocellular dysfunction developing after a shunting procedure carries a very grave prognosis, but is not always fatal, and the hyponatremia may reverse spontaneously. The prognosis is related primarily to the degree of reversibility of the hepatic disease, since renal function improves only in association with improved hepatic function. Death is often related to gastrointestinal bleeding, hepatic coma, and occasionally hyperkalemia. Treatment directed at correcting the renal failure itself is generally ineffective. Supportive measures, employed in hopes of allowing time for recovery of hepatic function, include restriction of fluid intake to prevent the dilutional state, restriction of sodium, and the avoidance of the use of paracentesis and diuretics in treatment of encephalopathy. In this regard, the substitution of another antibiotic for neomycin should be considered since absorption of small amounts of neomycin may have a nephrotoxic effect if renal function is impaired.[63] Dudrick, *et al.*[64] have reported the use of essential amino acids and hypertonic glucose hyperalimentation for patients with chronic renal failure. A positive nitrogen balance with a 50 percent reduction in the BUN level was achieved for periods up to 30 days.

Plasma volume expansion by intravenously administered albumin has provided little benefit. Dopamine has been used in an attempt to restore normal neurochemical transmitters, but this, too, has been ineffective.[65] Along similar lines, a beneficial effect of metaraminol, a direct-acting sympathomimetic amine, has been reported.[56,66] A proposed regimen[56] suggests the administration of metaraminol at rates of 200 to 1,000 micrograms per minute in order to raise the blood pressure arbitrarily by 30 to 40 mm. Hg. Each of the eight patients treated in this manner in one series[56] demonstrated increased peripheral vascular resistance, increased cardiac output, and increased sodium urinary excretion. Sugerman reported in the discussion following the presentation by Fischer and James[56] that three of six patients treated with metaraminol failed to respond, but three responded dramatically. The nonresponsive patients all had fulminating liver disease and markedly elevated serum bilirubin levels. The patients who did respond demonstrated increased renin substrate levels following therapy.

Late Postoperative Complications

Hemosiderosis. Although moderate hepatic hemosiderosis may develop in unshunted cirrhotic patients,[67] the portacaval shunt itself has been indicted as a cause of generalized hemosiderosis.[68,69] The full clinical picture of hemochromatosis has been noted to develop within three years of anastomosis in patients who had been free of hemosiderin at the time the shunt was constructed. Tisdale[68] reported that four of 20 shunted patients developed hemosiderosis, and a prospective study by Conn[70] recorded a 27 percent incidence of excessive hepatic hemosiderin accumulation in shunted patients as compared with only a 2 percent incidence in the nonshunted group. Pancreas, heart, adrenals, and kidneys also showed hemosiderin deposits in these patients. It has been suggested that this pathologic entity results from increased gastrointestinal absorption of dietary iron.[68] However, Doberneck, et al.[71] indicate that the increase in hepatic hemosiderin is more apparent than real, being due to weight loss, decline in red cell mass, and consequent hepatic storage of iron previously used in the production of hemoglobin. This is not supported by Conn's clinical observations,[70] which suggest that pancreatitis and hemolysis, the latter having been shown to cause hyperbilirubinemia following shunt,[72] contribute to increased iron absorption. Although Sherlock[43] has indicated that treatment, including chelating agents or phlebotomy, is rarely required, the fact that four of nine patients with post-shunt hemosiderosis in Conn's series[70] developed congestive heart failure and two developed diabetes suggests that therapy may be in order.

Peptic Ulcer. In the past, it had been an accepted fact that peptic ulceration occurred with greater frequency in cirrhotic patients and was further potentiated by an established shunt.[73,74,75,76] However, other reports have questioned a relationship between cirrhosis and the development of a peptic ulcer.[77,78,79] Thompson[80] collated several reported series and arrived at an incidence of 7.4 percent for peptic ulcer in nonshunted patients with cirrhosis.

The first evidence of an association between peptic ulceration and portacaval shunts was reported by Dubuque, et al.[81] who observed a 15 percent incidence of upper gastrointestinal ulceration in 60 patients following construction of the portacaval shunt. In Thompson's review of 14 papers,[80] an incidence of approximately 10 percent was noted following shunting procedures, but whether this represents an increase over the incidence for nonshunted cirrhotic patients was not established. A prospective evaluation by Orloff and associates[40] revealed a 12 percent incidence of peptic ulceration in cirrhotics, and all ulcers were located in the duodenum. The overall incidence in shunted patients was 27 percent, but the new ulcers in 12 of the 14 patients were superficial erosions of the acute stress ulcer type, and only two long-term survivors of the shunt operations developed chronic duodenal ulcers. In the combined and randomized series of Jackson, et al.,[19] there was no increase in ulcer disease in patients subjected to therapeutic portal-systemic shunts.

The effects of cirrhosis and portal-systemic shunting procedures on gastric secretions are as confusing as the incidence statistics. In 1933, Lebedinskaja[82] first noted increased acid output in dogs with Pavlov pouches following the construction of an Eck fistula. It was theorized that the shunting procedure prevented gastric secretagogues from being detoxified by the liver. Clarke and associates[83] demonstrated in experimentally prepared dogs that secretion of acid from a Heidenhain pouch was profoundly increased after portacaval transposition. Silen and Eiseman[84] presented evidence that histamine was responsible for the gastric hypersecretion occurring after shunting procedures. Ostrow, et al.[85] found no significant differences in the basal secretion, pepsin output, and the acid and pepsin responses to histamine in cirrhotic patients with shunts and in normal controls. Bendett, et al.[86] similarly reported no change in basal or histamine-stimulated secretion before and after shunting, while Schriefers, et al.[87] found no significant changes between basal and caffeine-stimulated gastric secretion before and after portacaval shunt. More recently, Orloff,, et al.[40] reported an enormous increase in acid secretion in shunted patients when food enters the stomach and postulated a potent intestinal hormone which stimulates the parietal cells of the stomach. In the nonshunted cirrhotic patients, the basal, food-stimulated and maximal histamine-stimulated acid secretions are all below normal.

The therapeutic implications of the incidence data and studies of gastric secretion raise the question whether any antacid regimen is required. The classic approach of placing patients on a diet generally prescribed for ulcer patients may not be appropriate.

Portal-Systemic Encephalopathy. Neuropsychiatric manifestations represent the most significant complication in the long-term management of patients after portal decompressive procedures. McDermott and Adams[88] were the first to draw attention to the relationship between a surgically created portacaval shunt and neuropsychiatric symptoms in man by reporting a patient in whom an Eck fistula had been constructed surgically after resection of the portal vein for invasive carcinoma of the pancreas. Portal-systemic encephalopathy is unusual in patients with portal hypertension secondary to obstruction of the extrahepatic portal venous system and is rarely seen before the age of 12.[89] The incidence in shunted cirrhotic patients has been reported to vary with etiology, age, patient selection, and operative procedure. It also varies with the criteria for establishing the diagnosis and the frequency of electroencephalography.

Voorhees and Price[90] reported an incident of postshunt encephalopathy of 44 percent in surviving patients and graded the complication as minimal in 10 percent, moderate in 23 percent, and severe in 11 percent. Minimal and moderate symptoms cleared either spontaneously or on medical therapy, but the severe symptoms failed to respond to treatment. The incidence was related to the duration of the follow-up period, with a 27 percent incidence reported for patients followed for less than five years and 56 percent incidence for patients followed longer. This has been substantiated by Sherlock and associates[43] who noted that while 42 percent of surviving patients developed encephalopathy during the first five years of follow-up, after that more than 72 percent of the patients had neuropsychiatric manifestations. Sherlock[91] noted an overall incidence of *significant* encephalopathy of about 20 percent. McDermott, *et al.*[92] reported neuropsychi-

atric manifestations in 19 percent of all shunted patients, but in only half of these were the symptoms incapacitating to any extent. Most patients responded promptly to protein restriction. Wantz and Payne[93] reported an encephalopathy incidence of 22 percent of shunted patients, while Zuidema, *et al.*[27] recorded an overall incidence of 21 percent.

Although Voorhees and Price[90] indicated the etiology of cirrhosis did not significantly influence the incidence of encephalopathy, Panke and associates[94] and Sherlock, *et al.*[43] reported higher incidences in the so-called cryptogenic and active chronic hepatitis groups compared with the alcoholic cirrhotics. Read and associates[53] stressed that more severe encephalopathy developed in older patients and were loath to suggest a shunt for patients over the age of 50. All studies have shown that encephalopathy occurs more frequently in patients who resume drinking, and the incidence also is significantly increased for diabetic patients.[19,90] As would be anticipated, postshunt encephalopathy occurs more frequently in patients with the greatest degree of hepatocellular dysfunction.[27,93]

Much controversy has centered around the relative effectiveness of various shunting procedures in reducing the incidence of postshunt encephalopathy. Following direct end-to-side portacaval anastomosis, the incidence ranges from 11 to 38 percent while portal encephalopathy has been reported in 5 to 19 percent of patients with splenorenal anastomoses.[89] Several authors[26,95,96] have stressed the fact that splenorenal shunts are associated with significantly lower incidences of encephalopathy than are portacaval shunts. By contrast, McDermott, *et al.*[92] noted approximately the same incidence of neurologic symptoms in patients subjected to the two types of shunts. In reference to portacaval shunts *per se*, Reynolds, *et al.*,[97] Panke, *et al.*,[94] and Zuidema, *et al.*[27] have reported the incidence of encephalopathy to be greater with side-to-side than with end-to-side portacaval shunts, while Voorhees and Price[90] noted no differences between the two procedures. The recent encouraging report from Warren's group[25] that, at most, only one patient had developed significant encephalopathy following a selective splenorenal decompressive procedure must be tempered by the fact that the number of patients, i.e., 31, is too small to provide significant statistical data.

The development of postshunt encephalopathy is related to the interaction of four major factors: (1) bacterial degradation of protein in the gastrointestinal tract, (2) hepatocellular impairment, (3) shunting of portal blood around the liver, and (4) status of the brain.

Dietary protein and blood present in the upper gastrointestinal tract are the major sources of intestinal nitrogen. These nitrogen-containing compounds are converted into ammonia by bacteria within the intestinal lumen. This usually occurs in the colon, but bacteria capable of producing ammonia and amines have been cultured from the small bowel as high as the jejunum in patients with cirrhosis.[98] In addition, some ammonia production from nonurea sources in the intestine occurs independent of bacterial action. The ammonia formed within the intestine is absorbed into the portal circulation, this occurring to the greatest extent in the colon. The portal circulation then carries the ammonia to the liver where it enters the Krebs-Henseleit ornithine-citrulline-arginine cycle and is converted into urea which is excreted by the kidney. The brain[99] and other tissues may contribute to detoxification of ammonia. In the cirrhotic patient, impaired hepatocellular function interferes with the conversion of ammonia into urea, and portal-systemic shunting of blood around the liver prevents action of the liver cell on ammonia and amines.

The clinical manifestations of portal-systemic encephalopathy include asterixis (liver flap), fetor hepaticus, tremor, abnormal behavior patterns, mental confusion, lapses of consciousness, and eventually the development of organic psychosis and coma. Certain objective tests may be used to evaluate the patient's condition. These include the serial 7 test, handwriting analysis, simple construction tests, plus the electroencephalogram and blood ammonia level determination.

Therapy is generally multifaceted and directed at the etiologic factors. The protein substrate on which bacteria can act may be initially reduced by using cathartics and enemas to purge the gastrointestinal tract. If active bleeding has occurred, infused pitressin plays a dual role in temporarily stopping the bleeding and also stimulating the motility and evacuation of the gut. Dietary protein intake should be reduced; in some instances 20 Gm. may be all that can be handled.

Bacteria within the bowel should be reduced by administering nonabsorbable antibiotics such as neomycin or kanamycin. In the presence of renal disease, kanamycin is preferred since there is less associated renal toxicity. In patients with severe renal impairment, chlortetracycline is more appropriate as it is not excreted primarily by the kidney.

Diuretics which may induce hypokalemia have been implicated in clinical deterioration since the hypokalemia may raise the blood ammonia level independent of the ammonia derived from the gastrointestinal tract. In this circumstance, the clinical manifestations are improved by the administration of potassium. Alkalosis, which frequently accompanies potassium depletion, also increases total ammonia production and shifts ammonia into tissues.

Results of lactulose treatment of hepatic encephalopathy have been encouraging.[100,101] This sugar acts as a mild cathartic and, in addition, the products of its oxidation by bacteria include lactic and acetic acids which lower the pH of the colon and interfere with ammonia transfer across colonic mucosa. Since the colon is the site of most of the bacterial degradation of protein and most of the ammonia absorption into the portal circulation, the initial suggestion of Atkinson, et al.[102] to surgically resect the colon in cases of intractable portal-systemic encephalopathy has logic. Voorhees and Price[90] collected 23 cases in which failure of medical treatment to control disabling neuropsychiatric symptoms prompted varying degrees of colectomy. The combined operative mortality of 26 percent and the effectiveness of more conservative approaches probably account for the relative infrequency of this operative approach. In 17 survivors of partial colectomy followed for 4 to 26 months, the symptomatic improvement was good to excellent in all instances, and the amount of dietary protein which was tolerated improved dramatically. Resnick, et al.[103] studied a matched group of 38 patients, randomly selecting half for colon bypass. The longevity figures for the two groups were identical, and the dietary protein tolerance and encephalopathy control slightly favored the bypass group.

The possibility of stimulating the liver's intrinsic mechanism for detoxifying ammonia has fostered the use of glutamic acid and arginine. Although success has been reported following the use of glutamic acid for patients in hepatic coma,[104] controlled studies have failed to demonstrate any consistent benefits such as lowered blood ammonia or neurologic improvements.[105,106,107] Similarly, although some investigators[108,109] indicate that arginine is effective, control studies have failed to demonstrate consistent clinical improvement or significant lowering of the blood ammonia.[110,111]

Attempts to dilute or remove toxic substances in the blood stream include hemodialysis, exchange transfusion, cross-circulation, isolated liver perfusion, and asanguineous hypothermic total body perfusion. Sherlock[112] was unable to demonstrate any permanent clinical benefits from hemodialysis. As mentioned previously, the other techniques depend on rapid regeneration of a normal liver, which essentially precludes their use for the cirrhotic patient.

The brain of the patient with liver disease is extremely sensitive to insult, and neuropathologic abnormalities, including widespread proliferation of protoplasmic astrocytes, have been demonstrated.[113] Opiates and barbiturates should be withheld since these drugs induce significant EEG changes in precomatose patients.

Prognosis and Justification of Shunting Procedures

The prognosis in reference to both 30-day postoperative mortality and long-term survival is related in large part to the extent of underlying liver disease. Of Child's Group A patients,[30] 90 percent were alive at five years and 70 percent survived ten years following an end-to-side shunt, while 50 percent were alive four years following a side-to-side shunt. For Group B patients, both the end-to-side and side-to-side shunts were associated with 80 percent survival at three years. Survival for the end-to-side group at seven years was 55 percent, but there were no long-term survival data for the side-to-side group. For Group C patients, the three-year survival of both end-to-side and side-to-side shunted patients was approximately 20 percent. Wantz and Payne[21] reported that 89 percent of Group A and B patients who survived 30 days after surgery were alive at the time of follow-up, 2 to 11 years after operation.

However, these data do not address themselves to the salient problem—whether the portacaval shunt is preferable to medical management. There is little question of the efficacy of the shunt in preventing rebleeding, but many have felt that the number of long-term survivors is disappointingly small, most patients dying of hepatic failure. Conn's review of more than 300 reported cases of emergency portacaval shunts[114] revealed a mortality rate ranging from 20 to 71 percent with an average of 39 percent, which compared favorably with 66 percent mortality generally expected for variceal hemorrhage. Orloff's compilation from many sources[31] reported that 73 percent of cirrhotics die during the hospitalization following the first hemorrhage from esophageal varices. In his own experience, the 30-day survival for the medically treated patients was 14 percent, as was the four-year survival rate. Of the patients subjected to emergency portacaval shunts, 53 percent left the hospital, and 43 percent were alive at four years.

Significant data comparing the relative efficacies of medical management and elective portacaval shunting, i.e., not performed at the time of bleeding, have been reported by only two series to date. Jackson, in the Veterans Administration Hospital series[19] considered male cirrhotic patients under the age of 65 who had bled and in whom bleeding had ceased. True randomization was carried out. Only 36 percent of the entire medical group had survived, while 57 percent of those with portacaval shunts were living. In the Discussion following Jackson's article, Malt reported the unpublished data of the Boston Inter-Hospital Liver Group. Although there were no initial differences between the medically and surgically treated patients, after 3½ years survival for patients with end-to-side anastomoses was 56 percent versus a 20 percent survival for those medically treated. This difference is significant at the 0.05 probability level.

In summary, this presentation has focused on the complications associated with portal-systemic shunting procedures. They are many and diverse, and they certainly demand the attention of surgeons performing these operations. At this point in time and considered in the light of statistically significant data, these complications do not negate the value of shunting procedures for esophagogastric varices which are actively bleeding or have bled. A sanguine (hopeful, not bloody) approach on the part of the surgeon is appropriate.

References

1. Whipple, A. O.: Problem of portal hypertension in relation to hepatosplenopathies. Ann. Surg., *122*:449, 1945.
2. Blakemore, A. H., and Lord, J. W.: The technic of using vitallium tubes in estab-

lishing portacaval shunts for portal hypertension. Ann. Surg., *122*:476, 1945.
3. Madden, J. L.: Conversion of the portal vein to an "outflow tract" is a misnomer. Surg. Gynec. Obstet., *117*:499, 1963.
4. Gliedman, M. L., Sellers, R. D., Burkle, J. S., and Enquist, I. F.: Cirrhosis with ascites: Hemodynamic observations. Ann. Surg., *155*:147, 1962.
5. Ekman, C. A.: Portal hypertension. Acta Chir. Scand. Suppl. 22, 1957.
6. Ferguson, D. J.: Hemodynamics in surgery for portal hypertension. Ann. Surg., *158*:383, 1963.
7. Longmire, W. P., Mulder, D. D., Mahoney, P. S., and Mellinkoff, S. W.: Side-to-side portacaval anastomosis for portal hypertension. Ann. Surg., *147*:881, 1958.
8. Britton, R. C., Voorhees, A. B., and Price, J. B.: Perfusion of the liver following side-to-side portacaval shunt. Surgery, *62*:181, 1967.
9. Kraft, R. O., and Fry, W. J.: Demonstration of hepatofugal flow following portacaval anastomosis. Surg. Gynec. Obstet., *118*:124, 1964.
10. Viamonte, M., Jr., Warren, W. D., Fomon, J. J., and Martinez, L. O.: Angiographic investigations in portal hypertension. Surg. Gynec. Obstet., *130*:37, 1970.
11. Warren, W. D., and Muller, W. H., Jr.: A clarification of some hemodynamic changes in cirrhosis and their surgical significance. Ann. Surg., *150*:413, 1959.
12. Britton, R. C.: Surgical treatment of complications of portal hypertension. Ann. N.Y. Acad. Sci., *170*:358, 1970.
13. Salam, A. A., Warren, W. D., LePage, J. R., Viamonte, M. R., Hutson, D., and Zeppa, R.: Hemodynamic contrasts between selective and total portal-systemic decompression. Ann. Surg., *173*:827, 1971.
14. Read, R. C., Thompson, B. H., Wise, W. S., and Murphy, M. L.: Mesocaval H venous homografts. Arch. Surg., *101*:785, 1971.
15. Drapanas, T. H.: To be published in Ann. Surg., 1972.
16. Warren, W. D., Zeppa, R., and Fomon, J. J.: Selective trans-splenic decompression of gastroespohageal varices by distal splenorenal shunt. Ann. Surg., *166*:437, 1967.
17. Child, C. G., and Turcotte, J. G.: Surgery and portal hypertension. *In* Child, C. G. (ed.): The Liver and Portal Hypertension, Vol. 1 in Major Problems in Clinical Surgery, Philadelphia, Saunders, 1964.

18. Mikkelsen, W. P., Turrill, F. L., and Pattison, A. C.: Portacaval shunt in cirrhosis of the liver. Amer. J. Surg., *104*:204, 1962.

19. Jackson, F. C., Perrin, E. B., Felix, W. R., and Smith, A. G.: A clinical investigation of the portacaval shunt: V. Survival analysis of the therapeutic operation. Ann. Surg., *174*:672, 1971.

20. Reynolds, T. B.: Hepatic circulatory changes after shunt surgery. Ann. N.Y. Acad. Sci., *170*:379, 1970.

21. Wantz, G. E., and Payne, M. A.: The emergency portacaval shunt. Surg. Gynec. Obstet., *109*:549, 1959.

22. Orloff, M. J.: Pathogenesis and surgical treatment of intractable ascites associated with alcoholic cirrhosis. Ann. N.Y. Acad. Sci., *170*:213, 1970.

23. Barker, H. G., and Reemtsma, K.: Portacaval shunt operation in patients with cirrhosis and ascites. Surgery, *48*:142, 1960.

24. Voorhees, A. B., Jr., Price, J. B., Jr., and Britton, R. C.: Portasystemic shunting procedures for portal hypertension: 26-year experience in adults with cirrhosis of the liver. Amer. J. Surg., *119*:501, 1970.

25. Warren, W. D.: Personal communication.

26. Hallenbeck, G. A., Wollaeger, E. E., Adson, M. A., and Gage, R. P.: Results after portal-systemic shunts in 120 patients with cirrhosis of the liver. Surg. Gynec. Obstet., *116*:435, 1963.

27. Zuidema, G. D., Kirsh, M. M., and Gaisford, W. D.: Hepatic encephalopathy. *In* Child, C. G. (ed.): The Liver and Portal Hypertension, vol. 1 in Major Problems in Clinical Surgery, Philadelphia, Saunders, 1964.

28. Maillard, J. N., Benhamou, J. P., and Rueff, B.: Arterialization of the liver with portacaval shunt in the treatment of portal hypertension due to intrahepatic block. Surgery, *67*:883, 1970.

29. Linton, R. R.: The selection of patients for portacaval shunts. Ann. Surg., *134*: 433, 1951.

30. Zuidema, G. D., and Child, C. G.: Current status of portal decompression. *In* Popper, H., and Schaffner, F. (eds.): Progress in Liver Diseases, vol. 1, New York, Grune & Stratton, 1961.

31. Orloff, M. J.: Emergency treatment of bleeding esophageal varices in cirrhosis. *In* Longmire, W. P. (ed.): Portal Hypertension, Current Problems in Surgery. Chicago, Year Book Publishers, 1966.

32. Warren, W. D., Fomon, J. J., Viamonte, M., and Zeppa, R.: Preoperative assessment of portal hypertension. Ann. Surg., *165*:999, 1967.

33. Warren, W. D., Restrepo, J. E., Respess, J. C., and Muller, W. H.: The importance of hemodynamic studies in management of portal hypertension. Ann. Surg., *158*: 387, 1963.

34. Grossi, C. E., Rousselot, L. M., and Panke, W. F.: Control of fibrinolysis during portacaval shunts. JAMA, *187*:1005, 1964.

35. Welling, R. E., and McDermott, W. V., Jr.: Combined caval and portal hypertension with cirrhosis of the liver: A problem in management. To be published.

36. Fonkalsrud, E. W., Linde, I., and Longmire, W. P., Jr.: Portal hypertension from idiopathic superior vena caval obstruction. JAMA, *196*:129, 1966.

37. Schwartz, S. I.: Liver. *In* Schwartz, S. I. (ed.): Principles of Surgery, New York, McGraw-Hill, 1969.

38. Nusbaum, M., Baum, S., Kuroda, K., and Blakemore, W. S.: Control of portal hypertension by selective mesenteric arterial drug infusion. Arch. Surg., *97*:1005, 1968.

39. Resnicoff, S. A., and Schwartz, S. I.: Portal decompressive surgery: Comparative evaluation of patients with Laennec's cirrhosis and other causes. Arch. Surg., *97*: 371, 1968.

40. Orloff, M. J., Chandler, J. G., Alderman, S. J., Keiter, J. E., and Rosen, H.: Gastric secretion and peptic ulcer following portacaval shunt in man. Ann. Surg., *170*:515, 1969.

41. Martin, L. W., and Bryant, L. R.: The use of fructose to determine the patency of portal-systemic shunts. Arch. Surg., *85*: 783, 1962.

42. Schwartz, S. I., and Greenlaw, R. H.: Evaluation of portal circulation by percutaneous splenic isotope injection. Surgery, *50*:833, 1961.

43. Sherlock, S., Hourigan, K., and George, P.: Medical complications of shunt surgery for portal hypertension. Ann. N.Y. Acad. Sci., *170*:392, 1970.

44. Orloff, M. J.: Surgical treatment of intractable cirrhotic ascites. *In* Longmire, W. P. (ed.): Portal Hypertension, Current Problems in Surgery. Chicago, Year Book Publishers, 1966.

45. Wolfman, E. F., Jr., Kowalczk, R. S., and Trevino, G.: Salt, water and adrenal steroid metabolism. *In* Child, C. G. (ed.):

The Liver and Portal Hypertension, Philadelphia, Saunders, 1964.

46. Schedl, H. P., and Bartter, F. C.: An explanation for and experimental correction of the abnormal water diuresis in cirrhosis. J. Clin. Invest., *39*:248, 1960.

47. Shaldon, S., and Sherlock, S.: Resistant ascites treated by combined diuretic therapy (spironolactone, mannitol and chlorothiazide). Gut, *1*:609, 1960.

48. King, H., Kaiser, G. C., King, R. D., and Lempke, R. E.: Ascitic fluid infusion: A method and apparatus for the treatment of ascites. JAMA, *184*:108, 1963.

49. Yamahiro, H. S., and Reynolds, T. B.: Effects of ascitic fluid infusion on sodium excretion, blood volume, and creatinine clearance in cirrhosis. Gastroenterology, *40*:497, 1961.

50. Wilkinson, P., and Sherlock, S.: The effect of repeated albumin infusions in patients with cirrhosis. Lancet, *2*:1125, 1962.

51. Mewett, J. W., and Schwartz, S. I.: Evaluation of portal circulation via subcutaneously translocated spleen. Surg. Forum, *18*:400, 1967.

52. Eisenmenger, W. J., and Nickel, W. F.: Relationship of portal hypertension to ascites in Laennec's cirrhosis. Amer. J. Med., *20*:879, 1956.

53. Read, A. E., Laidlaw, J., and Sherlock, S.: Neuropsychiatric complications of portacaval anastomosis. Lancet, *1*:961, 1961.

54. French, A. B., Barss, T. P., Fairlie, C. S., Bengle, A. L., Jones, C. M., Lenton, R. R., and Beecher, H. K.: Metabolic effects of anesthesia in man. V. A comparison of the effects of ether and cyclopropane anesthesia on the abnormal liver. Ann. Surg., *135*:145, 1952.

55. Crews, R. H., and Faloon, W. W.: The fallacy of a low-fat diet in liver disease. JAMA, *181*:754, 1962.

56. Fischer, J. E., and James, J. H.: Treatment of hepatic coma and hepatorenal syndrome: Mechanism of action of L-dopa and Aramine. Amer. J. Surg., *123*:222, 1972.

57. Trey, C., and Davidson, C. S.: The management of fulminant hepatic failure. *In* Popper, H., and Schaffner, F. (eds.): Progress in Liver Diseases, vol. III, New York, Grune & Stratton, 1970.

58. Eiseman, B., Liem, D. S., and Raffucci, T.: Heterologous liver perfusion in treatment of hepatic failure. Ann. Surg., *162*:329, 1965.

59. Abouna, G. M., Cook, J. S., Fisher, L. McA., Still, W. J., Costa, G., and Hume, D. M.: Treatment of acute hepatic coma by ex vivo baboon and human liver perfusions. *71*:537, 1972.

60. Klebanoff, G., Hollander, D., Cosimi, A. B., Stanford, W., and Kemmerer, W. T.: Asanguineous hypothermic total body perfusion (TBW) in the treatment of stage IV hepatic coma. J. Surg. Res., *12*:1, 1972.

61. Garrett, J. C., Voorhees, A. B., Jr., and Sommers, S. C.: Renal failure following portasystemic shunt in patients with cirrhosis of the liver. Ann. Surg., *172*:218, 1970.

62. Koppel, M. H., Cobrun, J. W., Matlock, M. M., Goldstein, H., Boyle, J. D., and Rubini, M. E.: Transplantation of cadaveric kidneys from patients with hepatorenal syndrome: Evidence for the functional nature of renal failure in advanced liver disease. New Eng. J. Med., *280*:1367, 1969.

63. Kunin, C. M., Chalmers, T. C., Leevy, C. M., Sebastyen, C., Lieber, C. S., and Finland, M.: Absorption of orally administered neomycin and kanamycin: With special reference to patients with severe hepatic and renal disease. New Eng. J. Med., *262*:380, 1960.

64. Dudrick, S. T., Steiger, E., and Long, J. M.: Renal failure in surgical patients: Treatment with intravenous essential amino acids and hypertonic glucose. Surgery, *68*:180, 1970.

65. Bernardo, D. E., Baldus, W. P., and Maher, F. T.: Effects of dopamine on renal function in cirrhosis. Gastroenterology, *58*:524, 1970.

66. Sugarman, H. J., Berkowitz, H. D., Davidson, D. T., and Miller, L. D.: Treatment of the hepatorenal syndrome with metaraminol. Surg. Forum, *21*:359, 1970.

67. Williams, R., Williams, H. S., Scheuer, P. J., Pitcher, C. S., Loiseau, E., and Sherlock, S.: Iron absorption and siderosis in chronic liver disease. Quart. J. Med., *36*:151, 1967.

68. Tisdale, W. A.: Parenchymal siderosis in patients with cirrhosis after portasystemic shunt surgery. New Eng. J. Med., *265*:928, 1961.

69. Schaefer, J. W., Amick, C. J., Oikawa, Y., and Schiff, L.: The development of haemochromatosis following portacaval shunt. Gastroenterology, *42*:181, 1962.

70. Conn, H. O.: Portacaval anastomosis and hepatic hemosiderin deposition: A prospective, controlled investigation. Gastroenterology, *62*:61, 1972.

71. Doberneck, R. C., Kline, D. G., Morse, A. S., and Berman, A.: Relationship of hemosiderosis to portacaval shunting. Surgery, *54*:912, 1963.

72. DaSilva, L. E., Jamra, M. A., Maspes, V., Pontes, J. F., Pieroni, R. R., and Cintra, A. B. deU.: Pathogenesis of indirect reacting hyperbilirubinemia after portacaval anastomosis. Gastroenterology, *44*:117, 1963.

73. Koide, S. S., Texter, E. C., Jr., and Bordon, C. W.: Perforation of peptic ulcer following paracentesis in patients with cirrhosis. Amer. J. Digest. Dis., *3*:24, 1958.

74. Fainer, D. C., and Halsted, J. A.: Sources of upper alimentary tract hemorrhage in cirrhosis of the liver. JAMA, *157*:413, 1955.

75. Swisher, W. P., Baker, L. A., and Bennett, H. D.: Peptic ulcer in Laennec's cirrhosis. Amer. J. Digest. Dis., *22*:291, 1955.

76. Clarke, J. S., Ozeran, R. S., Hart, J. C., Cruze, K., and Crevling, V.: Peptic ulcer following portacaval shunt. Ann. Surg., *148*:551, 1958.

77. MacDonald, R. A., and Mallory, G. K.: The neutral history of postnecrotic cirrhosis. A study of 221 autopsy cases. Amer. J. Med., *24*:334, 1958.

78. Thompson, J. C., and Peskin, G. W.: The intestinal phase of gastric secretion. Amer. J. Med. Sci., *241*:253, 1961.

79. Scobie, B. A., and Summerskill, W. H. J.: Reduced gastric acid output in cirrhosis: Quantitation and relationship. Gut, *5*:422, 1964.

80. Thompson, J. C.: Alterations in gastric secretion after portacaval shunting. Amer. J. Surg., *117*:854, 1969.

81. Dubuque, T. J., Jr., Mulligan, L. V., and Neville, E. C.: Gastric secretion and peptic ulceration in the dog with portal obstruction and portacaval anastomosis. Surg. Forum, *8*:208, 1958.

82. Lebedinskaja, S. I.: Gastric secretion in dogs with Eck's fistula. Ztschr. ges. exper. Med., *88*:264, 1933.

83. Clarke, J. S., McKissock, P. K., and Cruze, K.: Studies on the site of origin of the agent causing hypersecretion in dogs with portacaval shunt. Surgery, *46*:48, 1959.

84. Silen, W., and Eiseman, B.: The nature and cause of gastric hypersecretion following portacaval shunts. Surgery, *46*:38, 1959.

85. Ostrow, J. D., Timmerman, R. J., and Gray, S. J.: Gastric secretion in human hepatic cirrhosis. Gastroenterology, *38*:303, 1960.

86. Bendett, R. J., Fritz, H. L., and Donaldson, R. M.: Gastric acid secretion after parenterally and intragastrically administered histamine in patients with portacaval shunt. New Eng. J. Med., *268*:511, 1963.

87. Schriefers, K. H., Schreiber, H. W., and Esser, G.: Zur Frage der Magensaftsekretion und des Magen-Duodenalulcus beim Pfortaderhochdruck der Lebercirrhose und nach porto-cavalen Shunt-Operationen. Arch. klin. Chir., *302*:702, 1963.

88. McDermott, W. V., Jr., and Adams, R. D.: Episodic stupor associated with an Eck fistula in man, with particular reference to ammonia metabolism. J. Clin. Invest., *33*:1, 1954.

89. Schwartz, S. I.: Surgical Diseases of the Liver. New York, McGraw-Hill, 1964.

90. Voorhees, A. B., and Price, J. B., Jr.: Surgical treatment of hepatic encephalopathy. Ann. N.Y. Acad. Sci., *170*:259, 1970.

91. Sherlock, S.: Neuropsychiatric changes following porta-systemic shunting. *In* Colston, A. E. R. (ed.): The Liver, London, Butterworth, 1967, p. 241.

92. McDermott, W. V., Jr., Palazzi, H., Nardi, G. L., and Monde, A.: Elective portal systemic shunt: An analysis of 237 cases. New Eng. J. Med., *265*:419, 1961.

93. Wantz, G. E., and Payne, M. A.: Experience with portacaval shunt for portal hypertension. New Eng. J. Med., *265*:721, 1961.

94. Panke, W. F., Rousselot, L. M., and Burchell, A. R.: A sixteen-year experience with end-to-side portacaval shunt for variceal hemorrhage: Analysis of data and comparison with other types of portasystemic anastomoses. Ann. Surg., *168*:957, 1968.

95. Linton, R. R., Ellis, D. S., and Geary, J. E.: Critical comparative analysis of early and late results of splenorenal and direct portacaval shunts performed in 169 patients with portal cirrhosis. Ann. Surg., *154*:446, 1961.

96. Grace, N. D., Muench, H., and Chalmers, T. C.: The present status of shunts for portal hypertension in cirrhosis. Gastroenterology, *50*:684, 1966.

97. Reynolds, T. B., Hudson, N. M., Mikkelsen, W. P., Turrill, F. L., and Redeker,

A. C.: Clinical comparison of end-to-side and side-to-side portacaval shunt. New Eng. J. Med., *274*:706, 1966.

98. Martini, G. A., Phear, E. A., Ruebner, B., and Sherlock, S.: Bacterial content of small intestine in normal and cirrhotic subjects: Relation to methionine toxicity. Clin. Sci., *16*:35, 1957.

99. Sporn, M. B., Dingman, W., and Defalco, A.: Method for studying metabolic pathways in brain of intact animal: Conversion of proline to other amino acids. J. Neurochem., *4*:141, 1959.

100. Brown, H., Trey, C., and McDermott, W. V., Jr.: Lactulose treatment of hepatic encephalopathy in outpatients. Arch. Surg., *102*:25, 1971.

101. Price, J. B., Jr., Schwartz, G. F., Molavi, A., Britton, R. C., and Voorhees, A. B., Jr.: The mechanism and clinical significance of intestinal ammonia transport. Surg. Forum, *28*:331, 1967.

102. Atkinson, M., and Gligher, J. C.: Recurrent hepatic coma treated by colectomy and ileorectal anastomosis. Lancet, *1*:461, 1960.

103. Resnick, R. H., Chambers, T. C., Ishibara, A. M., Garceau, A. J., Callow, A. D., Schimmel, E. M., and O'Hara, E. T.: A controlled study of the prophylactic portacaval shunt. A final report. Ann. Intern. Med., *70*:675, 1969.

104. Eiseman, B., Bakewell, W., and Clark, G.: Studies in ammonia metabolism. I. Ammonia metabolism and glutamate therapy in hepatic coma. Amer. J. Med., *20*:890, 1956.

105. Summerskill, W. H. J., Wolfe, S. J., and Davidson, C. S.: The management of hepatic coma in relation to protein withdrawal of certain specific measures. Amer. J. Med., *23*:59, 1957.

106. Sherlock, S.: Pathogenesis and management of hepatic coma. Amer. J. Med., *24*:805, 1958.

107. Schwartz, R., Jr., Lehman, E., Hammond, J., Seibel, J. M., and Goldson, F.: Failure of monosodium glutamate in treatment of hepatic coma. Gastroenterology, *30*:869, 1956.

108. Najarian, J. S., and Harper, H. A.: Etiology and treatment of ammonia intoxication associated with disease of the liver. Surg. Gynec. Obstet., *106*:577, 1958.

109. Manning, R. T., and Delp, M.: Management of hepatocerebral intoxication. New Eng. J. Med., *258*:55, 1958.

110. Fazekas, J. F., Ticktin, H. E., and Shea, J. G.: Effects of L-arginine on hepatic encephalopathy. Amer. J. Med. Sci., *234*:462, 1957.

111. Reynolds, T. B., Redeker, A. G., and Davis, P.: Controlled study of effects of L-arginine on hepatic encephalopathy. Amer. J. Med., *25*:359, 1958.

112. Sherlock, S.: Hepatic coma. Gastroenterology, *41*:1, 1961.

113. Adams, R. D., and Foley, J. M.: The neurological disorder associated with liver disease. Res. Publ. Ass. Nerv. Ment. Dis., *32*:198, 1953.

114. Conn, H. O.: The prognosis and management of bleeding esophageal varices. Ann. N.Y. Acad. Sci., *170*:345, 1970.

Chapter 14

Cornelius Olcott IV, M.D.
F. William Blaisdell, M.D.

Postoperative Hemorrhage and Coagulation Disorders

Proper hemostasis is fundamental to all surgical operations. Bleeding or inappropriate clotting is responsible for the majority of the complications following vascular surgery. These complications may consist of massive hemorrhage at one extreme or immediate thrombosis of the vascular reconstruction on the other.

Some of the related complications are less obvious. Postoperative infection may result because of a wound hematoma. Pulmonary embolism can be catastrophic with cardiovascular collapse or may produce a subtle type of respiratory insufficiency which is recognized only upon careful physiologic monitoring. Many of the cardiovascular and respiratory derangements which were attributed previously to the "stress of the operation" are now recognized as being secondary to coagulation changes and thromboembolic phenomena.

Normally, hemostasis is assured by three factors: vascular reactivity, platelet function and coagulation. A number of factors related to vascular surgery may interfere with one or more phases of normal hemostasis. The use of anticoagulants will hinder normal coagulation, while synthetic arterial grafts lack a normal vessel's ability to vasoconstrict. The presence of liver disease may interfere with normal coagulation as it is the site of synthesis of all or most of the coagulation factors. Intravascular coagulation, a syndrome being recognized with increasing fre-

quency, may result in the increased utilization of platelets and clotting factors as well as the release of fibrin degradation products (FDP's) which may interfere with normal fibrin production and polymerization. Multiple transfusions, so frequently necessary in major vascular surgery, may result in impaired hemostasis secondary to abnormal platelet function and possibly abnormally low levels of coagulation factors.

Hence, the surgeon is absolutely dependent upon normal hemostasis to carry out successful vascular surgery and yet he may know surprisingly little about the fundamental assessment of bleeding and coagulation problems. This is the subject of this chapter.

The Normal Hemostatic Mechanism

The steps leading to normal hemostasis involve the following: (1) vasoconstriction; (2) platelet adhesion to the connective tissue of the injured vessel, followed by platelet aggregation; and (3) the formation of the fibrin clot.[1]

Vascular contraction is a poorly understood and primitive means of providing hemostasis. Arteries and arterioles with their inner elastic and muscular coats have the capacity to telescope inwardly as the intima and media of the blood vessel wall

Supported in part by NIH Grant GM-18470 and a Bay Area Heart Research Committee grant.

335

retract pulling the adventitial coat over the divided end of the vessel.

As for the smaller vessels, Quick has postulated that injury of the microcirculation results in a generation of cholinesterase. This hydrolyzes acetylcholine and abolishes the vasodilatory component of the autonomic nervous system, thereby making the vaso-constricting action of epinephrine dominant. The application of heat is presumed to shorten the bleeding time by enhancing the activation of cholinesterase, while cold lengthens the bleeding time by slowing cho-linesterase activation, hence the rationale for the application of warm packs to de-crease diffuse bleeding.[2]

Release of serotonin by platelets aggre-gating on the raw collagen of the vessel ends, and vasoactive peptides formed in the conversion of fibrinogen to fibrin may also enhance the local vasoconstriction and aid hemostasis.

The platelet is responsible for the initial hemostatic plug. Platelets adhere to the con-nective tissue underlying the injured en-dothelium. This leads to release of adenosine diphosphate (ADP) from the platelets which stimulates further platelet aggrega-tion resulting in a platelet plug. Several of the widely used medications are capable of interfering with normal platelet aggregation and therefore may interfere with primary

TABLE 14-1. INHIBITORS OF
PLATELET AGGREGATION

I. Anti-inflammatory Agents
  A. Aspirin
  B. Phenylbutazone

II. Antihistamines
  A. Cyproheptadine
  B. Diphenhydramine
  C. Pyrilamine maleate
  D. Chlorpheniramine maleate
  E. Promethazine hydrochloride

III. Local Anesthetics
  A. Cocaine
  B. Lidocaine
  C. Dibucaine

IV. Antidepressants and Tranquilizers
  A. Imipramine
  B. Desipramine
  C. Amitriptyline
  D. Nortriptyline
  E. Chlorpromazine
  F. Promethazine
  G. Diphenhydramine

V. Miscellaneous
  A. Dextran
  B. Dipyridamole
  C. Clofibrate
  D. Hematoporphyrin
  E. Fibrin degradation products

hemostasis (Table 14-1). This aspect of plate-let function may be measured at the bedside by means of the bleeding time or by specific tests for platelet adhesion (e.g., the Salzman glass bead test[3]) and aggregation.[4]

The platelets also furnish platelet factor 3 which is essential for the proper functioning of the coagulation system (Fig. 14-1). The fourth major function of the platelets is their role in clot retraction which is a function of their contractile protein, thrombosthenin.

Clot Formation. The coagulation system, which produces the fibrin clot, can be divided into two systems (Fig. 14-1). This intrinsic system is set off by the activation of Hageman Factor XII, which in turn results in the acti-vation of Factors XI, IX, VIII, and X, each as a result of a proteolytic reaction. This system is characteristically stimulated by contact of Factor XII with vessel-wall connective tis-sue and hence its action parallels the above

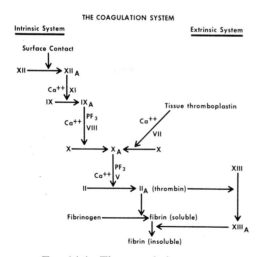

FIG. 14-1. The coagulation system.

described platelet activity. The extrinsic system is activated by the combination of tissue thromboplastin and Factor VII, which also results in the activation of Factor X. Activated Factor X, Factor V, calcium, and platelet Factor III together comprise the "prothrombin converting principle" which is responsible for the conversion of prothrombin to thrombin. Thrombin, also by a proteolytic action, attacks fibrinogen to release two pair of peptides and fibrin monomer. This fibrin monomer then normally polymerizes to form fibrin. Fibrin is subsequently broken down by the fibrinolytic enzyme plasmin to produce fibrin degradation products. The fibrin monomer molecule, in the absence of adjacent monomer, may join up with either a fibrinogen molecule or a fibrin degradation product to produce soluble fibrin monomer complexes (SFMC's).[5,6] As will be discussed below, identification of these large molecular weight substances may be important in detecting the "hypercoagulable state."[7]

Among the popular screening tests used to measure activity of the coagulation system are the prothrombin time and the activated partial thromboplastin time (PTT). The prothrombin time measures activity in the extrinsic system, particularly Factors V, VII, X, and II. The PTT measures activity in the intrinsic system.[1]

Factors Responsible for Thrombosis of Vascular Reconstructions

The primary problem which challenges successful vascular reconstruction is thrombosis. An enhanced tendency for thrombosis may be secondary to: (1) technical aspects of the operation; (2) presence of out-flow disease; (3) any of the factors which may function to enhance coagulation (e.g. raw surfaces, low flow, tissue damage, transfusions, sepsis, and shock). One or more of these factors may contribute to the unwanted thrombosis of the reconstruction.

Technical Aspects

In our experience, the most common cause of thrombosis of an arterial reconstruction is a technical error at the time of the vascular procedure. For the past ten years, therefore, we have routinely carried out angiography on the operating table following completion of the vascular repair. Inevitably, some technical factor is responsible for immediate graft thrombosis. "Spasm" is not a primary event; it should not be used to explain a poor result. When an operative arteriogram demonstrates a good technical result, postoperative spasm does not occur and failure of the reconstruction is rare. Usually the problem seen on the arteriogram is narrowing of the anastomosis, elevation of plaques, damage of the vessel lining from occluding clamps, peripheral thrombosis or embolism. For this reason thrombosis of a vascular reconstruction calls for immediate re-exploration, removal of the thrombus, correction of any technical defect, and re-establishment of flow. Operative arteriography is mandatory if the cause of the reconstruction failure is not immediately evident.

Outflow Disease

Vascular surgeons have long recognized the importance of outflow disease in contributing to failure of a vascular reconstruction. This is due primarily to decreased flow through the graft, leading to an increased tendency to thrombosis (see below). Complete pre-operative arteriographic evaluation including specific attention to outflow vessels is fundamental. This evaluation combined with selection of only those patients with adequate outflow to support the vascular reconstruction will prevent this complication.

Enhanced Coagulation

In addition to technical problems and the presence of other vascular disease, several interrelated factors may also contribute to thrombosis of the reconstruction.

Low flow tends to promote thrombosis due to build-up of platelet aggregates on raw or irregular arterial surfaces or on the synthetic graft. Rapid flow dilutes the local concentration of activated clotting factors and mechanically opposes the spread of the growing platelet mass.[8,9]

When low flow is combined with *metabolic acidosis,* which occurs in tissues deprived of an adequate blood flow and oxygenation, there is an increased clotting tendency.[10,11] As a result, when there is stasis, created by temporarily occluding the arterial flow for vascular surgery or secondary to poor perfusion from hypovolemia or poor cardiac function, combined with acidosis in the peripheral tissues, clotting is enhanced in the peripheral arterial and venous segments. In operations, such as those carried out for occlusive disease, where collateral flow has developed, distal thrombosis is rare. When surgery is performed for nonocclusive vascular disease, such as peripheral embolism or aneurysm, collateral flow is not well developed and hence low flow and acidosis may be expected. For this reason, systemic or local heparin should be utilized in vascular procedures associated with occlusion times longer than ten minutes or when the adequacy of peripheral collateral flow is in question. Absence of vigorous back-bleeding when the distal arterial clamp is removed can be used as a guide. When back-bleeding shows even a minor pulsatile component, collateral flow is excellent and no adjunctive measures to prevent distal thrombosis are necessary.

Shock is by definition a low flow state with inadequate tissue perfusion. It will produce a metabolic acidosis and stimulate catecholamine release. It can, if severe, produce tissue damage. Low flow, acidosis, catecholamines, and tissue damage all aggravate or directly produce a tendency for intravascular clotting. For this reason, shock associated with any vascular operation may result in intravascular coagulation. The ruptured abdominal aortic aneurysm is a classical example of this type of problem. If hypovolemia has been severe prior to operation, the vascular surgeon's best efforts to save the patient may be frustrated by the factors which promote intravascular coagulation and the full range of clotting and

bleeding complications which are associated with it.

Exposed collagen is the primary initiator of platelet adhesion, and a lining of platelets rapidly builds up on any raw surface exposed to the blood stream. If flow is good, the thickness of this lining is limited; however, low flow in the immediate postoperative period, or stasis during prolonged cross-clamping, may lead to excessive build-up of platelets and fibrin in ulcerated segments of arteries.[12]

Tissue damage, when present, as in those conditions associated with acute arterial ischemia, may release into the blood stream tissue factors which stimulate clotting. Tissue thromboplastins combined with a low flow state may lead to "hypercoagulability" or if severe, to intravascular clotting. For this reason, operations carried out to relieve an acute arterial occlusion, arterial embolism being a prime example, have a higher rate of postoperative thromboembolic complications than elective procedures. The surgical literature documents that the mortality rate of operations carried out for advanced ischemia approaches 25 percent.[13] We believe that much of this mortality and morbidity is due to unsuspected thromboembolic complications resulting from wash-out of small clots and by-products of coagulation from the distal vascular bed at the time of reperfusion of the ischemic extremity.[13]

Blood transfusions, especially if massive, introduce cellular debris and the risk of transfusion reaction with hemolysis.[11,14] Both are potentiators of clotting. Ordinarily, blood transfusion is benign. When circumstances require massive transfusion, however, the above factors may help to initiate intravascular clotting.

Infection, particularly septicemia, can produce intravascular coagulation.[15,16] Gram-negative endotoxin activates the coagulation system and many of the effects of septic shock may be related to the subsequent coagulation changes. When sepsis complicates a vascular reconstruction, or when surgery must be carried out in the face of sepsis, one must remain aware of the possibility of an increased clotting tendency.

The Spectrum of Intravascular Coagulation

Normal hemostasis is the result of a balanced interplay between the coagulation system, the function of natural inhibitors to clotting and clot lysis. Abnormal intravascular coagulation is usually prevented by circulating inhibitors to the various clotting factors and by the reticuloendothelial system, especially the liver, which functions to remove activated clotting factors from the circulation. The normal lytic mechanism (fibrinolysis) destroys any clot.

During vascular surgery, any of the factors described in the previous section may become operative, resulting in a breakdown of this delicate interrelationship and leading to various degrees of intravascular coagulation from the "hypercoagulable state" to frank disseminated intravascular coagulation. The latter has been defined by McKay as ". . . a biologic process involving many chemical substances and physiologic responses. It begins with the entry of a procoagulant material or activity into the circulating blood; it progresses to the stage of platelet aggregation and fibrin formation which may or may not result in thrombosis of capillaries, arterioles, and venules of various organs; it is associated with activation of the fibrinolytic enzyme system with dissolution of fibrin and fibrinogen and the release of fibrin-split products into the plasma; and it is not complete until the hemostatic mechanism and vasomotor apparatus have returned to normal and the last signicant amount of fibrin-split product has been cleared from the blood."[17,18]

In the mildest form of intravascular coagulation there may be *no discernible effect.* A small amount of thrombin released into the vascular system may produce fibrin monomer (Fig. 14-2) which in the absence of adjacent fibrin monomer may combine with fibrinogen or fibrin degradation products to form soluble fibrin monomer complexes. These complexes, while not actual clot, are analogous to a supersaturated solution which if given a slight additional stimulus, i.e. further fibrin monomer production, can then progress to normal fibrin polymerization and clot formation.

Thrombosis of the distal arterial bed may be present. This may occur if the period of arterial occlusion is prolonged without proper anticoagulation, particularly if there is any ulceration or irregularity of the normal endothelial lining. This usually results in immediate failure of the arterial reconstruction. Once good flow is re-established the clotting tendency is reversed and minor thrombotic defects seen on arteriograms will clear.

Thrombosis of the distal venous system may occur. Since stasis and acidosis are

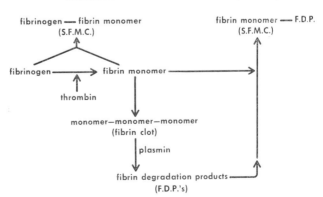

FORMATION OF FIBRIN DEGRADATION PRODUCTS (F.D.P.'s)
AND
SOLUBLE FIBRIN MONOMER COMPLEXES (S.F.M.C.'s)

FIG. 14-2. Formation of fibrin degradation products (F.D.P.'s) and soluble fibrin monomer complexes (S.F.M.C.'s).

greatest on the venous side, the tendency for thrombosis during vascular reconstruction or following arterial occlusion is probably greatest in this system. Thromboembolic events limited to the venous system may remain occult and hence less obvious than on the arterial side. Following reconstitution of arterial flow, any clot or by-product of coagulation may be washed into the venous circulation and carried to the lung.[13]

Undoubtedly, small amounts of clot are readily well tolerated by the venous system and even clot released into the circulation may be rapidly removed by the reticuloendothelial system and fibrinolysis or may be filtered out by normal lungs with minimal disability. On the other hand, the clot may organize and initiate thrombophlebitis and its sequelae, pulmonary embolism or late venous insufficiency.

Atelectasis has been a common complication of vascular surgery. This was ascribed to the length of the operation or the elderly status of the patient. Our observations suggest that this may be due to thromboembolism in many instances.[19] As clot is washed into the venous circulation and deposited into the pulmonary arterioles these fibrin-platelet aggregates, and the vasoactive substances they release, produce vasoconstriction and bronchoconstriction.[20] The latter may result in atelectasis. The closure of lung units subsequently increases stasis in the pul-

monary circulation with a tendency for pulmonary thrombosis to increase.

If the patient's pulmonary reserve is marginal or if the fibrinolytic or reticuloendothelial system is not functioning properly, the impact of the venous clot may be profound. The full syndrome of gross pulmonary embolism, or microembolism (Fig. 14-3) will result depending upon the age and size of the clot.

Thrombosis of other organ systems may also develop. Involvement of the kidneys may lead to renal cortical necrosis.[11] This is most apt to occur if the patient is hypovolemic and renal blood flow is decreased. This leads to renal failure which may be mild or severe. The ready availability of renal dialysis in most centers allows for support of these patients long enough to prevent mortality and to permit recovery of renal function. Prevention can usually be ensured by careful postoperative monitoring of the urine output and using renal function as a guide in volume replacement.

Thrombosis of the submucosal vessels of the gastrointestinal tract may also occur. The gastric mucosa is particularly vulnerable and intravascular coagulation in its submucosal vessels may result in superficial mucosal ulcerations, i.e. "stress ulcers." A recent review of the histologic sections from patients with stress ulcers seen at the San Francisco General Hospital revealed platelet-

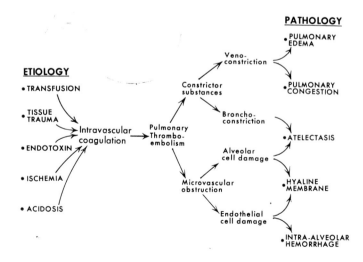

FIG. 14-3. Pathogenesis of the hemorrhagic lung syndrome secondary to intravascular coagulation. (Blaisdell, F. W., *et al.*: Surg., Gynec. & Obstet., *130*:15, 1970)

FIG. 14-4. Histological section of gastric mucosa demonstrating stress ulcer with fibrin thrombi in the mucosal capillaries. (PTAH stain, ×100)

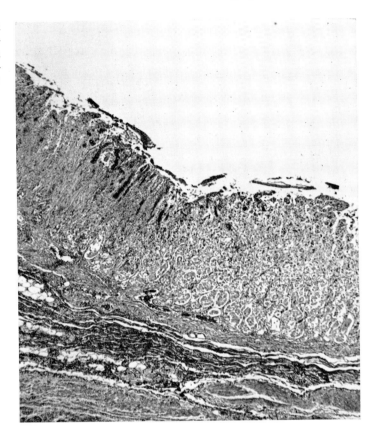

fibrin thrombi in 70 percent of sections taken through areas of gastric ulceration[21] (Fig. 14-4).

The liver can also be affected by intravascular coagulation. In fact, Regocczi and Brain found it to be the second most common site for fibrin deposition during experimental intravascular coagulation set off by a thrombin infusion.[22] This, of course, can trip off a vicious circle of events in that damage to the liver from thrombosis will lead to decreased synthesis of clotting factors and decreased phagocytic activity which is important for the removal of activated clotting factors and fibrin degradation products.[23,24]

Finally and paradoxically intravascular coagulation can lead to bleeding secondary to "anticoagulation" due to fibrin degradation products and/or consumption of clotting factors (see below).

Bleeding Syndromes

Etiology of Bleeding

Diffuse oozing may develop any time following the onset of the operation, especially in patients in whom shock has developed, e.g. hemorrhagic shock associated with a ruptured aneurysm or regional shock occurring in conjunction with severe ischemia. The source of bleeding may be *technical,* e.g. secondary to a slipped ligature or a defect in the vascular anastomosis, or secondary to a *hemostatic defect,* either congenital or acquired. Adult patients without an antecedent history of abnormal bleeding, particularly following surgery, can usually be relied upon not to have a congenital bleeding disorder.

If generalized bleeding develops immediately after the incision is made, anticoagulants may be responsible. Excluding anticoagulants, other reasons for an acquired hemostatic defect include: Multiple transfusions, platelet dysfunction, liver disease, vitamin K deficiency and intravascular coagulation. If unexplained bleeding develops, blood should be drawn for a hemostatic work-up. One tube should be left at the bedside to observe clot formation and retraction.

If laboratory studies can be obtained, a prolonged partial thromboplastin time suggests a defect somewhere in the intrinsic coagulation system (Fig. 14-1), while a prolonged prothrombin time suggests a defect in the extrinsic system. Alterations in both tests will reflect a defect in liver function and/or vitamin K deficiency.

A platelet count above 50,000 indicates an adequate level of platelets for primary hemostasis, provided platelet function is normal.[25] However, many factors affect platelet function. Many of the anti-inflammatory agents, particularly aspirin, block the platelet release reaction and hence interfere with platelet aggregation. A number of other drugs (Table14-1) also interfere with platelet aggregation including: certain local anesthetic agents, antihistamines, and dextran.[26,27] Therefore, effectively to rule out platelet dysfunction in the etiology of bleeding, specific studies of platelet function, as described earlier, should be carried out.

Massive blood transfusion can occasionally be incriminated as a contributing factor in bleeding. Ordinary blood transfused in the operating room is often days to weeks old. This blood may contain low levels of labile clotting Factors V and VIII and platelets. However, in the absence of intravascular coagulation critical deficiencies of Factors V and VIII rarely develop simply from multiple transfusions.[28,29] Most of the problems of massive transfusion relate to platelet deficiency or dysfunction and produce a defect in primary hemostasis.[28,29,30] Absence of platelets on a blood smear, platelet counts below 50,000, prolonged bleeding times, or poor clot retraction support this possibility. It should be kept in mind that the platelet count can be normal and platelet function remain faulty. Therefore, unless tests of platelet function are performed, this possibility cannot be excluded.

Generally speaking, any deficiency related to blood transfusion is rare when the transfusion does not exceed ten units of blood. Above this amount exchange transfusion can be considered to be well under way and continued transfusion with old blood can produce difficulty. As a result, we attempt to obtain at least two to four units of fresh blood if more than ten units of blood have to be administered.

Intravascular coagulation may occur following major vascular surgery and result in massive consumption of platelets and coagulation factors. Bleeding in these cases results from the decreased levels of platelets and coagulation factors and from the presence of fibrin degradation products, which will interfere with normal fibrin clot formation.[31,32] This type of coagulopathy is likely to occur in cases in which shock has occurred, the operation has been technically difficult, vascular occlusion time has been prolonged, and transfusion extensive. Should clotting factors and platelets drop to critical levels and/or fibrin degradation products increase, diffuse oozing can develop over all raw surfaces in the operative field.

Secondary hemorrhage may occur due to lysis of clot in the arterial graft interstices or at suture lines resulting in diffuse bleeding after initial hemostasis has appeared adequate. Primary fibrinolysis is a rare event, however, and any increased fibrinolysis is usually secondary to disseminated intravascular coagulation and treatment should be directed against the latter. For this reason the use of an antifibrinolytic agent, such as epsilon-aminocaproic acid, is contraindicated.

Treatment of Bleeding Syndromes

When diffuse bleeding becomes manifest in the operating room or in the immediate postoperative period, the first step should be to determine its cause. This essentially involves going through the differential diagnosis outlined above. Excluding a technical error, the most common cause for this problem in our experience is either multiple transfusions or intravascular coagulation.

If multiple transfusions are felt to be the problem, the primary defect probably lies in platelet function.[28,29] This can best be treated with either platelet packs or fresh, warm whole blood from walk-in donors. Blood which has been cooled or which is greater than eight hours old is defective in platelet function and therefore not useful in the treatment of this situation.[33,34] Only fresh blood will simultaneously correct platelet function and reinstitute hemostatic levels of the labile clotting factors.

If the diagnosis of intravascular coagulation is entertained, the first step is to remove the stimulus for clotting, e.g. shock and sepsis. In the meantime, if the episode is severe, heparin should be administered to prevent further intravascular coagulation, permit the clotting factors and platelets to return to normal levels, and allow clearance of the fibrin degradation products. During this time hemostasis will be dependent upon platelet function and hence platelet packs or fresh whole blood may be useful if platelet function is compromised. Heparin should be continued until the stimulus for clotting has been eliminated, the clotting factors have returned to normal levels, and the fibrin degradation products have been cleared. Following discontinuation of heparin, coagulation studies should be followed closely to ensure that intravascular coagulation does not recur.

Heparin. Heparin is an absolute anticoagulant. For this reason it is difficult to titrate relative degrees of partial anticoagulation with this drug. Most experts believe, however, that clotting times are indicated primarily to ensure that adequate doses of heparin have been given to accomplish anticoagulation. Lesser amounts may not prevent clotting. The problem is that the anticoagulation effect of heparin cannot be titered accurately by any of the common tests, including the Lee-White clotting time. This is particularly true when the coagulation system is being influenced by other factors such as multiple transfusions or intravascular coagulation. When we wish to anticoagulate a patient as therapy for a thromboembolic event, we prefer to err on the side of excess. Our usual anticoagulating dose is 10,000 units of heparin given intravenously followed by 2,000 units per hour. We prefer to give maintenance heparin by a continuous intravenous infusion. A constant infusion pump, such as is used in hyperalimentation, is a great asset in this regard. Our observations in cardiac and vascular surgery suggest that high doses of heparin are necessary to prevent further intravascular coagulation. There is some recent evidence, however, that when heparin is given prophylactically, smaller doses, e.g., 5,000 units every 12 hours, may be sufficient.[35,36] However, this may be useful only in those cases where heparin is begun prior to actual triggering of the coagulation system.

Three tests are commonly used in our hospital for routine determination of heparin activity. The first, and by far the least accurate, is the Lee-White clotting time. The second is the activated coagulation time (ACT) as described by Hattersley.[15] This test is carried out in pre-packaged tubes containing diatomaceous earth which immediately activates the intrinsic clotting system, thus obviating one of the variables in the Lee-White system. The normal ACT ranges from 1 min. 21 sec. to 2 min. 13 sec. The fully anticoagulated patient will have an ACT between three and a half to five minutes. This test has several advantages over the Lee-White method. It requires less time to carry out, it is performed in a constant temperature dry bath, and it has immediate activation of the intrinsic clotting system. It is also readily suitable for bedside use.

The third commonly used test is the partial thromboplastin time (PTT).[38,39] This test is easily performed in the routine clinical laboratory, and because it is performed by trained personnel under uniform conditions it is probably the most accurate.

When we desire to know the exact plasma

level of heparin, such as in cases of intravascular coagulation or when other clotting derangements are present, we utilize a protamine sulfate dilution technique described by Weiss.[40] In these cases we attempt to maintain a heparin level of one to two units per milliliter of plasma.

Regardless of the accuracy of control of heparin therapy, a few patients will develop a bleeding complication. The incidence of this can, however, be curtailed by ensuring that no platelet-paralyzing agents are given in conjunction with heparin (Table 14-1).

Heparin can be immediately counteracted at any time by the administration of protamine sulfate. We utilize 0.5 to 1.0 mg. protamine sulfate for each 100 units of heparin administered in the previous four to six hours. The calculated dose should be administered slowly over five to ten minutes intravenously.

Pre-Clotting Vascular Grafts

For elective vascular reconstruction we use grafts with the largest pore size compatible with reasonable hemostasis. The newer, light-weight knitted Dacron fabrics appear optimal in this regard. The appropriate graft is selected at the start of the procedure and when the major vessels are exposed, sufficient blood is aspirated to saturate the graft. This is particularly advantageous if one wishes to use heparin during the period of vascular occlusion. After completion of the first anastomosis of the by-pass or replacement graft, the graft is once again preclotted under pressure. The proximal occluding clamp is released by degrees until the anastomosis is dry and until the bleeding from the graft-to-artery anastomosis has subsided. At this point the proximal circulation is again occluded and clot is aspirated from the graft and the distal anastomosis is carried out.

When large grafts are required, such as those needed for aortic replacement, systemic heparin may be inadvisable because of the risk of extensive bleeding from the pores of the graft. In these instances, smaller doses (1,000 to 3,000 units) are injected into the distal vascular bed at the time of the arterial occlusion. When operations are performed for acute ischemia or aneurysm rupture, we believe that systemic anticoagulation is necessary. In this instance we use closely woven grafts for more secure hemostasis. Preclotting with blood drawn prior to anticoagulation is carried out if possible.

Summary

The scope and complexity of vascular surgery has increased immensely in the past two decades. With this, vascular surgeons have become more familiar with coagulation disorders following major surgery. As this chapter points out, these disorders can be broken down into two broad categories: increased thrombotic tendency, and bleeding. Both of these may arise from technical aspects of the operation, but in certain cases these may be secondary to derangements in the coagulation system. Only careful evaluation of both technique and changes in the hemostatic mechanism will allow the surgeon to properly diagnose the problem and treat it appropriately.

References

1. Macfarlane, R. G.: The hemostatic mechanism and its defects. Internatl. Rev. Exp. Path., *6*:55, 1968.
2. Quick, A. J.: Hemostasis in surgical procedures. Surg. Gynec. Obstet., *128*:523, 1969.
3. Salzman, E. W.: Measurement of platelet adhesiveness. J. Lab. Clin. Med., *62*:724, 1963.
4. Born, G. V. R., and Cross, M. J.: The aggregation of blood platelets. J. Physiol., *168*:178, 1963.
5. Kopec, M., Wegrzyhowicz, Z., and Latallo, Z. S.: Soluble fibrin complexes and a new specific test for their detection. Thromb. Diath. Haemorrh. Supp., *39*:219, 1970.
6. Lipinski, B. A., Wegrzyhowicz, Z., *et al.*: Soluble unclottable complexes formed in the presence of fibrin degradation products during the fibrinogen-fibrin conversion and their potential significance in pathology. Thromb. Diath. Haemorrh., *17*:65, 1967.
7. Fletcher, A. P., Akljaersig, N., O'Brien, J., and Tuleuski, V. G.: Blood hypercoagula-

bility and thrombosis. Trans. Ass. Amer. Phys., *83*:159, 1970.

8. Deykin, D.: Thrombogenesis. New Eng. J. Med., *276*:622, 1967.

9. Deykin, D.: Local and systemic factors in the pathogenesis of thrombosis. Calif. Med., *112*:31, 1970.

10. Broersma, R. J., Bullemer, G. D., and Mammen, E. F.: Acidosis induced disseminated intravascular microthrombosis and its dissolution by streptokinase. Thromb. Diath. Haemorrh., *24*:55, 1970.

11. Hardaway, R. M.: Syndromes of Disseminated intravascular coagulation. Springfield, Thomas, 1966.

12. Brinkhous, K. M., and Scarborough, D. E.: Some mechanisms of thrombin formation and hemorrhage following trauma. J. Trauma, *9*:684, 1969.

13. Stallone, R. J., Blaisdell, F. W., Cafferata, H. T., and Levin, S. M.: Analysis of morbidity and mortality from arterial embolectomy. Surgery, *65*:207, 1969.

14. Swank, R. L.: Alteration of blood on storage: Measurement of adhesiveness of "aging" platelets and leukocytes and their removal by filtration. New Eng. J. Med., *265*:728, 1961.

15. Clarkson, A. R., Sage, R. E., and Lawrence, J. R.: Consumption coagulopathy and acute renal failure due to gram-negative septicemia after abortion. Ann. Int. Med., *70*: 1191, 1969.

16. Corrigan, J. J., Ray, W. L., and May, N.: Changes in the blood coagulation system associated with septicemia. New Eng. J. Med., *279*:851, 1968.

17. McKay, D. G.: Disseminated Intravascular Coagulation. New York, Hoeber, 1965.

18. McKay, D. G.: Progress in disseminated intravascular coagulation. Calif. Med., *111*:186, 1969.

19. Blaisdell, F. W., Lim, R. C., and Stallone, R. J.: The mechanism of pulmonary damage following traumatic shock. Surg. Gynec. Obstet., *130*:15, 1970.

20. Rosoff, C. B., Salzman, E. W., and Gurewich, V.: Reduction of platelet serotonin and response to pulmonary emboli. Surgery, *70*:12, 1971.

21. Margaretten, W., and McKay, D. G.: Thrombotic ulcerations of the gastrointestinal tract. Arch. Int. Med., *127*:250, 1971.

22. Regoczzi, E., and Brain, M. C.: Organ distribution of fibrin in disseminated intravascular coagulation. Brit. J. Haemat., *17*:73, 1969.

23. Gans, H.: Preservation of vascular patency as a function of reticuloendothelial clearance. Surgery, *60*:1216, 1966.

24. Gans, H., and Lowman, J. T.: The uptake of fibrin and fibrin degradation products by the isolated rat liver. Blood, *29*:526, 1967.

25. Aggeler, P. M.: Physiologic basis for transfusion therapy in hemorrhagic disorders: A critical review. Transfusion, *1*:71, 1961.

26. Mustard, J. F., and Packham, M. A.: Factors influencing platelet function: Adhesion, release, aggregation. Pharm. Rev., *22*:97, 1970.

27. Packham, M. A., and Mustard, J. F.: Platelet reaction. Seminars Hemat., *8*:30, 1971.

28. Miller, R. D., Robbins, T. O., Tong, M. J., and Barton, S. L.: Coagulation defects associated with massive blood transfusion. Ann. Surg., *174*:794, 1971.

29. Wilson, R. F., Mammen, E., and Walt, A. J.: Eight years experience with massive blood transfusion. J. Trauma, *11*:275, 1971.

30. Krevans, J. R., and Jackson, D. P.: Hemorrhagic disorder following massive whole blood transfusion. JAMA, *159*:171, 1955.

31. Deykin, D.: The clinical challenge of disseminated intravascular coagulation. New Eng. J. Med., *283*:636, 1970.

32. Pitney, W. R.: Disseminated intravascular coagulation. Seminars Hemat., *8*:65, 1971.

33. Murphy, S., and Gardner, F. H.: Platelet preservation—Effect of storage temperature on maintenance of platelet viability—Deleterious effects of refrigerated storage. New Eng. J. Med., *280*:1094, 1969.

34. Murphy, S., and Gardner, F. H.: Platelet storage at 22 degrees centigrade; metabolic, morphologic and functional studies. J. Clin. Invest., *50*:370, 1971.

35. Kakkar, V. V., Field, E. S., Nicolaides, A. N., Fleete, P. T., Wessler, S., and Yin, E. T.: Low doses of heparin in prevention of deep venous thrombosis. Lancet, *2*:669, 1971.

36. Williams, H. T.: Prevention of postoperative deep vein thrombosis with perioperative subcutaneous heparin. Lancet, *2*:950, 1971.

37. Hattersley, P. G.: Activated coagulation time of whole blood. JAMA, *196*:436, 1966.

38. Marder, U. J.: A simple technique for the measurement of plasma heparin concentration during anticoalgulant therapy. Thromb. Diath. Haemorrh., *24*:230, 1970.

39. Spector, I., and Corn, M.: Control of heparin therapy with the activated thromboplastin time. JAMA, *201*:157, 1967.

40. Weiss, P. M.: Etude expérimentale des vitesses de disparition de l'héparine plasmatique après une injection intraveineuse. Hemostase., *6*:149, 1966.

Chapter 15 | Complications of

Charles H. Wray, M.D.
William H. Moretz, M.D.

Amputations

Surgeons have been most concerned with those aspects of amputation related to saving the patient's life and obtaining a healed wound. To attain these goals in the patient with an ischemic extremity often presents great challenges. With improved preoperative control of metabolic, cardiovascular and infectious problems, and with improved anesthetic and surgical techniques, mortality rates have steadily dropped and better wound healing has been obtained. The goals achieved have been very worthwhile, but to them must be added another—a successfully rehabilitated patient. A live patient with a perfectly healed stump is often quite an achievement, but confinement to a wheelchair in a darkened room is at the same time among the worst of complications. The plan of therapy from the beginning should be directed toward the successful use of a prosthesis.

Major advances in vascular reconstruction have increased the zeal of surgeons for restoring flow to salvage tissue. Decisions in older patients with advanced arterial disease for sympathectomy and reconstructive procedures must be made with care.[1] The patient's strongest desire is to walk without pain. If this can be accomplished by a timely amputation with early fitting of prosthesis, should the patient be subjected to operations with minimal chance of long-term success? The recent tendency toward reconstructions in the distal tibial vessels must be questioned since such procedures may jeopardize success of a below-knee amputation.[2]

The patient about to lose his leg faces many hazards. The loss of a part is a severe psychological blow to anyone, but to lose a limb and the independence afforded by ambulation may completely defeat an older person.

Amputation may be carried out at the wrong level. Amputation at or below the ankle for ischemic changes in the toes will not heal when diffuse occlusive disease is present (Fig. 15-1). Further pain and sickness then continue while further extirpation is accomplished. Amputation done at the mid-thigh level will heal, but the elderly patient may not be able to walk again.

The hazard of infection is ever present. Ischemia of the skin removes a barrier to the invasion of deeper tissues by the resident bacterial flora. If infection is not controlled by local measures, and if the technical aspects of the amputation are faulty, then the infection may move to a higher level.

Prolonged immobilization is a hazard to the older vascular amputee. If the patient is left in bed immobile, atrophy of mental and muscular faculties occurs to dispose him to depression and a host of metabolic and other vascular calamities.

While these hazards and others exist, techniques are available to the physician who would assist the patient to successful

347

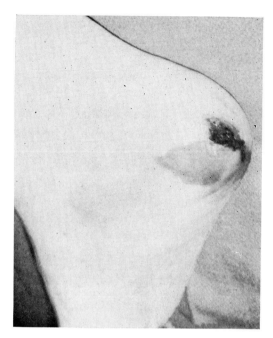

FIG. 15-1. Necrosis of the skin and deeper tissues of the heel. The patient could not walk because of pain. A below-knee amputation was performed because of popliteal artery occlusion and involvement of the heel.

rehabilitation following amputation. The accumulated experience of many centers where the elderly survive amputation to successfully walk can be utilized to meet each of the problems encountered. A discussion of complications tends to emphasize negative features but should lead to a clear understanding of problems to be overcome.

General Considerations

Most patients with infected ischemic tissue are poor risks for surgery. They are elderly with an average age of over 60 years. Since arteriosclerosis is a generalized disease, cardiac insufficiency, hypertension, cardiovascular accidents and renal disease are common. The incidence of diabetes mellitus is high.[3] Smoking and its accompanying chronic obstructive pulmonary disease are common. Usually one of these diseases is out of control at the time the patient requires amputation. At some centers, the need for amputation in such instances is considered urgent

and the tendency is to take the patient still in his precarious general status to the operating room to rid him of the offending extremity. Delay of the amputation for proper preparation of the patient may make the difference between survival and death.

In a series of 476 patients with an ischemic or infected extremity treated at the Medical College of Georgia Hospitals, 60 percent also had evidence of major cardiovascular disease. One-fourth of these patients were termed in "critical condition" in the anesthesia classification on admission. One-third of the patients demonstrated evidence of absorption of infected or toxic material from the extremity by fever, dehydration or leukocytosis. About one-third of these patients had diabetes. Although many were acidotic and had significant infection, the mortality rate in the diabetic group has been surprisingly low; 3.5 percent over a 15-year period as compared with 10 percent for the nondiabetic. Very few patients had amputation on the day of admission. The general policy has been to prepare the patient as well as possible for surgery. Their hospital stay has averaged 17 days.

Warren and Kihn, in a survey of 3,962 lower extremity amputations in the advanced age group found an overall mortality of 21.8 percent in V. A. hospitals.[4] The major causes of death were cardiac and pulmonary. Diabetes was present in more than 60 percent of those who had below-knee amputations and in only 31 percent of those who had above-knee amputations. In the presence of two associated diseases, the mortality was 31 percent, while with only one other disease the mortality was 8 percent. In Eidemiller's review of 436 patients with above-knee amputation for ischemia, the mortality was 19.7 percent as compared with a mortality of less than one-half percent for amputations done for trauma or tumor in young individuals.[5] This mortality which had remained stable from 1952 to 1967 was due, not to the trauma of operation itself, but to the increased age and the associated vascular disease. In Rosenberg's report on

176 major amputations performed between 1948 and 1961, 17 percent died in the total group, with a 23 percent mortality in diabetic and 10 percent mortality in nondiabetic patients.[6] Mid-thigh amputation was twice as lethal as mid-leg, and the mortality increased with age and obesity (Table 15-1). Urging special attention to the prevention of complications rather than treatment after they occur, he demonstrated a decrease in mortality with careful attention to the details of care.

Burgess at the University of Washington School of Medicine has reported 158 consecutive below-knee amputations in peripheral vascular amputees without a single "operative" death, although there were 10 deaths within 30 days of operation.[7] There has been a wide variation in the mortality of vascular amputees in recent years and mortality rates in excess of 25 percent are not uncommon.

The Choice of Amputation Site

In deciding upon the optimum site for amputation, many factors must be considered. All devitalized tissues must be removed up to a point where the blood supply will allow prompt healing. The lowest level compatible with a well-functioning prosthesis and within the area of acceptable blood supply is desirable.

Can the Amputation Be Too High? In the 1967 survey of lower extremity amputations in veterans hospitals, Warren and Kihn noted that above-knee amputations comprised the majority.[4] Approximately 20 percent of these patients with popliteal pulses were amputated below the knee with good healing rates. Surprisingly, many of the patients who did not have popliteal pulses also healed at the below-knee level. Prior to the 1960's, mid-thigh amputation was the rule for those who had no popliteal pulse. Eighty percent of patients would be candidates for the above-knee level if this single criterion were used alone.

Dissatisfaction with the above-knee level is related to the difficulties encountered in rehabilitation.[8] The loss of the knee joint increases the energy expenditure necessary for walking even though the above-knee prosthesis may fit quite satisfactorily.[9] If the level of amputation is above the mid-femoral level, many older patients are simply not able to control the prosthesis in a satisfactory manner. When the stump is short, the problems of suspension, the loss of a satisfactory fulcrum and the loss of the knee joint may require energy expenditures beyond the limits of the patient. Crutch walking consumes more energy than walking on an above-knee prosthesis.

When vascular occlusive disease leads to amputation, the likelihood of amputation of the remaining extremity also increases. Twenty to 30 percent may eventually lose both legs and diabetics are particularly prone to this unhappy circumstance.[10] If both amputations are done at the above-knee level then no older patients will walk. Some patients with one below-knee and one above-knee amputation will be sufficiently agile and strong to walk, and many with bilateral below-knee amputations will walk. The salvage of the knee joint at the time of the first amputation is therefore vital.

Can the Amputation Be Performed Too Low? There is very little mobility to the tissues of the foot. The tissues are composed of bone, fascia and tendons. The plantar surfaces are covered with a thick skin which overlies a fatty tissue that is separated by numerous fibrous septa. When the foot is ischemic, these tissues lose the ability to control satisfactorily infection and to promote wound healing. Particularly in diabetics, a

TABLE 15-1. VARIATIONS IN MORTALITY EFFECT OF DIABETES

Amputa-tion Level	Warren & Kihn 1967	Rosenberg 1970	E.T.M.H. 1970
Below-Knee	10%	9.9%	3.5%
Above-Knee	28%	21.9%	25%
Effect of Diabetes	None	Doubled	Lowered

* Eugene Talmadge Memorial Hospital.

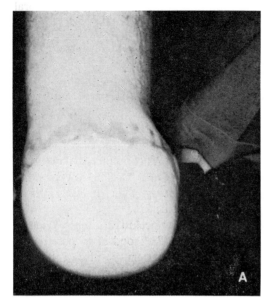

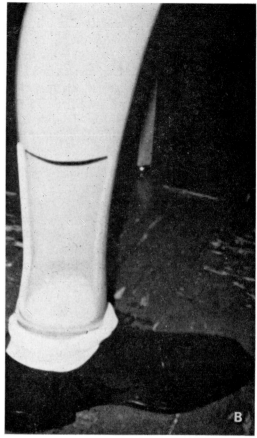

FIG. 15-2. (A) Syme stump with bulbous end; (B) Syme prosthesis.

very radical removal of all infected tissues is necessary. The skin frequently appears normal distal to areas of severe deep involvement. The presence of erythema and swelling in the plantar tissues usually belies an underlying, smouldering, hidden infection in the fat of these tissues. While these tissues will bleed because of inflammation, healing may not be accomplished until all of the involved tissue is removed.

In the majority of patients with arteriosclerosis, the blood supply to the foot is severely impaired and pulsatile flow is diminished at a level above the knee. Amputations in the foot, then, have little chance of success. For these reasons, less than 10 percent of the amputations performed in patients with vascular disease are below the ankle and of these around 40 percent do not heal and require higher revision.

Dr. James Syme discovered that the foot could be disarticulated at the ankle and he fortuitously fashioned a heel flap which led to a successful operation. Surgeons continue to be fascinated with this operation because of its potential of producing an end-bearing stump which allows walking without a prosthesis (Fig. 15-2). Recently, Rosenman has been successful with the Syme amputation in only 11 of 15 patients.[11] After careful selection, drainage and debridement, three weeks are allowed for the inflammed tissues to recover before the Syme amputation. Encouraged by successful below-knee amputation in vascular amputees, Sarmiento attempted the Syme amputation in a group of patients, but found that one-third of the patients did not heal and required higher amputation frequently at the above-knee level.[12] Poor healing rates and their attendant prolongation of illness and immobilization make this procedure of minimal use in vascular amputees.

Selection of Proper Level

Minor amputations of the toes or forefoot can be carried out in patients with vascular disease if there is well demarcated gangrene. If there is absolutely no evidence of spread of ischemia and if there is no pain in the foot indicating deeper ischemia, then these wounds will heal (Fig. 15-3). Many diabetics have excellent pulsatile flow in the foot that allows healing if infected and impaired tissues are removed.

The Syme amputation can also be used in those with good blood flow through the popliteal and posterior tibial arteries. In women, the bulbous end of the stump requires an unsightly prosthesis. The procedure should not be selected in patients with occlusive vascular disease in the older age group. Amputation through the knee joint, popular at one time because of the ease of performance in a relatively bloodless field, may be acceptable for the occasional patient who cannot be prepared for surgery and anesthesia.[13] But this level is undesirable because the necessary prosthesis has a joint at a level lower than the patient's knee, giving a very poor cosmetic effect especially apparent when sitting.

The preferred level of amputation is below-knee in 75 percent of the patients encountered. Prerequisites for the selection of this level are: (1) a patient who is expected to walk, (2) satisfactory skin at the level of the amputation, (3) the presence of a femoral pulse, (4) a patent deep femoral artery, and (5) an intact knee joint (Table 15-2).

Since the primary aim is to rehabilitate the patient, there is little need to consider a below-knee amputation for the patient expected to remain bedridden or with a short life expectancy. Incapacitation because of painful ischemia does not exclude a below-knee amputation.

The processes of gangrene and infection usually involve only the foot and seldom

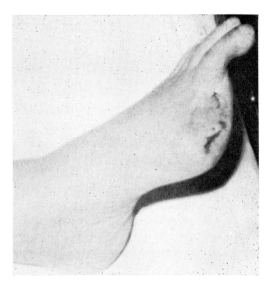

FIG. 15-3. Toe amputation will heal in patients with localized ischemia.

extend above the ankle. The presence of gangrenous skin near the level of amputation is associated with poor wound healing. The presence of deep pain in the calf musculature is associated with active necrosis at this level. Edema, even though extending to the knee, usually subsides with elevation and control of infection and should not exclude a B-K amputation.

Thorough knowledge of the distribution of the arterial disease in the affected extremity is vital. The popliteal pulse need not be present for successful below-knee amputation. The femoral pulse, however, is required in most instances. Moore[14] reported some successful below-knee amputations

TABLE 15-2. SELECTION OF CANDIDATES
FOR BELOW-KNEE AMPUTATION

1. Patient is expected to walk
   Not bed-ridden—has walked recently
2. Satisfactory condition of skin
   at level of incision
   Bleeding at surgery not a determinant
3. Presence of a femoral pulse
   Popliteal is not necessary
4. A patent deep femoral artery
   determined by arteriography or
   plethysmography
5. An intact knee joint

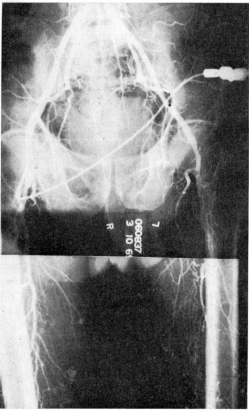

FIG. 15-4. Arteriogram from a left below-knee amputation failure. The patient had femoral pulses bilaterally. The left common femoral is patent. Both the superficial and deep femoral arteries are occluded. The medial femoral circumflex vessel is enlarged.

when both the superficial and deep femoral arteries were occluded or the iliac vessels were severely stenotic. Burgess states that the femoral pulse, but not the popliteal, must be present for satisfactory below-knee healing.[7]

Arteriograms are frequently performed to evaluate patients for vascular reconstruction and sympathectomy. DeBakey has emphasized that arteriograms should be done on all patients prior to the decision for amputation.[15] If reconstruction is not possible, then amputation may be elected. Meaningful data on which to base selection of the level for amputation is minimal. The statement is frequently made that arteriograms are not useful. However, our experience indicates that arteriography would be very helpful in selecting the site of amputation. Twenty-

eight arteriograms were performed in patients who had successful below-knee amputations. A normal deep femoral artery was demonstrated in each. The lower leg was supplied by collaterals frequently with refilling of segments of the popliteal and tibial vessels. Arteriograms on four below-knee failures, each with palpable femoral pulses at the time of amputation, revealed in each instance a completely occluded or severely diseased deep femoral artery (Fig. 15-4).

Plethysmographic techniques and skin temperature studies, likewise, have been evaluated in many patients, but no conclusions have been drawn. Winsor and Strandness have demonstrated that the levels of arterial occlusions can be predicted successfully with plethysmography.[16,17] In our own institution, segmental plethysmography has been used to delineate the level of obstruction. Forty-two patients had segmental plethysmography performed prior to amputation. In all cases in which the pulse amplitude at the upper thigh level was 12 mm. or above, there was satisfactory below-knee healing. In the four cases with proved deep femoral disease, the upper thigh values were less than 6 mm. amplitude. Continued observation with these and other techniques will yield helpful information for future use. Tentatively, we have concluded that a patent deep femoral artery detectable by either arteriography or plethysmography, is a prerequisite for successful below-knee amputation.

Around one-fifth of patients should be amputated at the above-knee level. These include the patient who is bedridden, those with diffuse occlusive disease and severe cardiopulmonary problems, those with no femoral pulse and those without a demonstrably patent deep femoral artery. The above-knee amputation is technically simple and heals well with an extremely low incidence of infection.

In 198 above-knee amputations performed in our institution, only 3 percent required re-amputations, of which only two were related to ischemia.[18] Because of this high degree of selectivity, mortality rates were high in the above-knee amputees. Many patients, however, will improve after above-knee amputation, and some will be energetic enough to walk.

Delayed Wound Healing

Despite excellent preoperative care, careful selection of the level of amputation and fine, meticulous technique, delay in wound healing may occur, particularly with the present emphasis on saving the knee joint. The early signs of poor healing include excessive edema with a peau d'orange skin, erythema and blistering of the skin. Focal areas of necrosis may appear near the suture line. There are usually no signs of systemic reaction. The severity of the pain usually parallels the severity of involvement. This complication is rare in the above-knee amputee and in the below-knee amputee with popliteal pulse, but occurs to some degree in nearly one-third of those seen with no popliteal pulse. If the stump is reasonably comfortable, no drastic measures are indicated. Instead, with continued observation, cautious re-wrapping and protection of the stump, most will go on to eventual healing.

Circumstances influence how the wound with delayed healing should be managed. Early re-amputation at a higher level should be considered for the very elderly patient with severe generalized arteriosclerosis who will not tolerate prolonged illness and bedrest. Others for whom further anesthesia and surgery would be particularly hazardous should be allowed more time to permit healing without re-amputation. From 10 to 15 percent of below-knee amputees require revision to a higher level. Since the diabetic patient so frequently loses the other extremity within two years, he should be given every opportunity to heal at the below-knee level, particularly in younger patients. Revision to a higher level should not be necessary in the diabetic in more than 5 percent. Scars and crevices incident to delayed healing do not affect the ability to wear the new plastic total contact type prosthesis. Even split-thickness skin grafts will remain intact (Fig. 15-5).

The usual surgical principles of debridement and excision of obviously necrotic tissue apply to these wounds. Obvious progression under observation of evidences of delayed healing such as spread of focal areas of necrosis, extension of blebs, and increasing deep pain indicate that further procrastination is unjustified. When entire flaps of skin and muscle are necrotic, when bone is exposed, or when there is obvious deep muscle necrosis, no delay in re-amputation is warranted.

When re-amputation is required because of failure to heal, the next higher election site is chosen. If the nonhealing wound is in the foot, a below-knee site is selected. Occasionally, as in the diabetic with a nonhealing toe amputation and with good foot pulses, a wedge resection of the involved ray, a transmetatarsal or a Syme amputation may be attempted. Such efforts hardly ever succeed in the elderly, nondiabetic patient with ischemic gangrene, and for those, such amputations are discouraged. In the below-knee amputee, nonhealing leads to an above-knee amputation. For the above-knee amputee, nonhealing requires usually a higher amputa-

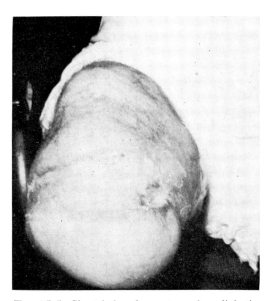

FIG. 15-5. Short below-knee stump in a diabetic. A split thickness skin graft is in place. The stump healed and has not required revision in three years.

tion through the femur or, very rarely, disarticulation of the hip.

In the absence of infection, prompt re-amputation at the next higher level with primary closure of the wound will usually be successful. With significant infection, systemic antibiotics are indicated and it is our preference to isolate the infected stump for a minimum of 72 hours before proceeding with re-amputation by physiologic amputation which is discussed below. Using this technique, re-amputation can be accomplished with primary wound closure with a higher degree of success.

Infection

In the ischemic extremity, the protective barrier of the skin is lost even before gangrene is obvious. Organisms find their way into the deeper tissues which because of decreased blood supply have decreased resistance to infection. Aided by the anatomic make-up of the tissues of the foot, organisms enter the lymphatics and move toward the blood stream. It is probable that bacterial invasion of some degree has occurred in most patients requiring amputation for ischemic changes, the main exception being those whose only indication is rest pain. Infection is an ever-present danger which, if not prevented, threatens not only the limb, but also the patient's life.

Infection is a major cause of death in the amputee. Prior to the advent of antibiotics, the mortality rates following amputation usually exceeded 40 percent. In recent years, the mortality rate has markedly improved due not only to the introduction of antibiotics, but also to advances in anesthesia, blood replacement and pre- and post-operative care. A failing myocardium encourages systemic infections: the edematous lung is susceptible to pneumonitis. In the series reported by Eidemiller, 28 percent died of pneumonia and nearly half of those had wound infections.[5] The organisms involved were principally staphylococi and staphylococci mixed with a variety of gram-negative organisms. In our own patients, nearly half had obvious signs of local or systemic infection on admission, and one-third had serious gross infection, spreading gangrene or sepsis. The organisms involved have been principally coagulase-positive staphylococcus and gram-negative organisms including *Escherichia coli,* Aerobacter, Klebsiella, Pseudomonas and clostridial organisms.

Should Antibiotics Be Used Prophylactically? The routine use of a predetermined drug at a set dosage for all patients needing amputation is not indicated. Thursby and Dunn reported a doubled incidence of primary wound infections when penicillin was used prophylactically, from 3½ percent to 7 percent.[19] The organisms recovered, except for clostridia, were not sensitive to penicillin.

When used widely, antibiotics are most helpful. Cultures of draining sites and of tissues removed at surgery should demonstrate the flora present and sensitivity studies should help determine the most logical drug to use. Sensitivity determinations are particularly needed in the many patients who were receiving antibiotics before admission. When immediate information is needed because of the clinical status of the patient, gram stain preparations may be helpful in evaluating the organisms present. The immediate use of antibiotics in patients who are septic is warranted. Much help in drug selection is provided by the information kept current by an infectious disease service and the general hospital laboratory on the prevalence of certain organisms within the hospital and their antibiotic sensitivities. Control of infection in these patients is vital. Between 1956 and 1966 at the

TABLE 15-3. CAUSES OF DEATH—
EUGENE TALMADGE MEMORIAL HOSPITAL

	1956 through 1960[20]	1961 through 1965[21]	1966 through 1970[18]
Cerebral	6	1	5
Myocardial	2	6	5
Renal	2	2	1
Pulmonary Embolus	1	4	1
Infection	3	5	0
Other	2	0	0

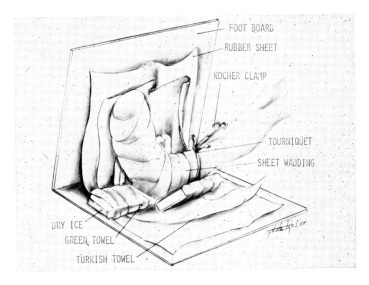

F<small>IG</small>. 15-6. During the technique of physiological amputation with dry ice, the foot is wrapped in sheet wadding below the tourniquet. The dry ice is wrapped in individual towels and further insulation is applied. The other foot is protected by the footboard.

Talmadge Memorial Hospital, eight amputee deaths occurred because of infection, while in the last five years no deaths were due to infection (Table 15-3). The use of antibiotics during both periods was similar in many ways, but in the recent period antibiotic agents were selected more intelligently.

While antibiotics have effectively reduced mortality, reduction in wound infections has been minimal. About half of the revisions to a higher level are necessitated by infection. Wound infections still occur in about 10 percent with a slightly higher incidence in diabetics than nondiabetics.

In addition to appropriate antibiotics, two other methods of controlling rampant or spreading infection must be considered. The first is surgical removal of the part, the second is preoperative physiologic amputation.

Many years ago, particularly in the diabetic, the infected foot was removed by the simplest surgical procedure possible—disarticulation at the ankle. This approach did not appreciably lower the mortality. The next simplest surgical procedure, a guillotine type amputation above the grossly infected area leaving the stump completely open, is relatively effective. When done at the site of the permanent stump, a granulating wound eventually develops which with skin traction sometimes aided by split-thickness grafts ultimately results in a completely healed stump. In addition to requiring a surgical procedure at a time when the patient is not optimally prepared, this method requires at least several weeks for healing during which time some degree of undesirable immobilization is necessary. A three-week delay, as recently advocated by Rosenman prior to a Syme amputation is likewise objectionable, if avoidable.[11]

Local hypothermia for the control of infection has been used by some since 1944 when the technique was described by Large and Heimbecker.[22] A very tight tourniquet and ice are used to isolate and cool the affected part. Pain is relieved since nerve conduction ceases at 25°C. Further breakdown of ischemic and necrotic tissues is prevented by hypothermia and absorption from the area is prevented by the tourniquet. Operative amputation is then carried out at a level higher than the tourniquet and hypothermia under appropriate anesthesia. Although this preoperative "physiologic amputation" has never been universally accepted, we have used it in those with severe local infections and sepsis (about half of the major amputations) since 1956 (Table 15-4).[20] Even in this high-risk group, mortality due to infections has been low and wound infections have been no more common than in those without infection on admission.

The technique of physiologic amputation

TABLE 15-4. INDICATIONS FOR PHYSIOLOGIC
AMPUTATION AND DURATION
IN 132 EXTREMITIES

	Number
Local infection	106
Mild	44
Severe	62
Need for treatment prior to surgery (coma, acidosis, septicemia, acute M.I. digitalis intoxication, pneumonia, uremia, etc.)	22
Pain	4

	Duration of Physiologic Amputation
Shortest (14 were for less than 24 hours)	9 Hours
Longest (21 were for 5 days or more)	15 Days
Average	78 Hours

allows careful preoperative preparation of the patient while effectively isolated from the infected tissue (Fig. 15-6). After 72 hours, the lymphatics and tissues above the level of physiologic amputation are cleared of offending chemicals and bacteria. Primary closure of the wound is allowed, thus materially shortening the period of immobilization.

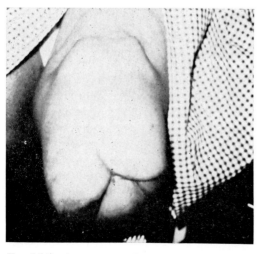

FIG. 15-7. Appearance of stump in a 74-year-old woman after delayed healing. The patient has worn a prosthesis without difficulty for two years.

Management of Infected Stump

Wound infections, like abscesses, require early and adequate drainage.[23] When the patient develops pain in the stump, particularly with fever and leukocytosis, the wound must be examined for signs of inflammation. Infection in the stump is a serious and urgent problem since the increased metabolic requirements of infected tissues cannot be met in tissue already deficient or marginal in blood supply. Infection must be drained and all necrotic tissue removed if infection is to be controlled. Delay in control may lead to excessive necrosis of tissue and require re-amputation at a higher level. Prompt recognition, drainage and any necessary debridement may permit healing without revision. Even though the scars may be unsightly, revision is not necessary for satisfactory prosthetic fitting (Fig. 15-7).

Often, however, in spite of our best efforts, sepsis occurs with evidence of infection spreading proximally from the wound. Amputation at a higher level may be mandatory. It is understood that our "best efforts" include appropriate wound and blood cultures for identification and sensitivity determinations of the offending organisms. It must be kept in mind that elderly, debilitated patients need not have high fever and marked leukocytosis with severe uncontrolled infections. When re-amputation at a higher level is required, this must be done through an area permeated with bacteria. A guillotine type of amputation may be selected leaving the wound completely open to heal later with time, skin traction, excessive scars and possibly some small skin grafts or the particular advantages of isolation of the infected part by physiologic amputation may be utilized for 72 hours followed by surgical re-amputation with primary closure.

Technical Considerations

Above-knee amputations are fairly well standardized, technically not difficult and, except for occasional wound infections, relatively free of complications. Excessive dissection of flaps should be avoided to prevent ischemia and delayed healing. The lateral end

FIG. 15-8. (A) Osteomyelitis in a diabetic with perforating necrotic sinus; (B) Appearance after removal of bone and infected soft tissue; (C) Appearance three weeks later near completion of healing.

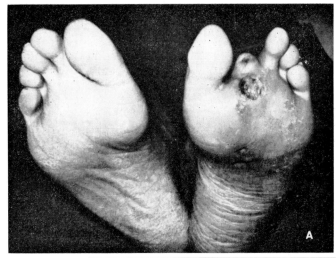

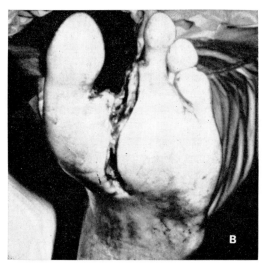

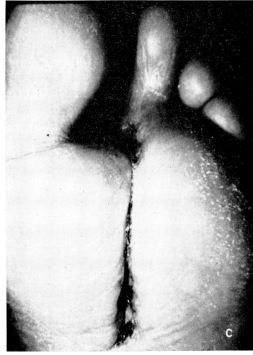

of the femur should be beveled to avoid pain which otherwise may occur when a sharp edge there presses against the prosthesis on ambulation. When myoplasty is not performed, the shape of the stump varies during ambulation making total contact in the socket difficult. With good meticulous surgery, minor alterations of technique have no apparent influence on subsequent complications.

Amputations at the ankle and in the foot are not complicated operations, but are associated with rather frequent complications relating chiefly to infection and failure to heal. These complications are related more to improper selection of procedure than to details of the procedure (Fig. 15-8). Failure to drain all infection and to excise all necrotic tissue inevitably leads to more infection and failure to heal and often to a higher reamputation. These procedures should rarely be performed in patients with ischemia.

Amputation at the below-knee level is now the most commonly chosen site for amputation for peripheral vascular disease. It is at this level also that meticulous attention to detail is most rewarding in preventing complications. The techniques used in younger patients for trauma cannot be transposed directly to the care of vascular patients. While, with old-style plug fit sockets, the scar should be on the end of the stump, with modern prosthetics the scar can be anywhere. With equal sized anterior and posterior flaps in vascular disease the most common complication is necrosis of the anterior flap. The blood supply to the skin overlying the anterior surface of the tissue is minimal even in normal young patients. In older patients, the skin along the anterior surface is thin and the subcutaneous tissue sparse. The periosteum is very close to the skin surface. With any anterior flap, division of the tibia at a proper level requires enough dissection and handling to further compromise its already poor blood supply. To avoid this, a clean transverse incision is made through skin and subcutaneous tissue down to periosteum, at a level about 2 cm. proximal to the anticipated tibia transection and is never elevated off the periosteum, the proximal skin and subcutaneous tissue.

By contrast to the anterior flap, the posterior flap usually has a relatively good blood supply even in those with advanced vascular disease, as do the muscles in the posterior compartment. The soleus muscle, which is more often subject to necrosis, is removed routinely by some in developing the long posterior flap. The vessels may be ligated lower to nourish the remaining muscle and skin of the long posterior flap which is left long enough to cover the end of the stump completely and be sutured without tension to the anterior skin edge (no flap) proximal to the ends of the tibia and fibula.

Warren and Burgess have advocated the use of no anterior flap in the vascular amputee.[24,25] This procedure, tested in many centers, has been found most satisfactory for primary wound healing and the stump holds up well in a total contact socket. Although the resultant scar is on the anterior surface of the tibia, no problems occur unless the scar becomes adherent to the bone because of infection or necrosis.

A technique of flapless below-knee amputation for arterial insufficiency has been tried, as recently advocated by Little.[26] A circular skin incision is made 5 cm. below the proposed level of bone section. The skin level is selected at a site of warmth and lack of serious color change. A tube of skin, subcutaneous tissue, deep fascia and periosteum is elevated upward. After the bone is transected, the skin is closed transversely. Although this technique has proved satisfactory in his hands, blood supply to the anterior skin is interfered with to some extent by the dissection required to transect the tibia at a level proximal to the anterior skin edge. In our hands, this circular no-flap technique is less successful than the no anterior, long posterior flap procedure.

Strict adherence to detail and fine meticulous technique are essential for successful below-knee amputations. The skin must be highly regarded and handled with the most delicate of techniques. The use of any instrument to grasp the skin must be avoided. During the necessary retraction of tissues, great care should be exercised not to contuse the wound. Sharp knife dissection is preferable. A thorough knowledge of anatomy and preoperative planning will minimize the need for handling of tissues during the operation. Hemostasis must be meticulous. Small hemostats should be carefully placed directly on bleeding vessels and only fine ligatures should be used. The posterior flap should be fashioned to fit nicely to the skin edge anteriorly. Of the deep tissues, only the fascia need be closed. Myoplasty and myodesis techniques advocated by some probably do not add to the successful use of the stump. The skin should be closed meticulously with fine suture, our preference being a continuous stitch of 5-0 monofilament nylon very accurately approximating the skin edges to provide an early barrier to infection and to achieve early complete epithelialization. Large bites can interfere with blood supply (Fig. 15-9).

Use of Drains

To drain or not to drain is a much debated issue. In spite of the most meticulous technique possible, some serum, lymph and blood appear in the wound. While small amounts of such fluid are well tolerated, significant accumulations delay healing and may cause pressure necrosis. If by meticulous technique and mild pressure bandaging, the quantity of fluid can be kept small, no drains are needed. If the quantity exceeds the minimum, drains may be inserted to allow egress of fluid. Even without drains, some fluid often escapes from wounds and some develop wound infection. And conversely, even with drains, some wounds develop hematomas or other fluid accumulations requiring attention.

While the presence of drains may allow entrance of bacteria from the skin, increasing the possibility of wound infection, this danger is minimized by removing the drains early. To remove the drains within 48 hours of surgery, the usual drain techniques require disturbing the dressing or cast at that time, which is undesirable. This disturbance may be minimized by using a closed technique with a suction catheter brought out through a lateral stab wound. These catheters need not be sutured in place and can be removed after 24 hours without disturbing the dressing or cast. This closed system probably subjects the wound to less danger of infection than Penrose drains.

Our preference is primary closure without any drains, the technique used in over 90 percent of the amputations performed at the Talmadge Memorial Hospital. We have been pleased with the results of this technique.

The detection of hematomas and seromas in the stump is difficult. Rosenberg reported a 4 percent incidence of hematoma.[6] Edema, common in the postoperative stump, makes it difficult to detect small amounts of fluid deep in the wound. Severe edema with very tense skin often means underlying serum or blood, and unless the swelling responds to pressure wrapping, aspiration is indicated for diagnosis and treatment. After thorough aspiration, re-accumulation of fluid is minimized by pressure of elastic dressings. If fluid continues to accumulate, it may be necessary to remove a few sutures to permit continued drainage.

Patient Mobilization

Mobilization of the entire patient must be the watchword from the beginning of illness throughout the period of rehabilitation. In many, the earliest lesion preceding amputation is a small area of gangrene sometimes associated with minor local trauma. Not infrequently, the onset is during a period of bedrest for something else. Cessation of walking, often erroneously advised by a physician, precipitates progression of gangrene. Prolonged delay of amputation after the need for it is obvious is unwise, although the patient may need some time to accept

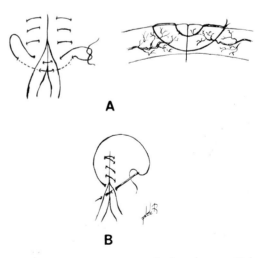

FIG. 15-9. (A) Large vertical mattress stitch interrupting the blood supply to the skin edge; (B) Continuous simple stitch placed near the skin edge.

this judgment. During delay, the patient frequently is in pain, taking narcotics and unable to rest well at night. He is relatively immobile and this immobilization in the elderly patient aggravates and accelerates pre-existing cardiovascular conditions, allowing pneumonia and thrombophlebitis to occur. Muscles atrophy and the patient is weakened by bedrest alone. Unless required, as in the diabetic patient with wet infected gangrene, immobilization should be minimized. If the lesion is dry and without infection, limited walking is safe, beneficial, and should be encouraged.

The patient should be encouraged to be physically active both in the pre-amputation period and in the early postoperative period and to care for himself as much as possible. The muscles of the arm and opposite leg should have strengthening exercises. Warren has suggested a regimen every two hours while awake: four sitting push-ups and four sitting pull-ups on an overhead trapeze attached to the bed.[24] Whenever possible, the opposite leg should be strengthened by bed exercises such as bicycle exercises and straight leg raising against a weight.

The patient who, on admission, is seriously ill with sepsis or heart failure cannot have this early emphasis on rehabilitation. His impressions of the serious nature of his illness may persist and interfere significantly with subsequent rehabilitation.

Additional specific measures may be needed to prevent contractures of the joint above, a frequent complication in amputations. Rehabilitation practices begun when the patient's therapy is first planned will minimize the need for other specific measures. Contracture of the knee joint after a below-knee amputation can be prevented by applying a cast or a posterior splint to the knee at the time of surgery. After recovery, extension exercise to the hip and knee should be performed daily. After above-knee amputation, the patient should lie on his face a part of each day to prevent hip flexion contractures. Contractures are not contraindications to the fitting of a prosthesis. The prosthesis may be fitted and readjusted as walking stretches the periarticular tissues.

Psychological Complications

The elderly patient frequently becomes disoriented as to time and place when moved into a new environment. Tranquilizers and narcotics further confuse the patient who may be already ill from the effects of gangrene. These acute brain syndromes may be mitigated somewhat by the judicious use of drugs. It is helpful to have members of the family in attendance to provide someone with whom the patient is familiar. The room should be well illuminated both day and night so that the patient can see well and not misinterpret shadows.

The patient who is suddenly confronted with the loss of limb frequently suffers a depressive reaction. The attitude of the physician and other health care personnel is very important at this point. It should be emphasized that the patient will soon have a better foot to walk on than he has at present. Exposure to patients of similar age who are successful prosthetic wearers will provide consolation and encouragement to the patient. If the patient is neglected and allowed to remain in bed, the depression may persist. A positive attitude toward rehabilitation from the beginning usually prevents such pyschological complications from becoming severe.

Care of the Stump

Early care of the postoperative stump is aimed primarily toward the prevention of edema, since edema interferes with blood supply and delays wound healing. Prevention of edema begins immediately after operation with application of a suitable dressing. Leaving the stump and wound opened to avoid pressure on the skin, as some prefer, is unnecessary and not in the best interest of healing. Those not subjected to immediate prosthetic casting should have compressive dressings from the beginning. For the below-knee amputation a posterior plaster splint helps with immobilization of the wound, decreases pain and prevents knee flexion. Care should be taken that these wrappings exert pressure from the distal end of the stump so there will be no choking by compressive dressings at a higher level. Compressive dressings are maintained at all times. Before the patient is discharged from the hospital he is carefully instructed in proper stump wrapping. He should be supervised until he understands and correctly wraps the stump with proper, even pressure. For the above-knee amputee, the wrapping needs to extend around the waist for suspension of the wrapping. The use of a snugly fitted elastic stump sock, or "stump shrinker" is to be preferred over the use of Ace bandages which can be misapplied causing proximal constriction. With satisfactory reduction of edema, the amputation stump should be ready for prosthetic fitting in four to six weeks. The presence of edema at this point delays fitting the prosthesis for at least two weeks.

Some, especially those with earlier extensive venous thrombosis have more edema than is easily controlled by wrapping. The use of intermittent pressure compression has been helpful in such situations. A convenient method is the use of an Intermittent Compression Unit made by Jobst, Inc. When used daily this may shorten appreciably the time required for edema reduction.

Complications of the Immediately Fitted Prosthesis

The technique of immediate fitting of prostheses has been adequately tested in vascular diseases. The combined series of Burgess, Condon, Sarmiento and Warren represents over 500 patients (Table 15-5). Satisfactory healing has been obtained in 92 percent of amputations. Mortality rates in these series have been low and rehabilitation rates have been high.

Immediate prosthetic fitting has many advantages. The immobilization of the limb and the reduction of edema encourages wound healing. The patient is psychologically comforted because he can achieve an erect posture early after operation.[28] While the technique is straightforward, there are many small points that need consideration. It is not wise to undertake this technique without prior special instructions such as that offered by several institutions in continuing education courses.

Most surgeons who are familiar with the technique of immediate fitting prostheses prefer to work simultaneously with a specially trained prosthetist who ideally should establish a relationship with the patient prior to amputation. The accurate fitting of the primary cast at the time of operation is of crucial importance in wound healing and should only be done by thoroughly experienced personnel. A casually applied elastic plaster cast used in immediate temporary prosthetic fitting can result in a failed below-knee amputation if improper pressure on the stump results.

The technique of immediate fitting was first used on younger patients suffering from trauma or tumor. When this technique was transposed to patients with vascular disease, it was found that early weight bearing prior to the first cast change at two weeks was unwise because the pressure exerted on the wound led to delayed healing. Most centers now allow the patient to be erect during this early period, but not to bear weight on the affected side. Standing and walking without weight bearing improves the patient's balance and boosts his morale. This activity must be supervised, preferably in the Physical Therapy Department. At two weeks, the cast is changed and if wound healing is satisfactory, graded weight bearing is allowed.

The application of the cast requires firm padding over bony prominences. This is

TABLE 15-5. HEALING WITH IMMEDIATE PROSTHESIS*

Total Patients	506	
Healed	469	92.7%
Failed	37	7.3%

(A summary of the experience of Burgess, Condon, Moore, Sarmiento and Warren.)[7,27,14,12,24]

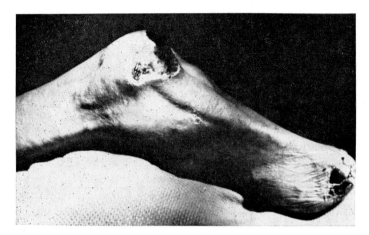

FIG. 15-10. Necrosis of skin of patella and distal stump caused by pressure from immediate fit prosthesis. No clinical signs suggested the lesion that was apparent when the cast was changed after two weeks.

particularly important around the patella and over the anterior tibial surfaces where improper pressure may cause skin necrosis (Fig. 15-10). If the patient complains about pain in the immediate postoperative period, the cast should be removed immediately and the wound inspected. Because edema reoccurs rapidly, the cast should be immediately replaced if no wound complications are noted.

Because of the continuous pressure the cast will prevent edema and reduce the muscle mass. The cast may become loose very rapidly in some patients who are especially active. A loose cast may damage the skin by rotating on the limb. To prevent harm, the fit of the cast should be noted frequently and if too loose, a new cast made.

Other complications that occur with use of this technique are common to all amputations. The few complications peculiar to this technique are entirely preventable by proper application of the cast.

Late Stump Complications

Neuroma. Many techniques for managing the cut-end of a nerve have been tried and advised for preventing neuromas. None seems to have particular advantage over others. All cut nerves heal with some bulging or neuroma formation at the nerve end. In general, these are symptomatic only if abnormal pressures are placed upon them.

During amputation, each major nerve should be isolated and severed at a high level away from positions subject to pressure when the patient wears a prosthesis. If the nerves are divided at the level of the skin flaps or at the level of the end of the bone they will remain near or attached to the scar. With a neuroma in this low position, pain may occur with motion or with pressure over the area.

Pain from a neuroma is usually well localized. Often the tender neuroma can be palpated near the incision or bone end. In the past, operations for excision of neuromas have been very common. At present, painful neuromas are less often seen and when they do occur they are usually successfully managed by adjusting the prosthesis to remove pressure from this area. Rarely is it necessary to operatively excise the nerve to a higher level.

Causalgia. Unusual vague but troublesome pains in the amputation site deserve early investigation and treatment. Causalgia is a diffuse burning type pain not localized to the distribution of a single nerve and often is worse at night. It is particularly annoying and soon causes severe psychological deterioration. Though rare, it seems to be more common in the introspective, neurosis-prone individual and those who have long-standing pain pre-operatively. The patient usually won't allow the stump to be touched, let alone wrapped and cared for. Excessive use of drugs for relief of this is a very real danger. Successful rehabilitation without relief of causalgia is impossible at this point.

When suspected, sympathetic block is indicated. A paravertebral lumbar sympathetic block is used and characteristically the pain is totally but transiently relieved. Several blocks may be curative and progressively lengthened periods of relief after each block suggest that operative sympathectomy will not be needed. However, if after two to four blocks, the period of relief is becoming shorter, operative sympathectomy should be elected.

Phenomenon of Phantom Limb Pain

Nearly all patients have some awareness of the presence of the lost extremity. This should be explained to the amputee to assure him that this is usual, otherwise he worries that he is imagining things and feels insecure. The explanation that the nerves at the end of the stump are sending signals that are misinterpreted by the brain usually suffices. If the pain has been present for a long time prior to amputation, "imprinting" may occur causing the pain to continue after the loss of the extremity. Early amputation when the need becomes obvious will prevent many such problems. This awareness usually dims with time. A rare patient suffers severe pain in the phantom limb. This may simulate his preoperative pain or it may be a new type of generalized pain. The patient may feel that the foot or leg is in a severely cramped position or that it is being burned or squeezed in a vise.

Frequently, these patients have not made a good psychological adjustment to the loss of the extremity. Positive efforts toward rehabilitation will help to reassure such a patient. The passage of time helps many. A very rare patient has persistent excruciating discomfort for which there is no known effective therapy short of a prefrontal lobotomy—an undesirable solution.[29] Lesser therapies which have been found to be successful include nerve sections, sympathectomies and cordotomies.

Late Vascular Complications

Very rarely, the patient's arterial disease may continue to progress and cause ischemia of the stump. One elderly patient developed sudden occlusion of his common femoral and superficial femoral artery about three months following amputation. He developed a cold painful stump and could not use his prosthesis. Since the previous status of his circulation had been well documented, thrombotic material was removed with Fogarty catheters restoring the stump to its previous state of health. Another patient who had an amputation early in life because of osteomyelitis, developed symptomatic arterial disease in the amputated leg and required sympathectomy for relief of pain and coldness of the stump. Only one of 500 has required amputation of both legs at a higher level because of progression of vascular disease in the stumps.

When arteries and veins are ligated together during any operation, subsequent necrosis at the site of the ligature may allow arteriovenous fistulas to develop. Such a complication is rare in amputation stumps, but must be handled surgically if discovered.

The loss of both extremities due to vascular disease is fairly common in amputees particularly among diabetics because of their susceptibility to infection, poor healing qualities, and severe vascular disease. In some series, bilateral amputations occur in nearly one-third of the patients. Because of this later development of ischemia or infection in the opposite extremity, prophylactic measures which may insure the wellbeing of the remaining extremity are indicated. The patient should be alerted to examine his remaining foot daily for evidence of minor infection and minor trauma. He should be told not to use chemicals which may be detrimental to the tissues and to use great care in trimming his nails. He should be told to protect the remaining foot at all times and to not walk about in the house, particularly at night, without his shoe on. The shoe should fit well so as to not damage the skin.

Because diabetics are particularly prone to lose the remaining extremity, it has been our policy to perform a lumbar sympathectomy on the contralateral side before the patient leaves the hospital after amputation. It is felt that, because sympathectomy abolishes sweating and increases the cutaneous blood supply, fungus infections are markedly deterred and superficial infections and minor trauma may heal better. We do not yet have statistical proof of the benefits of contralateral sympathectomy, and this procedure remains controversial in diabetic patients generally.

Bone Formation in the Stump. In children, the overgrowth of bone following amputation is common. In an adult with vascular disease, the lesion is uncommon but may cause severe pain. During amputation, care should be taken to incise the periosteum at the level of bone transection. Remnants of periosteum left hanging from bone ends may cause redeposition of osseous material and account for later symptoms.

Asymptomatic bone formation requires no treatment. If symptomatic, first consideration should be given to modifying the prosthesis to relieve pressure over the sites.[9] If unsuccessful or if bone growth continues and presents severe problems, operative removal of the tissue may be necessary.[30,31]

Failure of Rehabilitation

The impression is still too prevalent that elderly vascular amputees cannot walk. As long as the health team persists in this attitude, these patients will not walk. From the foregoing discussion, it is obvious that efforts must be made from the beginning to insure successful rehabilitation. In the last ten years, major rehabilitation efforts have been carried out in all types of hospitals and clinical settings. All observers are enthusiastic and demonstrate objectively that nearly all amputees can be rehabilitated. The beneficial effect of this change in attitude has been well demonstrated in our own hospital, where prior to 1966 very few patients who had amputations for vascular disease were

rehabilitated in the present meaning of the term. Most remained on crutches or in wheelchairs without useful prostheses. Since the institution of adequate rehabilitation efforts, 80 percent of the patients have achieved independence and walked well. Burgess, Warren, Kritter, Condon and Jordan have reported similar results. "Successful Rehabilitation" means for some, returning to work, for others becoming independent of other family members for their personal needs.

Among the 20 percent who are not rehabilitated are a few patients who are too feeble to walk, a few others who were confined to bed permanently prior to amputation and a very few patients who cannot walk because they think they cannot walk.

Successful rehabilitation is not dependent on the use of techniques for immediate fitting of the prosthesis. While this technique is desirable and helpful for some, the vast majority of amputees would benefit more from the less exacting and more important contributions possible through an improved philosophy and greater use of simple rehabilitation procedures which are within the reach of most surgeons and hospitals interested in the problem. Failure to achieve successful rehabilitation is still the most common complication of amputation for vascular disease, and is preventable by a properly organized, enthusiastic team approach.

References

1. Wheelock, F. C., Jr., and Filtzer, H. S.: Femoral grafts in diabetics. Resulting conservative amputations. Arch. Surg., *99*: 776, 1969.
2. Skversky, N., and Zislis, J. K.: Peripheral vascular disorders and the aged amputee. Geriatrics, *25*:142, 1970.
3. Cranley, J. J., Krause, R. J., and Strasser, E. S.: Below-knee amputation for arteriosclerosis obliterans, with and without diabetes mellitus. Arch. Surg., *98*:77, 1969.
4. Warren, R., and Kihn, R.: A survey of lower extremity amputations for ischemia. Surgery, *63*:107, 1968.
5. Eidemiller, L. R., *et al.*: Amputation of the ischemic extremity. Amer. Surg., *34*:491, 1968.

6. Rosenberg, N., and Adriate, E.: Mortality factors in major limb amputation for vascular disease: A study of 176 procedures. Surgery, *67*:437, 1970.

7. Burgess, E. M.: Below-knee amputations with immediate-fit prosthesis. *In* Management of Arterial Occlusive Disease. p. 49, Chicago, Yearbook, 1971.

8. Caine, D., and Klein, R.: Amputation site and morbidity in relation to circulatory disease. Med. J. Aust., *2*:259, 1967.

9. Hall, C. B.: Prosthetic socket shape as related to anatomy in lower extremity amputees. Clin. Orthop., *37*:32, 1964.

10. Ecker, M. L., and Jacobs, B. S.: Lower extremity amputation in diabetic patients. Diabetes, *19*:189, 1970.

11. Rosenman, L. D.: Syme amputation for ischemic disease in the foot. Amer. J. Surg., *118*:194, 1969.

12. Sarmiento, A.: "Modern Concepts in Surgery and Management of Lower Extremity Amputee." Postgraduate course. Miami, Florida, December 13-16, 1967.

13. Howard, R. R., Chamberlain, Jr., and MacPherson, A. I.: Through-knee amputation in peripheral vascular disease. Lancet, *2*:240, 1969.

14. Moore, W. W., Hall, A. D., and Wylie, E. J.: Below-knee amputation for vascular insufficiency. Experience with immediate postoperative fitting of prosthesis. Arch. Surg., *97*:886, 1968.

15. Garrett, H., and DeBakey, M.: Distal posterior tibial artery bypass with autogenous vein graft: A report of three cases. Surgery, *60*:283, 1966.

16. Winsor, T., and Hyman, C.: Methods of study. *In* Winsor, T., and Hyman, C. (eds.): A Primer of Peripheral Vascular Disease. Philadelphia, Lea and Febiger, 1965.

17. Strandness, D. E., Jr.: Chronic Arterial Occlusion. *In* Strandness, D. E., Jr. (ed.): Collateral Circulation in Clinical Surgery. Philadelphia, W. B. Saunders, 1969.

18. Wray, C. H., Still, J. M., Jr., and Moretz, W. H.: Present methods of amputation for peripheral vascular disease. Amer. Surg., *38*:87, 1972.

19. Thursby, P. F., and Dunn, R. M.: Amputations of the lower limb in a Reapt. hospital. Med. J. Aust., *1*:161, 1970.

20. Moretz, W. H., Voyles, W. R., and Thomas, C. F.: Value of preoperative physiologic amputation. Ann. Surg., *154*:851, 1961.

21. Still, J. M., Wray, C. H., and Moretz, W. K.: Selective physiologic amputation: A valuable adjunct in preparation for surgical operation. Ann. Surg., *171*:143, 1970.

22. Large, A., and Heimbecker, D.: Refrigeration in clinical surgery. Ann. Surg., *120*: 707, 1944.

23. Wangensteen, O. H.: Military surgeon and surgery, old and new: An instructive chapter in management of contaminated wounds. Surgery, *62*:437, 1970.

24. Warren, R.: Early rehabilitation of the elderly lower extremity amputee. Surg. Clin. N. Amer., *48*:807, 1968.

25. Burgess, E. M., Romano, R. L., and Zehn, J. K.: The Management of Lower Extremity Amputations. U. S. Government Printing Office, August, 1969.

26. Little, J., Stewart, G. R., *et al.*: A trial of flapless below-knee amputation for arterial insufficiency. Med. J. Aust., *1*:883, 1970.

27. Condon, R. E., and Jordan, P. R., Jr.: Immediate postoperative prostheses in vascular amputations. Ann. Surg., *170*:435, 1969.

28. Golbranson, F. L., *et al.*: Immediate postsurgical fitting and early ambulation. A new concept in amputee rehabilitation. Clin. Orthop., *56*:119, 1968.

29. Appenzeller, O., and Bicknell, J.M.: Effects of nervous system lesions on phantom experience in amputees. Proc. Roy. Soc. Med., *63*:71, 1970.

30. Hoover, R. M.: Problems and complications of amputees. Clin. Orthop., *37*:47, 1964.

31. Patrick, J. H.: Melorheostosis associated with arteriovenous aneurysm of the left arm and trunk. Report of a case with long follow-up. J. Bone Joint Surg. (Brit.), *51*: 126, 1969.

Chapter 16

Assessment of Immediate Postoperative Status in

William H. Moretz, M.D.
Charles H. Wray, M.D.

Peripheral Arterial Reconstruction

Whenever temporary occlusion of the aorta or a large artery is required, whether for treatment of an aneurysm, correction of occlusive disease or removal of an arteriovenous fistula, there is concern for the adequacy of peripheral circulation on restoration of blood flow. Although other types of complications such as hemorrhage, myocardial infarction, and pulmonary edema may also occur in the immediate postoperative period, we have focused here primarily on events which cause occlusion of an artery either in, or distal to, the operative area. This concern stems from unhappy experience wherein, after accomplishing the main objective of operation, such occlusive complications appear which may lead to loss of limb or life. These occlusive events include thrombosis, embolism, subintimal dissection, inadequate anastomosis and severe localized spasm. Despite all reasonable precautions, occlusive problems continue to occur during operative procedures on major arteries.

Assessment of the arterial circulation immediately after arterial surgery may be very easy or very difficult. If, after surgery, foot pulses are good and the extremity is warm and of good color, no significant occlusive complication has occurred. Often, however, especially in those patients with preexisting occlusion distal to the operative area, foot pulses are absent or equivocal. In these patients the possibility of an occlusive complication must be considered. Concern is increased when the extremity is cold and mottled, and either not improved or worse than before operation.

Immediately after operation, findings in the lower extremity distal to the operative site allow qualitative evaluation of the status of arterial circulation. By clinical observation the degree of restored circulation can be placed into one of three categories: *Good, Equivocal* or *Poor*. The *Good* status implies that no occlusive accident has occurred during operation. If the preoperative status was normal, the same should be evident postoperatively. Foot pulses are good, the skin is of good color and warmth, and sensation and movement are normal. The absence of foot pulses is sometimes compatible with *Good* status if pulses were absent before operation, the distal occlusion not surgically corrected, and color and temperature of the foot are normal.

An *Equivocal* status is disconcerting. Although often due to arterial spasm which may improve in a few hours, this status suggests the possibility of an occlusive complication. It is particularly common in those with uncorrected, preexisting occlusive disease distal to the area of operation. In this group foot pulses are reduced or absent, and the skin is cool or cold with mild cyanosis or pallor. Sensation and movement are usually present. Capillary filling time and venous filling time are slightly prolonged. Pain is usually absent.

367

TABLE 16-1. CLINICAL STATUS IMMEDIATELY POSTOPERATIVE

	Foot Pulses	*Skin*	*Capillary Refilling*	*Vein Refilling*	*Calf Musculature*	*Voluntary Movement*	*Sensation*	*Distal Pain*
GOOD	Clearly palable, may be absent if absent pre-op.	Good color — Warm	Normal < 2-3 sec.	Normal 5-15 sec.	Soft and supple	Normal	Normal	Absent
FAIR	Equivocal to Absent	Mild cyanosis or pallor — Cool to cold	Slightly prolonged (2-5 sec.)	10-45 sec.	Soft and supple	Normal	Normal	Absent
POOR	Absent	Cyanotic, pallid or mottled* Cold*	Prolonged usually > 6 sec.	> 45 sec.	Slightly spastic to rigid*	Normal, impaired,* or absent*	Normal — Reduced or absent*	Absent, mild or severe*

* Usually means there has been an occlusive accident.

A *Poor* status causes great concern. An intraoperative accident must be strongly considered and efforts made to substantiate or exclude this possibility. This status is characterized by absent foot pulses, and cold, mottled or pallid skin. Sensation and movement of the part are reduced, often with movement being painful, and markedly prolonged capillary and venous filling times are the rule. Particularly ominous are anesthesia, inability to move the foot, rigidity of calf muscles and constant pain in the part.

Table 16-1 briefly summarizes these criteria.

There are many causes for decreased circulation to an extremity in the immediate postoperative period. An occlusive complication may have occurred. Arteries may be constricted due to a decreased circulating blood volume. Blood loss may have been inadequately replaced. Vasoconstrictors may have been used. The smaller arteries may have developed spasm in response to hypotension distal to arterial clamping or possibly in response to the sudden increase in arterial pressure coincident with restoration of blood flow. This phenomenon is thought to occur more often in arteries acclimated to low pressure distal to chronic occlusion.

If the immediate postoperative status is *Equivocal* or *Poor,* the following questions should be answered. This information will form an appropriate background for decisions about further therapy.

1. Is the present circulation compatible with preexisting, uncorrected, distal arterial disease without a superimposed complication?

2. Is the present circulation explainable by peripheral vasoconstriction secondary to decreased circulating blood volume or the use of vasoconstrictors?

3. Will the extremity remain viable with its present amount of arterial inflow?

4. If a technical error was made, is it easily correctible or was the original procedure so difficult or so hazardous that even this degree of arterial circulation is satisfactory?

5. Would re-exploration be well tolerated or would it likely lead to even worse complications or a fatal outcome?

For many patients the most appropriate treatment is to correct any probable deficit in circulating blood volume and to observe them for a few hours. If the arterial status is still questionable, even if somewhat improved, intra-arterial injection of lidocaine, papaverine, or other vasodilators may bring further improvement which warrants continued observation. In some patients a paravertebral lumbar sympathetic block may be helpful.

For those who do not respond well to the above measures within a few hours, and for those with a *Poor* immediate postoperative status, development of an intraoperative occlusion must be strongly considered. The importance of early correction is well illustrated by DeWeese's report of successful operative management in 11 of 12 patients re-explored within 24 hours for failure of arterial reconstructive procedures.

Intraoperative Evaluation

It has been shown that most of the early occlusive phenomena noted after arterial surgery have their beginning during the operative procedure.[1-5] As experience has increased and techniques have improved these occlusions have become less frequent. Early failures in 4 to 29 percent have been noted after reconstruction. When they occur, detection prior to wound closure allows correction during the original operation. After the patient has reached the recovery room detection is not nearly as helpful, since reinduction of anesthesia and surgery with additional risks are required. For this reason, careful evaluation of restored circulation is desirable prior to completion of the original procedure.

Much attention has been paid to the degree of back bleeding occurring from the distal artery and pulses both in and distal to the operative field. Back bleeding is actually a sign of adequate collaterals about the operative area more than a sign of patent vessels distally beyond the re-entry point of collateral vessels. With good back bleeding, many surgeons assume since clotting has not occurred in the vessel immediately distal to the operative site, that vessels throughout the leg are patent. This is not a valid assumption. Evaluation of pulses in the operative field, in the graft, just below the distal anastomosis, or as far distally as the artery is exposed is subject to considerable error.

What is normal and what is subnormal is hard to quantify using only fingers as sensors. We have been fooled by a definitely palpable pulse distal to an anastomosis when no blood was flowing. The pulse was excellent because of dissection subintimally to a more distal point. Also, a fresh thrombus, still in a gel-like state, will transmit a normal-feeling pulse wave through an anastomosis or over the entire length of an arterial graft. Judging lumen adequacy by palpation after a tedious anastomosis is hazardous. Detection of foot pulses by a circulating assistant during operation is reassuring. But such assurance of arterial patency is lacking when pulses are equivocal or absent as in patients with distal, preexisting occlusive disease.

For these reasons, objective evidence obtained during operation of adequately restored circulation is highly desirable for recognition and treatment of complications before closing the wound. Various objective observations are practical either for routine use or for use when an accident is suspected. Much may be gained from routine intraoperative studies as demonstrated by arteriography, various types of monitoring and use of Fogarty catheters.

Routine Arteriography

Intraoperative arteriography has been used increasingly for specific indications since early experience in arterial surgery. Intraoperative arteriography as a means of routinely evaluating arterial status at the completion of operation was advocated in 1968.

Renwick, Royle and Martin[6] used operative angiography in femoropopliteal arterial reconstruction. Fifty-five patients who had arteriography performed at the end of operation were compared with 55 patients who did not have arteriography. Urografin 60 percent was injected through an 18-gauge needle into the vessel above the femoropopliteal reconstruction. Two films, placed under the extremity were then exposed. Repeated injections produced no adverse reactions, and no complications arose from puncture of the vessel wall. In 55 operative

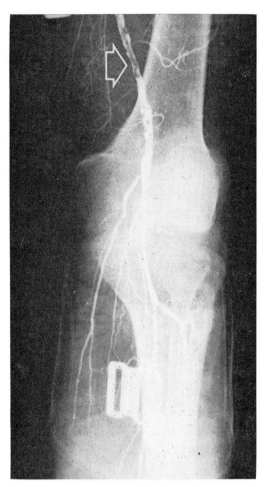

FIG. 16-1. During an aortoiliac graft segmental plethysmography was used as a monitoring device. The segmental cuff can be seen on the upper calf. After flow was restored, good pulses were detected on the right side but none on the left. The operative arteriogram shows a partially occluding thrombus in the distal superficial femoral artery (*arrow*). Operative arteriography is necessary in only one in twenty cases if segmental plethysmography is used.

angiograms, 15 (27%) revealed defects after endarterectomy, thrombus formation, or occlusion of a previously patent vessel requiring correction. These defects were detected often in reconstructions which seemed perfect to external inspection and palpation. Of these 55 none was returned to the operating room in the first 14 days following surgery. Two patients did require amputation within four weeks for progressive gangrene, but the

reconstructions were patent in each at the time of amputation. In the control group of 55 patients in whom operative angiography was not performed, 10 (18%) were returned to the operating room in the immediate postoperative period for failure. Of these, seven were readily cleared and remained patent, but three occluded again and came to amputation within a month. Patency rates at discharge were similar in both groups, but at three months, 91 percent of patients having angiography were patent as compared to 74.5 percent patency in the control group.

The following year Engleman, Clements and Herman[7] advised routine operative arteriography and presented seven cases illustrating the use of the technique in discovering operative errors. Common technical errors demonstrable by this method include: stenosis of the proximal or distal anastomosis, narrowing of arteriotomy closure following endarterectomy; axial twisting of a graft, too long a graft with narrowing or kinking, constricting adventitial bands in vein grafts, thrombus formation in distal arteries, embolism to distal arteries, evaluation of an intimal flap, and residual lumen irregularity particularly following endarterectomy. While many of these are avoidable and some are recognizable on direct inspection, all are apparent by arteriography.

We have reserved operative arteriography for those in whom segmental plethysmography demonstrates lack of satisfactory flow, and when examination of the vessels in the wound does not show a defect. Used in this way, only about 5 percent of those undergoing direct vascular reconstruction require operative arteriography to localize an area of difficulty.[8] The arteriographic technique can be quite simple, as demonstrated by Renwick and Engleman. One of our operating rooms is equipped with a special operating table that has a motorized film changer included in its understructure. The overhead tube is also mounted on a motorized track. The tube and film changer are synchronized to move down the table so that serial films can be made to include the area between the

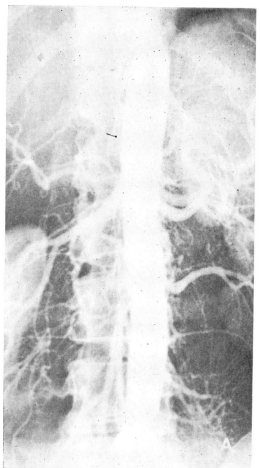 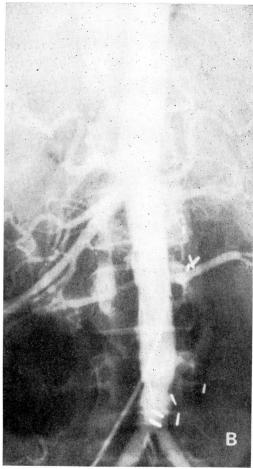

FIG. 16-2. (A) Preoperative arteriogram showing stenosis of left lower renal artery. A lower vessel did not fill from the aorta on the right. Branches to lower pole of right kidney are seen to refill through collaterals. (B) Intraoperative arteriogram. A plaque was found at the origin of the lower left renal artery. A lower pole vessel was found on the right with total occlusion by a plaque inside the aorta. Both plaques were removed and the right vessel was dilated with a Fogarty catheter. The right lower pole vessel is now filled. The patient is no longer hypertensive. There was an asymptomatic, but significant stenosis of the distal aorta in this 32-year-old woman which was corrected by endarterectomy.

abdominal aorta and the foot. Or the tube and film changer remain static for serial roentgenograms in renal artery, celiac and mesenteric artery reconstructions or portacaval anastomoses.

Intraoperative Monitoring

Two noninvasive techniques which can be repeated many times without danger to the extremity have been used for monitoring during the operative procedure. These are the digital and segmental types of plethysmography.

After a preliminary report in 1957,[9] specific reports and recommendations for intraoperative monitoring were made in 1961 using segmental plethysmography[2] and digital plethysmography.[10]

Digital Plethysmography. The mercury strain gauge plethysmography technique utilized a small loop of mercury-filled silastic tubing placed around a digit and connected

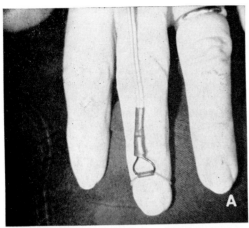

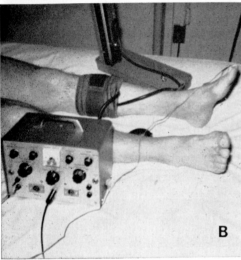

FIG. 16-3. (A) The simplicity of the mercury strain gauge is obvious. The selected gauge should have a diameter about 25 per cent below that of the digit. The gauges are very inexpensive so that a large variety can be on hand to fit any digit. (B) To measure calf pressure, a blood pressure cuff is placed on the calf, the mercury strain gauge on the left second toe. The gauge is connected to the strain gauge plethysmograph. A standard electrocardiograph can be used for recording.

to an amplifying device and recording system. The normal digital wave has a sharp systolic peak and a dicrotic wave on the down slope. Arterial obstruction is indicated by blunting of the systolic peak, decrease in amplitude, and loss of dicrotic notch. Blood pressure at any level in an extremity can be measured using a pneumatic cuff and the plethysmograph. The cuff pressure at which the digital pulse reappears is considered the systolic pressure at the cuff level. Normally the mean arterial pressure at the ankle approximates that of the arm. Arterial obstruction is indicated by the ankle systolic pressure being less than the systolic pressure in the arm, and by a difference of more than 20 mm. Hg between any two successive levels in the same extremity.[10]

In 1965, Dickson and Strandness[11] reported detecting 19 operative accidents in a total of 49 patients (55 reconstructive arterial procedures) monitored with digital plethysmography. They noted that back bleeding and a pulsating graft were unreliable as criteria for arterial patency, and that pedal pulses were of value only if definitely present. In aneurysm patients without preoperative occlusion, an occlusive accident was suspected if the pulse tracing and ankle pressure at the conclusion of the procedure did not equal the preoperative values. In other patients with primary occlusive disease, an intraoperative accident was suspected unless there was a distinct increase in ankle pressure and return of the digital pulse. Each of their early graft failures resulted from accidents which occurred during the operative procedure. Eleven of 19 patients with intraoperative accidents had patent arteries at the time of discharge, while eight were considered failures due to operative accidents incompletely corrected. There was no loss of limb. Of the 11 with patent arteries on discharge, seven had correction of occlusive accident by surgical intervention. How many of these were corrected during the initial operation was not stated, but in their illustrative case the accident was discovered in the recovery room, the patient being returned to surgery for operative correction. It is assumed that particularly in their early experience many of the occlusions were not identified until the patient was in the recovery room.

The technique of plethysmography has several advantages. The recording device required, an electrocardiograph, is available

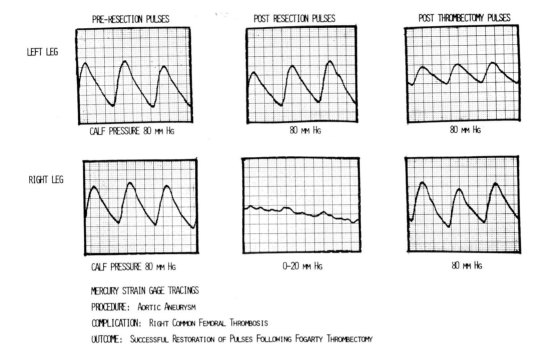

PRE-RESECTION PULSES   POST RESECTION PULSES   POST THROMBECTOMY PULSES

LEFT LEG

CALF PRESSURE 80 MM HG   80 MM HG   80 MM HG

RIGHT LEG

CALF PRESSURE 80 MM HG   0-20 MM HG   80 MM HG

MERCURY STRAIN GAGE TRACINGS

PROCEDURE: AORTIC ANEURYSM

COMPLICATION: RIGHT COMMON FEMORAL THROMBOSIS

OUTCOME: SUCCESSFUL RESTORATION OF PULSES FOLLOWING FOGARTY THROMBECTOMY

FIG. 16-4. An accident was detected in the operating room before wound closure. The lack of pulsations on the right required investigation. Correction of the defect resulted in return of the pulse at a slightly higher amplitude than on the normal side, presumably owing to reactive hyperemia.

in all hospitals and the mercury strain gauge plethysmograph is an inexpensive, easily operated instrument. In most patients it provides very satisfactory information. However, in patients with preexisting occlusive disease distal to the site of operation, the response after restoring blood flow is not reliable. Similarly, large blood loss during surgery, and poor cardiac output interfere with the response and make interpretation uncertain. Such patients comprise approximately one third of those requiring reconstructive arterial surgery.

Segmental Plethysmography. A two chan-

PRE-GRAFT PULSES   POST-GRAFT PULSES

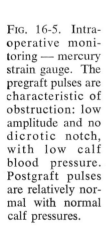

FIG. 16-5. Intraoperative monitoring — mercury strain gauge. The pregraft pulses are characteristic of obstruction: low amplitude and no dicrotic notch, with low calf blood pressure. Postgraft pulses are relatively normal with normal calf pressures.

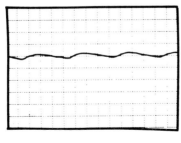
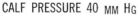
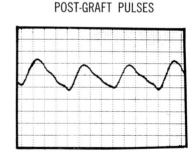

CALF PRESSURE 40 MM HG   CALF PRESSURE 100 MM HG

OPERATION: FEMOROPOPLITEAL VEIN BYPASS

RESULT: SUCCESSFUL RELIEF OF CLAUDICATION

TABLE 16-2. SUMMARY OF PROCEDURES

Procedure	Monitored	Not Monitored	Total
Aneurysmectomy			
Aorto-iliac	57	30	87
Femoropopliteal	4	11	15
Reconstructive Surgery			
Aorto-iliac	59	47	106
femoropopliteal	15	42	57
	135	130	265

nel segmental plethysmograph (Vasograph Electro-Medical Engineering Company, Burbank, California) can be used to measure pulsatile volume change in a segment of the limb. It is calibrated so that 1 cm. deflection equals a 1 ml. change in volume.[12] Although many features of the recording are of considerable value, only the height of maximum deflection has been used for intraoperative monitoring.

Segmental plethysmography is performed prior to operation, at the upper thigh, lower thigh, upper calf and lower calf levels bilaterally. For intraoperative monitoring, the cuffs are placed preferably on the lower calf level, but at a higher level if required to obtain at least a 3 mm. deflection. For most meaningful results at least a 3 mm. deflection preoperatively is required. Four level recordings are valuable postoperatively for following the results of surgery and natural

TABLE 16-3. INTRAOPERATIVE OCCLUSIVE PHENOMENA

	Monitored		Nonmonitored	
Thrombosis		11		14
Iliac	8		8	
Femoral	2		5	
Popliteal	1		1	
Embolism		3		2
Subintimal dissection		4		1
Inadequate anatomosis		1		1
Total		19		18

TABLE 16-4. COMPARISON OF MONITORED AND NONMONITORED GROUP

	Monitored	Non-monitored
Total No. of patients	135	130
Total No. of intra-operative accidents	19	18
Total No. of accidents detected during surgery	15	4
No. undergoing correction at same operation	11	2
No. of operative occlusions not corrected but apparent within 24 hrs.	8	16
No. reoperations required within 30 days for intra-operative occlusion	2*	8
No. deaths attributable to intraoperative occlusion	0	3
No. amputations required for intra-operative occlusion	2	10†

* For detectable but uncorrected intraoperative occlusion.
† 2 minor amputations, 8 A-K.

course of the disease. Our experience with intraoperative segmental plethysmography was reported in 1961[2] and most recently in 1971.[8] Of 265 direct arterial procedures, 135 were monitored and 130 were not monitored. The composition of the two groups is shown in Table 16-2.

Intraoperative occlusions were similar in the two groups and included thrombosis, embolism, subintimal dissection and inadequate anastomoses. Nineteen such events occurred in the 135 monitored patients and 18 in the 130 nonmonitored group, as outlined in Table 16-3. The difference in results of treatment of these accidents is important, and Table 16-4 summarizes this experience. Several points warrant emphasis. The improved prognosis resulting from detection of occlusive events during operation as opposed to detection postoperatively is significant.

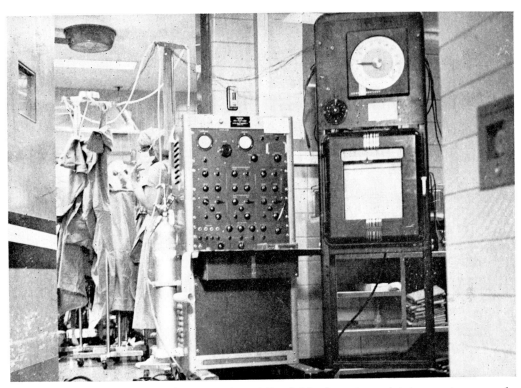

Fig. 16-6. The segmental plethysmograph and Leeds-Northrup ten-point temperature recorder outside the operating room. The pressure tubing and temperature leads course to the foot of the table and proceed under the drapes to the feet of the patient. Recordings can be made without interference with the operating team.

Amputation was later required in ten of the nonmonitored patients but in only two of those monitored. Death was attributed to intraoperative occlusion in three of the nonmonitored group and in none of the monitored group. The number of reoperations required within 30 days was markedly reduced in those monitored as was the number of occlusions becoming apparent within the first 24 hours after operation. Eleven monitored patients had correction of an occlusive event during the initial operation as compared to only two of the nonmonitored group.

Interpretation of intraoperative monitor responses was difficult at first. Experience has clarified some of the uncertainties and present results are highly reliable in most instances. A good plethysmographic response of greater than 1 mm. deflection after declamping was obtained in 86 per-

cent. No accident was identified in any patient with a "good response." A poor plethysmographic response of less than 1 mm. was obtained in 14 percent. These patients were divided into "accident" or "equivocal" categories depending upon the preclamping plethysmographic deflection. The "accident" response of less than 1 mm. in those whose preclamping deflection was 3 mm. or more, occurred in 7 percent and in each instance correctly indicated that occlusion had occurred. The "equivocal" response of less than 1 mm. in those whose preclamping deflection was less than 3 mm. occurred in 7 percent and was not diagnostic of an accident. Instead, further investigation either by arteriography or by passing a Fogarty catheter, was necessary. The significance of an "equivocal" response varied with the preoperative status of the distal run-off. Each of two patients with no significant

TABLE 16-5.

RESPONSES NOTED DURING SURGERY FOR
ANEURYSMAL AND OCCLUSIVE DISEASES

Type of Response	Aorto-iliac	Fem. Pop.	Total
Good	198 (44)*	18	216 (86%)
Poor			
Accident	17 (8)*	0	17 (7%)
Equivocal	17 (15)*	1*	18 (7%)
Total Limbs	232 (67)*	19	251

( )* No. with preexisting more distal occlusive disease, not being corrected.

preexisting occlusive disease distal to the site of operation had an intraoperative accident. Of the other 16 patients with significant preexisting occlusive disease distal to the site of operation, only three incurred an accident. Segmental plethysmography is a safe and reliable means of detecting intraoperative vascular occlusion.

Routine Exploration with Fogarty Catheter. Although not widely practiced, some surgeons routinely pass a Fogarty catheter into the distal arterial tree prior to comple-

tion of the distal anastomosis.[13,14] This maneuver is particularly useful in assuring patency of the main distal vessel when blood clots form toward the end of a procedure as heparin, given much earlier, is depleted. It is also applicable in patients not heparinized, or when clots return from the distal artery after flushing just prior to completing an anastomosis. It is usually desirable to instill dilute heparin distally in such situations prior to completing the anastomosis and re-establishing blood flow.

If the equipment needed for intraoperative monitoring is lacking, marked reassurance of successful restoration of blood flow is provided by passing the Fogarty catheter and finding no thrombus on withdrawal. In some situations this form of reassurance is easier to obtain than arteriography. Its usefulness is distinctly limited by preexisting distal occlusive disease not being corrected during the operation. Unfortunately, of the arteries below the knee, only the posterior tibial artery is easily checked by this method.

This useful technique has been accom-

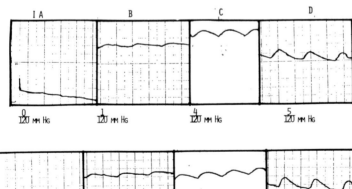

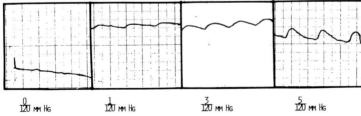

UPPER CALF LEVEL

AORTO-ILIAC OCCLUSIONS

A. NO DETECTABLE PULSES AFTER INDUCTION OF ANESTHESIA.
B. TWENTY MINUTES AFTER RESTITUTION OF FLOW, PULSATIONS ARE DETECTABLE.
C. ONE HOUR AFTER RESTITUTION OF FLOW, PULSATIONS HAVE INCREASED.
D. 24 HOURS FOLLOWING SURGERY, PULSATIONS ARE NORMAL.

FIG. 16-7. Operative monitoring with segmental plethysmograph. There was a definite but low amplitude pulse detected after correction of aorto-iliac occlusions. As time passed the amplitude of the pulse increased. This process may take several days. While this type of response may be due to "spasm" in vessels unaccustomed to high flows, it is also seen in hypovolemia and in patients who have a proximal aorto-iliac occlusion corrected but an uncorrected distal femoral block.

panied by few complications. Foster, *et al.*[15] reported 12 serious events such as rupture of an artery by the inflated balloon, perforation of an artery by the tip of the catheter, tear or disruption of the intima, and rupture of the balloon with embolization of a fragment of rubber. Hogg and MacDougall[16] as well as Krause and co-workers[17] have reported such complications. Rob and Battle have described formation of an arteriovenous fistula in the leg following use of a Fogarty catheter.[18]

The simplicity of the technique and a low incidence of complications make the use of balloon catheters for the removal of thrombi a useful procedure.[19]

Other Methods of Intraoperative Monitoring

Electromagnetic Flowmeter. Until very recently many difficulties were encountered in attempts to use electromagnetic flowmeters during reconstructive arterial surgery. Even now with much improved equipment and sensitive probes, the expense and expertise required markedly limit their use. Valuable information is being gained about flow rates in normal and abnormal vessels, before and after reconstructive procedures, and with augmentation of flow by sympathectomy or intra-arterial drugs.[20,21,22,23] Electromagnetic flowmeters will undoubtedly become more commonly used than at present, and hopefully will provide reliable information concerning blood flow and success of reconstructive surgery. Another limitation of their value for intraoperative monitoring is the necessity of having the artery surgically exposed.

Observed flow rates vary widely with changes in blood volume and blood pressure, making it difficult to establish criteria for diagnosis of occlusive accidents during arterial reconstruction.[24,25] Barner,[26] using the electromagnetic flowmeter in 26 patients, detected three faulty distal anastomoses in 29 femoropopliteal bypass operations. His positive criteria included lack of increased absolute blood flow and failure of rate of flow to increase after intra-arterial papaverine.

FIG. 16-8. Operative monitoring with segmental plethysmograph. An intraoperative accident was detected and corrected. After restoration of flow, no pulse was detected on the right. This drop from 12 mm. to 0 mm. was significant and could not be ignored for an occlusion had occurred. If examination of the operative area is not helpful, then arteriograms or insertion of Fogarty catheters should be done. Note that on the left the pulse is slightly lower than at the beginning of the operation. This finding is frequently associated with long operating times or unreplaced blood loss. The pulse on the right was not as high after extraction of the thrombus but was a normal response. Within an hour the pulse had returned to the preoperative level.

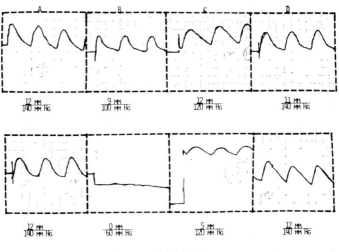

UPPER CALF LEVEL

AORTIC ANEURYSM

A. AFTER INDUCTION OF ANESTHESIA, PULSATIONS REMAINED AT THE PREOPERATIVE LEVEL.

B. AFTER INSTALLATION OF THE GRAFT, PULSATIONS WERE PRESENT ON THE LEFT, BUT ABSENT ON THE RIGHT.

C. AFTER EXTRACTION OF THROMBUS FROM THE COMMON FEMORAL ARTERY, PULSATIONS RETURN, BUT NOT AT THE PREOPERATIVE LEVEL.

D. ONE HOUR LATER PULSES ARE EQUAL AGAIN.

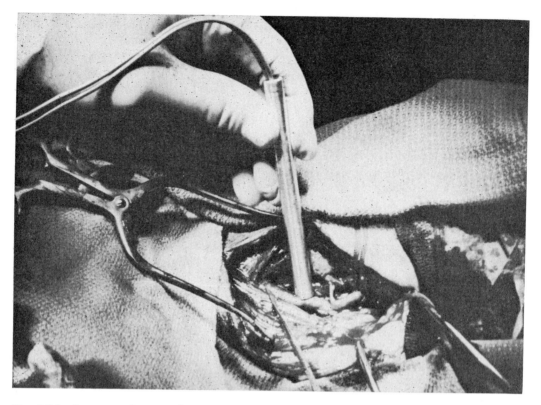

FIG. 16-9. Intraoperative use of Doppler during carotid endarterectomy; a sterile Doppler probe is shown on the carotid artery.

Sheinen and Inbert[27] studied 53 patients during arterial surgery and concluded that flow studies would be helpful in selecting those who would benefit from sympathectomy.

This method, perhaps with an implanted probe allowing continued monitoring in the early postoperative period, may become more widely used in the future.[6,28,29,30] Potential infection constitutes a restraint on enthusiasm for this technique, however.

Pressure Determinations. Measurement of intra-arterial pressure proximal and distal to areas of obstruction has been used to determine the significance of partial occlusions and to show satisfactory correction of occlusions. This method has been used most in renal and carotid arteries, but is less helpful in arteries of the extremities. In the extremities, elimination of one gradient by operation has less meaning because a more distal oc-

clusion may also affect the arterial pressure by increasing resistance to outflow. For the same reason, this method is not effective for detecting possible occlusive accidents distal to the operative area.

Doppler Flowmeter. Instruments based on the Doppler principle detect movement of blood within underlying vessels and produce output which varies with velocity of blood flow. Sterile probes may be used within the operative field, and probes can be used over the course of distal vessels. With experience, areas of occlusion or narrowing may be detected. Our experience with this instrument for intraoperative monitoring is relatively limited, but it has accurately located an embolic occlusion in the common femoral artery following aortoiliac reconstruction. It has also correctly indicated the absence of intraoperative occlusive accidents in many instances. Since the

Doppler flowmeter detects flow rather than a pulse, it is often more useful than simple palpation of a vessel.

Early Postoperative Evaluation

At the conclusion of an arterial reconstructive procedure the status of the arterial tree and the clinical appearance of the extremity should be definitely established. Any subsequent change in the extremity can be meaningfully compared to this baseline observation. If the status of the arterial tree is not known, information vitally needed for sound conclusions and logical treatment is lacking in those patients with *Equivocal* or *Poor* status. In these patients we need to know whether or not an occlusive accident has occurred. If one has, we must decide whether it should be operatively corrected. In all of those with less than a *Good* status, an occlusive accident is suspected. Careful observations are begun aimed at differentiating those with occlusion from those with vasospasm without an occlusive accident.

An *Equivocal* status, most often seen in those with uncorrected preexisting distal occlusive disease, may also be due to a partially occluding accident in a major artery or a completely occluding accident in a less major artery. Immediate efforts should be made to correct causes of vasoconstriction. Correction of blood volume deficit and improvement in cardiac output will often lead to early improvement in vasoconstriction. Intra-arterial injection of lidocaine or papaverine or a paravertebral lumbar sympathetic block may also be effective. In the extremity which has not shown the improvement expected from correcting an occlusion, these general measures should bring prompt improvement unless an occlusive accident has occurred. Evaluation during this critical period is aided materially by objective tests such as plethysmography and the Doppler flowmeter. Continued gradual improvement supports the impression that vasoconstriction was an important cause of the *Equivocal* response and suggests continuing these general measures.

If improvement from these general mea-

RIGHT POSTERIOR TIBIAL ARTERY   LEFT POSTERIOR TIBIAL ARTERY

 INTRAOPERATIVE PRIOR TO EMBOLECTOMY

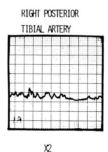 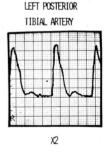

x2   x2

INTRAOPERATIVE AFTER EMBOLECTOMY

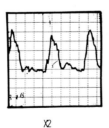 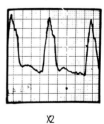

x2   x2

PAPER SPEED 50 mm/sec.

Fig. 16-10. Intraoperative application of Doppler flowmeter. There was absent flow in the right leg preoperatively. Immediately after extraction of the embolus and closure of the arteriotomy, normal flow was immediately detected at the ankle. This instrument may detect flow before the pulse is easily palpable and gives accurate information without need of arteriogram.

OPERATION: Right Femoral Embolectomy

There was no detectable signal prior to embolectomy. Following extraction of the embolus, an audible and recordable signal was recorded. The uninvolved left side remained the same.

sures is lacking, suspicion of an occlusive accident is strengthened and the need for re-exploration must be considered.

Arteriography is valuable in determining the presence and nature of an occlusion. Occlusion may also be located by the abrupt cessation of blood flow detected by a Doppler flowmeter or by the abrupt reduction of blood pressure at a level detected by plethysmography. The disappearance of a previously present femoral or foot pulse is ominous. In these situations, an accurate intraoperative appraisal of the status of the major arteries at the end of the procedure is invaluable in determining the need for reoperation.

In those with a *Poor* status, unless considerable improvement occurs within a few hours with restoration of blood volume and other measures used to overcome vasoconstriction, an occlusive accident must be presumed. Arteriography and plethysmographic and Doppler flowmeter studies may be informative and the response to heparin, if not contraindicated, or to dextran may be noted. However, since early correction of occlusion gives superior results, reoperation is indicated without delay when the clinical picture fits an occlusive complication.

A *Poor* status postoperatively may be a continuation of a situation known to exist at the time the original procedure was completed. In most such instances, every reasonable effort to improve the circulation by operation will have already been made. Thus, there usually is little more than can be done operatively, however individualization is required. Thrombosis may have occurred at a questionable anastomosis or in an endarterectomized segment. Arteriography or repeated plethysmography may be needed to provide additional information.

Early reoperation can be decided upon after carefully weighing the overall condition of the patient, the known or suspected arterial status of the extremity, the chance of improving the arterial supply by re-exploration, and the probable fate of the extremity if no operative intervention is attempted.

Often, the original procedure helps to foretell the site and nature of the occlusion. For example, if after resection of an aortic aneurysm in a patient with good foot pulses preoperatively, absence of a foot pulse is noted in the presence of a femoral pulse, the probability of an embolus to the popliteal artery is great. Or, if after experiencing marked difficulty during anastomosis of a prosthesis to the left common iliac artery the left femoral pulse disappears, thrombosis or possibly a subintimal dissection at that anastomosis, would be strongly suspected.

Decision to Reoperate in Early Postoperative Period

Absolute criteria for reoperation are difficult to establish, since many individual factors must be considered. These factors include: overall general condition of the patient; the preoperative status of the arteries of the extremity, the nature and magnitude of the initial surgery, the anticipated viability of the part if not subjected to reoperation, the location and nature of the occlusion, the magnitude of surgery necessary to correct it, and the local response to elimination of vasospasm and restoration of blood volume during immediate postoperative period.

This decision is less often required and much easier to make in those patients who have had intraoperative studies, whether by arteriography, plethysmographic monitoring, or some other reliable method. Knowing the arterial status at completion of operation permits better understanding of findings in the extremity and better interpretation of subsequent changes. If occlusion had occurred, a decision concerning operative correction is required. When this decision involves considerable risk to life, it can be an extremely difficult one.

If it appears that the limb will be nonviable, and the patient is in good general condition, and if the occlusive accident is easily correctible, then obviously reoperation is indicated. An example of this would be a 45-year-old man who had an endarterectomy for Leriche syndrome who immediately after operation was noted to have good femoral pulses, but a cold, mottled right foot and lower leg. The embolus or thrombosis in the popliteal artery should be easily correctable by either direct exposure of the popliteal artery or more likely by a Fogarty catheter passed from the common femoral artery.

At the opposite extreme, if the initial operation was a very difficult resection of a ruptured aneurysm in a poor risk, 70-year-old hypertensive man who had had a myocardial infarction two months previously, reoperation would be a very serious undertaking and would require very strong indications. In such an individual, a nonviable foot would be accepted if the alternative meant a second laparotomy. If correctable by a transfemoral Fogarty catheter under local anesthesia, restoration of flow should be attempted.

If a nonviable extremity can be salvaged by a simple procedure it usually should be attempted. A viable but moderately ischemic extremity also should usually have corrective surgery if the surgery required is simple and not an undue risk to life. If at the initial femoropopliteal bypass, the distal anastomosis was the best possible, although poor, and there was no other acceptable artery distally, nothing would be accomplished by trying it again. If it is felt that the distal anastomosis, now thrombosed, could be improved upon, re-exploration would be indicated.

Innumerable situations are encountered with different degrees of ischemia, all varieties of patient status, and many magnitudes of surgery necessary for correction of the occlusive accident. Judgments must be made after considering all aspects of the situation. The risk to the limb must be weighed against the risk of life, and in most instances a live patient with one leg is preferable to a dead one with two.

Summary

Evaluation of the status of the lower extremities in the early postoperative period remains a complex problem. The problem is materially simplified by accurate assessment of the peripheral arterial blood flow during initial surgery. For many patients accurate assessment requires specific objective evidence as provided by arteriography, plethysmography or other means.

Occlusive complications most often occur during operation and are best corrected during the initial procedure. For those not detected during operation, best results are obtained by recognition and correction as soon as possible in the postoperative period. To accomplish this, occlusion should be suspected in those whose extremities have a questionable status immediately after surgery. Confirmation or exclusion by specific tests is needed in those who do not respond favorably to measures directed at elimination of fluid deficits and vasospasm.

Occlusions should be corrected promptly unless contraindicated by overriding factors.

References

1. DeWeese, J. A.: Early failures in arterial reconstruction. Arch. Surg., *85*:901, 1962.
2. Belisle, C. A., and Moretz, W. H.: Detection of vascular complications by plethysmography during direct vessel surgery. Ann. Surg., *154*:839, 1961.
3. Crawford, E. S., DeBakey, M. D., Morris, G. C., Jr., and Garrett, E.: Evaluation of late failures after reconstructive operations for occlusive lesions of the aorta and iliac, femoral and popliteal arteries. Surgery, *47*: 79, 1960.
4. Dale, W. A., DeWeese, J. A., and Scott, W. J. H.: Autogenous venous shunt grafts. Surgery, *46*:145, 1959.
5. Haimovici, H.: Stenosing arterial thrombosis. Surgery, *36*:1075, 1954.
6. Renwick, S., Poyle, J. P., and Martin, P.: Operative angiography after femoropopliteal arterial reconstruction—Its influence on early failure rate. Brit. J. Surg., *55*:134, 1968.
7. Engelman, R. M., Clements, J. M., and Herrman, J. B.: Routine operative arteriography following vascular reconstruction. Surg. Gynec. Obstet., *128*:745, 1969.
8. Griffin, L. H., Jr., Wray, C. H., Vaughan, B. L., and Moretz, W. H.: Detection of vascular occlusions during operation by segmental plethysmography and skin thermometry. Ann. Surg., *173*:389, 1971.

9. Creech, O., Jr., DeBakey, M. D., and Culotta, R.: Digital blood flow following reconstructive arterial surgery. Arch. Surg., *74*:5, 1957.

10. Radke, H. M., Bell, J. W., Strandness, D. E., Jr., and Jesseph, J. E.: Monitor of digit volume changes in angioplastic surgery: Use of strain gauge plethysmography. Ann. Surg., *154*:818, 1961.

11. Dickson, A. H., Strandness, D. E., Jr., and Bell, J. W.: The dectection and sequelae of operative accidents complicating reconstructive arterial surgery. Amer. J. Surg., *109*:143, 1965.

12. Winsor, T.: The segmental plethysmograph. Angiology, *8*:87, 1957.

13. Fogarty, T. J., and Cranley, J. J.: Catheter technic for arterial embolectomy. Ann. Surg., *161*:325, 1965.

14. Fogarty, T. J., Cranley, J. J., Krause, R. J., Strasser, E. S., and Hafner, C. D.: A method for extraction of arterial emboli and thrombi. Surg. Gynec. Obstet., *116*:241, 1963.

15. Foster, J. H., Carter, J. W., Graham, C. P., Jr., and Edwards, W. H.: Arterial injuries secondary to the use of the Fogarty catheter. Ann. Surg., *171*:971, 1970.

16. Hogg, G., and MacDougall, J. T.: An accident of embolectomy associated with the use of the Fogarty catheter. Surgery, *61*:716, 1967.

17. Krause, R. J., Cranley, J. J., Strasser, E. S., Hafner, C. D., and Fogarty, T. J.: Further experience with a new embolectomy catheter. Surgery, *59*:81, 1966.

18. Rob, C. R., and Battle, S.: Arteriovenous fistula following use of the Fogarty balloon catheter. Arch. Surg., *102*:144, 1971.

19. Baker, L. D., Leshin, S. J., Mathur, V. S., and Messer, J. V.: Routine Fogarty thrombectomy in arterial catheterization. New Eng. J. Med., *279*:1203, 1968.

20. Cronestrand, R., and Ekestrom, S.: Blood flow after peripheral arterial reconstruction. Scand. J. Thor. Cardiov. Surg., *4*:159, 1970.

21. Cronestrand, R., Ekestrom, S., and Hambraeus, G.: The value of blood flow measurements in acute arterial surgery. Scand. J. Thor. Cardiov. Surg., *3*:48, 1969.

22. Lee, B. Y., Madden, J. L., and McDonough, W. B.: Use of square-wave electromagnetic flowmeter during direct arterial surgery, before and after lumbar sympathectomy in peripheral vascular surgery. Vasc. Surg., *3*:218, 1969.

23. Little, J. M., Sheil, A. G. R., Lowenthal, J., and Goodman, A. H.: Prognostic value of intraoperative blood-flow measurements in femoropopliteal bypass vein-grafts. Lancet, *2*:648, 1968.

24. Kirkpatrick, J. R., and Miller, D. R.: Effects of decreased arterial inflow and runoff on vein graft patency. Surgery, *69*:870, 1971.

25. Kouchoukos, N. T.: Pulsatile blood flow patterns in femoropopliteal venous bypass grafts. Surg. Forum, *18*:192, 1967.

26. Barner, H. B., Judd, D. R., Kaiser, G. C., Willman, V. L., and Hanlon, C. R.: Blood flow in femoropopliteal bypass vein grafts. Arch. Surg., *96*:619, 1968.

27. Schenin, T. M., and Inberg, M. V.: Determination of blood flow in arterial surgery. Acta Chir. Scand., *134*:55, 1968.

28. Cronestrand, R., Ekestrom, S., and Hambraeus, G.: Pre- and postoperative flow measurements after femoral-popliteal arterial reconstructions. Scand. J. Thor. Cardiov. Surg., *2*:128, 1968.

29. Mauderly, J. L.: Chronic implantation of electromagnetic flow probes on major abdominal vessels in the dog. Lab. Animal Care, *20*:662, 1970.

30. Renwick, S., Gabe, I. T., Shillingford, J. P., and Martin, P.: Blood flow after reconstructive arterial surgery measured by implanted electromagnetic flow probes. Surgery, *64*:544, 1968.

Chapter 17 | Anesthesia for

T. Crawford McAslan, M.D. | # Vascular Surgery

The chapters in this book deal with surgical management of localized manifestations of a disease process involving the entire cardiovascular system, albeit the process has proceeded at different rates in different parts of the arterial tree. For this reason most patients warrant much more detailed management than that afforded to the routine elective surgical procedure. There is much to be said in favor of handling such patients in special centers with complete facilities and specialized teams. The anesthesiologist should function as an integral part of such a team where physicians, pooling their knowledge and skills, can develop a unified approach to pre-, intra-, and postoperative management. In emergencies, such a relationship of mutual respect and understanding allows the team to swing smoothly into action. This chapter outlines those aspects of clinical management which have proven most important in insuring the comfort and safety of the patient, and in providing the best operating conditions contributing to the successful outcome of surgery.

Preoperative Evaluation

A detailed clinical history is necessary, with a diligent search for clues indicative of cerebral, coronary, or renal insufficiency. The frequent association of atherosclerosis with obesity, diabetes mellitus and hypertension should be borne in mind. Close attention should be directed to the pulmonary system

and to smoking and drinking habits. In the past, statistics have been presented showing high mortality rates in surgery performed within three to six months of myocardial infarction.[2,19,23] The enthusiastic direct surgical attack on the coronary arteries in recent years would suggest that fear of anesthesia and surgery in this group of patients may not have been fully justified. The probability of a second infarction would appear more related to the degree of coronary artery obstruction, and to the presence of collaterals, than to the time relationship of a recent attack.[25] Obviously, common sense must prevail and decisions should be based on the urgency of the proposed surgery.

A detailed knowledge of the drug history is necessary to allow anticipation of interdrug reactions. Few drugs require discontinuing prior to surgery, with the possible exception of propranolol, which should be stopped at least 24 hours before operation. Despite the discontinuance of propranolol, isoproterenol should still be immediately at hand during anesthesia. The presence of heart failure dictates the use of digitalis, and the author recommends its use, if time allows, in all patients who have coronary artery disease and are about to undergo major surgery. A complete physical examination should include inspection of the optic fundi and comparison of blood pressure and pulses in both arms as well as in the upper and lower limbs.

383

An ECG, preferably before and following exercise, should be required in all of these patients regardless of their age, both for diagnostic purposes and as a baseline. The presence of a history of cerebral or coronary insufficiency merits consideration of the need for additional angiographic studies. A preoperative chest x-ray is mandatory.

In addition to routine blood studies, baseline blood gas/acid-base values obtained from an arterial blood sample are of great value. Ventilation function screening studies are also highly desirable.

Physiological Considerations During Anesthesia

Despite the absence in the history or in investigative studies of evidence of involvement of the cerebral, coronary or renal circulations, the potential existence of such involvement should be assumed in patients undergoing vascular surgery. Attention must then be directed to the insurance of adequate uptake, transportation and delivery of oxygen to the tissues of the brain, heart and kidney without disrupting the delicate autoregulatory mechanism in each organ. Preservation of regional blood flow is the goal without sacrificing the splanchnic bed or limbs by excessive redistribution of circulating blood volume. The minimizing of venous stasis is an important additional consideration.

During the transportation of the patient to and from the operating room, the optimal position for breathing should be selected, with continuance of uninterrupted oxygen administration when necessary. Compulsive attention should be paid to position on the operating table. Arms are best placed by the side and not abducted, feet supported by an adequate table length, the head placed on a pillow in neutral position and pressure points and the application of tight straps avoided. The serious consequences of infection demand the strictest sterile techniques in cannulation.

Oxygen Availability

The quantity of oxygen transferred to tissues per minute, the "oxygen flux," may be expressed in the simplified form of the oxygen transport equation.[15]

$$\text{Available oxygen} = \frac{\text{Hb. conc.}}{100} \times 1.39$$
$$\times \frac{\text{Hb. satn.}}{100}$$
$$\times \text{Cardiac Output}$$

$$= \frac{15}{100} \times 1.39$$
$$\times \frac{95}{100} \times 5000$$

$$= 1000 \text{ ml/min.}$$

Consciousness is lost when the internal jugular venous PO_2 falls below about 20 torr. During general anesthesia the minimum oxygen compatible with life is believed to be in the region of 125 ml/minute. Consideration of the oxygen transport equation will show that cardiac output is the only significant compensatory mechanism available for deficiencies, however brief, in hemoglobin concentration and hemoglobin saturation. It is therefore desirable to secure the optimal hemoglobin value before surgery.

Hemoglobin

In addition to the importance of hemoglobin in maintaining the adequacy of available oxygen, the concentration of erythrocytes is an important determinant of the viscosity of blood. Richardson and Guyton have shown that cardiac output varies inversely with the hematocrit and that maximum oxygen delivery is obtained at hematocrits of 35 to 40 percent.[17] Where blood vessels are partly obstructed by atheromatous plaques, the untoward effects of increased viscosity will be compounded. Transient falls in perfusion pressure will further add to the influence of viscosity on local blood flow.[11]

Hemoglobin Saturation and Arterial Oxygen Tension

The alveolar/arterial PO_2 difference is a major factor influencing the arterial PO_2. The A-aDO_2 in turn is influenced by: 1) venous admixture ("shunt"), 2) ventilation/perfusion ratios, 3) cardiac output, 4) alveolar PO_2 and 5) blood hemoglobin, pH, and temperature.

The major cause of oxygen desaturation seen in the hospital course of surgical patients is venous admixture resulting from mixed venous blood perfusing nonventilated alveoli. In the past decade it has become apparent that success of the ventilation of a patient during and after surgery cannot be measured by the isolated observation of the arterial blood gases. In 1958, Campbell, Nunn, and Peckett[4] reported findings of increased alveolar/arterial oxygen tension differences in the presence of normal or decreased arterial PCO_2 values in patients during general anesthesia. Similar findings were reported in the early postoperative period by Nunn and Payne in 1962.[16]

The explanation for the development of these large venous admixtures has only recently been established. The resting end-expiratory position, the Functional Residual Capacity (F.R.C.), is the equilibrium point reached by the elastic recoil of the lungs balanced by the elastic recoil of the thoracic cage. In awake, healthy subjects in the upright position, at total lung capacity all alveoli are equally filled.[21] In the same posture at F.R.C. the terminal airways throughout the lung are still open, although the apices remain relatively more expanded than the basilar lung zones.[10] However, at residual volume (maximal expiration) many airways at the bottom of the lung will have closed, with a resultant perfusion of nonventilated alveoli with resultant venous admixture effect.[3] The critical lung volume at which the terminal airways begin to close has been designated as the closing volume (C.V.). Normally F.R.C. is greater than C.V. Any

mechanism tending to reduce F.R.C. or increase C.V. will therefore promote airway closure. It has been shown that with increasing age,[1,9] obesity,[5] smoking, asthma, bronchitis, the supine position,[6,7,14] severe trauma, general anesthesia,[8] kyphoscoliosis and cirrhosis of the liver, airway closure may occur at F.R.C. due to either an increase in closing volume, a decrease in F.R.C. or a combination of both. Following airway closure, absorption atelectasis will occur, the rate and degree of atelectasis being greater if high concentrations of oxygen are being administered. It should be noted that it is the resting expiratory position that is the determinant of airway closure and not the magnitude of the tidal volume.

The key to management is prevention. This is achieved by preoperative attention to weight reduction, discontinuance of smoking, postural drainage and physical therapy to "dry" the lungs and by the use of appropriate antibiotics where specific pulmonary infection has been demonstrated. Before surgery the patient should be mobilized, when possible, until the evening before and as soon as possible after surgery. During surgery anesthetic gases should be delivered with adequate heated humidification and attention directed to more sophisticated ventilatory patterns. Gaseous distribution can be secured in this group of patients by the use of volume limited mechanical ventilators with a sine wave flow pattern, or better, an initial sine wave followed by an inspiratory hold which allows equilibration of fast and slow alveoli. The latter pattern is provided in the Engstrom and Drager ventilators. The F.R.C. may be reestablished above C.V. by the use of a positive end-expiratory pressure, a value of $5cm.H_2O$ usually proving adequate. The actual level to be used should, however, be determined by its effect on the A-a oxygen gradient. The increasing circulatory effects and risk of mediastinal emphysema must be borne in mind as one raises the mean airway pressure. The risk of mediastinal emphysema is more associated with maldistribution of gases than the mean airway pressure, and occurs more frequently, particularly in the postoperative period, if the patient is allowed to get "out of phase" with the ventilator. The use of a positive end-expiratory pressure is contraindicated in patients suffering from emphysema where the F.R.C. is already increased. In these patients an added expiratory resistance (retard) should be substituted.

Serious consideration should be given to the continuance of mechanical ventilation, using the patterns described, for the first evening after intra-abdominal, intrathoracic or prolonged surgery on the extremities. This may be continued for longer periods if the postoperative course is complicated by abdominal distention, as may be anticipated after surgery of the abdominal aorta, or where there is evidence of progressive increase in the A-a oxygen difference. Mechanical ventilation has the additional advantage of allowing the provision of adequate narcotic and sedative administration and significantly reducing the oxygen consumption of these patients. If the patient is allowed to breathe spontaneously postoperatively, nasal oxygen should be administered for the first 48 hours and the arterial gases monitored.[16]

Cardiac Output

Myocardial oxygen requirement is increased by bradycardia, which necessitates the maintenance of an increased tension in the myocardial wall, and by tachycardia due to the reduction of diastole. Katz and Feinberg have shown that oxygen consumption of the heart is a function of the product of heart rate and peak systolic pressure.[12] Reduction of peak systolic pressure by judicious and cautious reduction of peripheral resistance may therefore be desirable. The mean arterial pressure is a better guide of perfusion pressure, the actual value being determined by that required to insure basal urine output. It bears repetition that the most important determinant of cardiac output in the supine position is the filling pressure of the heart

and this can usually be obtained by providing adequate circulating blood volume.

Blood Volume

Bearing in mind the necessity of maintaining an optimal hematocrit, the preservation of colloid pressure and avoidance of excessive sodium load, the volume and type of fluids administered should be carefully managed. Measurement of blood loss in prolonged surgery can lead to considerable error. Estimates should therefore be substantiated by the response of the heart to intermittent volume challenges. In the past, the response of the central venous and arterial blood pressures have been the main guides to the heart's ability to handle the venous return. The Swann-Ganz catheter,[22] which allows convenient placement in the pulmonary artery using pressure waveforms, has made available pulmonary artery and wedge pressures. Experience has shown these measurements to be of great value in patients where there is concern over cardiac function. The use of this catheter is recommended in such patients during intra- and postoperative management.

Renal Function

Provided inadequacy of circulatory volume, and colloid pressures are excluded and catheter placement and patency have been checked, the persistent reduction of urine output below 30 ml per hour will require the use of a diuretic. Furosemide, by virtue of its small volume and rapid potent action has much to commend its use. Mannitol is still widely used and is probably the most popular choice in aortic surgery when administered prior to clamping for its protective effect. Where such diuresis is promoted, appropriate attention must be directed to electrolyte balance.

Cerebral Function

In health, the blood flow to cerebral tissue is autoregulated, responding to local hypercarbia, acidosis, hypoxia or hypotension by vasodilatation, and to hypocarbia and hypertension by vasoconstriction. In the presence of carotid artery disease, blood vessels in or near ischemic areas of brain lose this autoregulatory mechanism, developing a state of vasomotor paralysis and are probably maximally dilated. These vessels no longer respond to the vasoconstrictor influences noted above. Adjoining areas of healthy brain tissue retain their vosomotor response. It may be reasoned that if reactive blood vessels constrict, the ischemic areas with their nonreactive vessels will have blood diverted to them, and conversely, if response of the circulation of ischemis areas will be subjected to an intracerebral steal.[13] In practice it has been shown that the response of the circulation of ischemic areas of brain to changes in blood pressure or carbon dioxide tension cannot be accurately predicted, particularly when the effects of anesthetic agents and intermittent positive pressure ventilation are superimposed.[24] It is therefore not surprising that there is no uniformity of opinion as to the anesthetic and ventilatory management of these patients.[18] Until practical techniques of preoperatively demonstrating the response of blood flow in ischemic areas of the brain in a particular patient to changes in arterial PCO_2 or systemic blood pressure, a middle course, striving to maintain normal PCO_2, normal PO_2 and normal blood pressure by the combination of appropriate controlled ventilation with light anesthetic techniques seems wise.

Monitoring

Patients undergoing vascular surgery merit special consideration, and it follows that they require close monitoring during and immediately after operation. In addition to applying four-lead electrocardiogram electrodes, any major vascular surgery suggests the use of percutaneous radial and central venous cannulae prior to the induction of anesthesia. Frequently a Swann-Ganz catheter placed in the pulmonary artery provides a better al-ternative to the central venous catheter. A baseline ECG is obtained in the induction room along with mean arterial, mean central venous, and where available, mean pulmonary artery and wedge pressures. Central arterial and mixed venous gases with the patient breathing room air are also obtained. Close monitoring of ECG, pressures, arterial and venous gases are continued throughout surgery and into the postoperative phase.

Where cardiac dysfunction is apparent or suspected, cardiac output determinations using the dye dilution method are performed as a guide to therapy, both in the operating room and at the bedside. During the postoperative management of carotid endarterectomy, hypertension attributed to denervation of the carotid sinus may be a troublesome complication. This has been observed developing suddenly intra-operatively during light anesthesia. The availability of intra-arterial and central venous monitoring allows for easier management of these patients, particularly if the use of ganglionic blocking agents is considered. Warm blood should always be used during replacement in the course of major vascular surgery. Alert correction of acid-base abnormalities as blood determinations indicate is critically important. With these measures, close attention to volume replacement, and slow release occluding arterial clamps, the occurrence of hypotension following declamping has been a rarity.

Detailed discussions of anesthetic technique have been deliberately avoided in this chapter. Today, the anesthesiologist has agents available which enable him to provide ideal operating conditions with the minimum of general "blanket" depression of past decades. The selection of particular agents will rarely be the determinant of complications by themselves. Rather, attention to circulatory and respiratory management during and after surgery, based on physiological considerations will be helpful in prevention of complications to which vascular surgical patients are particularly liable.

References

1. Anthonisen, N. R., Danson, J., Robertson, P. C., et al.: Airway closure as a function of age. Resp. Physiol., 8:58, 1969.
2. Arkins, R., Smessaert, A., and Hicks, R. G.: Mortality and morbidity in surgical patients with coronary artery disease. JAMA, 190:485, 1964.
3. Burger, E. J., and Macklem, P.: Airway closure: demonstration by breathing 100% O_2 at low lung volumes and by N_2 washout. J. Appl. Physiol., 25:139, 1968.
4. Campbell, E. J. M., Nunn, J. F., and Peckett, B. W.: A comparison of artificial ventilation and spontaneous respiration with particular reference to ventilation—blood-flow relationships. Br. J. Anaesth., 30:166, 1958.
5. Couture, J., Picken, J., Trop, D., et al.: Airway closure in normal, obese, and anesthetized supine subjects. Fed. Proc., 29:269, 1970.
6. Craig, D. B., Wahba, W. M., and Don, H. F.: Airway closure and lung volumes in surgical patients. Can. Anaesth. Soc. J., 18:92, 1971.
7. Craig, D. B., Wahba, W. H., Don, H. F., et al.: "Closing Volume" and its relationship to gas exchange in seated and supine positions. J. Appl. Physiol., 31:717, 1971.
8. Don, H. F., Wahba, W. M., and Craig, D. B.: Airway closure, gas trapping, and the functional residual capacity during anesthesia. Anesthesiology, 36:533, 1972.
9. Holland, J., Milic-Emili, J., Macklem, P. T., et al.: Regional distribution of pulmonary ventilation and perfusion in elderly subjects. J. Clin. Invest., 47:81, 1968.
10. Hughes, J. M. B., Rosenzweig, D. Y., and Kivitz, P. B.: Site of airway closure in excised dog lungs: histologic demonstration. J. Appl. Physiol., 29:340, 1970.
11. Johansson, B., Linder, E., and Seeman, T.: Effect of haematocrit and blood viscosity on myocardial blood flow during temporary coronary occlusion in dogs. Scand. J. Thorac. Cardiovasc. Surg., 1:165, 1967.
12. Katz, L. N., and Feinberg, H.: Relation of cardiac effort to myocardial O_2 consumption and coronary flow. Circ. Res., 6:656, 1958.
13. Lassen, N. A., and Palvölgyi, R.: Cerebral steal during hypercapnia and the inverse reaction during hypocapnia observed by the 13 3 Xenon technique in man. Scand. J. Clin. Lab. Invest. 22, Suppl. 102:13D, 1968.
14. Leblanc, P., Ruff, F., and Milic-Emili, J.: Effects of age and body position on "airway closure" in man. J. Appl. Physiol., 28:448, 1970.
15. Nunn, J. F., and Freeman, J.: Problems of oxygenation and oxygen transport during haemorrhage. Anesthesia, 19:206, 1964.
16. Nunn, J. F., and Payne, J. P.: Hypoxaemia after general anesthesia. Lancet, 2:631, 1962.
17. Richardson, T. Q., and Guyton, A. C.: Effects of polycythemia and anemia on cardiac output and other circulatory factors. Amer. J. Physiol., 197:1167, 1959.
18. Sabawala, B. S., Strong, M. J., and Keats, A. S.: Surgery of the aorta and its branches. Anesthesiology, 33:229, 1970.
19. Skinner, J. F., and Pearce, M. L.: Surgical risk in the cardiac patient. J. Chronic Dis., 17:57, 1964.
20. Soloway, M., Nadel, W., Albin, M. S., and White, R. J.: The effect of hyperventilation on subsequent cerebral infarction. Anesthesiology, 29:975, 1968.
21. Sutherland, P. W., Katsura, J., and Milic-Emili, J.: Previous volume history of the lung and regional distribution of gas. J. Appl. Physiol., 25:566, 1968.
22. Swan, H. J. C., Ganz, W., et al.: Catheterization of the heart in man with use of a flow directed balloon-tipped catheter. N. Engl. J. Med., 283:447, 1970.
23. Topkins, M. J., and Artusio, J. F., Jr.: Myocardial infarction and surgery. A five year study. Anesth. Analg., 43:716, 1964.
24. Wollman, H.: Editorial View. Anesthesiology, 33:379, 1972.
25. Wynands, J. E., Sheridan, C. A., Batra, M. S., Palmer, W. H., and Shanks, J.: Coronary artery disease. Anesthesiology, 33:260, 1970.

Index

Numerals in italics indicate a figure and "t" following a page number indicates tabular material concerning the subject.

Abscess, in peritoneal cavity, as complication in abdominal aortic surgery, 60

Acidosis, metabolic, and low flow, in thrombosis of arterial reconstruction, 338

Adhesions, from previous operations, as complication in abdominal aortic surgery, 60
 intestinal obstruction from, as early postoperative complication of abdominal aortic surgery, 63

Airway closure, 385

Allografts, venous, from cadavers, in arterial reconstruction, 91

Amputation(s), above-knee, 352-353
 rehabilitation difficulties associated with, 349
 technical considerations in, 356-357
 at ankle, complications of, 357
 Syme technique in, 350, *350*
 below-knee, prerequisites for, 351-352, 351t
 technical considerations in, 358-359, *359*
 bilateral, 363-364
 complications of, 347
 delayed wound healing in, 353
 management of, 353-354
 in diffuse occlusive disease, 347, *348*
 drains in, 359
 in foot, 349-350
 complications of, 357, *357*
 goals of, 347
 immediately fitted prosthesis in, advantages of, 361
 complications of, 362, *362*
 healing with, 361, 361t
 technique of, 361-362
 immobilization in, 347
 infection and, 347, 354
 antibiotics in prophylaxis in, 354-355
 immediate surgery in, 355
 mortality in, 354
 preoperative physiologic amputation in, 355-356, *355*, 356t
 in stump, 356, *356*

Amputation(s) (*continued*)
 late vascular complications of, 363-364
 level of, selection of, 351-353
 lower extremity, popliteal pulses and, 349
 mobilization of patient in, 359-360
 mortality in, 348-349, 354, *354*
 effect of diabetes on, 349t
 infection and, 354
 patients for, 348
 physiologic, 355-356, *355*
 primary, 114, *114*
 psychological complications of, 360
 rate, and arterial repair, since World War II, 103
 in evaluation of arterial injury repair, 118, 118t
 re-amputation, 353-354
 in stump infection, 356
 rehabilitation following, 364
 site of, choice of, 349-353
 stump, bone formation in, 364
 care of, 360-361
 edema of, 359
 infection of, 356, *356*
 late complications involving, 362-363
 Syme, 350-351, *350*
 toe, 351, *351*
 too high, 349
 too low, 349-350

Anastomosis(es), bleeding from, in renal revascularization, 186-187, *186*
 cobra hood, in renal revascularization, 184-185, *184*
 stenosis at, incorrect angle of anastomosis causing, 182-183, *183*
 suturing techniques causing, 183-184, *184*
 in venous bypass graft, 76, *75*

Anesthesia(s), and hepatic damage, 324
 regional nerve, hazards of, 212
 hemometakinesia following, 211-212
 in postoperative stump causalgia, 363
 precautions in use of, 212
 in sympathectomy, 211-212
 technical dangers in, 211
 for vascular surgery, cerebral function and, 386-387
 monitoring during, 387
 oxygen availability and, 384-386

Anesthesia(s), for vascular surgery (*continued*)
 physiological considerations during, 384
 preoperative evaluation in, 383-384
 renal function and, 386

Aneurysm(s), of abdominal aorta. *See* Aorta, abdominal, aneurysm of
 of aortic arch. *See* Aorta, arch of, aneurysm of
 false, as complication of arterial reconstruction, causes of, 81
 incidence of, 80-81
 management of, 81
 as late postoperative complication of abdominal aortic surgery, 64-65
 as postoperative complication of internal carotid artery endarterectomy, 162
 bruit associated with, 123
 delayed recognition of, 119-120
 diagnosis of, 122-123, *123*
 involving major vessels, 122, 122t
 preoperative complications of, 123-124, *124*
 recognition of, historical note on, 121
 signs and symptoms of, 123
 surgical management of, 125, 126t
 thoracic aortic. *See* Aorta, thoracic, descending, aneurysm of
 thoracoabdominal. *See* Aorta, aneurysm of, thoracoabdominal
 true, as complication of arterial reconstruction, 81-83, *82*, *83*, *84*

Angina, abdominal, 193

Angiographer, responsibilities of, 26-27, 35-37

Angiography. *See also* Arteriography; Phlebography
 in diagnosis of arteriovenous fistula and false aneurysm, 123, *123*
 Seldinger technique in. *See* Seldinger technique in angiography

Ankle, amputation at, complications of, 357
 Syme technique in, *350-351*

389